OPHTHALMOLOGY

SECRETS

IN COLOR

Third Edition

James F. Vander, MD
Attending Surgeon, Retina Service
Wills Eye Institute
Clinical Professor of Ophthalmology
Thomas Jefferson University
Philadelphia, Pennsylvania

Janice A. Gault, MD, FACS
Associate Surgeon, Cataract and Primary Eye Care Service
Wills Eye Institute
Assistant Clinical Professor of Ophthalmology
Thomas Jefferson University
Philadelphia, Pennsylvania
Eye Physicians PC
Voorhees, New Jersey

MOSBY

ELSEVIER

MOSBY
ELSEVIER

1600 John F. Kennedy Boulevard, Suite 1800
Philadelphia, PA 19103-2899

Ophthalmology Secrets in Color   ISBN-13: 978-0-323-03469-2
Third Edition   ISBN-10: 0-323-03469-1

NOTICE

Knowledge and best practice in this field are constantly changing. As new research and experience broaden our knowledge, changes in practice, treatment and drug therapy may become necessary or appropriate. Readers are advised to check the most current information provided (i) on procedures featured or (ii) by the manufacturer of each product to be administered, to verify the recommended dose or formula, the method and duration of administration, and contraindications. It is the responsibility of the practitioner, relying on his or her own experience and knowledge of the patient, to make diagnoses, to determine dosages and the best treatment for each individual patient, and to take all appropriate safety precautions. To the fullest extent of the law, neither the Publisher nor the Editor assumes any liability for any injury and/or damage to persons or property arising out or related to any use of the material contained in this book.

Library of Congress Cataloging-in-Publication Data

Ophthalmology secrets in color / [edited by] James F. Vander, Janice A. Gault. – 3rd ed.
   p.; cm. – (The secrets series)
  Rev. ed. of: Ophthalmology secrets.
  Includes bibliographical references and index.
  ISBN-13: 978–0–323–03469–2   ISBN-10: 0–323–03469–1
  1. Ophthalmology–Miscellanea. 2. Eye–Diseases–Miscellanea. I. Vander, James F., 1960- II. Gault, Janice A. III. Ophthalmology secrets. IV. Series.
  [DNLM: 1. Eye Diseases–Examinatiion Questions. WW 18.2 O612 2007]
  RE48.O666 2007
  617.7′0076–dc22

                             2006046682

Senior Acquisitions Editor: James Merritt
Developmental Editor: Stan Ward
Project Manager: Mary Stermel
Marketing Manager: Alyson Sherby

Working together to grow
libraries in developing countries

www.elsevier.com | www.bookaid.org | www.sabre.org

ELSEVIER   BOOK AID International   Sabre Foundation

Printed in China.

Last digit is the print number: 9   8   7   6   5   4   3   2

DEDICATION

To Caroline Anna, William Henry, and Eliza Avery

CONTENTS

Top 100 Secrets 1

I. GENERAL

1. Clinical Anatomy of the Eye 9
   Kenneth B. Gum, MD

2. Anatomy of the Orbit and Eyelid 16
   Edward H. Bedrossian, Jr., MD

3. Optics and Refraction 19
   Janice A. Gault, MD

4. Color Vision 33
   Mitchell S. Fineman, MD

5. Ophthalmic and Orbital Testing 41
   Caroline R. Baumal, MD, and Patric De Potter, MD

6. Visual Fields 59
   Janice A. Gault, MD

II. CORNEA AND EXTERNAL DISEASES

7. The Red Eye 77
   Janice A. Gault, MD

8. Corneal Infections 90
   Sherman W. Reeves, MD, MPH, Elisabeth J. Cohen, MD, and Terry Kim, MD

9. Ophthalmia Neonatorum 101
   Janine G. Tabas, MD

10. Topical Antibiotics and Steroids 106
    Stephen Y. Lee, MD

11. Dry Eyes 116
    Janice A. Gault, MD

12. Corneal Dystrophies 120
    Sadeer B. Hannush, MD, and Lorena Riveroll, MD

13. Keratoconus 129
    Irving Raber, MD

14. Refractive Surgery..137
    Brandon D. Ayres, MD, and Christopher J. Rapuano, MD

III. GLAUCOMA

15. Glaucoma...149
    Mary Jude Cox, MD, and George L. Spaeth, MD

16. Angle-Closure Glaucoma..157
    Anup K. Khatana, MD, and George L. Spaeth, MD

17. Secondary Open-Angle Glaucoma..................................174
    Janice A. Gault, MD

18. Medical Treatment of Glaucoma..................................181
    Jeffrey D. Henderer, MD, and Richard P. Wilson, MD

19. Trabeculectomy Surgery..190
    Marlene R. Moster, MD, and Augusto Azuara-Blanco, MD, PhD

20. Traumatic Glaucoma and Hyphema 199
    Douglas J. Rhee, MD

IV. CATARACTS

21. Cataracts..213
    Richard Tipperman, MD

22. Techniques of Cataract Surgery..................................218
    Sydney Tyson, MD, MPH

23. Complications of Cataract Surgery...............................225
    John D. Dugan, Jr., MD, and Robert S. Bailey, Jr., MD

V. OCULAR DEVIATIONS

24. Amblyopia..231
    Steven E. Brooks, MD

25. Esodeviations..237
    Scott E. Olitsky, MD, and Leonard B. Nelson, MD

26. Miscellaneous Ocular Deviations.................................243
    Janice A. Gault, MD

27. Strabismus Surgery..251
    Bruce M. Schnall, MD

28. Nystagmus...256
    Robert D. Reinecke, MD

VI. NEURO-OPHTHALMOLOGY

29. The Pupil 261
   Barry Schanzer, MD, and Peter J. Savino, MD

30. Diplopia 266
   Julian D. Perry, MD

31. Optic Neuritis 274
   Barry Schanzer, MD, and Peter J. Savino, MD

32. Miscellaneous Optic Neuropathies and Neurologic Disturbances 278
   Janice A. Gault, MD

VII. OCULOPLASTICS

33. Tearing and the Lacrimal System 287
   Nancy G. Swartz, MS, MD, and Marc S. Cohen, MD

34. Proptosis 293
   David G. Buerger, MD

35. Thyroid-Related Ophthalmopathy 298
   Robert B. Penne, MD

36. Orbital Inflammatory Diseases 304
   Roberta E. Gausas, MD, and Madhura Tamhankar, MD

37. Ptosis 309
   Carolyn S. Repke, MD

38. Eyelid Tumors 315
   Janice A. Gault, MD

VIII. UVEITIS

39. Uveitis 321
   Tamara R. Vrabec, MD, Caroline R. Baumal, MD, Vincent F. Baldassano, Jr., MD, Vinay N. Desai, MD, and Jay S. Duker, MD

IX. RETINA

40. Toxic Retinopathies 341
   Sobha Sivaprasad and Philip G. Hykin

41. Coats Disease 348
   William Tasman, MD

42. Fundus Trauma 353
   Jeffrey P. Blice, MD

43. Age-Related Macular Degeneration....................................361
   Joseph I. Maguire, MD

44. Retinopathy of Prematurity...368
   J. Arch McNamara, MD

45. Diabetic Retinopathy...376
   James F. Vander, MD

46. Retinal Arterial Obstruction.......................................384
   Jay S. Duker, MD

47. Retinal Venous Occlusive Disease...................................390
   Vernon K. W. Wong, MD

48. Retinal Detachment 396
   Michael J. Borne, MD, and James F. Vander, MD

49. Retinoblastoma..405
   Carol L. Shields, MD

50. Pigmented Lesions of the Ocular Fundus............................412
   Jerry A. Shields, MD

X. NEOPLASMS

51. Ocular Tumors..417
   Ralph C. Eagle, Jr., MD

52. Orbital Tumors...429
   Jurij R. Bilyk, MD

INDEX..435

CONTRIBUTORS

Brandon D. Ayres, MD
Corneal Associates PC, Wills Eye Institute, Philadelphia, Pennsylvania

Augusto Azuara-Blanco, MD, PhD, FRCS(Ed)
Consultant Ophthalmic Surgeon and Honorary Senior Lecturer, Aberdeen Royal Infirmary,
University of Aberdeen, Aberdeen, United Kingdom

Robert S. Bailey, Jr., MD
Department of Ophthalmology, Jefferson Medical College of Thomas Jefferson University;
Attending Surgeon, Wills Eye Institute; Attending Surgeon, Chestnut Hill Hospital, Philadelphia,
Pennsylvania

Vincent F. Baldassano, Jr., MD
Department of Ophthalmology, Temple University, Philadelphia, Pennsylvania

Caroline R. Baumal, MD
Department of Ophthalmology, Tufts University School of Medicine; Residency Director,
Division of Vitreoretinal Diseases and Surgery, New England Eye Center, Boston, Massachusetts

Edward H. Bedrossian, Jr., MD
Associate Clinical Professor, Department of Ophthalmology, Jefferson Medical College of
Thomas Jefferson University; Chief, Oculoplastic and Reconstructive Surgery Division, Temple
University Hospital; Associate Surgeon, Oculoplastic Surgery Department; Founding Director,
Fascia Lata Bank, Wills Eye Institute, Philadelphia, Pennsylvania

Jurij R. Bilyk, MD
Oculoplastic and Orbital Surgery Service, Wills Eye Institute; Parkview Eye Care Center,
Philadelphia, Pennsylvania

Jeffrey P. Blice, MD
Uniformed Services Health Sciences University; National Naval Medical Center,
Bethesda, Maryland

Michael J. Borne, MD
Department of Ophthalmology, University of Mississippi School of Medicine,
Jackson, Mississippi

Steven E. Brooks, MD
Eye Consultants of Augusta, Martinez, Georgia

David G. Buerger, MD
Department of Ophthalmology, University of Pittsburgh Medical Center; Pittsburgh Oculoplasty
Associates, Pittsburgh, Pennsylvania

Elisabeth J. Cohen, MD
Corneal Associates PC, Wills Eye Institute, Philadelphia, Pennsylvania

Marc S. Cohen, MD
Associate Surgeon, Wills Eye Institute, Philadelphia, Pennsylvania

Mary Jude Cox, MD
Instructor, Glaucoma Service, Wills Eye Institute, Philadelphia, Pennsylvania; Eye Physicians PC, Voorhees, New Jersey

Patric De Potter, MD
Professor and Chairman, Department of Ophthalmology, Cliniques Universitaires St.-Luc, Université Catholique de Louvain, Brussels, Belgium

Vinay N. Desai, MD
Department of Ophthalmology, Washington Hospital Center, Washington, DC

John D. Dugan, Jr., MD
Associate Surgeon and Codirector Refractive Surgery Department, Wills Eye Institute, Philadelphia, Pennsylvania; Eye Physicians PC, Voorhees, New Jersey

Jay S. Duker, MD
New England Eye Center, Boston, Massachusetts

Ralph C. Eagle, Jr., MD
Director, Department of Pathology, Noel T. and Sara L. Simmonds Professor of Ophthalmic Pathology, Wills Eye Institute; Professor of Ophthalmology and Pathology, Thomas Jefferson University, Philadelphia, Pennsylvania

Mitchell S. Fineman, MD
Assistant Surgeon, Wills Eye Institute; Assistant Professor of Ophthalmology, Thomas Jefferson University, Philadelphia, Pennsylvania

Janice A. Gault, MD, FACS
Associate Surgeon, Cataract and Primary Eye Care Service, Wills Eye Institute; Assistant Clinical Professor of Ophthalmology, Thomas Jefferson University, Philadelphia, Pennsylvania; Eye Physicians PC, Voorhees, New Jersey

Roberta E. Gausas, MD
Department of Ophthalmology, University of Pennsylvania Medical School; Scheie Eye Institute, Philadelphia, Pennsylvania

Kenneth B. Gum, MD
Section Chief, Department of Ophthalmology, Munson Medical Center, Transverse City, Michigan

Sadeer B. Hannush, MD
Department of Ophthalmology, Jefferson Medical College of Thomas Jefferson University; Cornea Service, Wills Eye Institute, Philadelphia, Pennsylvania

Jeffrey D. Henderer, MD
Assistant Professor of Ophthalmology, Thomas Jefferson University School of Medicine; Assistant Surgeon, Wills Eye Institute Glaucoma Service, Philadelphia, Pennsylvania

Philip G. Hykin, FRCS, FRCOphth
Surgeon, Medical Retina Service, Moorfields Eye Institute, London, United Kingdom

Anup Khatana, MD
Cincinnati Eye Institute, Cincinnati, Ohio

Terry Kim, MD
Associate Professor of Ophthalmology, Duke Medical Center; Director of Fellowship Programs, Duke University Eye Center, Durham, North Carolina

Stephen Y. Lee, MD
Cornea Service, Wills Eye Institute; Jefferson Medical College of Thomas Jefferson University, Philadelphia, Pennsylvania

Joseph I. Maguire, MD, FACS
Assistant Professor, Thomas Jefferson University Hospital; Wills Eye Institute, Philadelphia, Pennsylvania

J. Arch McNamara, MD
Retinovitreous Associates, Ltd., Wyndmoor, Pennsylvania

Marlene R. Moster, MD
Wills Eye Institute Glaucoma Service, Philadelphia, Pennsylvania

Leonard B. Nelson, MD
Associate Professor of Ophthalmology and Pediatrics, Jefferson Medical College of Thomas Jefferson University; Codirector of Pediatric Ophthalmology, Wills Eye Institute, Philadelphia, Pennsylvania

Scott E. Olitsky, MD
Children's Mercy Hospital and Clinics, Kansas City, Missouri

Robert B. Penne, MD
Associate Professor of Ophthalmology, Jefferson Medical College of Thomas Jefferson University; Codirector of Oculoplastic Surgery Department, Wills Eye Institute; Chief of Ophthalmology, Lankenau Hospital, Philadelphia, Pennsylvania

Julian D. Perry, MD
Section Head, Department of Ophthalmic Plastic and Orbital Surgery, The Cole Eye Institute, Cleveland Clinic Foundation, Cleveland, Ohio

Irving Raber, MD
Clinical Assistant Professor of Ophthalmology, Scheie Eye Institute at Presbyterian Medical Center, University of Pennsylvania School of Medicine; Clinical Assistant Professor of Ophthalmology, Thomas Jefferson University School of Medicine; Clinical Associate Professor of Ophthalmology, Drexel University College of Medicine, Philadelphia, Pennsylvania

Christopher J. Rapuano, MD
Corneal Associates, Wills Eye Institute, Philadelphia, Pennsylvania

Sherman W. Reeves, MD, MPH
Minnesota Eye Consultants, Minneapolis, Minnesota

Robert D. Reinecke, MD
Professor of Ophthalmology, Jefferson Medical College of Thomas Jefferson University; Wills Eye Institute, Philadelphia, Pennsylvania

Carolyn S. Repke, MD
Philadelphia Eye Associates, Philadelphia, Pennsylvania

Douglas J. Rhee, MD
Assistant Professor, Massachusetts Eye and Ear Infirmary, Harvard Medical School, Boston, Massachusetts

Lorena Riveroll, MD
Department of Ophthalmology, Cornea Service, Asociación Para Evitar la Ceguera en Mexico, Mexico City, Mexico

Peter J. Savino, MD
Professor of Ophthalmology, Jefferson Medical College of Thomas Jefferson University; Director, Neuro-ophthalmology Service, Wills Eye Institute, Philadelphia, Pennsylvania

Barry Schanzer, MD
Department of Ophthalmology, Jefferson Medical Center, Philadelphia, Pennsylvania

Bruce M. Schnall, MD
Associate Surgeon, Pediatric Ophthalmology, Wills Eye Institute, Philadelphia, Pennsylvania; Clinical Assistant Professor, Department of Surgery, Robert Wood Johnson Medical School, Piscataway, New Jersey

Carol L. Shields, MD
Attending Surgeon, Ocular Oncology Service, Wills Eye Institute; Professor of Ophthalmology, Jefferson Medical School of Thomas Jefferson University, Philadelphia, Pennsylvania

Jerry A. Shields, MD
Director, Oncology Service, Wills Eye Institute; Professor of Ophthalmology, Jefferson Medical School of Thomas Jefferson University, Philadelphia, Pennsylvania

Sobha Sivaprasad, FRCS
Moorfields Eye Institute, London, United Kingdom

Nancy G. Swartz, MS, MD
Associate Surgeon, Wills Eye Institute, Philadelphia, Pennsylvania

George L. Spaeth, MD
Attending Surgeon, Glaucoma Service, Wills Eye Institute; Professor of Ophthalmology, Jefferson Medical College of Thomas Jefferson University, Philadelphia, Pennsylvania

Janine G. Tabas, MD
Cataract and Primary Eye Care Service, Wills Eye Institute, Philadelphia, Pennsylvania

Madhura Tamhankar, MD
Department of Ophthalmology, University of Pennsylvania Medical School; Scheie Eye Institute, Philadelphia, Pennsylvania

William Tasman, MD
Ophthalmologist-in-Chief, Wills Eye Institute; Professor and Chairman, Department of Ophthalmology, Jefferson Medical College of Thomas Jefferson University, Philadelphia, Pennsylvania

Richard Tipperman, MD
Cataract and Primary Eye Care Service, Wills Eye Institute, Philadelphia, Pennsylvania

Sydney Tyson, MD, MPH
Attending Surgeon, Cataract and Primary Care Eye Care Service, Wills Eye Institute, Philadelphia, Pennsylvania

James F. Vander, MD
Attending Surgeon, Retina Service, Wills Eye Institute; Clinical Professor of Ophthalmology, Thomas Jefferson University, Philadelphia, Pennsylvania

Tamara R. Vrabec, MD
Associate Eye Surgeon, Wills Eye Institute; Associate Professor, Jefferson Medical College of Thomas Jefferson University, Philadelphia, Pennsylvania; Lehigh Eye Specialists PC, Allentown, Pennsylvania

Richard P. Wilson, MD
Professor of Ophthalmology, Thomas Jefferson University School of Medicine; Attending Surgeon and Codirector, Wills Eye Institute Glaucoma Service, Philadelphia, Pennsylvania

Vernon K. W. Wong, MD
Assistant Clinical Professor, Division of Ophthalmology, Department of Surgery, University of Hawaii School of Medicine, Honolulu, Hawaii

PREFACE

Much of the information in this book can be found in a number of other ophthalmology textbooks. The table of contents is similar to that of many other books already in print. So why bother to write a new ophthalmology text? The value of the book is in the unique manner in which the material is presented, continuing the tradition the *Secrets Series*® has established in numerous other specialties. The question-and-answer "Socratic method" format reflects the process by which a large portion of clinical medical education actually takes place. Our purpose is not to displace the comprehensive textbooks of ophthalmology from the shelves of clinicians and students. Instead, we hope that we have filled a useful spot beside them. We greatly appreciate the efforts of the talented contributors who have shared their wisdom and experiences to help fill this void.

We have received much positive feedback on the first two editions of this book. This third edition includes many more color figures as well as the helpful study aids of the Top 100 Secrets and Key Points. We have enjoyed updating *Ophthalmology Secrets,* and we hope that clinicians and students will enjoy this book and find it valuable.

James F. Vander, MD
Janice A. Gault, MD, FACS

TOP 100 SECRETS

These secrets are 100 of the top board alerts. They summarize the concepts, principles, and most salient details of ophthalmology.

1. Corneal opacification in a neonate has a differential diagnosis of **STUMPED: s**clerocornea, **t**rauma, **u**lcers, **m**etabolic disorder, **P**eter's anomaly, **e**ndothelial dystrophy, and **d**ermoid.

2. A break in Bruch's membrane is necessary for a choroidal neovascular membrane to form.

3. Posterior fractures most commonly occur in the posteromedial orbital floor.

4. Eyelid trauma that reveals orbital fat has, by definition, violated the orbital septum.

5. The goal of refractive correction is to place the circle of least confusion on the retina.

6. To find the spherical equivalent of an astigmatic correction, add half the cylinder to the sphere.

7. Recheck the axial lengths if the A-scan measures less than 22 mm or more than 25 mm, or if there is more than a 0.3 mm difference between the two eyes. For each 1 mm in error, the calculation is off by 2.5 diopters (D). Recheck keratometry readings if the average K power is <40 D, >47 D, or if there is a difference of more than 1 D between eyes. For every 0.25 D error, the calculation is in error of 0.25 D.

8. According to Kollner's rule, retinal diseases cause acquired blue-yellow color vision defects, whereas optic nerve diseases affect red-green discrimination.

9. Ultrasound findings of low-to-medium internal reflectivity and collar-button shape can confirm diagnosis of a choroidal melanoma and differentiate it from other choroidal lesions.

10. A junctional scotoma is a unilateral central scotoma associated with a contralateral superotemporal field defect and is caused by compression of the contralateral optic nerve near the chiasm.

11. False-negative errors cause a visual field to appear worse than it actually is. False-positive errors cause a visual field to look better than it actually is.

12. Lesions anterior to the optic chiasm cause unequal visual acuity, a relative afferent papillary defect, and color abnormalities. The optic disc may also have asymmetric cupping and pallor.

13. Always check the pressure in the contralateral eye in a patient with ocular trauma. Asymmetrically low intraocular pressure may be an important clue to a potential ruptured globe.

14. A drop of 2.5% neosynephrine is a simple test to distinguish between episcleritis (these vessels will blanch) and scleritis (these vessels do not)—two entities with very different prognoses and evaluations. Because 50% of patients with scleritis have systemic disease, referral to an internist is necessary for further evaluation.

15. A patient with a corneal abrasion from a dirty source (contact lens use, tree branch) is at risk for a corneal ulcer and should not be patched while healing.

16. Immediately irrigate any patient with a chemical ocular injury from an alkali or acid, even before checking visual acuity.

17. Recurrent subconjunctival hemorrhages should be evaluated to rule out uncontrolled hypertension or blood dyscrasias.

18. A corneal ulcer is infectious until proven otherwise. You are never wrong to culture an ulcer, and any ulcer not responding to therapy should be recultured.

19. Systemic treatment is necessary for gonococcal, chlamydial, and herpetic neonatal conjunctivitis due to the potential for serious disseminated disease. The mother and her sexual partners must be evaluated for other sexually transmitted diseases.

20. Treatments that are effective for prophylaxis of gonococcal and chlamydial neonatal conjunctivitis include 1% silver nitrate, 0.5% erythromycin, and 1% tetracycline. Silver nitrate is rarely used, however, due to its potential for causing chemical conjunctivitis.

21. Topical steroids may promote herpetic keratitis if viral shedding is coincident with administration.

22. Steroid-induced increases in intraocular pressure occur in about 6% of patients on topical dexamethasone. This risk is higher in patients with known glaucoma or a family history of glaucoma.

23. Ask about gastric bypass procedures in patients who have recent severe dry eye with no discernible cause. Vitamin A deficiency may be the reason.

24. Treat patients for dry eye if they are symptomatic even if their exam is normal. Rose bengal stain will show signs of dry eye earlier than fluorescein stain.

25. If a patient presents with symptoms consistent with recurrent corneal erosion syndrome but no findings of the same, look for an underlying dystrophy, specifically epithelial basement membrane dystrophy.

26. If a patient with a corneal dystrophy is undergoing corneal transplantation but also has a clinically significant cataract, consider staging the cataract extraction a few months after the corneal transplant, offering the patient the advantage of better intraocular lens power calculation and postoperative refractive result. Alternatively, Descemet stripping endothelial keratoplasty (DSEK), which does not alter corneal contour, may be combined with cataract surgery with a predictable refractive outcome.

27. Keratoconus is found more frequently in atopic and Down syndrome patients, possibly related to eye rubbing. All keratoconus patients should be advised to avoid eye rubbing.

28. Most patients with keratoconus can be managed successfully with contact lens wear. Corneal transplantation is highly successful in treating keratoconus patients whose visual needs cannot be satisfied by spectacle or contact lens correction.

29. If there are significant complications with refractive surgery in the first eye, do not proceed with refractive surgery in the fellow eye on the same day.

30. As many as 30–50% of individuals with glaucomatous optic nerve damage and visual field loss have an initial intraocular pressure measurement less than 22 mmHg.

31. The treatment of both primary open-angle glaucoma (POAG) and low tension glaucoma (LTG) aims to preserve vision and quality of life through the lowering of intraocular pressure.

32. When evaluating a patient with angle closure glaucoma, it is important to look at the fellow eye. Except for cases of marked anisometropia, the fellow eye should have a similar anterior chamber depth and narrow angle. If it does not, consider other nonrelative papillary block mechanisms of angle closure.

33. Lens-induced glaucoma includes phacomorphic, phacolytic, phacoanaphylactic, and lens-particle glaucoma.

34. Patients with sporadic inheritance of aniridia need to be evaluated for Wilms' tumor, which is associated with 25% of cases.

35. The prostaglandin analogs are the most potent topical intraocular pressure-lowering medications, have a favorable side-effect profile, and are easy to use. However, prostaglandin analogs and miotics are contraindicated in any type of inflammatory glaucoma.

36. Topical medication allergy can present months to years after starting the drop.

37. If a patient's glaucoma continues to worsen, even with seemingly reduced intraocular pressure during office visits, think noncompliance.

38. Adrenergic agonists except for apraclonidine are absolutely contraindicated in infants. Apraclonidine should be used only as a last resort in healthy infants.

39. Before trabeculectomy surgery, detect high risk patients in whom sudden hypotony should be avoided: those with angle-closure glaucoma, shallow anterior chambers, very high preoperative IOP, or elevated episcleral venous pressure or high myopia. Hemorrhagic choroidals and expulsive hemorrhages are more likely.

40. Patients with traumatic ocular injuries must be evaluated for systemic injuries as well.

41. Patients recovering from a traumatic hyphema are at increased risk for glaucoma and retinal detachments in the future. They need ongoing ophthalmic evaluation for the rest of their lives.

42. Complete evaluation by a pediatrician is mandatory for any infant with a congenital cataract.

43. Patients must have a documented interference in quality of life from a visual standpoint before cataract surgery is indicated.

44. Topical anesthesia allows the surgical patient to recover functional vision more quickly and decreases the risk of some complications compared with retrobulbar anesthesia.

45. Glare testing can reveal significant functional visual problems not noted by Snellen testing.

46. When complications result in the unplanned decision to place an intraocular lens in the ciliary sulcus, remember to lower the power of the implant approximately 0.5 D from what was chosen for capsular fixation to compensate for the more anterior location of the lens.

47. If amblyopia is associated with an afferent pupillary defect, a lesion of the retina or optic nerve should be suspected and ruled out.

48. Although amblyopia is most effectively treated prior to age 6 years, treatment can be successful at older ages if compliance is good. Atropine penalization can be as effective as patching in the treatment of mild and moderate amblyopia.

49. Treat amblyopia prior to surgery for esotropia.

50. Early treatment for congenital esotropia gives the best chance for the development of binocular vision. Be certain that a patient with a partial accommodative esotropia is wearing the maximum tolerated hyperopic prescription.

51. Check the light reflex test and cover test to determine if a true deviation exists. If the light reflex is in the appropriate place and there is no refixation on cover testing, the patient is orthophoric.

52. A young patient with asthenopia should be evaluated for exophoria at near (convergence insufficiency) as well as checking his or her cycloplegic refraction for undercorrected hyperopia (accommodative insufficiency).

53. Any patient with chronic progressive external ophthalmoplegia needs an electrocardiogram to rule out heart block. These patients may need a pacemaker to prevent sudden death.

54. A patient with acute onset of any combination of III, IV, V, and VI cranial nerve palsies; extreme headache; and decreased vision must be immediately placed on intravenous steroids and referred to neurosurgery for pituitary apoplexy.

55. The signs of endophthalmitis typically appear 1–4 days after strabismus surgery and include lethargy, asymmetric eye redness, eyelid swelling, and fever.

56. When performing a recess-resect procedure, the recession should be done first.

57. Try for fusion of all patients with nystagmus. Aim for exophoria with fusion.

58. All patients with anisocoria need to have their pupils measured in both dim and bright illumination.

59. Smoking is a controllable risk factor for thyroid eye disease.

60. All patients with optic neuritis should experience some improvement in vision. However, 5% of patients who presented with visual acuity of less than 20/200 were still 20/200 or less at 6 months.

61. An abnormal MRI in a patient with optic neuritis is the strongest predictor of developing multiple sclerosis (MS). Fifty-six percent of patients with optic neuritis and a white matter lesion on MRI will develop MS at 10 years.

62. The closer a patient stands to a visual-field testing screen, the smaller the field should be. This is helpful in determining a malingering patient.

63. Any patient suspected of giant cell arteritis should immediately be started on intravenous steroids to prevent involvement of the other eye even if the temporal artery biopsy cannot be done beforehand.

64. The primary causes of tearing are dry eyes, lower eyelid laxity, and blockage of the lacrimal system.

65. Dacryocystitis must be treated emergently to prevent cellulitis or intracranial spread.

66. CT scanning is superior to MRI in most cases of orbital disease due to better bone-tissue delineation.

67. The most common cause of unilateral or bilateral proptosis is thyroid eye disease (Graves' ophthalmopathy).

68. A child with rapidly progressive proptosis, inferior displacement of the globe, and upper eyelid edema should have immediate neuroimaging followed by an orbital biopsy to rule out rhabdomyosarcoma.

69. Suspect thyroid-related ophthalmopathy (TRO) in patients with nonspecific redness and inflammation of the eyes even if there is no history of a systemic thyroid imbalance.

70. Most patients with TRO will not require surgery for their disease; it will burn out with time and multiple office visits.

71. Surgical drainage should be undertaken in orbital cellulitis if sinuses are completely opacified, response to antibiotics is poor by 48–72 hours, vision decreases, or an afferent pupillary defect presents.

72. Mild ptosis associated with miosis and neck or facial pain should raise suspicion of a carotid artery dissection, prompting an urgent workup.

73. Acute ptosis and ocular misalignment mandate a careful evaluation of the pupil to rule out pupil-involving third-nerve palsy. A dilated pupil requires neurologic evaluation for a compressive aneurysm.

74. Basal cell carcinoma is the most common malignant eyelid tumor. It has a 3% mortality rate because of invasion to the orbit and brain via the lacrimal drainage system, prior radiation therapy, or clinical neglect.

75. Squamous cell carcinoma may metastasize systemically.

76. Keratoacanthomas often resolve spontaneously but should be removed surgically if near the lid margin to prevent permanent deformity.

77. A patient with a recurrent chalazion in the same spot must be evaluated for sebaceous cell carcinoma.

78. Young patients with xanthelasma should be evaluated for diabetes mellitus and hypercholesterolemia.

79. All patients who have anterior uveitis must have a dilated examination to exclude associated posterior segment disease.

80. Masquerade syndromes should be considered in the very young or elderly and in patients who have uveitis that does not respond to treatment. Uveitis in patients with AIDS is almost invariably part of a disseminated systemic infection. Lymphoma may masquerade as retinitis.

81. Early signs of chloroquine retinopathy are perifoveal retinal pigment epithelium changes.

82. Never aspirate subretinal exudates for diagnostic purposes in a patient with potential Coats disease unless retinoblastoma has been absolutely ruled out.

83. The five trauma-related breaks are horseshoe tears, operculated tears, dialyses, retinal dissolution, and macular holes.

84. The globe is most likely to rupture at the limbus, underneath a rectus muscle, or at a previous surgical site.

85. Age-related macular degeneration (ARMD) is the leading cause of legal blindness in the Western world. The leading epidemiologic risk factors for ARMD are increasing age, smoking, and genetic predisposition.

86. In the treatment of ARMD, therapeutic paradigms are shifting from destructive laser-based modalities to physiologic pharmacologic therapies such as inhibitors of vascular endothelial growth factor (VEGF).

87. Threshold disease of retinopathy of prematurity (ROP) is five contiguous or eight cumulative clock hours of stage 3 ROP in zone I or II in the presence of plus disease.

88. Patients who weigh <1500 grams at birth and/or are ≤28 weeks' gestational age should be screened for ROP at 4–6 weeks after birth or 31–33 weeks postconceptual age.

89. The most common cause of vision loss in diabetic retinopathy is macular edema.

90. Clinically significant macular edema (CSME) is defined as one of the following: retinal thickening within 500 microns of the center of the fovea, hard yellow exudate within 500 microns of the fovea and adjacent retinal thickening, or at least one disc area of retinal thickening, any part of which is within 1 disc diameter of the center of the fovea.

91. Most central retinal artery obstructions are thrombotic; most branch retinal artery obstructions are embolic. Systemic disease must be ruled out in any patient with retinal artery obstruction.

92. Perform iris examination and gonioscopy prior to dilation in a patient with a central retinal vein occlusion. Neovascular glaucoma is the most feared complication of a central retinal vein occlusion.

93. The classic symptoms of a retinal break are flashes and floaters. Pigmented cells or blood in the vitreous strongly suggests the possibility of a retinal break.

94. Risk factors for rhegmatogenous retinal detachments include previous cataract surgery, lattice degeneration, and myopia.

95. Retinoblastoma is the leading eye cancer in children. Over 95% of children with retinoblastoma in the United States and developed nations survive due to early detection and proper management.

96. Most children with unilateral retinoblastoma are managed with enucleation. Most children with bilateral retinoblastoma are managed with chemoreduction.

97. The presence of dilated, tortuous episcleral blood vessels warrants a complete exam to rule out an underlying ciliary body or peripheral choroidal tumor.

98. Uveal melanomas with epithelioid cells have a poorer prognosis. Seventy percent of uveal metastases are from breast or lung cancer.

99. The most common cause of unilateral proptosis in children is orbital cellulitis; in adults, thyroid-related ophthalmopathy (Graves' ophthalmopathy).

100. Based on recent data, the treatment of choice for optic nerve sheath meningioma is stereotactic radiotherapy.

I. GENERAL

CLINICAL ANATOMY OF THE EYE

Kenneth B. Gum, MD

1. **Name the seven bones that make up the bony orbit and describe which location is most prone to damage in an orbital blow-out fracture.**
   The seven orbital bones are the frontal, zygoma, maxillary, sphenoid, ethmoid, palatine, and lacrimal. A true blow-out fracture most commonly affects the orbital floor posteriorly and medially to the infraorbital nerve. The ethmoid bone of the medial wall is often broken.

2. **Which nerves and vessels pass through the superior orbital fissure? Which motor nerve to the eye lies outside the annulus of Zinn, leaving it unaffected by retrobulbar injection of anesthetic?**
   The superior orbital fissure transmits the third, fourth, and sixth cranial nerves as well as the first division of the fifth cranial nerve, which has already divided into frontal and lacrimal branches. The superior ophthalmic vein and sympathetic nerves also pass through this fissure. The fourth cranial nerve, supplying the superior oblique muscle, lies outside the annulus. This position accounts for residual intorsion of the eye sometimes seen during retrobulbar anesthesia (Fig. 1-1).

3. **A 3-year-old is referred for evaluation of consecutive exotropia after initial bimedial rectus recessions for esotropia performed elsewhere. Review of the operative notes discloses that each muscle was recessed 4.5 mm for a 30-prism diopter deviation. Unfortunately, the child had mild developmental delay and presents with a 25-prism diopter exotropia. You decide to advance the recessed medial rectus of each eye back to its original insertion site. Where is this site in relation to the limbus? Identify the location of each of the rectus muscle insertion sites relative to the limbus.**
   Reattach each medial rectus muscle 5.5 mm from the limbus. Insertion of the inferior rectus is 6.5 mm from the limbus; the lateral rectus is 6.9 mm from the limbus; and the superior rectus, 7.7 mm. The differing distances of rectus-muscle insertions from the limbus make up the spiral of Tillaux. An important caveat in developmentally delayed children is to postpone muscle surgery until much later, treating any amblyopia in the interim. Early surgery frequently leads to overcorrection.

4. **What is the most common cause of both unilateral and bilateral proptosis in adults?**
   Thyroid orbitopathy is the most common cause. Many signs are associated with thyroid eye disease, which is probably caused by an autoimmune reactivity toward the epitope of thyroid-stimulating hormone (TSH) receptors in the thyroid and orbit. The order of frequency of extraocular muscle involvement in thyroid orbitopathy is as follows: inferior rectus, medial rectus, lateral rectus, superior rectus, and obliques. There is enlargement of the muscle belly with sparing of the tendons.

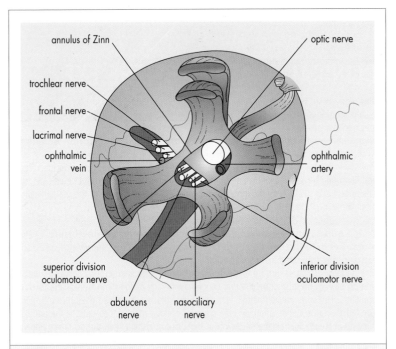

Figure 1-1. The annulus of Zinn and surrounding structures. (From Campolattaro BN, Wang FM: Anatomy and physiology of the extraocular muscles and surrounding tissues. In Yanoff M, Duker JS [eds]: Ophthalmology, 2nd ed. St. Louis, Mosby, 2004.)

5. **You have just begun a ptosis procedure. A lid crease incision was made, and the orbital septum has been isolated and opened horizontally. What important landmark should be readily apparent? Describe its relation to other important structures.**

   The orbital fat lies directly behind the orbital septum and directly on the muscular portion of the levator (Fig. 1-2). A separate medial fat pad often herniates through the septum in later years.

6. **To what glands do the lymphatics of the orbit drain?**

   There are no lymphatic vessels or nodes within the orbit. Lymphatics from the conjunctivae and lids drain medially to the submandibular glands and laterally to the superficial preauricular nodes.

7. **What is the orbital septum?**

   The septum is a thin sheet of connective tissue that defines the anterior limit of the orbit. In the upper lid it extends from the periosteum of the superior orbital rim to insert at the levator aponeurosis, slightly above the superior tarsal border (see Fig. 1-2). The lower lid septum extends from the periosteum of the inferior orbital rim to insert directly on the inferior tarsal border.

8. A 70-year-old patient presents with herpes zoster lesions in the trigeminal nerve distribution. Classic lesions on the side and tip of the nose increase your concern about ocular involvement. Why?

This sign, called Hutchinson's sign, results from involvement of the infratrochlear nerve. The infratrochlear nerve is the terminal branch of the nasociliary nerve, which gives off the long ciliary nerves (usually two) that supply the globe.

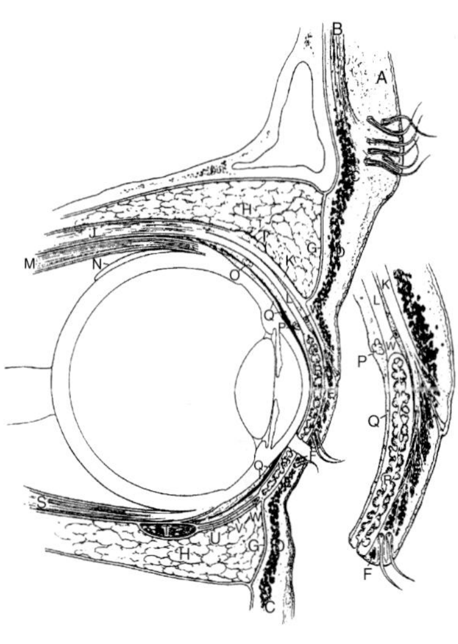

9. Where is the sclera the thinnest? Where are globe ruptures after blunt trauma most likely to occur?

The sclera is thinnest just behind the insertion of the rectus muscles (0.3 mm). Scleral rupture usually occurs opposite the site of impact and in an arc parallel to the limbus at the insertion of the rectus muscles or at the equator. The most common site of rupture is near the superonasal limbus.

10. Describe the surgical limbus and Schwalbe's line.

The surgical limbus can be differentiated into an anterior bluish zone that extends from the termination of Bowman's layer to Schwalbe's line, which is the

Figure 1-2. Schematic cross-section of eyelids and anterior orbit. A, skin; B, frontalis muscle; C, orbicularis muscle (orbital portion); D, orbicularis muscle (preseptal, portion); E, orbicularis muscle (pretarsal portion); F, orbicularis muscle (muscle of Riolan); G, orbital septum; H, orbital fat; I, superior transverse ligament; J, levator muscle; K, levator aponeurosis; L, Müller's muscle; M, superior rectus muscle; N, superior oblique tendon; O, gland of Krause; P, gland of Wolfring; Q, conjunctiva; R, tarsus; S, inferior rectus muscle; T, inferior oblique muscle; U, inferior tarsal muscle; V, capsulopalpebral ascia; W, peripheral arterial arcade. (From Beard C: Ptosis, 3rd ed. St. Louis, Mosby, 1981.)

termination of Descemet's membrane. The posterior white zone overlies the trabecular meshwork and extends from Schwalbe's line to the scleral spur.

11. You are preparing to do an argon laser trabeculoplasty. Describe the gonioscopic appearance of the anterior chamber angle.

The ciliary body is a visible concavity anterior to the iris root. The scleral spur appears as a white line anterior to the ciliary body. Above this are the trabecular meshwork and canal of Schlemm. Treatment is applied to the anterior trabecular meshwork.

12. After a filtering procedure, your patient develops choroidal effusions. Explain the distribution of these fluid accumulations based on uveal attachments to the sclera.

The uveal tract is attached to the sclera at the scleral spur, the optic nerve, and the exit sites of the vortex veins. The fluid dissects the choroid from the underlying sclera but retains these connections.

13. Describe the structure of Bruch's membrane. Name two conditions in which defects develop in this structure spontaneously.

Bruch's membrane consists of five layers: internally, the basement membrane of the pigment epithelium, the inner collagenous zone, a central band of elastic fibers, and the outer collagenous zone; externally, the basement membrane of the choriocapillaris. Pseudoxanthoma elasticum and myopia may cause spontaneous defects in this membrane, making the patient prone to development of choroidal neovascularization.

KEY POINTS: BRUCH'S MEMBRANE

1. Composed of five layers.

2. Spontaneous breaks can occur in pseudoxanthoma elasticum and myopia.

3. Defect in Bruch's membrane in age-related macular degeneration may lead to the exudative form.

4. Trauma may cause a break in the membrane, leading to a choroidal neovascular membrane.

14. **Less laser power is required for photocoagulation in darkly pigmented fundi. What determines this pigmentation?**
   The pigmentation of the fundus seen ophthalmoscopically is largely determined by the number of melanosomes in the choroid. The darker macular area results from taller pigment epithelial cells that contain more and larger melanosomes than the periphery.

15. **What is the blood-retinal barrier?**
   The inner blood-retinal barrier consists of the retinal vascular endothelium, which is nonfenestrated and contains tight junctions. The outer blood-retinal barrier is the retinal pigment epithelium. Bruch's membrane is permeable to small molecules.

16. **Name the 10 classically described anatomic layers of the retina and the cells that make up the retina.**
   The retina may be divided into 10 layers, starting just above the choroids and extending to the vitreous:
   - Retinal pigment epithelium
   - Outer segments of the photoreceptors
   - External limiting membrane
   - Outer nuclear layer
   - Outer plexiform layer
   - Inner nuclear layer
   - Inner plexiform layer
   - Ganglion cell layer
   - Nerve fiber layer
   - Internal limiting membrane
   Within these layers lie the photoreceptors, horizontal cells, bipolar cells, amacrine cells, retinal interneurons, ganglion cells, and the glial cells of the retina, the Müller cells.

17. **Which retinal layer is referred to as the fiber layer of Henle in the macular region?**
   The outer plexiform layer, which is made up of connections between photoreceptor synaptic bodies and horizontal and bipolar cells, becomes thicker and more oblique in orientation as it deviates away from the fovea. At the fovea this layer becomes nearly parallel to the retinal surface and accounts for the radial, or star-shaped, patterns of exudate in the extracellular spaces under pathologic conditions causing vascular compromise, such as hypertension.

18. **What are three clinically recognized remnants of the fetal hyaloid vasculature?**
Mittendorf's dot, Bergmeister's papilla, and vascular loops (95% of which are arterial).

19. **A patient presents with a central retinal artery occlusion and 20/20 visual acuity. How do you explain this finding?**
Fifteen percent of people have a cilioretinal artery that supplies the macular region. Thirty percent of eyes have a cilioretinal artery supplying some portion of the retina. These are perfused by the choroidal vessels, which are fed by the ophthalmic artery and thus are not affected by central retinal artery circulation.

20. **Where do branch retinal vein occlusions occur? Which quadrant of the retina is most commonly affected?**
Branch retinal vein occlusions occur at arteriovenous crossings, most commonly where the vein lies posterior to the artery. The superotemporal quadrant is most often affected because of a higher number of arteriovenous crossings on average.

21. **Discuss the organization of crossed and uncrossed fibers in the optic chiasm.**
Inferonasal extramacular fibers cross in the anterior chiasm and bulge into the contralateral optic nerve (Willebrand's knee). Superonasal extramacular fibers cross directly to the opposite optic tract. Macular fibers are located in the center of the optic nerve. Temporal macular fibers pass uncrossed through the chiasm, whereas nasal macular fibers cross posteriorly. However, in albinism, many temporal fibers also cross.

22. **Describe the location of the visual cortex.**
The visual cortex is situated along the superior and inferior lips of the calcarine fissure. This area is called the striate cortex because of the prominent band of geniculocalcarine fibers, termed the stria of Gennari after its discoverer.

23. **What is the most likely anatomic location of pathology associated with downbeat nystagmus?**
Downbeat nystagmus is usually indicative of cervicomedullary structural disease. The most common causes are Arnold-Chiari malformation, stroke, multiple sclerosis, and platybasia. Any patient with this finding should have neuroimaging studies done.

24. **A patient presents with a chief complaint of tearing and ocular irritation. As she dumps the plethora of eye drops from her purse, she explains that she has seen seven different doctors and none has been able to help her. The exam shows mild inferior punctate keratopathy but a normal tear lake and normal Schirmer's test. Of interest, she had blepharoplasty surgery 6 months previously. What is the diagnosis?**
You are already patting yourself on the back as you ask if the irritation is worse in the morning or evening. She replies emphatically that it is much more severe upon awakening. You ask her to close her eyes gently and see two millimeters of lagophthalmos in each eye. This is a frequently overlooked cause of tearing in otherwise normal eyes.

25. **During orbital surgery, a patient's lacrimal gland is removed. Afterward, there is no evidence of tear deficiency. Why not?**
Basal tear production is provided by the accessory lacrimal glands of Krause and Wolfring. Krause's glands are located in the superior fornix, and the glands of Wolfring are located above the superior tarsal border. They are cytologically identical to the main lacrimal gland.

26. **Describe the anatomy of the macula and fovea.**
The macula is defined as the area of the posterior retina that contains xanthophyllic pigment and two or more layers of ganglion cells. It is centered approximately 4 mm temporal and 0.8 mm inferior to the center of the optic disc. The fovea is a central depression of the inner retinal surface and is approximately 1.5 mm in diameter.

27. **Fluorescein angiography typically shows perfusion of the choroid and any cilioretinal arteries prior to visualization of the dye in the retinal circulation. Why?**
Fluorescein enters the choroid via the short posterior ciliary arteries, which are branches of the ophthalmic artery. The central retinal artery, also a branch of the ophthalmic artery, provides a more circuitous route for the dye to travel, resulting in dye appearance in the retinal circulation 1–2 seconds later.

28. **Explain why visual acuity in infants does not reach adult levels until approximately 6 months of age, based on retinal differentiation.**
The differentiation of the macula is not complete until 4–6 months after birth. Ganglion cell nuclei are initially found directly over the foveola and gradually are displaced peripherally, leaving this area devoid of accessory neural elements and blood vessels as neural organization develops to adult levels by age 6 months. This delay in macular development is one factor in the inability of newborns to fixate, and improvement in visual activity parallels macular development.

29. **A neonate presents with an opacification in her left cornea. What is the differential diagnosis?**
Neonatal cloudy cornea usually falls into one of the following categories (which can easily be recalled by using the mnemonic **STUMPED**): **s**clerocornea, **t**rauma, **u**lcers, **m**etabolic disorder, **P**eters' anomaly, **e**ndothelial dystrophy, and **d**ermoid.

30. **Describe the innervation of the lens.**
The lens is anatomically unique because it lacks innervation and vascularization. It depends entirely on the aqueous and vitreous humors for nourishment.

31. **Describe the innervation of the cornea.**
The long posterior ciliary nerves branch from the ophthalmic division of the trigeminal nerve and penetrate the cornea. Peripherally, 70–80 branches enter the cornea in conjunctival, episcleral, and scleral planes. They lose their myelin sheath 1–2 mm from the limbus. The network just posterior to Bowman's layer sends branches anteriorly into the epithelium.

32. **What are the three layers of the tear film? Where do they originate?**
   - The **mucoid layer** coats the superficial corneal epithelial cells and creates a hydrophilic layer that allows for spontaneous, even distribution of the aqueous layer of the tear film. Mucin is secreted principally by the conjunctival goblet cells but also from the lacrimal gland.
   - The **aqueous layer** is secreted by the glands of Kraus and Wolfring (basal secretion) and the lacrimal gland (reflex secretion). The aqueous layer contains electrolytes, immunoglobulins, and other solutes, including glucose, buffers, and amino acids.
   - The **lipid layer** is secreted primarily by the meibomian glands and maintains a hydrophobic barrier that prevents tear overflow, retards evaporation, and provides lubrication for the lid/ocular interface.

33. **What are the differences in the structure of the central retinal artery and retinal arterioles?**
The central retinal artery contains a fenestrated internal elastic lamina and an outer layer of smooth muscle cells surrounded by a basement membrane. The retinal arterioles have no

internal elastic lamina and lose the smooth muscle cells near their entrance into the retina. Hence, the retinal vasculature has no autoregulation.

34. **Where is the macula represented in the visual cortex?**
Macular function is represented in the most posterior portion at the tip of the occipital lobe. However, there may be a wide distribution of some macular fibers along the calcarine fissure.

35. **What is macular hole formation?**
Macular hole formation is a common malady that can result in rapid loss of central vision. Approximately 83% of cases are idiopathic, and 15% are due to some sort of trauma.

36. **Describe the stages of macular hole formation as proposed by Gass, as well as the changes in our understanding of the disease process since the development of optical coherence tomography (OCT).**
Gass's theory proposed that the underlying causative mechanism was centripetal tangential traction by the cortical vitreous on the fovea. He also proposed the following stages:
- **Stage 1a:** Tractional elevation of the foveola with a visible yellow dot
- **Stage 1b:** Enlargement of the tractional detachment with foveal elevation. A yellow ring becomes visible
- **Stage 2:** Full-thickness retinal defect less than 400 μm
- **Stage 3:** Full-thickness retinal defect larger than 400 μm
- **Stage 4:** Stage 3 with complete posterior vitreous detachment

OCT analysis has revealed that some patients have perifoveal vitreous detachment with a remaining attachment of the fovea. Occasionally patients may develop an intraretinal split with formation of a foveal cyst. This cyst may evolve into a full-thickness hole with disruption of the inner retinal layer and opening of the foveal floor. These findings suggest a complex array of both anterior-posterior and tangential vector forces as an etiology for molecular hole formation. Clearly the classification of macular holes will need to be reworked in light of these new findings.

BIBLIOGRAPHY

1. American Academy of Ophthalmology: Basic and Clinical Science Course, Section 2. San Francisco, American Academy of Ophthalmology, 1993–1994.
2. Burde RM, Savino PJ, Trobe JD: Clinical Decisions in Neuro-ophthalmology. St. Louis, Mosby, 1985.
3. Fine BS, Yanoff M: Ocular Histology, 2nd ed. Hagerstown, MD, Harper & Row, 1979.
4. Gass JDM: Stereoscopic Atlas of Macular Diseases, 4th ed. St. Louis, Mosby, 1997.
5. Guyer DR, Yannuzzi LA, Chang S, et al: Retina-Vitreous-Macula. Philadelphia, W.B. Saunders, 1999.
6. Jaffe NS: Cataract Surgery and its Complications, 5th ed. St. Louis, Mosby, 1990.
7. Justice J, Lehman RP: Cilioretinal arteries: A study based on review of stereofundus photographs and fluorescein angiographic findings. Arch Ophthalmol 94:1355–1358, 1976.
8. Miller NR: Walsh and Hoyt's Clinical Neuro-Ophthalmology, vol. 1, 4th ed. Baltimore, Williams & Wilkins, 1982.
9. Spaide RF: Optical Coherence Tomography: Interpretation and Clinical Applications. Course #590, AAO Annual Meeting, Chicago, 2005.
10. Stewart WB: Surgery of the Eyelid, Orbit, and Lacrimal System. Ophthalmology Monographs, vol. 1. San Francisco, American Academy of Ophthalmology, 1993.
11. Weinberg DV, Egan KM, Seddon JM: The asymmetric distribution of arteriovenous crossing in the normal retina. Ophthalmology 100:31–36, 1993.

CHAPTER 2

ANATOMY OF THE ORBIT AND EYELID
Edward H. Bedrossian, Jr., MD

ORBIT

1. **Name the bones of the orbit.**
   - **Medial wall:** Sphenoid, ethmoid, lacrimal, maxillary
   - **Lateral wall:** Zygomatic, greater wing of sphenoid
   - **Roof:** Frontal, lesser wing of sphenoid
   - **Floor:** Maxillary, zygomatic, palatine
   See Fig. 2-1.

2. **What are the weak spots of the orbital rim?**
   - Frontozygomatic suture
   - Zygomaticomaxillary suture
   - Frontomaxillary suture

3. **Describe the most common location of blow-out fractures.**
   The posteromedial aspect of the orbital floor.

4. **What is the weakest bone within the orbit?**
   The lamina papyracea portion of the ethmoid bone.

5. **Name the divisions of cranial nerve V that pass through the cavernous sinus.**
   - Ophthalmic division (V1)
   - Maxillary division (V2)

6. **What is the annulus of Zinn?**
   The circle defined by the superior rectus muscle, inferior rectus muscle, lateral rectus muscle, and medial rectus muscle (see Fig. 2-1).

7. **What nerves pass through the superior orbital fissure but outside the annulus of Zinn?**
   Frontal, lacrimal, and trochlear nerves.

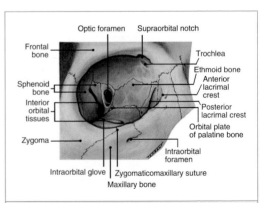

Optic foramen   Supraorbital notch
Frontal bone
Trochlea
Ethmoid bone
Anterior lacrimal crest
Sphenoid bone
Interior orbital tissues
Posterior lacrimal crest
Orbital plate of palatine bone
Zygoma
Intraorbital foramen
Intraorbital glove   Zygomaticomaxillary suture
Maxillary bone

Figure 2-1. Anatomy of the orbit. (From Kanski JJ: Clinical Ophthalmology: A Systematic Approach, 5th ed. New York, Butterworth-Heinemann, 2003.)

EYELID

8. **List the factors responsible for involutional entropion.**
   - Lower lid laxity
   - Override of the preseptal orbicularis oculi muscle onto the pretarsal orbicularis oculi muscle
   - Dehiscence/disinsertion of the lower lid retractors
   - Orbital fat atrophy

9. **Describe the sensory nerve supply to the upper and lower eyelids.**
   - The ophthalmic nerve (V1) provides sensation to the upper lid.
   - The maxillary nerve (V2) provides sensation to the lower lid.

10. **What are the surgical landmarks in locating the superficial temporal artery during temporal artery biopsies?**
    The superficial temporal artery lies deep to the skin and subcutaneous tissue but superficial to the temporalis fascia.

11. **What structures would you pass through during a transverse blepharotomy 3 mm above the upper eyelid margin?**
    - Skin
    - Pretarsal orbicularis muscle
    - Tarsus
    - Palpebral conjunctiva

    See Fig. 2-2.

12. **What is meant by the term *lower lid retractors*?**
    The lower lid retractors consist of the capsulopalpebral fascia and the inferior tarsus muscle. The capsulopalpebral fascia of the lower lid is analogous to the levator complex in the upper lid. The inferior tarsus muscle of the lower lid is analogous to Müller's muscle in the upper lid.

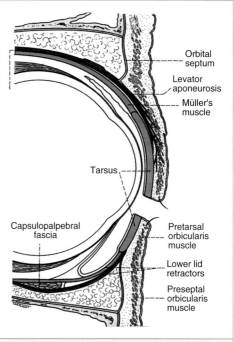

Labels: Orbital septum; Levator aponeurosis; Müller's muscle; Tarsus; Capsulopalpebral fascia; Pretarsal orbicularis muscle; Lower lid retractors; Preseptal orbicularis muscle

Figure 2-2. Eyelid structures. (From Kanski JJ: Clinical Ophthalmology: A Systematic Approach, 5th ed. New York, Butterworth-Heinemann, 2003.)

13. **What structures would be cut in a full-thickness lower-lid laceration 2 mm below the lower tarsus?**
    - Skin
    - Preseptal orbicularis oculi muscle
    - Conjoint tendon (fused orbital septum and lower lid retractors)
    - Palpebral conjunctiva

14. **What structures would be cut in a full-thickness lower-lid laceration 6 mm below the lower tarsus?**
    - Skin
    - Preseptal orbicularis oculi muscle
    - Orbital septum
    - Fat
    - Lower lid retractors (capsulopalpebral fascia and inferior tarsus muscle)
    - Conjunctiva

15. **Discuss the bony attachments of Whitnall's superior suspensory ligament.**
    Medially, it attaches to the periosteum of the trochlea. Laterally, the major attachment is to the periosteum at the frontozygomatic suture. It also sends minor attachments to the lateral orbital tubercle.

16. **What structure separates the medial fat pad from the central (also called the preaponeurotic) fat pad in the upper eyelid?**
    The superior oblique tendon.

17. **Lester Jones divided the orbicularis oculi muscle into three portions. Name them.**
    - Orbital portion
    - Preseptal portion
    - Pretarsal portion

18. **What portions of the orbicularis oculi muscle are important in the lacrimal pump mechanism?**
    The preseptal and pretarsal portions.

BIBLIOGRAPHY

1. Anderson R, Dixon R: The role of Whitnall's ligament in ptosis surgery. Arch Ophthalmol 97:705–707, 1979.
2. Bedrossian EH Jr: Embryology and anatomy of the eyelids. In Tasman W, Jaeger E (eds): Foundations of Clinical Ophthalmology. Lippincott, Williams & Wilkins, 1998, pp 1–22.
3. Bedrossian EH Jr: Surgical anantomy of the eyelids. In Della Rocca RC, Bedrossian EH Jr, Arthurs BP (eds): Opthalmic Plastic Surgery: Decision Making and Techniques. Philadelphia, McGraw-Hill, 2002, pp 163–172.
4. Dutton J: Atlas of Clinical and Surgical Orbital Anatomy. Philadelphia, W.B. Saunders, 1994.
5. Gioia V, Linberg J, McCormick S: The anatomy of the lateral canthal tendon. Arch Ophthalmol 105:529–532, 1987.
6. Hawes M, Dortzbach R: The microscopic anatomy of the lower eyelid retractors. Arch Ophthalmol 100:1313–1318, 1982.
7. Jones LT: The anatomy of the lower eyelid. Am J Ophthalmol 49:29–36, 1960.
8. Lemke B, Della Rocca R: Surgery of the Eyelids and Orbit: An Anatomical Approach. Norwalk, CT, Appleton & Lange, 1990.
9. Lemke B, Stasior O, Rosen P: The surgical relations of the levator palpebrae superioris muscle. Ophthal Plast Reconstr Surg 4:25–30, 1988.
10. Lockwood CB: The anatomy of the muscles, ligaments and fascia of the orbit, including an account of the capsule of tenon, the check ligaments of the recti, and of the suspensory ligament of the eye. J Anat Physiol 20:1–26, 1886.
11. Meyer D, Linberg J, Wobig J, McCormick S: Anatomy of the orbital septum and associated eyelid connective tissues: Implications for ptosis surgery. Ophthal Plast Reconstr Surg 7:104–113, 1991.
12. Sullivan J, Beard C: Anatomy of the eyelids, orbit and lacrimal system. In Stewart W (ed): Surgery of the Eyelids, Orbit and Lacrimal System. American Academy of Ophthalmology Monograph no. 8, 1993, pp 84–96.
13. Whitnall SE: The levator palpebrae superioris muscle: The attachments and relations of its aponeurosis. Ophthalmoscope 12:258–263, 1914.
14. Whitnall SE: The Anatomy of the Human Orbit and Accessory Organs. London, Oxford Medical Publishers, 1985.

OPTICS AND REFRACTION

Janice A. Gault, MD

CHAPTER 3

1. **What is the primary focal point (f)?**
   The point along the optical axis at which an object must be placed for parallel rays to emerge from the lens. Thus, the image is at infinity (Fig. 3-1).

2. **What is the secondary focal point (f′)?**
   The point along the optical axis at which parallel incoming rays are brought into focus. It is equal to 1/lens power in diopters (D). The object is now at infinity (Fig. 3-2).

3. **Where is the secondary focal point for a myopic eye? A hyperopic eye? An emmetropic eye?**
   The secondary focal point for a **myopic eye** is anterior to the retina in the vitreous (Fig. 3-3A). The object must be moved forward from infinity to allow the light rays to focus on the retina. A **hyperopic** eye has its secondary focal point posterior to the retina (Fig. 3-3B). An **emmetropic** eye focuses light rays from infinity onto the retina.

4. **What is the far point of an eye?**
   The term *far point* is used only for the optical system of an eye. It is the point at which an object must be placed along the optical axis for the light rays to be focused on the retina when the eye is not accommodating.

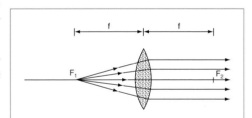

Figure 3-1. The primary focal point (F₁), which has an image at infinity. (From Azar DT, Strauss L: Principles of applied clinical optics. In Albert DM, Jakobiec FA [eds]: Principles and Practice of Ophthalmology, vol. 6, 2nd ed. Philadelphia, W.B. Saunders, 2000, pp 5329–5340.)

5. **Where is the far point for a myopic eye? A hyperopic eye? An emmetropic eye?**
   The far point for a **myopic** eye is between the cornea and infinity. A **hyperopic** eye has its far point beyond infinity or behind the eye. An **emmetropic** eye has light rays focused on the retina when the object is at infinity.

6. **How do you determine which lens will correct the refractive error of the eye?**
   A lens with its focal point coincident with the far point of the eye allows the light rays from infinity to be focused on the retina. The image at the far point of the eye now becomes the object for the eye.

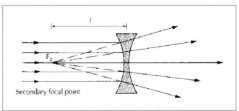

Secondary focal point

Figure 3-2. The secondary focal point (F₂), which also has an object at infinity. (From Azar DT, Strauss L: Principles of applied clinical optics. In Albert DM, Jakobiec FA [eds]: Principles and Practice of Ophthalmology, vol. 6, 2nd ed. Philadelphia, W.B. Saunders, 2000, pp 5329–5340.)

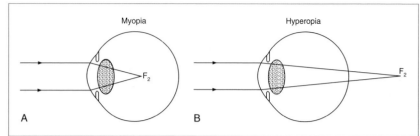

Figure 3-3. *A,* The secondary focal point of a myopic eye is anterior to the retina in the vitreous. *B,* In hyperopia, the secondary focal point is behind the retina. (From Azar DT, Strauss L: Principles of applied clinical optics. In Albert DM, Jakobiec FA [eds]: Principles and Practice of Ophthalmology, vol. 6, 2nd ed. Philadelphia, W.B. Saunders, 2000, pp 5329–5340.)

7. **What is the near point of an eye?**
   The point at which an object will be in focus on the retina when the eye is fully accommodating. Moving the object closer will cause it to blur.

8. **Myopia can be caused in two ways. What are they?**
   - **Refractive myopia** is caused by too much refractive power due to steep corneal curvature or high lens power.
   - **Axial myopia** is due to an elongated globe. Every millimeter of axial elongation causes about 3 D of myopia.

9. **The power of a proper corrective lens is altered by switching from a contact lens to a spectacle lens or vice versa. Why?**
   Moving a minus lens closer to the eye increases effective minus power. Thus, myopes have a weaker minus prescription in their contact lenses than in their glasses. Patients near presbyopia may need reading glasses when using their contacts but can read without a bifocal lens in their glasses (see question 45). Moving a plus lens closer to the eye decreases effective plus power. Thus, hyperopes need a stronger plus prescription for their contact lenses than for their glasses. They may defer bifocals for a while. The same principle applies to patients who slide their glasses down their nose and find that they can read more easily. They are adding plus power. This principle works for both hyperopes and myopes.

10. **What is the amplitude of accommodation?**
    The total number of diopters that an eye can accommodate.

11. **What is the range of accommodation?**
    The range of clear vision obtainable with accommodation only. For an emmetrope with 10 D of accommodative amplitude, the range of accommodation is infinity–10 cm.

12. **How does a diopter relate to meters?**
    A diopter is the reciprocal of the distance in meters.

13. **What is the near point of a 4-D hyperope with an amplitude of accommodation of 8?**
    The far point is 25 cm ($\frac{1}{4}$ D) behind the cornea. The patient must use 4 D of accommodation to overcome hyperopia and focus the image at infinity on the retina. Thus, he or she has 4 D to accommodate to the near point, which is 25 cm ($\frac{1}{4}$ D) anterior to the cornea. However, when wearing a +4.00 lens, he or she has the full amplitude of accommodation available. The near point is now 12.5 cm ($\frac{1}{8}$ D).

14. **What is the near point of a 4-D myope with an amplitude of accommodation of 8?**
The far point is 25 cm ($\frac{1}{4}$ D) in front of the eye. The patient can accommodate 8 D beyond this point. The near point is 12 D, which is 8.3 cm ($\frac{1}{12}$ D) in front of the cornea.

15. **When a light ray passes from a medium with a lower refractive index (n) to a medium with a higher refractive index (n′), is it bent toward or away from the normal?**
It is bent toward the normal (Fig. 3-4).

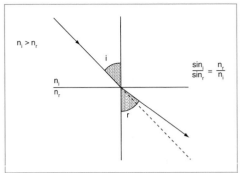

Figure 3-4. When light passes from a medium with lower refractive index (n_i) to a medium of higher refractive index (n_r), it slows down and is bent toward the normal to the surface. Snell's law determines the amount of bending. i = angle of incidence, r = angle of refraction. (From Azar DT, Strauss L: Principles of applied clinical optics. In Albert DM, Jakobiec FA [eds]: Principles and Practice of Ophthalmology, vol. 6, 2nd ed. Philadelphia, W.B. Saunders, 2000, pp 5329–5340.)

16. **What is the critical angle?**
The incident angle at which the angle of refraction is 90 degrees to normal. The critical angle occurs only when light passes from a more dense to a less dense medium.

17. **What happens if the critical angle is exceeded?**
Total internal reflection. The angle of incidence equals the angle of reflection (Fig. 3-5).

18. **Give examples of total internal reflection.**
Total internal reflection at the tear-air interface prevents a direct view of the anterior chamber. To overcome this limitation, the critical angle must be increased for the tear-air interface by applying a plastic or glass goniolens to the surface. Total internal reflection also occurs in fiberoptic tubes and indirect ophthalmoscopes.

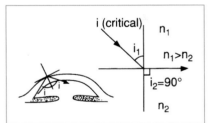

Figure 3-5. Total internal reflection occurs when the critical angle is exceeded. (From Azar DT, Strauss L: Principles of applied clinical optics. In Albert DM, Jakobiec FA [eds]: Principles and Practice of Ophthalmology, vol. 6, 2nd ed. Philadelphia, W.B. Saunders, 2000, pp 5329–5340.)

19. **What is the formula for vergence?**

$$U + P = V$$

Where U is the vergence of light entering the lens, P is the power of the lens (the amount of vergence added to the light by the lens), and V is the vergence of light leaving the lens. All are expressed in diopters. By convention, light rays travel left to right. Plus signs indicate anything to the right of the lens, and minus signs indicate points to the left of the lens.

20. **What is the vergence of parallel light rays?**
    Zero. Parallel light rays do not converge (which would be positive) or diverge (which would be negative). Light rays from an object at infinity or going to an image at infinity have zero vergence.

21. **What is the image point if an object lies 25 cm to the left of a +5.00 lens?**
    Everything must be expressed in diopters: 25 cm is 4 D (1/0.25 m). Because the image is to the left of the lens,

$$U = -4\,D$$
$$P = +5\,D$$
$$-4 + 5 = 1$$

    The vergence of the object is +1 D. Converted to centimeters, the object lies 1 m to the right of the lens (1/1 D = 1 m = 100 cm).

22. **Draw the schematic eye with power (P), nodal point (np), principal plane, primary (f) and secondary (f′) focal points, refractive indices (n, n′), and respective distances labeled.**
    See Fig. 3-6.

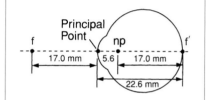

Figure 3-6. The reduced schematic eye. (From Azar DT, Strauss L: Principles of applied clinical optics. In Albert DM, Jakobiec FA [eds]: Principles and Practice of Ophthalmology, vol. 6, 2nd ed. Philadelphia, W.B. Saunders, 2000, pp 5329–5340.)

23. **How is the power of a prism calculated?**
    The power of a prism is calculated in prism diopters (Δ) and is equal to the displacement in centimeters of a light ray passing through the prism measured 100 cm from the prism. Light is always bent toward the base of the prism. Thus, a prism of 15 Δ displaces light from infinity 15 cm toward its base at 100 cm.

24. **What is Prentice's rule?**

$$\Delta = hD$$

    The prismatic power of a lens (Δ) at any point on the lens is equal to the distance of that point from the optical axis in centimeters (h) multiplied by the power of the lens in diopters (D). It follows that a lens has no prismatic effect at its optical center; a light ray will pass through the center undeviated (Fig. 3-7).

25. **How is Prentice's rule used in real life?**
    In a patient who has anisometropia, the reading position may cause hyperdeviation of one eye due to the prismatic effect.

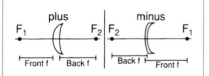

Figure 3-7. Prismatic effect of a lens according to Prentice's rule. d = induced prism (measured in prism diopters), h = distance from optical center in centimeters, and D = power of lens in diopters. (From Azar DT, Strauss L: Principles of applied clinical optics. In Albert DM, Jakobiec FA [eds]: Principles and Practice of Ophthalmology, vol. 6, 2nd ed. Philadelphia, W.B. Saunders, 2000, pp 5329–5340.)

KEY POINTS: ALLEVIATION OF SYMPTOMATIC ANISOMETROPIA

1. Contact lenses
2. Lowering optical centers
3. Slab-off

26. **How can the prismatic effect be alleviated?**
    - Contact lenses move with the eye and allow patients to see through their optical center, preventing the prismatic effect.
    - Lowering the optical centers decreases the h of Prentice's rule.
    - Slab-off (removing the prism inferiorly from the more minus lens) helps to counteract the prismatic effect.

27. **How does Prentice's rule affect the measurement of strabismic deviations when the patient is wearing glasses?**
    Plus lenses decrease the measured deviation, whereas minus lenses increase the measured deviation. The true deviation is changed by approximately 2.5 D% where D is the spectacle power. The plus lenses have the base of the prism peripherally, whereas the minus lenses have the base of the prism centrally.

28. **Bifocals can cause significant problems induced by prismatic effect. What is the difference between image jump and image displacement?**
    - **Image jump** is produced by the sudden introduction of the prismatic power at the top of the bifocal segment. The object that the patient sees in the inferior field suddenly jumps upward when the eye turns down to look at it. If the optical center of the segment is at the top of the segment, there is no image jump. Image jump is worse in glasses with a round-top bifocal because the optical center is far from the distance lens' optical center. A flat-top bifocal is better because the optical center is close to the distance optical center.
    - **Image displacement** is the prismatic effect induced by the addition of the bifocal and the distance lenses in the reading position. Image displacement is more bothersome than image jump for most people. A flat-top lens is essentially a base-up lens whereas a round-top lens is a base-down lens. A myopic distance lens has base-up prismatic power in the reading position; thus, image displacement is worsened with a flat-top lens. The prism effects are additive. Similarly, a hyperopic correction is a base-down lens in the reading position; thus, a round-top lens makes image displacement an issue.

29. **Should a hyperope use a round-top or flat-top reading lens?**
    A plus lens will have significant image displacement with a flat-top lens. Image displacement is lessened with a round-top lens. Although image jump will be present, it is the less disturbing of the two.

30. **Should a myope use a flat-top or round-top reading lens?**
    A round-top lens has significant image displacement with a minus lens. A flat-top lens minimizes image displacement and image jump.

31. **What is the circle of least confusion?**
    Patients with astigmatism have two focal lines formed by the convergence of light rays. The first focal line is nearer the cornea and created by the more powerful corneal meridian. The second focal

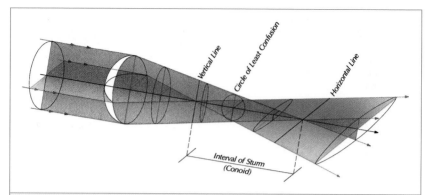

Figure 3-8. The circle of least confusion. (From Azar DT, Strauss L: Principles of applied clinical optics. In Albert DM, Jakobiec FA [eds]: Principles and Practice of Ophthalmology, vol. 6, 2nd ed. Philadelphia, W.B. Saunders, 2000, pp 5329–5340.)

line is further away, created by the less powerful meridian. The circle of least confusion is the circular cross-section of Sturm's conoid, dioptrically midway between the two focal lines (Fig. 3-8). The goal of refractive correction is to choose a lens that places the circle of least confusion on the retina.

32. **What is the spherical equivalent of –3.00 + 2.00 × 125?**
    Take half the cylinder and add it to the sphere. The spherical equivalent is –2.00 sphere.

33. **Change the following plus cylinder refraction to minus cylinder form: –5.00 + 3.00 × 90.**
    First, add the sphere and cylinder to each other. Then change the sign of the cylinder, and add 90 degrees to the axis. Thus, the minus cylinder form is –2.00 – 3.00 × 180.

34. **After cataract surgery, a patient has the following refraction: +1.00 + 3.00 × 100. Does the patient have with-the-rule or against-the-rule astigmatism?**
    With-the-rule astigmatism is corrected with a plus cylinder at 90 degrees (±15–20 degrees). Against-the-rule astigmatism is corrected with a plus cylinder at 180 degrees (±15–20 degrees). The patient has with-the-rule astigmatism.

35. **How should you proceed with the patient's care?**
    Check the remaining sutures. Cutting the 11:00 suture will relax the wound and decrease the amount of astigmatism.

36. **What if a postoperative patient has a refraction of +2.00 – 2.00 × 90? Where should you cut the suture?**
    Changing the refraction to plus cylinder form, you see that the patient is plano + 2.00 × 180 and has against-the-rule astigmatism. You cannot cut any sutures to relax the astigmatism. The only option is to do a relaxing incision of the cornea, but it is likely that the patient will tolerate glasses, especially if the refraction is close to the preoperative correction. Also, check the preoperative keratometry. The patient may have had against-the-rule astigmatism before surgery.

37. **Thick lenses have aberrations. List them.**
    ■ **Spherical aberration:** The rays at the peripheral edges of the lens are refracted more than the rays at the center, thus causing night myopia. The larger pupil at night allows more spherical aberration than the smaller pupil during daylight.

- **Coma:** A comet-shaped blur is seen when the object and image are off the optical axis. Coma is similar to spherical aberration but occurs in the nonaxial rays.
- **Astigmatism of oblique incidence:** When the spherical lens is tilted, the lens gains a small astigmatic effect that causes curvature of the field (i.e., spherical images produce curved images of flat objects). This effect is helpful in the eye because the retina has a similar curvature (Fig. 3-9).
- **Chromatic aberration:** Each wavelength has its own refractive index; the shortest wavelengths are bent the most (Fig. 3-10).
- **Distortion:** The higher the spherical power, the more significantly the periphery is magnified or minified in relation to the rest of the image. A high plus lens produces pincushion distortion; a high minus lens produces barrel distortion.

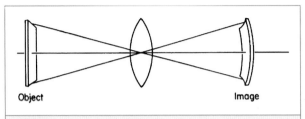

Figure 3-9. The aberration caused by the astigmatism of oblique incidence is helpful in the eye because the curvature of the field that it induces is almost identical to the retinal curvature.

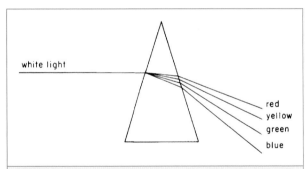

Figure 3-10. Because each wavelength has a different refractive index, light passing through a prism will reveal the characteristic visible spectrum. (From American Academy of Ophthalmology: Basic and Clinical Science Course. Section 3. Optics, Refraction, and Contact Lenses. San Francisco, American Academy of Ophthalmology, 1992.)

38. **Are red or green light rays refracted more by a plus lens?**
   The shorter green rays are bent more than the longer red rays. This distinction causes chromatic aberration and is the basis for the red-green duochrome test. Green rays are focused 0.50 D closer to the lens than red rays. When a corrected myopic patient is fogged to prevent accommodation, the red letters should be clearer than the green. Slowly add more minus in 0.25 increments until the green and red letters are equal in clarity. This technique prevents overcorrection of myopia.

39. **A myopic patient tilts his glasses to see in the distance. What does this tell you?**
   The patient is using the principle of astigmatism of oblique incidence to strengthen the power of his glasses. He needs a refraction. Tilting a minus lens induces a minus cylinder with axis in the

axis of tilt. Tilting a plus lens induces a plus cylinder with axis in the axis of tilt. A small amount of additional sphere of the same sign is induced as well.

40. **What measurements are necessary in determining the intraocular lens implant calculation?**
Axial length in millimeters and keratometry readings in diopters. The desired postoperative refraction is also necessary. The SRK formula is commonly used. For emmetropia, the formula is $P = A - 2.5$ (axial length) $- 0.9$ (K_{avg}), where P equals the implant power, A is the implant constant as determined by the manufacturer, and K_{avg} is the average of the keratometry readings. The A constant also can be individualized by analysis of previous cases. For each diopter of desired ametropia, add 1.25–1.50 D. For example, if the SRK formula reveals a calculation of $+18.0$ D for emmetropia, implant a $+19.50$ D lens for -1.00 D.

41. **How does an axial error that is incorrect by 0.1 mm affect the intraocular lens calculation?**
For every 0.1 mm error, the calculation is impacted by 0.25 D. Recheck the A scan if the axial length is less than 22 mm or more than 25 mm, or if there is more than a 0.3 mm difference in the measurement between the two eyes.

42. **How does an error in keratometry readings affect the intraocular lens calculation?**
For every error of 0.25 D, the calculation is in error by 0.25 D. Recheck the keratometer measurements if the average corneal power is less than 40 D or more than 47 D. Also check if there is a difference of more than 1 D in the average keratometer readings between eyes.

43. **What is the formula for transverse magnification?**
Also known as linear or lateral magnification, transverse magnification equals $I/O = v/u$, where I is the size of the image, O is the size of the object, v is the distance from the lens to the image, and u is the distance of the object from the lens. All are measured in millimeters.

44. **What is the formula for axial magnification?**
The square of the transverse magnification. Magnification along the visual axis causes distortion in three-dimensional images.

45. **What is the effect of axial magnification on accommodative requirements for a given near-viewing distance?**
Hyperopes must accommodate more through glasses than through contact lenses, because the stronger plus prescription required in the contact lens provides more axial magnification of the image compared with the prescription for glasses. Conversely, myopes must accommodate less through glasses than through contact lenses. This effect can be clinically significant in early presbyopic years. The effect is greatest with high refractive errors. For example, a -5.00 myope may be able to read without bifocal glasses but require reading glasses with contact lenses. Conversely, a hyperope may be able to forego reading glasses with contact lenses but need bifocal glasses.

46. **What is angular magnification?**
The magnification of a simple magnifier, such as viewing something with an eye or a single lens. Magnification is D/4, where D is the power of the lens used.

47. **What is the magnification of a direct ophthalmoscope?**
The examiner uses the optics of the patient's eye as a simple magnifier. Estimating the power of the eye as $+60$ D, the magnification is $15\times$. Thus, the retina appears 15 times larger than it is.

48. **Does an astronomic telescope form an upright or an inverted image?**
An inverted image, which has few uses in ophthalmic optics.

49. **Does a Galilean telescope form an upright or an inverted image?**
An upright image, which is used often in ophthalmic optics. An aphakic eye corrected with spectacles or a contact lens is an example. The eyepiece is the aphakic eye estimated to be −12.50 D, and the objective is the corrective lens.

50. **What is the magnification formula for a telescope?**

$$\text{Magnification} = D \text{ eyepiece}/D \text{ objective}$$

This formula applies to both astronomic and Galilean telescopes. For the aphakic eye with a spectacle correction of +10.00 D, the magnification is 1.25 or 25%. For a contact lens, this translates to +11.75 D, accounting for the vertex distance of 10 mm. Magnification now is 1.06 or 6%. Thus, aniseikonia with a contact lens is better tolerated than aniseikonia with glasses if the patient needs less powerful correction in the other eye.

51. **When using the direct ophthalmoscope, which patient provides the larger image of the retina—the hyperope or the myope?**
The myope functions as a Galilean telescope and provides extra magnification. The eyepiece (spectacle lens) is a minus lens, and the objective (the patient's own lens) is a plus lens. The hyperope functions as a reverse Galilean telescope and provides minification in comparison. In this situation, the eyepiece is a plus lens, and the objective is a minus lens.

52. **What do you need to determine the best low-vision aid for a patient?**
Best refraction, visual acuity, visual field, and practical needs of the patient.

53. **What are the advantages and disadvantages of using a high add in a bifocal for a low-vision aid?**
The advantages include a large field of view. Disadvantages include a short reading distance, as well as significant cost.

54. **What are the advantages and disadvantages of using a high-power single-vision lens as a low-vision aid?**
High-power single-vision lenses come in monocular and binocular forms. They also afford a large field of view but have a short reading distance.

55. **How do you estimate the strength of plus lens needed to read newspaper print without accommodation?**
The reciprocal of the best Snellen acuity is equal to the plus power of the lens required. For example, if a patient can read 20/60, a +3.00 D will suffice. The reciprocal of the diopter power gives the reading distance (i.e., 33 cm).

56. **What adjustment is necessary when a binocular high-power single-vision lens is used?**
Base in prisms to augment the natural ability to converge. Otherwise, patients develop exotropia at near when looking through high plus lenses.

57. **What are the advantages and disadvantages of hand-held magnifiers for low-vision aids?**
Hand-held magnifiers have a variable eye-to-lens distance and are easily portable. They enjoy a high rate of acceptability. However, they have a small field of view when the lens is held far from

the eye and are difficult to manipulate by patients with tremors and arthritis. A stand magnifier may be more useful for such patients.

58. **What are the advantages and disadvantages of using loupes as a low-vision aid?**
Loupes are basically prefocused telescopes. They allow a long working distance and keep the hands free. But they have a small field of view, limited depth of field, and are expensive.

59. **The devices mentioned thus far are for magnifying at near. What is available for distance aids?**
The only magnifying device for distance is a telescope. Telescopes are monocular or binocular and can be hand-held or mounted on glasses. They also have an adjustable focus. Unfortunately, they have a restricted field of view (approximately 8 degrees). Thus, the object of regard may be difficult to find.

60. **Do convex mirrors add plus or minus vergence?**
Convex mirrors add minus vergence like minus lenses. Concave mirrors add plus vergence like plus lenses. Plane mirrors add no vergence.

61. **What is the reflecting power in diopters of a mirror?**
$D = 2/r$, where r is the radius of curvature. The focal length is one half the radius.

62. **What instrument uses the reflecting power of the cornea to determine its readings?**
The keratometer uses the reflecting power of the cornea to determine the corneal curvature. The formula is $D = (n - 1)/r$, where D is the reflecting power of the cornea and n is the standardized refractive index for the cornea (1.3375).

63. **How much of the cornea is measured with a keratometer?**
Only the central 3 mm. A peripheral corneal scar or defect may be missed by using a keratometer instead of a cornea map.

64. **Why does a keratometer use doubling of its images?**
To avoid the problems of eye movement in determining an accurate measurement. Doubling is done with prisms.

65. **What is a Geneva lens clock?**
A device to determine the base curve of the back surface of a spectacle. It is often used clinically to detect plus cylinder spectacle lenses in a patient used to minus cylinder lenses. It is specifically calibrated for the refractive index of crown glass. A special lens clock is available for plastic lenses.

66. **Do you measure the power of spectacles in a lensmeter with the temples toward you or away from you?**
The distance is measured with the temples facing away from you (back vertex power). The add is measured with the temples pointing toward you (front vertex power). You must measure the difference between the top and bottom segments, especially if the patient has a highly hyperopic prescription.

67. **If you obtain "with" movement during retinoscopy, is the far point of the patient in front of the peephole, at the peephole, or beyond the peephole?**
Beyond the peephole. The goal is neutralization of the light reflex so that the patient's far point is at the peephole. The light at the patient's pupil fills the entire space at once. More plus must be added to the prescription to move the far point to neutralization. "Against" movement means that the far point is in front of the peephole; more minus must be added to move the far point to neutralization.

68. **What does a pachymeter measure?**
The corneal thickness or anterior chamber depth.

69. **How does the Hruby lens give an upright or inverted image?**
A Hruby lens is −55 D and gives an upright image. The Goldman lens is −64 D and also provides an upright image. The Volk 90 D lens provides an inverted image.

70. **Why does the indirect ophthalmoscope provide a larger field of view than the direct ophthalmoscope?**
The condensing lens used with the indirect ophthalmoscope captures the peripheral rays to give a field of view of 25 degrees or more depending on the lens power used. The direct ophthalmoscope does not use the condensing lens and thus provides only a 7-degree field of view.

71. **What are the wavelengths of the spectrum of visible light?**
The range is from 400 nm for violet light to 700 nm for red light. Anything shorter than 400 nm is considered ultraviolet, and anything longer than 700 nm is in the infrared spectrum.

72. **Antireflective coatings on spectacle lenses are based on what principle?**
Interference. Antireflective coatings use destructive interference. The crest of one wavelength cancels the trough of another.

73. **What is the most effective pinhole diameter?**
A pinhole diameter of 1.2 mm neutralizes up to 3 D of refractive error. A 2 mm pinhole neutralizes only 1 D. An aphakic patient may need a +10 D lens in addition to the pinhole to obtain useful visual acuity.

74. **When is a cycloplegic refraction indicated?**
- Patients younger than 15 years, especially if they have strabismus. Make sure to measure the deviation before cycloplegia.
- Hyperopes younger than 35 years, especially if they experience asthenopia.
- Patients with asthenopia suggestive of accommodative problems.

Note: Check accommodative amplitudes and reading adds before cycloplegia.

75. **Which cycloplegic agent lasts the longest? The shortest?**
Atropine lasts for 1–2 weeks. Watch for toxic effects in small children and elderly patients. Tropicamide (Mydriacyl) lasts 4–8 hours and is not strong enough for cycloplegia in children. One or two D of hyperopia may remain. Cyclogyl lasts 8–24 hours; homatropine, 1–3 days; and scopolamine, 5–7 days.

76. **What are the signs and symptoms of systemic intoxication from cycloplegic medications? How are they treated?**
Dry mouth, fever, flushing, tachycardia, nausea, and delirium. Treatment includes counteraction with physostigmine.

77. **When is it important to measure the vertex distance in prescribing glasses?**
When the patient has a strong prescription of more than ±5.00 D.

78. **What is the threshold for prescribing glasses in a child with astigmatism?**
When visual acuity is not developing properly, as noted by amblyopia or strabismus. Give the full correction. Children tolerate full correction better than adults. Most often, amblyopia or strabismus occurs with at least 1.50 D of astigmatism. Anisometropia that presents with 1.00 D or more of hyperopic asymmetry also requires full correction.

79. **What may cause monocular diplopia?**
    - Corneal or lenticular irregularity
    - Decentered contact lens
    - Inappropriate placement of reading add
    - Transient sensory adaptations after strabismus surgery
    - Distortion from retinal lesions (rare)

80. **What conditions may give a false-positive reading with a potential acuity meter?**
    Macular scotomas in a patient with amblyopia or retinal disease, such as age-related macular degeneration. Acute macular edema also may elevate the reading, but the elevation disappears with chronic edema. An irregular corneal surface can falsely improve the potential acuity; however, wearing a contact lens may help.

81. **What do you check when patients complain that their new glasses are not as good as their previous pair?**
    - Ask specifically what the complaint is. Distance reading? Near problems? Asthenopia? Diplopia? Pain behind the ears or at the nose bridge from ill-fitting glasses?
    - Read the new and old glasses on the lensmeter and compare. Make sure that the old glasses did not have any prism. Check the patient for undetected strabismus with cover testing.
    - Refract the patient again, possibly with a cycloplegic agent if the symptoms warrant.
    - Check the optical centers in comparison with the pupillary centers.
    - Check whether the reading segments are in the correct position-level with the lower lid.
    - Make sure that the new glasses fit the patient correctly.
    - Check whether the old glasses were made with plus cylinder by using the Geneva lens clock.
    - Check whether the base curve has changed with the Geneva lens clock.
    - Evaluate the patient for dry eye.
    - If the patient has a high prescription, check the vertex distance. Often it is easier to refract such patients over their old pair of glasses to keep the same vertex distance.
    - Check the pantoscopic tilt. Normally the tilt is 10–15 degrees so that when the patient reads, the eye is perpendicular to the lens. If the tilt is off, especially in relation to the old glasses, the patient may notice.
    - With postoperative glasses, evaluate for diplopia in downgaze due to anisometropia.
    - Perhaps the add is too strong or too weak. Check the patient using trial lenses and reading material.
    - Sometimes if the diameter of the lens is much larger in the newer frames, the patient notices significant distortion in the peripheral lens. Encourage a small frame. However, too small a frame can make progressive bifocals very difficult. It is best to keep a frame size fairly consistent.
    - Did the patient change bifocal types? Round top, flat top, executive style, and progressives all require different adaptations. Patients often have trouble when changing styles.
    - Above all, try to test the new prescription in trial frames with a walk around the office. You do not want to go through this process again.

82. **If after repeat refraction the patient suddenly develops more hyperopia than you previously noted, what do you look for?**
    A cause of acquired hyperopia, such as a retrobulbar tumor, central serous retinopathy, posterior lens dislocation, or a flattened cornea from a contact lens.

KEY POINTS: CAUSES OF MONOCULAR DIPLOPIA

1. Corneal or lenticular irregularity

2. Decentered contact lens, intraocular implant, or refractive surgery

3. Inappropriate placement of reading add

4. Sensory problems after strabismus surgery

5. Retinal lesions (very rare)

83. **What if the patient has more myopia than previously noted?**
Check the cycloplegic refraction to make sure that it is true. Acquired myopia may be caused by diabetes mellitus, sulfonamides, nuclear sclerosis, pilocarpine, keratoconus, a scleral buckle for retinal detachment, and anterior lens dislocation.

84. **What about acquired astigmatism?**
Lid lesions such as hemangiomas, chalazions, and ptosis may cause acquired astigmatism. A pterygium or keratoconus may reveal a previously undetected astigmatism. And, of course, healing cataract wounds may change the previous astigmatism.

85. **If the astigmatism has changed and the patient has difficulty with tolerating the new prescription, what are the options?**
If the astigmatism is oblique, try rotating the axis toward 90 or toward the old axis. The astigmatic power may be reduced, but keep the spherical power the same. Sometimes a gradual change in prescription over time may allow the patient to adapt. For example, if a patient's prescription is $-3.00 + 2.00 \times 110$, a possibility is $-2.50 + 1.00 \times 90$. The spherical equivalent of -2.00 D has been maintained.

86. **What does laser stand for?**
Light amplification by stimulated emission of radiation.

87. **To steepen a contact lens fit, do you increase the diameter of the lens or the radius of curvature?**
Increasing the diameter of the lens or decreasing the radius of curvature will steepen the lens (Fig. 3-11). This information is useful for lenses that fit too tightly.

88. **How many seconds of arc does the "E" on the 20/20 line of the Snellen eye chart subtend?**
Five seconds. The Snellen eye chart measures the minimal separable acuity.

89. **When the Jackson cross is used to define the astigmatic axis, is the handle of the lens parallel to the axis or 45 degrees from it?**
Parallel. To define the astigmatic power, the handle is 45 degrees to the axis. Define the axis before the power.

90. **A 25-year-old patient has a manifest refraction of +0.50 OU and complains of asthenopia. What do you do?**
Check the patient's accommodative amplitude and look for an exophoria at near to evaluate for convergence insufficiency. Then do a cycloplegic refraction to check for undercorrection. On exam, the amplitude of accommodation is 3 D OU. Because this value is low for a young person,

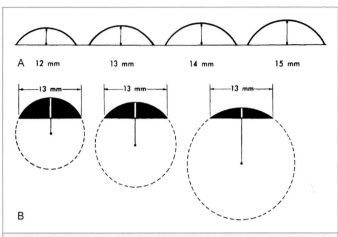

Figure 3-11. **A,** When the radius of curvature is kept constant while the diameter of the contact lens is increased, the fit steepens. **B,** Conversely, increasing the radius of curvature while maintaining the same diameter allows a flatter fit. (From American Academy of Ophthalmology: Basic and Clinical Science Course. Section 3: Optics, Refraction, and Contact Lenses. San Francisco, American Academy of Ophthalmology, 1992.)

suspect undercorrection of hyperopia. Indeed, the cycloplegic refraction is +2.50 OU. The patient has accommodative spasm. Try giving one half of the cycloplegic findings. Sometimes atropine is needed to break the spasm.

91. **What instrument is useful to measure the accommodative amplitude?**
    Prince rule.

92. **A 35-year-old man has 20/40 uncorrected vision. With +0.50 glasses, he is 20/20. He will remain 20/20 with a +1.50 manifest refraction. With cycloplegia, he has a refraction of +4.00. Define absolute hyperopia, facultative hyperopia, manifest hyperopia, and latent hyperopia.**
    - **Total hyperopia:** Found by cycloplegia, +4.00
    - **Manifest hyperopia:** Found without cycloplegia; more plus will blur vision, +1.50
    - **Latent hyperopia:** Total minus manifest hyperopia, +2.50
    - **Absolute hyperopia:** The minimal correction that the patient needs to see distances, +0.50
    - **Facultative hyperopia:** Manifest minus absolute hyperopia; compensation accomplished by accommodation, +1.00

BIBLIOGRAPHY

1. American Academy of Ophthalmology: Basic and Clinical Science Course. San Francisco, American Academy of Ophthalmology, 1992.
2. Milder B, Rubin ML: The Fine Art of Prescribing Glasses Without Making a Spectacle of Yourself, 2nd ed. Gainesville, FL, Triad Publishing, 1991.
3. Rubin ML: Optics for Clinicians, 3rd ed. Gainesville, FL, Triad Publishing, 1993.

COLOR VISION

Mitchell S. Fineman, MD

CHAPTER 4

1. **What are photons?**

   Atoms consist of a nucleus (composed of protons and neutrons) and electrons, which revolve around the nucleus of orbits of more or less fixed diameter. An electron can move to a higher orbit if it receives energy from an external source (e.g., heating). However, it remains in the higher orbit for only one-hundred-millionth of a second. As it falls back to its original lower orbit, it releases its excess energy by emitting a small "packet" of energy called a quantum or a photon.

2. **Describe the physical properties of photons.**

   In a vacuum, all photons move at the speed of light. As they travel, they vibrate, causing measurable electric and magnetic effects (wave properties). The further an electron falls to reach its original lower orbit, the greater its frequency of vibration, and the shorter its wavelength (λ), which is the straight-line distance a photon moves during one complete vibration. Frequency and wavelength are related by the formula $f = c/\lambda$, where f = frequency of vibration, λ = wavelength, and c = speed of light. Thus, f and λ are inversely proportional (i.e., as frequency increases, wavelength decreases). For example, gamma rays have a very high frequency and a very short wavelength, and radio waves have a very low frequency and a rather long wavelength.

3. **What is the electromagnetic spectrum?**

   Light, x-rays, gamma rays, and radio waves are all forms of electromagnetic energy. When photons (quanta) are classified according to their wavelength, the result is the electromagnetic spectrum. The photons with the longest wavelengths are radio and television waves; those with the shortest are gamma rays. The photons we see (visible light) are near the middle of the spectrum.

4. **Why can we "see" light, but not other types of electromagnetic energy?**

   The rods and cones of the retina (photoreceptors) contain pigments that preferentially absorb photons with wavelengths between 400 nm and 700 nm (a nanometer is a billionth of a meter) and convert their energy into a neuronal impulse that is carried to the brain. Wavelengths longer than 700 nm and shorter than 400 nm tend to pass through the sensory retina without being absorbed (Fig. 4-1).

5. **What is the light spectrum?**

   Photons can be classified not only by their wavelength but also by the sensation they cause when they strike the retina. Photons of the shortest wavelengths that we can see are perceived as blue and green; those of longer wavelengths are perceived as yellow, orange, and red.

6. **How does a prism break white light into the colors of the rainbow?**

   Photons travel at the speed of light in a vacuum, but if they enter a denser medium, such as glass, their wavelength and speed decrease. The frequency of vibration remains the same. The shorter the wavelength, the more the speed is decreased. For example, imagine two photons traveling through a vacuum, one of wavelength 650 nm and the other of wavelength 450 nm. As long as they remain in a vacuum, they keep pace with one another. When they strike the glass

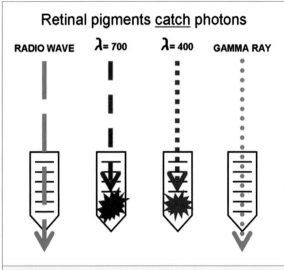

Figure 4-1. Photoreceptors are stimulated only by certain wavelengths of light.

perpendicularly, the 450 nm photon is slowed down more than the 650 nm photon. If they enter the glass obliquely, their paths are bent in proportion to how much their speed is slowed. In other words, the shorter the wavelength, the greater the bending. The blue is bent more and is separated from the red.

7. **How do rods differ from cones?**
Both rods and cones are photoreceptors, which are defined as retinal cells that initiate the process of vision. Rods function best when the eye is dark-adapted (i.e., for night vision). They cannot distinguish one color from another. Cones, on the other hand, function when the retina is light-adapted (i.e., for day vision).

8. **What are the visual pigments?**
There are four visual pigments: rhodopsin, which is present in rods, and the three cone pigments. All visual pigments are made up of 11-cis retinal (vitamin A aldehyde) and a protein called an opsin. When a photon is absorbed, the 11-cis retinal is converted to the all-trans form and is released from the opsin, initiating an electrical impulse in the photoreceptor that travels toward the brain. The eye then resynthesizes the rhodopsin.

9. **Describe the three cone pigments.**
Our ability to distinguish different colors depends on the fact that there are three different kinds of cone pigment. All visual pigments use retinal, but each has a different opsin. The function of the different opsins is to rearrange the electron cloud of retinal, thereby changing its ability to capture photons of different wavelengths. Red-catching cones (R cones) contain erythrolabe, which preferentially absorbs photons of long wavelengths. It is best stimulated by 570-nm photons, but also absorbs adjoining wavelengths. Blue-catching cones (B cones) contain cyanolabe, which absorbs the shortest wavelengths best. Its maximal sensitivity is at 440 nm. Green-catching cones (G cones) contain chlorolabe, which is most sensitive to the intermediate wavelengths. Its maximal sensitivity is at 540 nm.

10. **How does the sensation of light get to the brain?**
The electrical signals initiated by absorption of photons by the photoreceptors are transmitted to bipolar cells and then to ganglion cells. Horizontal and amacrine cells modify these messages. For example, if a cone is strongly stimulated, it sends inhibitory messages by way of a horizontal cell to neighboring cones, thereby reducing "noise" and sharpening up the message the brain receives. Bipolar cells send similar inhibitory messages by way of amacrine cells. The axons of ganglion cells form the optic nerve, which carries information to the brain. In the brain is the "hue center" (Fig. 4-2), which adds up the information from the different color channels and determines which color we see. In general, the hue we see depends on the relative number of photons of different wavelength that strike the cones.

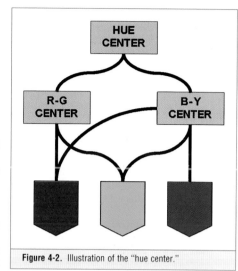

Figure 4-2. Illustration of the "hue center."

11. **What three attributes are necessary to describe any color?**
To accurately describe any color, one must specify three attributes: hue, saturation, and brightness.

12. **What is hue?**
Hue is synonymous with "color" and is the attribute of color perception denoted by blue, red, purple, and so forth. Hue depends largely on what the eye and brain perceive to be the predominant wavelength present in the incoming light. In simplest terms, this means that if light of several wavelengths strikes the eye and more light of 540 nm is present than is light of other wavelengths, we will see green.

13. **What is saturation?**
Saturation (chroma) corresponds to the purity or richness of a color. When all the light seen by the eye is the same wavelength, we say that a color is fully saturated. Vivid colors are saturated. If we add white to a saturated color, the hue does not change, but the color is paler (desaturated). For example, pink is a desaturated red.

14. **What is brightness?**
Brightness (luminance, value) refers to the quantity of light coming from an object (the number of photons striking the eye). If we place a filter over a projector or gradually (with a rheostat) lower its intensity, the brightness decreases.

15. **What are complementary colors?**
When equal quantities of complements are added, the result is white. Blue-green and red are complements as are green and magenta. (We are talking of colored lights, not paints.)

16. **What is the color wheel?**
The color wheel is made up of all hues arranged in a circle so that each hue lies between those hues it most closely resembles and complementary hues lie opposite each other. Using the color wheel,

we can predict the color that will result when two different lights are mixed. When noncomplements are mixed, the resultant color lies between the two original colors. The exact color seen depends on the quantity of each color used. For example, equal quantities of red and green result in yellow, whereas a large quantity of red and a relatively small quantity of green result in orange.

17. How does the eye differ from the ear?

Unlike the ear, which can distinguish several musical instruments playing at once, our eye and brain cannot determine the composition of a color we see. For example, if we present the eye with a light composed purely of 589 nm photons, the eye sees yellow. However, if we mix green and red lights in the proper proportions, the eye also sees yellow and cannot differentiate this from the other. Similarly, when two complements are mixed, we see white and cannot distinguish this white from the white seen when equal quantities of all wavelengths are present. Further, if we add white light to our original 589 nm yellow, the eye still sees yellow. Similarly, a light composed only of 490 nm photons is seen as blue-green and cannot be distinguished from an appropriate mixture of blue and green.

18. What are the primary colors?

When speaking of colored lights, the primary hues (also called the additive primaries) are red, green, and blue. Any color, including white, can be produced by overlapping red, green, and blue lights on a screen in the proper proportions. The reflecting screen can be regarded as a composite of an infinite number of tiny projectors. The eye, bombarded by all these photons, "adds up" their relative contribution. The color we see is determined by how many quanta of each wavelength reach the eye. Color television relies on this ability of the eye to add up tiny adjacent points of light. If one looks at a color television from 6 inches away, one sees tiny dots of only three colors: red, green, and blue. If one then backs away, the full range of colors becomes apparent and the eye can no longer distinguish the tiny dots. It synthesizes (adds up) the adjacent colors (e.g., tiny dots of red and blue = purple, red and green = yellow, red and green and blue = white, and so forth).

19. Where is the final determination of color made?

The hue center, localized in the cortex, synthesizes information it receives from two "intermediate centers": the R-G center and the B-Y center. The information sent to the hue center from the R-G center depends on the relative stimulation of the R and G cones. For example, when light of 540 nm strikes the retina, it will stimulate both R and G cones. However, because the G cones are stimulated much more than the R cones, the message received by the hue center is predominantly "green." On the other hand, if light of 590 nm strikes the retina, the R cones are stimulated more than the G cones and we see yellow. When light of 630 nm strikes the retina, the G cones are not stimulated at all and we see red. The B cones send information to the B-Y center. The Y information does not come from Y cones because there are no Y cones. Information from R and G cones has the effect of yellow in the B-Y center.

20. Why is brown, which is definitely a color, not on the color wheel?

Because brown is a yellow or orange of low luminance.

21. Describe the Bezold-Brucke phenomenon.

As brightness increases, most hues appear to change. At low intensities, blue-green, green, and yellow-green appear greener than they do at high intensities, when they appear bluer. At low intensities, reds and oranges appear redder and at high intensities, yellower. The exceptions are a blue of about 478 nm, a green of about 503 nm, and a yellow of about 578 nm. These are the wavelengths of invariant hue.

22. What is the Abney effect?

As white is added to any hue (desaturating it), the hue appears to change slightly in color. All colors except a yellow of 570 nm appear yellower.

23. **What are the relative luminosity curves?**
   The relative luminosity curves illustrate the eye's sensitivity to different wavelengths of light. They are constructed by asking an observer to increase the luminance of lights of various wavelength until they appear to be equal in apparent brightness to a yellow light whose luminance is fixed. When the eye is light-adapted, yellow, yellow-green, and orange appear brighter than do blues, greens, and reds. The cones' peak sensitivity is to light of 555 nm. A relative luminosity curve can also be constructed for the rods in a dark-adapted eye, even though the observer cannot name the various wavelengths used. The rods' peak sensitivity is to light of 505 nm (blue).

24. **Define lateral inhibition.**
   As mentioned above, as cones of one kind (e.g., R cones) are stimulated, they may send an inhibitory message by way of horizontal and amacrine cells to adjacent cones of the same kind (e.g., other R cones). Therefore, when a purple circle is surrounded by a red background, the R cones in the purple area are inhibited, making the purple (a combination of red and blue) appear bluer than it really is. If the purple is surrounded by blue, it appears redder.

25. **What are afterimages?**
   If one stares at a color for 20 seconds, it begins to fade (desaturate). Then, if one gazes at a white background, the complement of the original color (afterimage) appears (Fig. 4-3). These two phenomena depend on the fact that even when cones are not being stimulated, they spontaneously send a few signals toward the brain. For example, when red light is projected onto the retina, the eye sees red because the R cones are stimulated much more than the G cones and B cones. The G and B contribution to the hue center is far outweighed by the R. After several seconds, the red color fades (becomes desaturated) because the red cones, being more strongly stimulated, cannot regenerate their pigment fast enough to continue to send such a large number of signals (fatigue). Now the G and B cone contribution to the hue center increases relative to that of the R cones and the brain "sees" a desaturated or paler red. It is as if we added blue-green light to the red. (Recall that blue-green is the complement of red and that mixing complements yields white). When the red light is turned off, the frequency of the spontaneous messages sent to the brain by the fatigued R cones is far less than that sent by the G and B cones, so the brain sees blue-green, or cyan, the complement of red (Fig. 4-4).

26. **Why are white flowers white?**
   The color of any object that is not white or black depends on the relative number of photons of each wavelength that it absorbs and reflects. Our ambient light, derived from the sun, contains approximately equal numbers of all the photons that make up the light spectrum. White paint reflects all photons equally well, so white flowers appear white.

27. **Why is charcoal black?**
   Charcoal absorbs most of the light that strikes it. Because very few photons are reflected toward the eye, the photoreceptors are not stimulated and no color is seen.

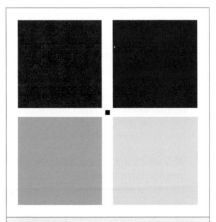

Figure 4-3. Stare at the black dot for 30 seconds and then look at a blank white area. The afterimage seen is the complement of each color.

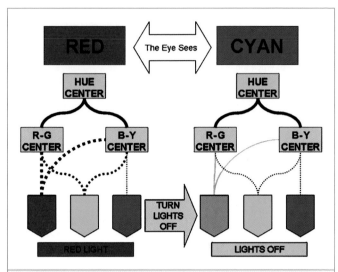

Figure 4-4. Afterimages are formed when certain photoreceptors cannot regenerate pigment quickly enough, allowing other photoreceptors to appear relatively more stimulated.

28. **Why are blue flowers blue?**
   The pigments in blue flowers absorb red and yellow photons best, green next best, and blue least of all; therefore, more blue photons are reflected than others, and the eye sees blue. A green leaf is green because chlorophyll strongly absorbs blue and red and reflects green.

29. **Why does mixing red and blue-green lights result in white, but mixing red and green paint results in brown?**
   Oil paints are made by mixing (suspending) tiny clumps of pigment in an opaque medium (the binder). Pigments reflect and absorb some wavelengths of light better than others. The dominant wavelength reflected is the color of the paint. When two lights are mixed, we speak of an "additive" mixture. But when two paints are mixed, each pigment subtracts some of the light the other would reflect. The resultant mixture is darker than either of the two originals. Red paint mixed with green paint results in brown because enough light is subtracted that the eye sees a yellow of low luminance.

30. **Why does mixing paints yield unpredictable results?**
   An artist or home decorator never knows the exact absorption spectrum of the originals. Two greens may appear to be the same but, because their pigments are not identical, do not yield the same color when mixed with the same yellow.

31. **Why do colors appear different under fluorescent light as opposed to incandescent lights?**
   Tungsten (incandescent) light bulbs emit relatively more photons of the longer (red) wavelengths than of the shorter (blue) wavelengths, whereas fluorescent light bulbs emit relatively more light in the blue and green wavelengths. A shopper who picks out material for drapes in a store that has fluorescent lighting may be surprised to find out that the material looks quite different at home. A purple dress appears redder under incandescent light than it does under fluorescent light.

KEY POINTS: COLOR VISION

1. Rods function best in the dark-adapted state and cones function in the light-adapted state.

2. Any color can be produced by overlapping red, green, and blue lights in the proper proportions.

3. Afterimages appear as the complement of the original color.

4. Deuteranopes and tritanopes have difficulty distinguishing red from green.

5. All red-green disorders are inherited in an X-linked recessive pattern.

32. Why is the sky blue?
The sun emits light of all of the spectral colors. If an astronaut in space looks at the sun, it appears white. If the astronaut looks away from the sun, he sees that the outer space is black, because the photons not coming directly at him pass through space unhindered and are not reflected toward him. On Earth, the atmosphere, which contains ozone, dust, water droplets, and many other reflecting molecules and substances, is interposed between the sun and our eyes. The atmosphere scatters blue light more than it does green, yellow, or red. Therefore, if during the daytime we look away from the sun, we see the blue photons that are being bent toward us and the sky appears to be blue.

33. Why is the sunset red?
At dusk, in order to reach us, the light from the sun has to pass through much more of the Earth's atmosphere than it does during the daytime. Therefore, even more of the blue and green photons are bent away from the atmosphere. The red and yellow photons penetrate better. If some of these are eventually reflected toward us by clouds or dust, we see a red sky. Similarly, the sun appears red.

34. Define trichromats.
Trichromats are the 92% of the population who have "normal" color vision. They have all three different kinds of cones, normal concentration of the cone pigments, and normal retinal wiring.

35. What is congenital dichromatism?
In dichromats, the cones themselves are normal, but one of the three contains the wrong pigment. For example, in deuteranopes, the "G" cones are normal in every way except that they contain erythrolabe (red pigment) instead of chlorolabe (green pigment). In protanopes, the "R" cones are normal in every way except that they contain chlorolabe (green pigment) instead of erythrolabe (red pigment). Tritanopia is a defect of "B" cones.

36. Why do deuteranopes have difficulty in distinguishing red from green?
In deuteranopia, because both R and G cones contain the same pigment, when red light strikes the retina, the R and G cones are stimulated equally and send an equal number of messages to the R-G center. Similarly, there is an increased R input to the B-Y center, where the R input now equals the G input. In other words, the hue center thinks that equal quantities of red and green light are striking the retina. When green or blue-green light strikes the retina, the R and G cones are again stimulated equally. An accurate analysis of the mechanics of color vision abnormalities would require a computer, but it should be apparent that because both red and green light stimulate the R and G cones equally, the information the hue center receives from the R-G center is not useful and the deuteranope would have difficulty distinguishing red from green. Similarly, protanopes also have difficulty seeing red from green.

37. **What is anomalous trichromatism?**

In anomalous trichromatism, two of the three cone pigments are normal, but the third functions suboptimally. Depending on which pigment is abnormal, the affected persons are termed **protanomalous, deuteranomalous,** or **tritanomalous**. Anomalous trichromats can distinguish between fully saturated colors but have difficulty distinguishing colors of low saturation (pastels) or low luminance (dark colors), or both. Deuteranomaly is present in approximately 5% of the population; deuteranopia, protanopia, and protanomaly in 1% each; and tritanopia or tritanomaly in only 0.002%.

38. **How is abnormal color vision inherited?**

All red-green disorders are inherited in a sex-linked recessive pattern. This means that men almost exclusively manifest the disorder. Women are carriers. In other words, the women have perfectly normal color vision, but approximately 50% of their sons are abnormal. Both men and women can have the tritan disorders, which are inherited as autosomal dominant traits (Table 4-1).

TABLE 4-1. INHERITED COLOR VISION DEFECTS		
Defect	Incidence	Inheritance
Deuteranomaly	5% (of males)	XR
Deuteranopia	1% (of males)	XR
Protanomaly	1% (of males)	XR
Protanopia	1% (of males)	XR
Tritanomaly and tritanopia	0.002%	AD

AD = autosomal dominant, XR = x-linked recessive.

39. **What is Kollner's rule?**

As a very general rule, the errors made by persons with optic nerve disease tend to resemble those made by protans and deutans, whereas those made by persons with retinal disease resemble those made by tritans.

WEBSITE

http://retina.umh.es/webvision/

BIBLIOGRAPHY

1. Boynton RM: Color, hue and wavelength. In Carterette EC, Friedman MP (eds): Handbook of Perception, vol. V. New York, Academic Press, 1975, pp 301–350.

2. Gerritsen F: Theory and Practice of Color. New York, Van Nostrand, 1974.

3. Krill AE: Hereditary retinal and choroidal diseases. In Krill AE (ed): Evaluation of Color Vision. Hagerstown, MD, Harper & Row, 1972, pp 309–340.

4. Linksz A: Reflections, old and new, concerning acquired defects of color vision. Surv Ophthalmol 17:229–240, 1973.

5. Rubin ML, Walls GL: Fundamentals of Visual Science. Springfield, IL, Charles C. Thomas, 1969.

6. Smith VC: Color vision of normal observers. In Potts AM (ed): The Assessment of Visual Function. St. Louis, Mosby, 1972, pp 105–135.

CHAPTER 5

OPHTHALMIC AND ORBITAL TESTING

Caroline R. Baumal, MD, and Patric De Potter, MD

1. **What is the electroretinogram?**
   The electroretinogram (ERG) is a recording of the electrical discharges from the retina elicited by a flash of light. This response occurs secondary to transretinal movement of ions induced by the light stimulus.

2. **How is an ERG performed?**
   Light is delivered uniformly to the entire retina. This is called Ganzfeld or full-field stimulation, which is achieved with a bowl perimeter. The light-induced electrical discharges are recorded from the eye with a corneal contact lens electrode. There is international standardization of the full-field ERG technique.

KEY POINTS: COMPONENTS OF THE FULL-FIELD ERG

1. The **a wave** is the initial negative ERG waveform arising from photoreceptor cells.

2. The positive **b wave** following the a wave is generated by the Müller cells and bipolar cells in the outer retina.

3. **Oscillatory potentials** are small wavelets that may be superimposed on the b wave and arise from cells in the midretinal layers (Fig. 5-1).

4. Under certain recording conditions, additional waveforms may be noted, such as the **c wave** following the b wave, which reflects electrical activity at the level of the retinal pigment epithelium and is recorded in the dark-adapted eye.

5. The **early receptor potential** (ERP) is a rapid transient waveform that occurs immediately after a light stimulus, and this response originates from the bleaching of photopigments at the level of the photoreceptor outer segments.

3. **What parameters are measured during evaluation of the ERG?**
   Two major ERG parameters, **amplitude** and **implicit time,** are measured. The amplitude (in microvolts) of the a wave is measured from baseline to the trough of the a wave, and the b wave amplitude is measured from the trough of the a wave to peak of the b wave. The implicit time (in milliseconds) is the time from the stimulus onset to peak of the response.

4. **How is the ERG amplitude affected in retinal disorders?**
   The **full-field light-evoked** ERG is a mass response reflecting activity from the entire retina. The amplitude of the ERG is proportional to the area of functioning retina stimulated and is abnormal only when large areas of the retina are functionally impaired.

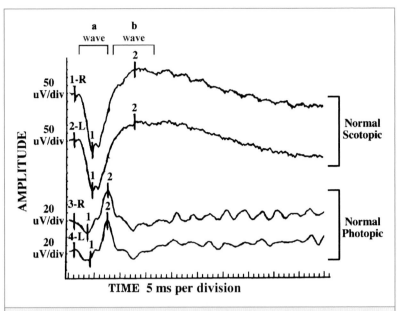

Figure 5-1. Nocturnal scotopic (dark-adapted) and photopic ERG responses to a high-intensity (0 dB) light flash demonstrating the a wave and b wave. Oscillatory potentials are present on the ascending limb of the b wave. The implicit time is measured from the stimulus onset to the peak of the a wave (1) or b wave (2). The a-wave amplitude is measured from the baseline to the trough of the a wave, and the b-wave amplitude is measured from the trough of the a wave to the peak of the b wave.

5. **Describe different stimulus conditions and the associated photoreceptor response.**

   Certain light stimuli allow the isolation of either the cone or rod responses so that each photoreceptor type can be studied independently (Table 5-1 and Fig. 5-2). After sufficient dark adaptation (known as scotopic conditions), the rod responses are optimized. Under the light-adapted or photopic conditions, the rods are sufficiently dampened so that the response is primarily from the cones.

6. **What five responses are evaluated during a standard full-field ERG?**
   - Rod response (dark-adapted)
   - Maximal combined rod-cone response (dark-adapted)
   - Oscillatory potentials
   - Single flash cone response (light-adapted)
   - 30-Hz flicker cone response

7. **How is the ERG affected in age-related macular degeneration?**

   The entire retina is stimulated by the bright flash in the Ganzfeld. Thus, the full-field ERG is not affected if small areas of the retina are damaged. In age-related macular degeneration with small localized retinal lesions, the full-field ERG is normal.

8. **What does the ERG demonstrate in retinal ganglion cell disease?**

   Because the ganglion cells do *not* play a role in generation of the full-field ERG, disorders primarily affecting ganglion cells, such as glaucoma, do not alter the full-field ERG. On occasion,

TABLE 5-1. PHOTORECEPTOR RESPONSE ASSOCIATED WITH DIFFERENT STIMULUS CONDITIONS

State of Adaptation	Light Stimulus	Photoreceptor Response
Scotopic	Dim white (24 dB)	Rod
Scotopic	Dim blue (10 dB)	Rod
Scotopic	Bright white (0 dB)	Mixed response: maximal rod and cone
Scotopic	Red (0 dB)	Mixed response: early cone, late rod
Scotopic	Bright white (0 dB)	Cone oscillatory potentials
Photopic	Bright white (0 dB)	Cone
Photopic	White flicker at 30 Hz	Pure cone

dB = decibels, Hz = hertz.

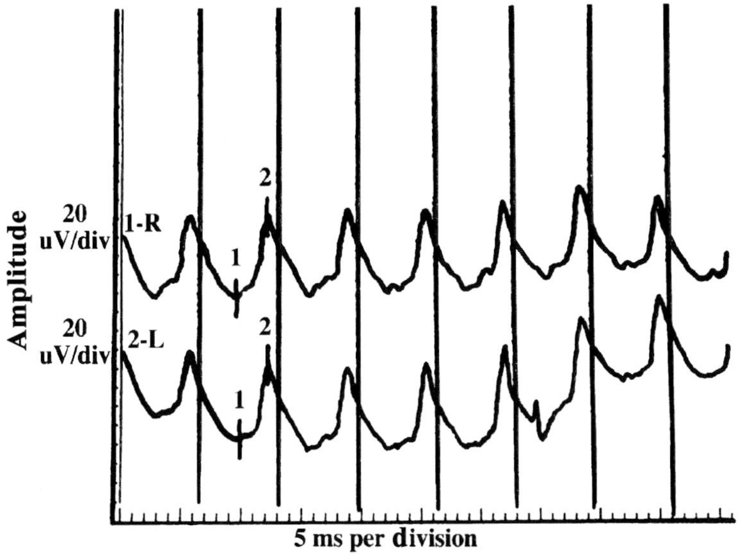

Figure 5-2. The normal cone response to a flicker light stimulus at 30 Hz.

the b wave may be reduced in optic atrophy or central retinal artery occlusion, which is postulated to result from trans-synaptic degeneration from ganglion to the bipolar cell layer.

9. Describe the clinical situations where the ERG is utilized.
   - To diagnose a generalized degeneration of the retina
   - To assess family members for a known hereditary retinal degeneration
   - To assess decreased vision and nystagmus present at birth
   - To assess retinal function in the presence of opaque ocular media or vascular occlusion
   - To evaluate functional visual loss

10. **List the retinal degenerations in which the ERG can help clarify the diagnosis.**
    - Retinitis pigmentosa and related hereditary retinal degenerations
    - Retinitis pigmentosa sine pigmento
    - Retinitis punctata albescens
    - Leber's congenital amaurosis
    - Choroideremia
    - Gyrate atrophy of the retina and choroid
    - Goldman-Favre syndrome
    - Congenital stationary night blindness
    - X-linked juvenile retinoschisis
    - Achromatopsia
    - Cone dystrophies
    - Disorders mimicking retinitis pigmentosa

11. **What are the clinical and ERG features of retinitis pigmentosa?**
    Retinitis pigmentosa (RP) is an inherited retinal disorder of the photoreceptors and other retina cell layers. Inheritance may be autosomal dominant, autosomal recessive, or X-linked. Both the rods and, to a lesser extent, the cones are abnormal in retinitis pigmentosa. Clinical features include decreased night vision (nyctalopia), visual field loss, and abnormal ERG (Fig. 5-3).

    Ocular features include waxy pallor of the optic nerve, attenuated retinal vessels, mottled retinal pigment epithelium with bone-spicule pigmentation, cellophane maculopathy, cystic macular edema, pigment cells in the vitreous, and cataracts.

    The ERG shows reduced amplitude (usually b wave) and prolonged photopic implicit time in early RP. Over time, the ERG becomes extinguished with no detectable rod or cone responses to bright white light.

12. **What does the ERG demonstrate in female carriers of X-linked retinitis pigmentosa?**
    Female carriers of X-linked retinitis pigmentosa may have either a normal retinal examination or demonstrate milder retinal findings without subjective complaints. ERG abnormalities are

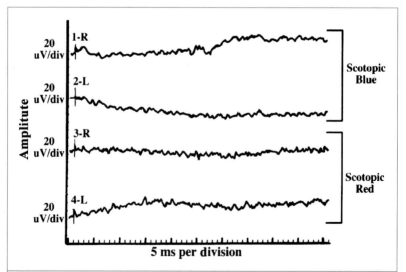

Figure 5-3. The ERG in retinitis pigmentosa reveals an extinguished response to scotopic blue and scotopic red light stimuli.

noted in the majority of female carriers, even without fundus abnormalities with prolonged photopic b wave implicit time and/or a reduction in the amplitude of the scotopic b wave in the dark-adapted eye.

13. **What does the ERG reveal in congenital rubella syndrome?**
Diffuse pigmentary retinal changes in congenital rubella syndrome may be confused with retinitis pigmentosa. However, the ERG is normal in congenital rubella. Other ocular signs of rubella include deafness and congenital cataracts.

14. **Describe the ERG in X-linked retinoschisis.**
Clinical findings include peripheral retinoschisis cavities in 50% of cases and foveal cystic changes in almost all cases. ERG reveals reduced scotopic and photopic b-wave amplitude, reflecting widespread midretinal changes.

15. **What does the ERG demonstrate in a progressive cone dystrophy?**
There is a markedly reduced photopic flicker response and a normal rod scotopic response. This disorder initially affects peripheral cones with progression to involve central cones. When the central cones are intact, the visual acuity and color vision are good; however, the ultimate acuity falls to the 20/200 range.

16. **Why is the ERG useful in patients with congenitally decreased vision?**
Three disorders characterized by nystagmus, congenitally reduced vision, and normal retinal examination can be diagnosed with an ERG:
   - **Achromatopsia** (also known as rod monochromatism) is a nonprogressive autosomal recessive near absence of cones. The ERG reveals absent cone function and normal rod function.
   - **Leber's congenital amaurosis** is a congenital autosomal recessive form of retinitis pigmentosa. The ERG is markedly reduced or extinguished with profound visual impairment.
   - The ERG in **congenital stationary nightblindness** reveals normal photoreceptors with a normal a wave, but an abnormal bipolar cell region as demonstrated by the absent b wave.

17. **How can the ERG measure retinal function in the presence of opaque ocular media?**
The full-field ERG can be used to assess the retinal function when the retina cannot be visualized, due to cataracts, or corneal or vitreous opacities. A normal ERG provides information regarding the overall retinal function, but does not indicate whether central vision is normal because macular degeneration and optic atrophy typically do not affect the ERG amplitude. A cataract or corneal opacity may act as a diffuser of light, on occasion producing a "supernormal" ERG.

18. **List the disorders that may demonstrate an extinguished ERG.**
   - Retinitis pigmentosa and related disorders
   - Ophthalmic artery occlusion
   - Diffuse unilateral subacute neuroretinitis (DUSN)
   - Metallosis
   - Total retinal detachment
   - Drugs such as phenothiazines or chloroquine
   - Cancer-associated retinopathy

19. **List the disorders that may demonstrate normal a-wave and reduced b-wave amplitude.**
   - Central stationary nightblindness

- X-linked juvenile retinoschisis
- Central retinal vein or artery occlusion
- Myotonic dystrophy
- Oguchi's disease
- Quinine intoxication
- Transsynaptic degeneration from the ganglion to the bipolar cell layer (i.e., secondary to optic atrophy or central retinal artery occlusion)

20. **List the disorders characterized by an abnormal photopic ERG and a normal scotopic ERG.**
    - Achromatopsia (also known as rod monochromatism)
    - Cone dystrophy

21. **What are new variations of the standard ERG?**
    - The **focal electroretinogram** (FERG) is induced by a focal-directed flash of light and measures the response from central cone photoreceptors and outer retina. It can be used to evaluate focal macular disorders.
    - The **pattern electroretinogram** (PERG) measures the electrical response to an alternating pattern stimulus that has a constant overall retinal luminance, and the response appears to be localized to retinal ganglion cells. This was determined because the PERG was extinguished after transection of the optic nerve while the full-field was not altered. The PERG may be used to diagnose or monitor disorders such as glaucoma, ocular hypertension, optic neuritis, optic atrophy, and amblyopia. Although ganglion cells appear to generate the PERG, normal functioning retinal cells distal to the ganglion cells are required for a normal PERG. Thus, abnormal PERG responses can occur with retinal degenerations that affect the photoreceptor cells.
    - The **multifocal ERG** provides an objective equivalent to the visual field by simultaneously assessing the retinal electrical response at multiple locations. The resultant local responses contain components from all levels of the retina.

22. **What is an electro-oculogram?**
    The **electro-oculogram** (EOG) is an indirect measure of the standing potential of the eyes (Fig. 5-4). This standing potential exists because of a voltage difference between the inner and outer retina. The EOG is measured by placing electrodes near the medial and lateral canthi of each eye and having a patient move the eyes back and forth over a specific distance.
    The clinical measurement of the EOG relies on the fact that the amplitude of the response changes when the luminance conditions are varied. After dark adaptation, the response progressively decreases, reaching a trough in 8–12 minutes. With light adaptation, there is a progressive rise in amplitude, reaching a peak in 6–9 minutes. The greatest EOG amplitude achieved in light (light peak) is divided by the lowest amplitude in the dark (dark trough). This calculated ratio is the **Arden ratio**. Normal subjects have an **Arden ratio** value of 1.80 or greater, while a ratio of less than 1.65 is distinctly abnormal.

23. **In what retinal location is the EOG response generated?**
    This electrical response in the EOG is generated by the retinal pigment epithelium, with the light peak being produced by a depolarization of the basal portion of the retinal pigment epithelium. To generate the EOG potential, it is necessary to have intact photoreceptors in physical contact with the retinal pigment epithelium. Like the full-field ERG, the EOG reflects activity from the entire retina.

24. **What are the clinical uses for the EOG?**
    The normalcy of the EOG is dependent on the total number of functioning photoreceptors. The EOG is often abnormal in any condition in which the ERG is abnormal. A patient with an

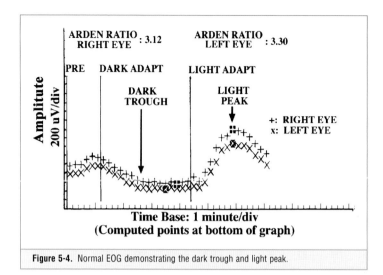

Figure 5-4. Normal EOG demonstrating the dark trough and light peak.

extinguished ERG due to retinitis pigmentosa will show little or no EOG light rise, and this is similarly noted in any disorder with widespread generalized degeneration of the photoreceptor cells.

However, an abnormal ERG and a normal EOG may be noted in some disorders. In congenital stationary nightblindness and X-linked retinoschisis, there may be an abnormality in neural transmission in the bipolar cell region, and the EOG may be normal due to normal functioning rods. The EOG light rise is almost completely dependent on rod function, so it is normal in disorders of cone dysfunction.

25. **What does the EOG demonstrate in pattern dystrophies?**
The EOG light peak–dark trough ratios in pattern dystrophy are usually either normal or minimally subnormal. This distinguishes pattern dystrophy from Best's disease, where the EOG is abnormal.

26. **How does optic nerve disease affect the EOG?**
Primary disease of the optic nerve does not affect the EOG light peak-to-dark trough Arden ratio.

27. **How is the EOG affected by rhegmatogenous retinal detachment?**
The degree of retinal detachment is reflected in a progressively abnormal EOG ratio. This pattern is similar to the effect of retinal detachment on the ERG. The abnormal ratio indicates the necessity of maintaining the physical contiguity of the rod-and-cone outer segments as well as the retinal pigment epithelium (RPE) for proper generation of EOG responses.

28. **How are the ERG and EOG affected by chloroquine and hydroxychloroquine?**
Abnormal findings in the EOG and ERG, such as a reduced light peak-to-dark trough ratio and reduced amplitudes, have been reported in patients receiving these antimalarial drugs, which are used more frequently for arthritis or related disorders. Electrophysiologic changes tend to occur after prolonged administration, and many patients have coexisting funduscopic evidence of foveal or even peripheral pigmentary changes. Thus these tests are not very useful to identify signs of early retinal toxicity before notable funduscopic changes occur.

29. **What are the characteristics of dark adaptation?**
    Dark adaptometry measures the absolute threshold of cone and rod sensitivity and is tested on an instrument known as the Goldmann-Weekers adaptometer. Initially, the subject is adapted to a bright background light, which is then extinguished. In the dark, the patient is presented with a series of dim lights. The threshold at which the light is just perceived is plotted against time. The normal dark adaptation curve (Fig. 5-5) is biphasic, where the first curve represents the cone threshold and is reached in 5–10 minutes, and the second curve represents the rod threshold and is reached after 30 minutes. The rod-cone break is a well-defined point between these two curves. Dark adaptometry is useful to evaluate retinal disorders with nightblindness and some conditions with cone dysfunction.

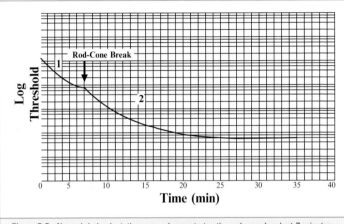

Figure 5-5. Normal dark adaptation curve demonstrates the rod-cone break at 7 minutes, separating the cone threshold (1) and the rod threshold (2).

30. **What are the indications for ophthalmic ultrasonography?**
    - Evaluation of the anterior or posterior segment in eyes with opaque ocular media
    - Assessment of the dimensions of ocular tumors as well as their tissue characteristics, such as calcium in retinoblastoma or choroidal osteoma
    - Evaluation of orbital disorders
    - Detection and localization of intraocular foreign bodies
    - Measurement of distances within the eye and orbit (also known as biometry)

31. **What frequency is used for standard ophthalmic ultrasonography?**
    Ultrasound is an acoustic wave that consists of an oscillation of particles within a medium. By definition, ultrasound waves have a frequency greater than 20 kHz. In standard ophthalmic ultrasound, frequencies are in the range of 8–10 MHz. This high frequency produces short wavelengths, which allow precise resolution of small ocular structures. In contrast, abdominal ultrasound typically uses a lower frequency in the range of 1–5 MHz, which produces longer wavelengths that permit deeper penetration into tissues. Resolution of structures is decreased, although resolution is less critical because the structures in the abdomen are much larger than those within the eye.

32. **What are the principles of ultrasonography?**
    Ultrasound is based on physical principles of tissue-acoustic impedance mismatch and pulse-echo technology. As the acoustic wave is propagated through tissues, part of the wave may be

reflected toward the source of the emitted wave (i.e., the probe). This reflected wave is referred to as an echo. Echoes are generated at adjoining tissue interfaces that have differential acoustic impedance. The greater the difference in acoustic impedance, the stronger the echo. For example, strong reflections occur at the interface between retinal tissue and vitreous, which is essentially water. When adjoining tissue interfaces have relatively small differences in acoustic impedance (e.g., vitreous gel and mild vitreous hemorrhage or clumped intravitreal white blood cells), weak reflections are seen. Pulse-echo technology uses synthetic crystal transducers to produce ultrasonic wavefront pulses and to retrieve echoes for electronic display processing.

33. **How is the clinical ophthalmic ultrasound displayed?**
The reflected echoes are received, amplified, electronically processed, and displayed in visual format as an A-scan or a B-scan (Fig. 5-6):
- **A-scan ultrasonography**, or the A-mode, is a one-dimensional, time-amplitude display. The horizontal baseline represents the distance and depends on the time required for the sound beam to reach a given interface and for its echo to return to the probe. In the vertical dimension, the height of the displayed spike indicates the amplitude or strength of the echo.
- **B-scan ultrasonography**, or the B-mode, produces a two-dimensional, cross-sectional display of the globe and orbit. The image is displayed in variable shades of gray, and the shade depends on the echo strength.

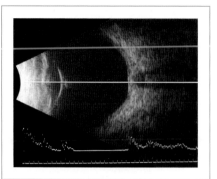

Figure 5-6. A-scan (bottom) and B-scan (top) of the normal globe. A cross-sectional anterior-posterior view is presented in the B-scan. The lens capsule is seen toward the left of the display, and the optic nerve is seen toward the right. A vector line through the B-scan demonstrates the position of the A-scan information.

Strong echoes appear white, and weaker reflections are seen as gray.
The A-scan is used predominantly for tissue characterization, whereas the B-scan is used to obtain architectural information. A-scans are also helpful in determining intraocular lens calculations for cataract surgery (see question 41).

34. **What lesion features are evaluated during the ultrasound examination?**
1. The **topography** (location, configuration, and extension) of a lesion is evaluated most often by the two-dimensional B-scan.
2. The **quantitative features** include the reflectivity, internal structure, and sound attenuation of a lesion.
   - The **reflectivity** of a lesion is evaluated by observing the height of the spike on the A-scan and the signal brightness on the B-scan. The internal reflectivity refers to the amplitude of echoes within a lesion and correlates with its histologic architecture.
   - The **internal structure** refers to the degree of variation in the histologic architecture within a mass lesion. Regular internal structure indicates a homogeneous architecture and is noted by minimal or no variation in the height of spikes on the A-scan and a uniform appearance of echoes on the B-scan. In contrast, an irregular internal structure is noted in a lesion with a heterogeneous architecture and is characterized by variations in the echo appearance.
   - **Sound attenuation** occurs when the acoustic wave is scattered, reflected, or absorbed by a tissue and is noted by a decrease in the strength of echoes either within or posterior to a lesion. It is indicated by a decrease in spike height on the A-scan or a decrease in

the brightness of echoes on the B-scan. Sound attenuation may produce decreased signal strength and a void posterior to the lesion that is referred to as shadowing. Substances such as bone, calcium, and foreign bodies typically produce sound attenuation (Fig. 5-7).

35. **The dynamic features of or within a lesion can be detected on the B-scan.**
    - **Aftermovement** is determined by observing the motion of lesion echoes after cessation of eye movements. The rapid movement of a vitreous hemorrhage is distinguished from the slower, undulating movement of the retina in an acute rhegmatogenous retinal detachment.
    - **Vascularity** is indicated by spontaneous motion of echoes within a lesion and represents blood flow within vessels.

36. **How is ultrasound used in preoperative cataract evaluation?**
    The A-scan is used to measure the axial length of the globe, which is required in the formula to calculate the intraocular lens power. The B-scan is useful if the ocular media are opaque to assess for a retinal disorder that may affect visual outcome after cataract surgery.

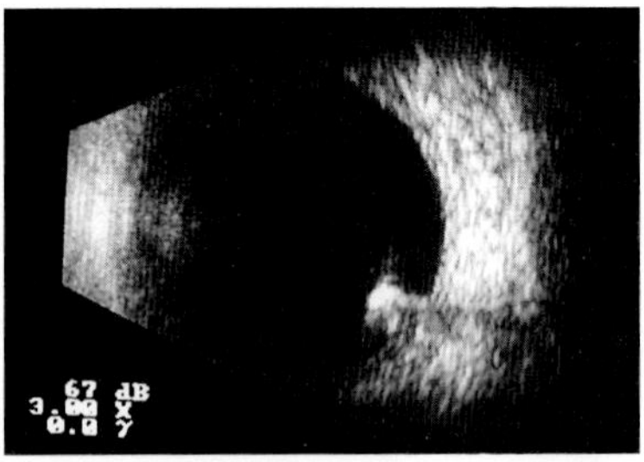

37. **How is ultrasound used to assess intraocular tumors?**
    Ultrasound may be used for diagnosis, to plan treatment, and to evaluate tumor response to therapy. Specifically the tumor shape, dimensions (such as thickness and basal diameter), and tissue characteristics are evaluated, along with the presence of extraocular extension.

Figure 5-7. B-scan image of a metallic foreign body located on the surface of the retina. A bright echo is produced by the foreign body with shadowing of the structures posteriorly.

38. **What are the characteristic features of a choroidal melanoma on ultrasound?**
    - Collarbutton or mushroom shape on B-scan (Fig. 5-8)
    - Low-to-medium internal reflectivity on A-scan (Fig. 5-8)
    - Regular internal structure
    - Internal blood flow (vascularity)

39. **Describe the ultrasound patterns in the differential diagnosis of choroidal melanoma.**
    Ultrasound is often used in the evaluation of choroidal melanoma, choroidal hemangioma, metastatic choroidal carcinoma, choroidal nevus, choroidal hemorrhage, and a disciform lesion. It should be combined with clinical information because there are more tumor types than differentiating ultrasound patterns (Table 5-2).

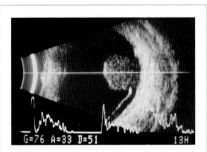

Figure 5-8. A-scan and B-scan of choroidal melanoma. The B-scan reveals a collarbutton-shaped mass with a regular internal structure. A serous retinal detachment extends from the margin of the tumor. The A-scan reveals a strong initial echo from the retinal tissue overlying the tumor followed by a rapid decline in the A-scan echo amplitude (low internal reflectivity) within the tumor tissue. High reflectivity is noted again at the level of the sclera and orbital fat.

TABLE 5-2. ULTRASOUND PATTERNS IN THE DIFFERENTIAL DIAGNOSIS OF CHOROIDAL MELANOMA

Lesion	Location	Shape	Internal Reflectivity	Internal Structure	Vascularity
Melanoma	Choroid and/or ciliary body	Dome or collarbutton	Low to medium	Regular	Yes
Choroidal hemangioma	Choroid, posterior pole	Dome	High	Regular	No
Metastatic carcinoma	Choroid, posterior pole	Diffuse, irregular	Medium to high	Irregular	No
Choroidal nevus	Choroid	Flat or mild thickening (usually <2 mm)	High	Regular	No
Choroidal hemorrhage	Choroid	Dome	Variable	Variable	No
Disciform lesion	Macula	Dome, irregular	High	Variable	No

40. **Describe the ultrasound features of a choroidal hemangioma.**
    Within a choroidal hemangioma, the adjoining cell and tissue layers have marked differences in acoustic impedance (acoustic heterogeneity), which create large echo amplitudes at each interface. The A-scan reveals high internal reflections within the tumor, and lesions appear solid white on the B-scan.

41. **Describe the ultrasound features of a retinal detachment.**
    A detached retina produces a bright, continuous, folded appearance on B-scan (Fig. 5-9). When detachment is total or extensive, the retina inserts into both the optic nerve and ora serrata. The A-scan reveals a 100% high spike. There is motion of the detached retina with voluntary eye movement; however, it is less mobile than with posterior vitreous detachment. Chronic retinal detachment may show calcification, intraretinal cysts, or cholesterol debris in the subretinal space.

    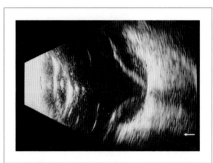

    Figure 5-9. B-scan of a total retinal detachment. An anteroposterior view reveals the characteristic V-shaped appearance with attachment to the optic nerve. A cataract is also present.

42. **Describe the ultrasound features that differentiate retinal detachment, posterior vitreous detachment, and choroidal detachment.**
    See Table 5-3.

TABLE 5-3. ULTRASOUND FEATURES THAT DIFFERENTIATE RETINAL DETACHMENT, POSTERIOR VITREOUS DETACHMENT, AND CHOROIDAL DETACHMENT

Ultrasound Features	Retinal Detachment	Posterior Vitreous Detachment	Choroidal Detachment
Topographic (B-scan)	Smooth or folded surface	Smooth surface	Smooth, dome, or flat surface
	Open or closed funnel with insertion at optic nerve	Open funnel with or without optic disc or fundus insertion	No optic nerve insertion
	Inserts at ora serrata		Inserts at ora serrata or ciliary body
	With or without intraretinal cysts	Inserts at ora serrata or ciliary body	
Quantitative (A-scan)	Steep 100% high spike	Variable spike height that is <100%	Steeply rising, thick, double-peaked 100% high spike
Mobility after eye move-ment	Moderate to none	Marked to moderate	Mild to none

43. **What ocular conditions may demonstrate calcification on ultrasound?**
    - Tumors (retinoblastoma, choroidal osteoma, optic nerve sheath meningioma, choroidal hemangioma, choroidal melanoma)
    - Toxocara granuloma
    - Chronic retinal detachment
    - Optic nerve head drusen
    - Disciform retinal lesion
    - Vascular occlusive disease of the optic nerve
    - Phthisis bulbi
    - Intumescent cataractous lens

44. **When is ultrasound used to evaluate ocular trauma?**
    Ultrasound may be used to evaluate the position of the lens and the status of the retina if visualization is impeded by an opaque cornea, hyphema, or vitreous hemorrhage resulting from trauma. It also may diagnose a posterior rupture site in the globe and assess for an intraocular foreign body.
    The globe should be evaluated visually by slit lamp technique before ultrasonography to determine whether ocular integrity has been severely disrupted and whether ultrasound examination is indicated.

45. **What are the ultrasound findings with an intraocular foreign body?**
    Ultrasound may diagnose and localize an intraocular foreign body (see Fig. 5-7), although ultrasound examination alone is not sufficient to exclude a foreign body. It is particularly useful with a nonmetallic intraocular foreign body that may not be visible radiographically. Although computerized tomography is often used for localization, it may not be able to define the exact position of a foreign body that lies close to the ocular wall.
    Foreign bodies have high reflectivity when the ultrasound probe beam is perpendicular to a reflective surface of the foreign body. On the B-scan, a metallic foreign body produces a bright echo that persists when the gain of the ultrasound output is decreased. Small, spherical, metallic foreign bodies may demonstrate ringing, which is a string of reflections that extends posterior to the foreign body and is produced by reflections of the acoustic pulses within the foreign body. Shadowing is often present behind a foreign body because of nearly complete reflection of the examining probe beam.

46. **What is ultrasound biomicroscopy?**
    Ultrasound biomicroscopy (UBM) is a new B-scan method that uses high frequencies in the range of 50–100 MHz. The depth of penetration is in the range of 5–7 mm. This technique produces high-resolution images of anterior segment structures (Fig. 5-10) and has been useful for characterizing the mechanism of secondary glaucoma.

47. **How is color-Doppler ultrasonography used in ophthalmologic evaluation?**
    Color-Doppler ultrasonography is a noninvasive approach to evaluate ocular blood flow. It is useful for assessing morphologic and velocimetric data from the ophthalmic artery, central retinal artery, central retinal vein, and posterior ciliary vessels. This technique has been

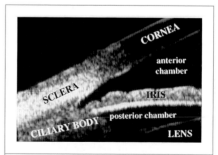

Figure 5-10. Ultrasound biomicroscopic image of the anterior segment angle structures.

used to evaluate many ocular disorders, including glaucoma, optic nerve disorders, diabetes, hypertension, and ocular ischemia.

48. **What is required when you order orbital MRI studies?**
    - Surface coil (orbital or head coil) for better visualization of structures of the orbit
    - Precontrast axial, coronal, and sagittal T1-weighted images
    - Axial, coronal T2-weighted images (fast spin-echo sequences)
    - Postcontrast axial coronal T1-weighted images with fat suppression techniques
    - Sedation in children

49. **What are paramagnetic agents?**
    Paramagnetic agents produce proton relaxation enhancement by shortening the intrinsic T1 and T2 relaxation times of the tissues in which they are present. Therefore, tissues containing paramagnetic agents will present with increased signal intensity, best seen on T1-weighted images. Melanin, methemoglobin, protein, and gadolinium are the most common paramagnetic agents. For example, a dermatoid cyst with a high proteinaceous content shows a higher signal intensity on T1- and T2-weighted images than a clear inclusion cyst does.

50. **Which ocular and orbital tissues do not normally enhance on postcontrast MRI studies?**
    - Lens
    - Vitreous
    - Retina
    - Sclera
    - Orbital fat
    - Optic nerve sheath complex
    - Peripheral nerve
    - Tendon
    - High-flow blood vessels

51. **Which ocular and orbital tissues do normally enhance on postcontrast MRI studies?**
    - Choroid
    - Ciliary body
    - Extraocular muscles
    - Lacrimal gland
    - Nasal: sinus mucosa
    - Cavernous sinus
    - Low blood-flow vessels

52. **What is the strategy in ordering imaging studies in a child with leukocoria and total retinal detachment?**
    First perform B-scan ultrasonography. It is cheap and easy to perform in the office without sedation. The goal is to identify calcification, which favors the diagnosis of retinoblastoma.
    If calcification is documented by ultrasonography, MRI studies are the second imaging step in order to assess the optic nerve and orbital structures and to rule out extraocular retinoblastoma. MRI studies are also helpful in evaluating the pineal gland and parasellar region, particularly in patients with bilateral and/or familial retinoblastoma.
    If calcification is not visualized by ultrasonography, orbital computed tomography (CT) should be the second imaging step because MRI cannot easily detect minor calcification.

53. **What is the strategy in ordering imaging studies in an adult with the diagnosis of intraocular neoplasm?**
A- and B-scan ultrasonography is the first imaging step in evaluating an adult presenting with an intraocular tumor. The role of CT is limited because of its poor histologic specificity. Therefore, there is no indication for CT in the evaluation of an elevated choroidal or subretinal mass. If ultrasonography, fluorescein angiography, and indocyanine green angiography do not help in the differential diagnosis, pre- and postcontrast-enhanced MRI studies with fat suppression techniques are most helpful in detecting and diagnosing intraocular lesions.

54. **In which clinical situation are contrast-enhanced MRI studies most helpful in the evaluation of a child with leukocoria?**
When you are distinguishing between retinoblastoma from Coats disease.

55. **In which clinical situations are contrast-enhanced MRI studies most helpful in the evaluation of an adult with vitreous hemorrhage?**
When you are distinguishing between a malignant melanoma of the choroid and a hemorrhagic retinal detachment in age-related macular/extramacular degeneration. Although in precontrast studies both lesions may show the same MRI features, choroidal melanoma shows enhancement after contrast injection, whereas hemorrhagic retinal detachment does not.

56. **What are the indications for ordering CT orbital studies as a first choice?**
   - Evaluation of orbital trauma
   - Detection of foreign body
   - Detection of calcification
   - Evaluation of a patient with proptosis presumably produced by a lacrimal gland tumor
   - Evaluation of a patient with proptosis presumably produced by a paranasal and/or sinus tumor
   - Evaluation of orbital soft tissue lesion with suspicion of bony erosion or detection
   - Contraindication to MRI

57. **What are the indications for ordering MRI orbital studies as a first choice?**
   - Acute proptosis (to differentiate cystic and/or hemorrhagic lesions from solid tumors)
   - Optic disc swelling or atrophy (to differentiate optic nerve from optic nerve sheath lesions)
   - Intraocular tumor with extraocular extension
   - Detection of wooden foreign body
   - Contraindications to CT

KEY POINTS: SUMMARY OF MODALITIES FOR OPHTHALMIC IMAGING

1. Evaluation of ocular structure
   - Ultrasound (A scan, B scan, UBM)
   - Optical coherence tomography
   - CT scan
   - MRI
   - Corneal topography

2. Evaluation of function
   - Angiography (fluorescein, indocyanine green)
   - Doppler blood flow

58. **Name the most common orbital lesions showing a well-circumscribed and sharply delineated appearance on CT and MRI.**

Children	Adults
1. Dermoid cyst	1. Cavernous hemangioma
2. Lymphangioma	2. Neurofibroma
3. Rhabdomyosarcoma	3. Neurilemoma
4. Optic nerve glioma	4. Fibrous histiocytoma
5. Hemangiopericytoma	
6. Lymphoma	

59. **Name the most common orbital lesions showing an ill-defined appearance on CT and MRI.**

Children	Adults
1. Capillary hemangioma	1. Idiopathic orbital inflammation
2. Idiopathic orbital inflammation	2. Metastasis
3. Plexiform neurofibroma	3. Leukemic infiltrate
4. Leukemic infiltrate	4. Primary malignant tumor
5. Eosinophilic granuloma	5. Lymphoproliferative disorders

60. **In which clinical situations are contrast-enhanced MRI studies most helpful in the evaluation of a patient with proptosis?**
In general, the soft tissue definition of MRI does not allow an accurate histopathologic diagnosis. In a growing lesion-related proptosis, however, MRI studies may differentiate true mitotic growth from mucinoid degeneration and hemorrhagic process.

Pre- and postcontrast MRI studies are also very helpful in patients diagnosed with a well-circumscribed lesion because they can differentiate a solid (enhancing) tumor from a cystic (nonenhancing) tumor. In a young patient with acute proptosis, MRI studies can differentiate a hemorrhagic lymphangioma from a growing rhabdomyosarcoma.

In suspected orbital inflammation, MRI characteristics of the ill-defined inflammatory tissues may predict the therapeutic response to steroids. Lesions showing high signal on T2-weighted images and marked contrast enhancement respond better to steroids than lesions presenting with lower signal intensity on T2-weighted images and/or with minimal or no contrast enhancement.

61. **What are the indications for orbital ultrasonography in imaging orbital lesions?**
Orbital ultrasonography is of little help because of its poor histologic specificity and the rapid sound attenuation in the retro-ocular structures. It may be useful to evaluate extraocular extension of an intraocular tumor, the proximal portion of the optic nerve, and extraocular muscles adjacent to the sclera.

62. **What are the indications for MRI angiography and carotid angiography in imaging orbital lesions?**
None. MRI angiography and carotid angiography are indicated only when clinical examination and MRI studies favor the diagnosis of carotid-cavernous sinus fistula or arteriovenous malformation.

63. **How can you differentiate optic nerve lesions from optic nerve sheath lesions with CT and MRI studies?**

Differentiation is almost impossible with CT except that optic nerve sheath meningioma may sometimes show linear calcifications best seen on CT. MRI studies are most relevant. First, a normal optic nerve does not demonstrate any enhancement on MRI studies after contrast injection. The localization of the enhancement (best seen on T1-weighted images with fat suppression techniques) helps to differentiate a true optic nerve lesion (neoplastic or inflammatory) from an optic nerve sheath process. An optic nerve tumor or inflammation demonstrates enhancement with the core of the optic nerve, whereas an optic nerve sheath neoplasm or inflammation demonstrates peripheral and/or eccentric enhancement. A cystic or hemorrhagic lesion does not enhance.

64. **Summarize the MRI features of normal ocular and orbital tissues.**

See Table 5-4.

TABLE 5-4. MRI FEATURES OF NORMAL OCULAR AND ORBITAL TISSUES			
Location	Signal Intensity T1-Weighted Images	Signal Intensity T2-Weighted Images	Enhancement After Gadolinium-DTPA Injection
Lens	High	Low	−
Vitreous	Low	High	−
Choroid	High	High	+++
Retina	Not detected	Not detected	−
Sclera	Low	Low	−
Optic nerve	Low	Low	−
Orbital fat	High	Low	−
Extraocular muscle	Low	Low	+++
Lacrimal gland	Low	Low	+++
Cortical bone	Low	Low	−

+++ = significant enhancement with gadolinium, − = no enhancement with gadolinium.

BIBLIOGRAPHY

1. Baumal CR: Clinical applications of optical coherence tomography. Curr Opin Ophthalmol 10:182–188, 1999.
2. Berson EL: Retinitis pigmentosa and allied diseases: Applications of electroretinographic testing. Int Ophthalmol 4:7–22, 1981.
3. Carr RE, Siegel IM: Electrodiagnostic Testing of the Visual System: A Clinical Guide. Philadelphia, F.A. Davis, 1990.
4. De Potter P, Flanders AE, Shields JA, et al: The role of fat-suppression technique and gadopentetate dimeglumine in magnetic resonance imaging evaluation of intraocular tumors and simulating lesions. Arch Ophthalmol 112:340–348, 1994.
5. De Potter P, Shields JA, Shields CL: Computed tomography and magnetic resonance imaging of intraocular lesions. Ophthalmol Clin North Am 7:333–346, 1994.

6. De Potter P, Shields JA, Shields CL: MRI of the Eye and Orbit. Philadelphia, J.B. Lippincott, 1995.

7. De Potter P, Shields CL, Shields JA, Flanders AE: The role of magnetic resonance imaging in children with intraocular tumors and simulating lesions. Ophthalmology 103:1774–1783, 1996.

8. Deramo VA, Shah GK, Baumal CR, et al: Ultrasound biomicroscopy as a tool for detecting and localizing occult foreign bodies after ocular trauma. Ophthalmology 106:301–305, 1999.

9. Fishman GA, Birch DG, Holder GE, Brigell MG: Electrophysiologic Testing in Disorders of the Retina, Optic Nerve, and Visual Pathway, 2nd ed. Ophthalmology Monograph, San Francisco, American Academy of Ophthalmology, 2001.

10. Hee MRI, Baumal CR, Puliafito CA, et al: Optical coherence tomography of age-related macular degeneration. Ophthalmology 103:1260–1270, 1996.

11. Marmor MF, Arden GB, Nilsson SEG, Zrenner E, International Standardization Committee: Standard for clinical electroretinography. Arch Ophthalmol 107:816–819, 1989.

12. Newton TH, Bilaniuk LT: Radiology of the Eye and Orbit. New York, Raven, 1990.

13. Sutter EE: Imaging visual function with the multifocal m-sequence technique. Vision Res 41:1241–1255, 2001.

14. Trope GE, Pavlin CJ, Bau A, et al: Malignant glaucoma: Clinical and ultrasound biomicroscopic features. Ophthalmology 101:1030–1035, 1994.

CHAPTER 6

VISUAL FIELDS

Janice A. Gault, MD

1. **What are the main types of visual field tests?**
   - **Confrontation visual fields** are a crude, qualitative method of determining gross defects in the peripheral field. The test is performed with the examiner facing the patient and asking if the patient can see fingers in all four quadrants while looking directly at the examiner, testing one eye at a time. A defect noted by confrontation fields can be described more accurately with formal field testing.
   - In **kinetic perimetry,** a stimulus is chosen and moved throughout the visual field. The area within which a given target is perceived is known as that target's isopter. They may be marked with different colors to easily differentiate them. The Goldmann perimeter and tangent screen are examples of kinetic techniques. Highly trained personnel are needed to administer these tests, but they can be helpful in patients who require significant supervision to complete visual-field testing.
   - With **static perimetry,** a test site is chosen and the stimulus intensity or size is changed until it is large enough or bright enough for the patient to see it. The Humphrey and Octopus machines are examples of static perimetry.
   - **Amsler grids** can be used to detect central and paracentral scotomas. If held at one third of a meter, each square subtends one degree of visual field.

2. **What is full-threshold testing?**
   Full-threshold testing refers to static visual-field testing in which the exact threshold of the eye is measured at every point tested. This technique differs from suprathreshold testing where test objects are presented at a fixed intensity. Suprathreshold testing is used mainly in screening programs and may miss early defects. Also, shallow defects will appear the same as an extremely deep defect.

3. **You order a Goldmann visual field, and the isopters are labeled with notations such as I2e and V4e. What do these notations mean?**
   The target size and intensity are indicated by a Roman numeral (I–V), an Arabic numeral (1–4), and a lowercase letter (a–e). The Roman numeral represents the size of the target in square millimeters. Each successive number is an increase by a factor of four. The Arabic numeral represents the relative intensity of the light presented. Each successive number is 3.15 times brighter than the previous one. The lowercase letter indicates a minor filter. The "a" is the darkest, and each progressive letter is an increase by 0.1 log unit.

4. **Where is the physiologic blind spot located?**
   In the temporal visual field. The fovea is the center of the visual field. The blind spot is 15 degrees temporal and just below the horizontal plane. On the Humphrey visual field, it is marked by a triangle.

5. **When looking at a visual field, how do you differentiate the right eye from the left eye?**
   By noting where the blind spot is located. The right eye has the blind spot on the right side in its temporal field, and the left eye has the blind spot on the left in its temporal field. If the field loss is so great that the blind spot cannot be identified, the top of the printout should say which eye was tested.

6. **What is a scotoma?**
    An area of lost or depressed vision within the visual field surrounded by an area of less depressed or normal visual field.

7. **What are causes of fixation errors? What can be done to decrease them?**
    - Poor patient fixation
    - "Trigger-happy" patient
    - Mistake in locating the blind spot
      Try replotting the blind spot, reinstructing the patient, or change the fixation diamond to one that does not require central vision in patients with macular disease or central scotoma. If fixation losses are greater than 20%, the test is not reliable. Small defects may be missed and the depth of large defects can be underestimated.

8. **What are false-negative errors?**
    False negatives occur when a stimulus brighter than threshold is presented in an area where sensitivity has already been determined and the patient does not respond. The patient is usually inattentive and the field will appear worse than it actually is. They may also occur in patients with tremendously dense defects.

9. **What are false-positive errors?**
    Most projection perimeters are fairly noisy, and there is an audible click or whirring while the machine moves from one position to another in the field. False positives occur when the projector moves as if to present a stimulus but does not and the patient responds. The patient is "trigger-happy," and the field will look better than it actually is.

10. **What are false field defects? What are some of their causes?**
    False field defects occur when the interpreter overlooks physical factors and interprets them as true field defects:
    - Ptosis and dermatochalasis can cause loss in the upper parts of the field. Taping the lid up will clear these defects.
    - A tilted optic disc can cause local variations in retinal topography, giving the impression of a field defect for refractive reasons alone. When a patient has bilateral tilted discs, the effect can mimic a bitemporal visual field loss.
    - A small pupil may give a false impression of true field loss. Dilation of the pupil will clear these defects. This is especially important in patients on miotic therapy (Fig. 6-1).
    - The rim of the trial lens will give a defect in the periphery of the central visual field. This will be noted if the patient pulls the head back from the machine while taking the test (Fig. 6-2).
    - Media opacities: cornea, lens, and vitreous opacities may cause routine test objects to be invisible. Using larger, brighter test objects may help clarify this problem.

KEY POINTS: CAUSES OF FALSE-POSITIVE FIELD DEFECTS

1. Ptosis

2. Tilted optic disc

3. Small pupil

4. Rim defect

5. Media opacities

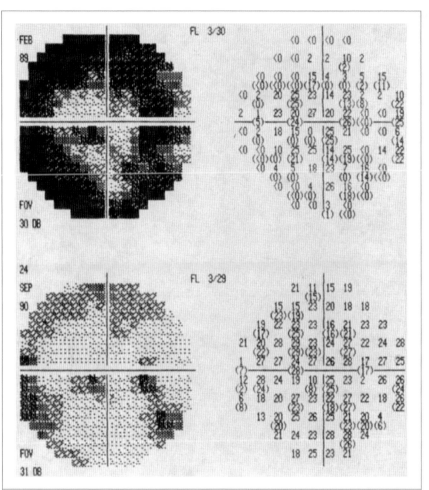

Figure 6-1. A small pupil can create a false impression of visual-field defects. Note a majority of the defects disappear or lessen when the pupil is dilated from 2 mm to 8 mm. (From Gross R: Clinical Glaucoma Management. Philadelphia, W.B. Saunders, 2001.)

11. **What is hemianopia?**
Hemianopia is defective vision or blindness in half of the visual field of one or both eyes.

12. **Define the terms homonymous and congruous in relation to visual-field defects.**
- **Homonymous:** pertaining to the corresponding vertical halves of the visual field of both eyes. In plain language, the term is used for defects that occur after neurologic insults that cause loss of a portion of the visual field subsumed by both eyes. A completely homonymous hemianopia is nonlocalizing.
- **Congruous:** Matched visual field defects. The more congruous the defect, the more posterior the lesion.

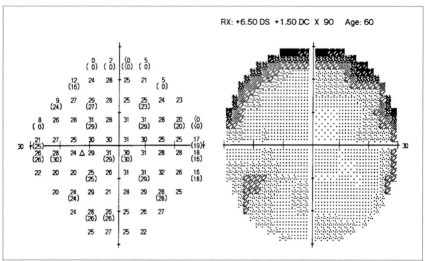

RX: +6.50 DS +1.50 DC X 90   Age: 60

Figure 6-2. Rim artifact caused by the lens and lens carrier. This is most commonly seen in patients on whom a hyperopic correction is being used. A clue to the presence of a rim artifact is the abrupt change from a fairly normal reading to a sensitivity of 0 dB. (From Alward WLM: Glaucoma: The Requisites in Ophthalmology. St. Louis, Mosby, 2000.)

13. **How do you describe a visual-field defect?**
   1. **Position:** Central (defined as the central 30 degrees), peripheral, or a combination of both. Note if the defects are unilateral or bilateral.
   2. **Shape:** Very helpful diagnostically. Visual-field defects can be monocular or binocular. The most common form of monocular sector defect is found in glaucoma. The shape is determined by physiologic interruption of nerve fiber bundles. The typical binocular sector defect is a hemianopia, which can be subdivided as follows:
      - **Homonymous, total:** Loss of temporal field in one eye and nasal field of the other eye. The vertical midline is respected. The fixation point may be included or spared. This defect implies total destruction of the visual pathway beyond the chiasm unilaterally, anywhere from the optic tract to the occipital lobe.
      - **Homonymous, partial:** The most common visual-field defect. It may be caused by injury to postchiasmal pathways. Again, it can result from damage at any point from the optic tract to the occipital lobe (Fig. 6-3).
      - **Homonymous quadrantanopia:** This is a form of partial homonymous hemianopia.
      - **Bitemporal:** May vary from a loss of a small amount of the temporal field to complete temporal hemifield loss. This defect signifies damage in the optic chiasm.
      - **Binasal:** This defect signifies an interruption of the uncrossed fibers in both lateral aspects of the chiasm, both optic nerves, or both retinas.
      - **Crossed quadrantanopia:** A rare defect in which the upper quadrant of one field is lost along with the lower quadrant of the opposite visual field. It can occur as part of the chiasmal compression syndrome where the chiasm is compressed from beneath against a contiguous arterial structure. This produces pressure simultaneously from above and below.
      - **Altitudinal:** This defect can be unilateral or bilateral. A unilateral defect is prechiasmal. Bilateral lesions may be produced by lesions that press the chiasm up, wedging the optic nerve, such as an olfactory groove meningioma (Fig. 6-4).

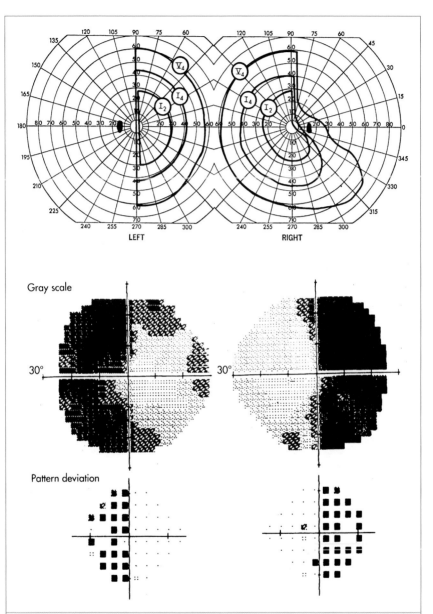

Figure 6-3. Bitemporal hemianopia: incongruous noted on both the Goldmann perimeter (above) and the Humphrey perimeter (below). (From Burde RM, Savino PJ, Trobe JD: Clinical Decisions in Neuro-Ophthalmology, 2nd ed. St. Louis, Mosby, 1992.)

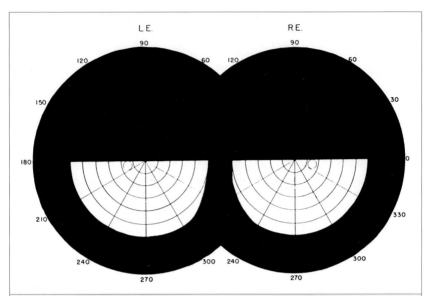

Figure 6-4. Bilateral altitudinal hemianopia. (From Harrington DO, Drake MV: The Visual Fields: Text and Atlas of Clinical Perimetry, 6th ed. St. Louis, Mosby, 1990.)

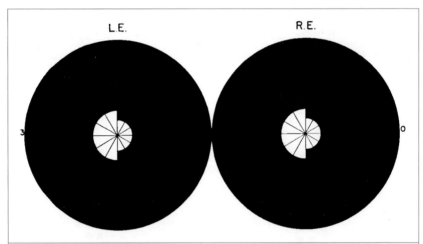

Figure 6-5. Double homonymous hemianopia. (From Harrington DO, Drake MV: The Visual Fields: Text and Atlas of Clinical Perimetry, 6th ed. St. Louis, Mosby, 1990.)

- **Double homonymous hemianopia:** A result of lesions of the occipital area. There is a loss of all peripheral vision with a remaining small area of central vision representing the spared macula of both eyes. Most are vascular in origin, but they can result from trauma, anoxia, carbon monoxide poisoning, cardiac arrest, and exsanguination (Fig. 6-5).
- **Macula sparing:** This is the rule in occipital damage. The central visual acuity can remain normal.

- **Macula splitting:** Uncommon and difficult to detect because patient will refixate often during the test. This defect occurs with homonymous hemianopia, caused by lesions in the anterior portion of the postchiasmal pathway.
3. **Intensity:** This refers to the depth of the defect.
4. **Uniformity:** This refers to the depth of the defect throughout the defect.
5. **Onset and course:** This is determined by serial visual fields.

14. **Describe the visual pathway.**
The first-order neuron is the photoreceptor, a rod or a cone. They synapse with the second-order neurons, the bipolar cells. These synapse with the third-order neurons, the ganglion cells. Axons from these cells cross the retina as the nerve fiber layer and become the optic nerve. The arrangement of these fibers determines the visual-field defects seen in glaucoma and other optic nerve lesions.

At the chiasm, the temporal fibers are uncrossed, but the nasal fibers cross. The optic tracts begin posterior to the chiasm and connect to the lateral geniculate body on the posterior of the thalamus. Crossed fibers go to laminae 1, 4, and 6. Uncrossed fibers terminate in laminae 2, 3, and 5. The retinal ganglion cell fibers synapse to cells that then connect to the occipital cortex (area 17) via optic radiations in the temporal and parietal lobes.

15. **What visual-field defects are characteristically seen in neuro-ophthalmologic disorders?**
The pattern of visual-field loss in these patients can often be used to locate very precisely the area of the visual system involved (Fig. 6-6 and Table 6-1).

16. **Describe the visual-field defect in Fig. 6-7. What are its major causes?**
This is a bitemporal hemianopia. Lesions of the chiasm cause bitemporal hemianopia because they damage the crossing nasal nerve fibers. Masses in this area include pituitary tumors, pituitary apoplexy, meningiomas, aneurysms, infection, cranio-pharyngiomas, gliomas, and other less

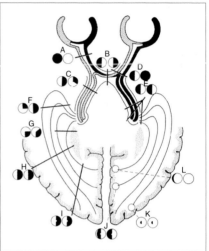

Figure 6-6. Diagram of the visual pathway with sites of nerve fiber damage and corresponding visual fields produced by this damage. *A*, Optic nerve: blindness on involved side with normal contralateral field. *B*, Chiasm: bitemporal hemianopia. *C*, Optic tract: contralateral incongruous homonymous hemianopia. *D*, Optic nerve-chiasmal junction: junctional scotoma. *E*, Posterior optic tract, external geniculate ganglion, posterior limb of internal capsule: contralateral homonymous hemianopia, complete or incomplete incongruous. *F*, Optic radiation, anterior loop in temporal lobe: incongruous contralateral homonymous hemianopia or superior quadrantopia. *G*, Medial fibers of optic radiation: contralateral incongruous inferior homonymous quadrantopia. *H*, Optic radiation in parietal lobe: contralateral homonymous hemianopia, may be mildly incongruous, minimal macular sparing. *I*, Optic radiation in posterior parietal lobe and occipital lobe: contralateral congruous homonymous hemianopia with macular sparing. *J*, Midportion of calcarine cortex: contralateral congruous homonymous hemianopia with wide macular sparing and sparing of contralateral temporal crescent. *K*, Tip of occipital lobe: contralateral congruous homonymous hemianoptic scotomas. *L*, Anterior tip of calcarine fissure: contralateral loss of temporal crescent with otherwise normal visual fields. (Adapted from Harrington DO, Drake MV: The Visual Fields: Text and Atlas of Clinical Perimetry, 6th ed. St. Louis, Mosby, 1990.)

TABLE 6-1. SUMMARY OF NEURO-OPHTHALMOLOGIC VISUAL-FIELD DEFECTS	
Lesion	Visual Field
Optic nerve	Central and cecocentral scotomas (i.e., optic neuritis, compressive lesions)
	Altitudinal defects (i.e., optic nerve drusen, chronic papilledema, ischemic optic neuropathy, optic nerve colobomas)
Optic chiasm	Anterior chiasm or posterior optic nerve: junctional scotoma
	Body and posterior chiasm: bitemporal hemianopia
Optic tract	Incongruous homonymous hemianopia with or without central scotoma
Optic radiations	Internal capsule: congruous homonymous hemianopia
	Temporal lobe: superior quadrantanopia
	Parietal lobe: inferior quadrantanopia
Occipital lobe	Posterior: highly congruous homonymous hemianopia
	Anterior: monocular contralateral temporal defect
	Macular or extreme temporal fields may be spared

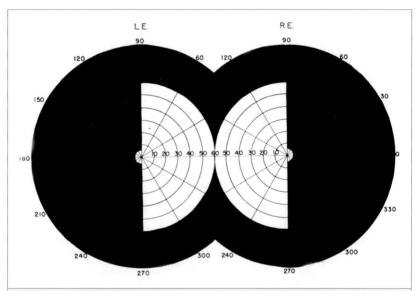

Figure 6-7. Bitemporal hemianopia. (From Harrington DO, Drake MV: The Visual Fields: Text and Atlas of Clinical Perimetry, 6th ed. St. Louis, Mosby, 1990.)

common tumors. In addition, the chiasm may be damaged by trauma (typically causing a complete bitemporal hemianopia), demyelinating disease, and inflammatory diseases such as sarcoidosis, and rarely, ischemia.

17. **What causes binasal hemianopia?**
Most nasal field defects are due to bilateral arcuate scotomas from glaucoma. True binasal hemianopias are rare, but they are never a result of chiasmal compression. They may be due to pressure upon the temporal aspect of the optic nerve and the anterior angle of the chiasm or near the optic canal. Causes include aneurysm, tumors such as pituitary adenomas, and vascular infarction.

18. **Where would you expect the lesion causing an homonymous hemianopia without optic atrophy to be located?**
Posterior to the lateral geniculate body. Any lesion anterior to the lateral geniculate body would cause the ganglion axon cells to degenerate.

19. **Does visual acuity help to locate the cause of a visual-field defect?**
Patients with isolated retrochiasmatic lesions do not have decreased visual acuity unless the lesions are bilateral, and then the visual acuity should be equal. Thus, unequal visual acuity would locate the lesion at or before the chiasm. This can be supported with color plate abnormalities and a relative afferent pupillary defect. Also examine the patient for optic disc abnormalities such as pallor, cupping, and drusen.

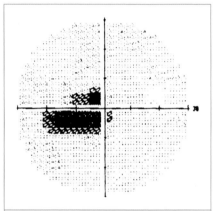

20. **Describe the visual-field defect in Fig. 6-8. What causes this?**
This is a cecocentral lesion defined as a lesion involving both the blind spot and the macular area (to the 25-degree circle). Four primary causes are typically cited: dominant optic atrophy, Leber's optic atrophy, toxic/nutritional optic neuropathy (i.e., tobacco, alcohol, lead, multiple medications), and congenital pit of the optic nerve with a serous retinal detachment. Optic neuritis also may cause cecocentral lesions.

Figure 6-8. Cecocentral scotoma. (From Burde RM, Savino PJ, Trobe JD: Unexplained visual loss. In Burde RM, Savino PJ, Trobe JD [eds]: Clinical Decisions in Neuro-Ophthalmology, 3rd ed. St. Louis, Mosby, 2002, pp 1–26.)

21. **Describe the visual-field defect in Fig. 6-9. Where is the lesion? Are there any coexistent symptoms?**
A "pie-in-the-sky" lesion is a homonymous quadrantanopia involving the superior quadrant. The term indicates a lesion in the optic radiations through the temporal lobe, but similar defects can be seen with occipital lobe lesions as well. These patients often have coexistent seizures and visual hallucinations.

22. **Describe the visual-field defect in Fig. 6-10. Where is the lesion? Are there any coexistent symptoms?**
A "pie-on-the-floor" lesion is a homonymous quadrantanopia involving the inferior quadrant. The term indicates a lesion in the parietal lobe. These patients often have coexistent spasticity of conjugate gaze (tonic deviation of eyes opposite to the side of the lesion when attempting Bell's phenomenon) and optokinetic asymmetry (diminished or absent response with rotation of optokinetic objects toward the side of the lesion).

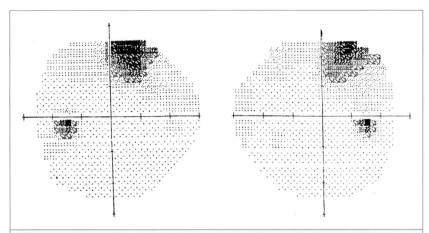

Figure 6-9. Congruous right superior homonymous quadrantanopia following left temporal lobectomy for epilepsy. (From Burde RM, Savino PJ, Trobe JD: Clinical Decisions in Neuro-Ophthalmology, 3rd ed. St. Louis, Mosby, 2002.)

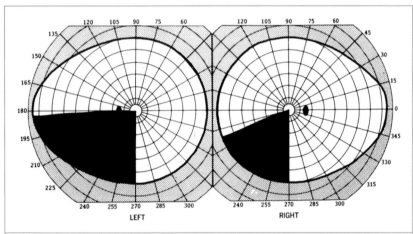

Figure 6-10. Left inferior quadrantanopia in a patient with a right parietal lobe lesion. (From Kline LB, Bajandas FJ: Neuro-Ophthalmology Review Manual, 4th ed. Thorofare, NJ, Slack, 1996.)

23. **Describe the visual-field defect seen in Fig. 6-11.**
A junctional scotoma is a unilateral central scotoma associated with a contralateral superior temporal field defect. Thus, in a patient that comes in with poor vision in one eye, it is very important to check the contralateral visual field for superior temporal field loss.

24. **What is the anatomic explanation for a junctional scotoma?**
Inferonasal retina fibers cross in the chiasm, passing into the contralateral optic nerve (Willebrand's knee). The contralateral optic nerve is compressed near the chiasm. These patients have decreased visual acuity and a relative afferent visual defect.

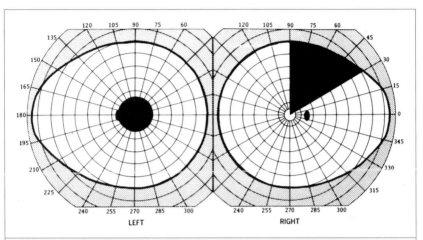

Figure 6-11. Junctional scotoma from a lesion at the left optic nerve and anterior chiasm. (From Kline LB, Bajandas FJ: Neuro-Ophthalmology Review Manual, 4th ed. Thorofare, NJ, Slack, 1996.)

25. **What is an optic-tract syndrome?**
Mass lesions of the optic tract are usually large enough to compromise the optic nerve and chiasm as well. Patients have an incongruous homonymous hemianopia (Fig. 6-12), bilateral optic disc atrophy, often in a "bow-tie" pattern, and a relative afferent defect on the side opposite the lesion (i.e., the eye with temporal field loss).

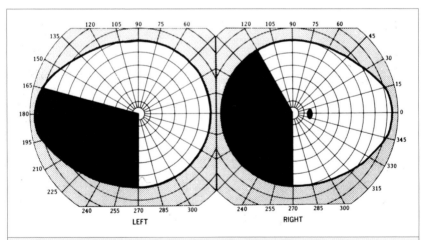

Figure 6-12. Incongruous left homonymous hemianopia from a right optic-tract lesion. (From Kline LB, Bajandas FJ: Neuro-Ophthalmology Review Manual, 4th ed. Thorofare, NJ, Slack, 1996.)

26. **What are the most common visual-field findings in glaucoma?**
Glaucoma is a disease characterized by loss of retinal ganglion cells with characteristic optic nerve findings. The classic defects are determined by the anatomy of retinal ganglion cells as

they travel to the optic nerve. The axons circle around the fovea in an arc. With damage to the nerve bundles, the classic findings include a nasal step, an arcuate defect within 15 degrees of fixation (also known as a Bjerrum defect), or a Siedel scotoma (a comma-shaped extension of the blind spot; Fig. 6-13). Such a defect obeys the horizontal midline (in contrast to neurologic field defects, which obey the vertical midline). The exam of the optic nerve is helpful in making the diagnosis in less clear cases. Defects in the optic nerve will predict the visual-field loss (e.g., a superior notch of the nerve will be manifested by an inferior arcuate field defect). Usually, the central field is retained until a late stage of the disease. When the central field is lost, a small temporal island may remain.

27. **When has the visual field of a person with glaucoma progressed?**
The answer remains controversial. First, do not base a diagnosis of glaucoma on one field. If there the patient has clear optic nerve damage and corresponding visual-field defects, one can make the diagnosis, but the baseline field needs to be repeated because of the general tendency of people to improve after taking the test several times. Improved fixation can also cause field

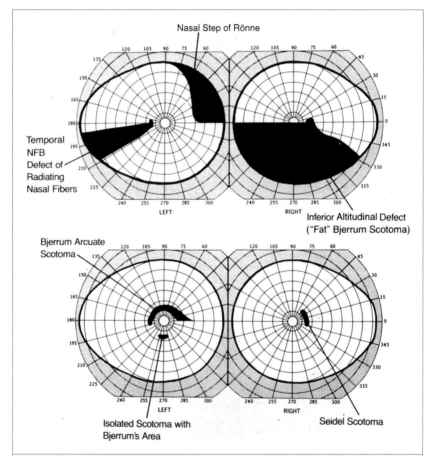

Figure 6-13. Common visual-field findings in glaucoma. (From Kline LB, Bajandas FJ: Neuro-Ophthalmology Review Manual, 4th ed. Thorofare, NJ, Slack, 1996.)

defects to appear more clearly. Persons with glaucoma tend to have more variable visual fields than normal subjects; thus, a single visual field showing worsening should be confirmed with a repeat field. One study concluded that to be certain of progression, one needs a minimum of 5 years of annual visual fields. However, use of clinical correlation can help (Fig. 6-14). Ongoing research is trying to improve our ability to determine which patients are progressing.

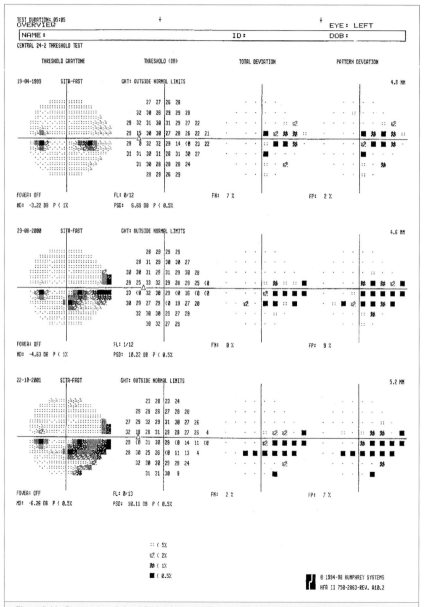

Figure 6-14. Progression of visual-field defects over 3 years. (From Kanski JJ: Clinical Ophthalmology: A Systematic Approach, 5th ed. New York, Butterworth-Heinemann, 2003.)

28. **Describe the visual field in Fig. 6-15. What is your differential diagnosis?**
This is a ring scotoma. Severe glaucoma, retinitis pigmentosa, panretinal photocoagulation, vitamin A deficiency, other retinal and/or choroidal diseases affect the peripheral retina selectively. Aphakic patients may have a prominent ring scotoma from lens-induced magnification of the central field. Clinical exam should differentiate the above easily. Functional visual loss from hysteria or malingering may reveal a ring scotoma on visual-field testing. A Goldmann visual field may be helpful in this situation, as spiraling where an isopter of greater luminance overlaps one that is dimmer can rule out organic disease (Fig. 6-16).

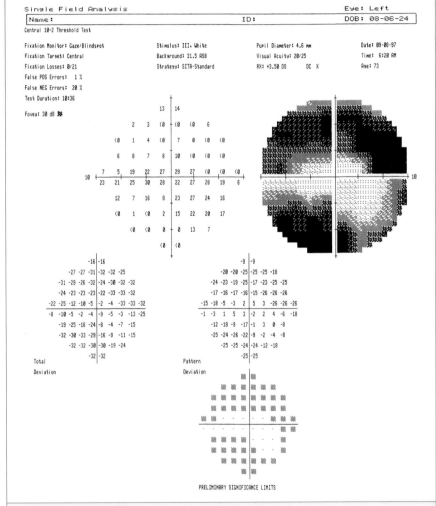

Figure 6-15. Ring scotoma. (From Gross R: Clinical Glaucoma Management. Philadelphia, W.B. Saunders, 2001.)

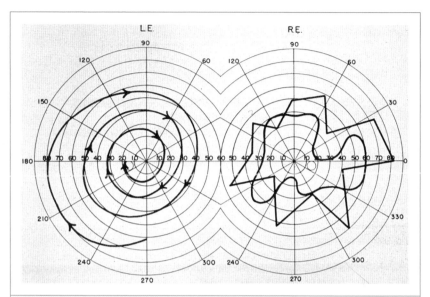

Figure 6-16. Visual fields in a hysterical patient. The left eye shows spiraling. The right eye shows a fatigue field in which a star-shaped interlacing field results from testing opposite ends of the various meridians. (From Harrington DO, Drake MV: The Visual Fields: Text and Atlas of Clinical Perimetry, 6th ed. St. Louis, Mosby, 1990.)

29. **What is the differential diagnosis of general depression of the field without localized field defects?**

    This is a general sign without diagnostic value, but can be an indication of glaucoma, media opacities, small pupils, refractive error, and/or an inexperienced or inattentive patient.

30. **What clinical findings might mimic a neurologic defect?**

    An altitudinal defect can be seen with a hemibranch artery or vein occlusion (Fig. 6-17). Peripapillary atrophy will reveal an enlarged blind spot. A disciform macular scar will show a

KEY POINTS: USING VISUAL FIELDS TO DETERMINE CAUSE

1. Monocular defects are prechiasmal except that the far temporal visual field is seen only by one eye. Watch this in an anterior occipital infarct, which can produce a monocular temporal defect.

2. Lesions posterior to the chiasm do not cross the vertical meridian by more then 15 degrees.

3. Patients with postchiasmal defects typically have normal visual acuity, normal pupils, and a normal exam of the ocular fundus. Papilledema, however, may be seen in patients with space-occupying lesions.

4. Use clinical correlation to interpret fields.

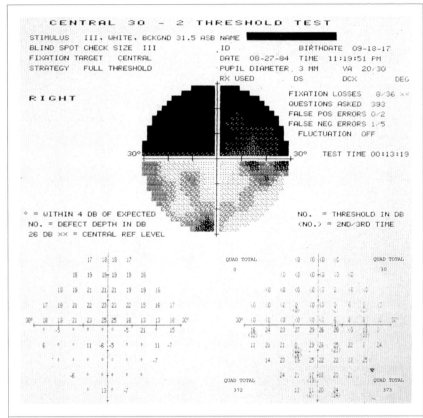

Figure 6-17. A patient with a retinal artery obstruction in the left eye, manifesting a unilateral altitudinal field defect. The patient has count fingers vision in this eye with a plaque in the central retinal artery with diffuse retinal edema over the posterior pole with a narrowing of the arterial blood column. (From Haley MJ [ed]: The Field Analyzer Primer, 2nd ed. San Leandro, CA, Allergan Humphrey, 1987.)

central scotoma (Fig. 6-18). Retinal detachment will show a correlating visual-field defect, even after it has been repaired.

31. **What does the future hold for visual-field testing?**
    The three important advances in visual-field testing are faster algorithms that decrease test time, short wavelength automated perimetry (SWAP), and frequency-doubling perimetry. The new algorithm uses previous patient responses to help choose the testing threshold and thus takes less time. Test times are approximately 5 minutes per eye, as opposed to 15 minutes with the older algorithms. SWAP may detect field loss earlier than traditional white-on-white perimetry. SWAP uses standard static threshold-testing strategies with a blue test object on a yellow background. Early results indicate that visual-field defects may be detected several years earlier with SWAP than with standard static testing. Finally, frequency-doubling perimetry is in the early stages of development but may be extremely useful as a screening tool in the future.

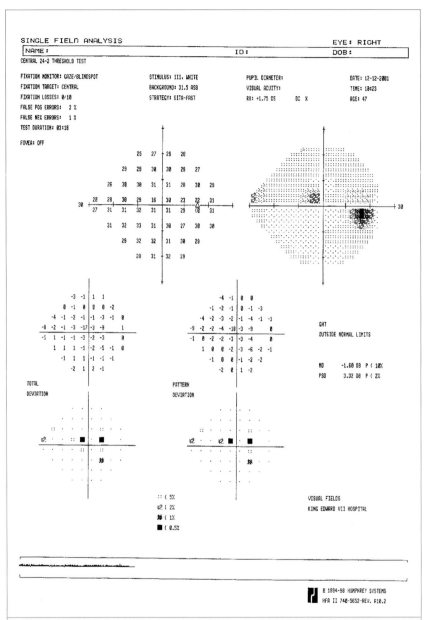

Figure 6-18. Paracentral scotoma. (From Kanski JJ: Clinical Ophthalmology: A Systematic Approach, 5th ed. New York, Butterworth-Heinemann, 2003.)

BIBLIOGRAPHY

1. Anderson DA: Automated Static Perimetry. St. Louis, Mosby, 1992.

2. Burde RM, Savino PJ, Trobe JD: Clinical Decisions in Neuro-Ophthalmology, 2nd ed. St. Louis, Mosby, 1992.

3. Haley MJ (ed): The Field Analyzer Primer, 2nd ed. San Leandro, CA, Allergan Humphrey, 1987.

4. Harrington DO, Drake MV: The Visual Fields: Text and Atlas of Clinical Perimetry, 6th ed. St. Louis, Mosby, 1990.

5. Johnson CA, Brandt JD, Khong AM, Adams AJ: Short-wavelength automated perimetry in low-, medium-, and high-risk ocular hypertensive eyes. Arch Ophthalmol 113:70–76, 1995.

6. Johnson CA: Screening for glaucomatous visual field loss with frequency-doubling perimetry. Invest Ophthalmol Vis Sci 38:413–425, 1997.

7. Katz J, Tielsch JM, Quigley HA, Sommer A: Automated perimetry detects field loss before manual Goldmann perimetry. Ophthalmology 102:21–26, 1995.

8. Kline LB, Bajandas FJ: Neuro-Ophthalmology Review Manual, 4th ed. Thorofare, NJ, Slack, 1996.

9. Miller NR: Walsh and Hoyt's Clinical Neuro-Ophthalmology, vol. 1. Baltimore, Williams & Wilkins, 1982.

10. Smith SD, Katz J, Quigley HA: Analysis of progressive changes in automated visual fields in glaucoma. Invest Ophthalmol Vis Sci 37:1419–1428, 1996.

II. CORNEA AND EXTERNAL DISEASES

THE RED EYE

Janice A. Gault, MD

1. **Name the main causes of a red eye.**
   - Conjunctivitis
   - Episcleritis
   - Subconjunctival hemorrhage
   - Scleritis
   - Corneal disease and trauma
   - Dry eye
   - Anterior uveitis
   - Acute glaucoma
   - Blepharitis

2. **A 40-year-old woman complains of watery, itchy eyes with swollen lids. How should you proceed?**
   In the differential diagnosis of a red eye, the history is often helpful. By asking more questions, you find that she has been mowing the grass; subsequently, her hay fever worsened and her eyes flared. Examination reveals red, edematous lids, chemosis, conjunctival papillae, and mucous strands in the cul-de-sac. A preauricular node is not palpable. Appropriate treatment includes systemic medications such as loratadine (Claritin) or diphenhydramine (Benadryl). Options for topical medications include:
   - Mast cell inhibitors
     - Lodoxamide (Alomide)
     - Cromolyn sodium (Crolom)
     - Pemirolast (Alamast)
   - H_1 receptor antagonists
     - Levocabastine (Livostin)
     - Emedastine (Emadine)
   - Combination H_1 antagonists/mast cell inhibitors
     - Ketotifen (Zaditor)
     - Olopatadine (Patanol)
     - Nedocromil sodium (Alocril)
     - Azelastine hydrochloride (Optivar)
     - Nedocromil (Alocril)
   - Nonsteroidal anti-inflammatory drugs (NSAIDs)
     - Diclofenac (Voltaren)
     - Ketorolac (Acular)
   - Low-dose steroid (only for short-term use or under close supervision): loteprednol (Alrex, Lotemax)
   - Antihistamine/decongestant
     - Naphazoline/pheniramine (Opcon-A, Naphcon A, Visine A)
     - Naphazoline/antazoline (Vasocon A)

   A patient who is allergic to a medication used in or around the eyes presents in a similar fashion. Typical offenders include aminoglycosides, sulfa medications, atropine, epinephrine agents, apraclonidine, trifluorothymidine (Viroptic), pilocarpine, and any ophthalmic medication with preservatives. Immediate cessation of the offending agent as well as cool compresses and preservative-free artificial tears or a topical antiallergy medication are appropriate. Impress on the patient that lid rubbing will worsen the condition. If the lid reaction is severe, an ophthalmic steroid cream may be prescribed. Some patients are affected severely enough to develop an ectropion of their lower lids.

3. **What might you expect to see in a patient with "pink eye?"**
Examination may reveal tarsal conjunctival follicles as well as a preauricular node. In more severe cases, the patient may have membranes or pseudomembranes. Often the condition may begin in one eye and spread to the other. Viral conjunctivitis may precede, accompany, or follow an upper respiratory infection. This condition is contagious, and patients need to be warned not to leave any contaminated material in a place where others may touch it. Frequent handwashing is crucial. The physician's exam room needs to be washed down thoroughly, because an epidemic may occur among other patients as well as staff. Patients should not return to work or school until the eyes stop weeping, often as long as 2 weeks. The condition typically worsens in the first week before improving over the course of 2–3 weeks. Treatment is mainly supportive with artificial tears and cool compresses. Only in select cases should steroid therapy be used. Examples include subepithelial infiltrates that reduce vision and membranes or pseudomembranes. Steroids may help in the short term but often increase the duration of the disease. Topical NSAIDs may alleviate discomfort without prolonging the disease course.

4. **A 25-year-old man states that his eyes have been dripping with discharge over the past 8 hours. You notice significant purulent discharge, a preauricular node, and marked chemosis. What is the next step?**
This condition is an emergency. The most likely diagnosis is gonococcal conjunctivitis. An immediate Gram stain and conjunctival scrapings for culture and sensitivities are imperative. Cultures should be done on blood agar, on chocolate agar at 37°C and 10% CO_2, and a Thayer-Martin plate.

5. **What are you looking for on the Gram stain?**
Gram-negative intracellular diplococci.

6. **How should the patient be treated?**
    1. Ceftriaxone, 1 gm IM in a single dose. However, if corneal involvement exists or you are unable to visualize the cornea because of chemosis and lid swelling, the patient should be hospitalized and treated with ceftriaxone, 1 gm IV every 12–24 hours. *Neisseria gonorrhoeae* can perforate an intact cornea quickly. Penicillin-allergic patients can be treated orally with 500 mg of ciprofloxacin or 400 mg of ofloxacin, both as single doses.
    2. Topical bacitracin or erythromycin ointment four times/day or ciprofloxacin drops every 2 hours.
    3. Eye irrigation with saline four times/day until the discharge is gone.
    4. Doxycycline, 100 mg twice a day for 7 days, or azithromycin, 1 gm orally as a single dose for chlamydial infection, which often coexists. Use erythromycin or clarithromycin if the patient is pregnant or breast feeding because of the risk of teeth staining.
    5. Referral of the patient and sexual partners to family doctors for evaluation of other sexually transmitted diseases.

7. **A 35-year-old man complains of pain in his left eye for several days, watery discharge, and blurred vision. He thinks he has had the same symptoms before. He admits to stress on the job as well as a recent cold sore. What do you expect to see?**
Herpes simplex virus (HSV). With fluorescein staining of the eye, you can see a dendritic ulcer with terminal bulbs (Fig. 7-1). It is placed centrally, accounting for the decrease in vision. The patient may also have some anterior chamber cell and flare. He needs a topical antiviral

such as trifluorothymidine (Viroptic) or vidarabine (Vira-A) and a cycloplegic drop if photophobia and anterior chamber reaction are significant. Topical steroids should be tapered. Oral antivirals such as famvir and acyclovir have not been shown to be beneficial in the prevention of stromal disease or iritis in HSV infection, but they are beneficial if iritis is already present. Long-term, oral antiviral prophylaxis such as acyclovir 400 mg twice a day may be indicated if the patient has had multiple episodes of herpetic epithelial or stromal disease.

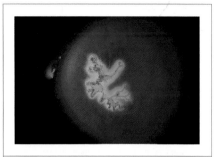

Figure 7-1. A dendrite typical of herpes simplex keratitis with epithelial ulceration, raised edges, and terminal bulbs. (From Kanski JJ: Clinical Ophthalmology: A Synopsis. New York, Butterworth-Heinemann, 2004.)

Herpetic Eye Disease Study Group: Acyclovir for prevention of recurrent herpes simplex virus eye disease. N Engl J Med 339:300–306, 1998.

Herpetic Eyes Disease Study Group: Oral acyclovir for herpes simplex virus eye disease: Effect on prevention of epithelial keratitis and stromal keratitis. Arch Ophthalmol 118:1030–1036, 2000.

Langston DP: Oral acyclovir suppresses recurrent epithelial and stromal herpes simplex. Arch Ophthalmol 117:391–392, 1999.

8. **An 80-year-old woman complains of red eyes that constantly tear and burn. She also feels foreign-body sensation and reports that her vision is not as clear as before. The vision varies with tear blink. She has noticed this condition over the past several years. What may you find?**

On exam, you may find a poor tear film filled with debris, a low tear meniscus, superficial punctate keratopathy inferiorly or throughout the cornea, and, if severe, mucus filaments adherent to the cornea. A normal meniscus is 1 mm in height in a convex shape. A Schirmer's test can quantify her tearing. Rose bengal stains the cornea and conjunctiva (Fig. 7-2). Make sure that she can close her eyes completely, because lagophthalmos may cause similar symptoms. The condition may be due to an eyelid deformity from scarring, tumor, or Bell's palsy. Patients may have trouble closing their eyes after ptosis surgery.

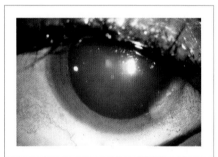

Figure 7-2. Dry eye syndrome with rose bengal staining. (From Tu EY, Rheinstrom S: Dry eye. In Yanoff M, Duker JS [eds]: Ophthalmology. 2nd ed. St. Louis, Mosby, 2004, pp 520–524.)

9. **What may cause superficial punctate keratopathy (SPK)?**

Blepharitis, trauma from eye rubbing, exposure, topical drug toxicity, ultraviolet burns (welder's flash, snow blindness), foreign body under the upper lid, mild chemical injury, trichiasis, floppy-lid syndrome, entropion, and ectropion may cause bilateral SPK. Treatment consists of lubrication and eliminating the cause. Thygeson's SPK consists of bilateral stellate, whitish-gray corneal opacities that are slightly elevated with minimal to no staining. Tears are usually the only required treatment, with occasional topical steroids for severe cases. Thygeson's SPK has a chronic course with remissions and exacerbations.

10. **An 83-year-old man has crusty lids and red eyes and complains of "sand in my eyes." What is your diagnosis?**

A common scenario indeed. Blepharitis manifests with crusty, red, thickened eyelid margins with prominent blood vessels (Fig. 7-3). Inspissated oil glands at the lid margins cause meibomianitis. Patients often have both and complain of red, tearing eyes. The lids may be significantly swollen. Patients often have trouble opening their eyes in the morning because of the amount of crusting. SPK is common.

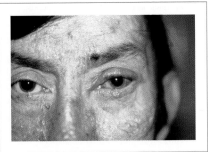

Figure 7-3. Blepharitis. (From Kanski JJ: Clinical Ophthalmology: A Test Yourself Atlas, 2nd ed. New York, Butterworth-Heinemann, 2002.)

This chronic condition requires treatment indefinitely. Warm compresses four times/day for 10 minutes at a time, baby shampoo on a washcloth or commercial lid scrubs to scrub the eyelid margins twice a day, and artificial tears as needed will help. It may take a week or two of compliance before improvement is seen. Once the condition is under better control, the regimen can be reduced to once a day or as needed. However, when the condition flares, the regimen needs to be increased. In severe cases, a topical antibiotic/steroid combination may be helpful in the short term, but make sure that the patient understands the risks of long-term use of steroids (e.g., cataracts, glaucoma, increased risk of infection).

Patients also may have trichiasis or misdirected lashes that scratch the cornea and conjunctiva. If this condition is found, the lashes can be epilated. If they become a recurring problem, electrolysis or cryotherapy may provide a more permanent solution.

11. **A 45-year-old man with red, weepy eyes complains of foreign-body sensation, which has been occurring for a while. Of note, you realize he has a bulbous nose and telangiectasias across both cheeks. What is your diagnosis? How do you treat?**

Acne rosacea is a disease of the eyes and the skin. Pustules, papules, telangiectasias, and erythema develop on the nose, cheeks, and forehead. Rhinophyma occurs in the later stages of the disease. Telangiectasias of the eyelid margin and chalazia are common, as are blepharitis and meibomianitis. Dry eye, SPK, phlyctenules, and staphylococcal hypersensitivity may occur. In severe cases, the cornea may develop vascularization and even perforate.

Treatment for blepharitis and meibomianitis with warm compresses and lid scrubs may be all that is necessary. If the patient does not respond, tetracycline or doxycycline for several weeks may relieve the symptoms. However, some patients require a low dose indefinitely. Erythromycin should be substituted in pregnant or nursing women and children. A low-dose antibiotic/steroid combination may be useful if SPK or staphylococcal hypersensitivity is a problem; staphylococcal exotoxins may be the cause. However, patients also develop infected corneal ulcers; thus, scrapings for smears and cultures may be necessary in patients with "sterile" corneal ulcers before steroids are used.

12. **An 18-year-old contact lens wearer presents with her hand over her right eye. She noticed that her eye was somewhat red and irritated 2 days ago but believes that it has gotten worse even though she took out her lens at that time. What are you concerned about?**

Whenever a contact lens wearer complains of a red, irritated eye that does not improve over a few hours, a corneal ulcer is high on the differential. After a corneal anesthetic such as proparacaine is instilled, the patient feels some relief and can tolerate examination. You notice a corneal infiltrate with an overlying epithelial defect and anterior chamber cell and flare. See the chapter on corneal infections for the necessary workup and treatment.

13. **What else is in the differential diagnosis of a red eye in a contact lens wearer?**

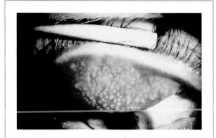

- Hypersensitivity reactions to preservatives in solution. The patient may develop an allergy or may not be rinsing the enzyme off completely before placing the lens in the eye.
- Giant papillary conjunctivitis (Fig. 7-4). Patients have large conjunctival papillae on upper lid eversion. Patients may need to discontinue lens wear for several weeks, change to a disposable lens regimen, and/or use topical medications such as nonsteroidal anti-inflammatory medications, mast-cell inhibitors, or antihistamines. Increased enzyme use and discontinuation of overnight wear also help.

Figure 7-4. A typical case of giant papillary conjunctivitis in a contact lens wearer. (From Rubenstein JB, Jick SL: Disorders of the conjunctiva and limbus. In Yanoff M, Duker JS [eds]: Ophthalmology, 2nd ed. St. Louis, Mosby, 2004, pp 397–412.)

- Contact lens deposits. Old lenses should be replaced.
- Tight lens syndrome. Lenses shrink with age. On exam, the patient may have significant chemosis around the lens, and the lens will not move with a blink. In severe cases, a sterile hypopyon can develop.
- Corneal abrasion.

14. **A young mother enters with her infant child. Her left eye is tearing profusely, and she has trouble keeping it open. She states that she was changing the child's diaper when he scratched her eye with his fingernail. What treatment do you recommend?**

At the slit lamp, you see a fairly large, central corneal abrasion with no sign of an infiltrate. The upper lid is everted, and no foreign body is seen. The abrasion will heal fairly quickly regardless of treatment; the goals are comfort and prevention of infection. Some patients desire a pressure patch, but they should not be used in patients who wear contact lenses or who have had trauma from a fingernail or vegetable matter (e.g., a dirty nail or tree branch). Such injuries have a higher chance of contamination and need to be observed for the development of a corneal ulcer. Patching may increase the rate of infection in these patients. A cycloplegic drop, such as cyclopentolate 2%, may relieve the discomfort of ciliary spasm. An antibiotic such as erythromycin or trimethoprim/polymyxin (Polytrim) four times/day is a reasonable choice. If the infection is considered "dirty," tobramycin or ciprofloxacin is a better choice for *Pseudomonas* sp. coverage. A topical anti-inflammatory decreases pain, and some evidence suggests that it may promote healing. However, long-term use of NSAIDs has been associated with corneal melts.

If the abrasion is large, central, or in a contact lens wearer, the patient should return the next day to make sure that no infection is developing and that the lesion is healing. A contact lens wearer can resume lenses after the defect has healed and the eye feels normal for 3 or 4 days. Examine the patient while he or she is wearing the lenses to ensure that they fit well. Make sure that the lens does not have a tear or significant deposits, which may have contributed to the abrasion.

KEY POINTS: CAUSES OF RED EYE IN A CONTACT LENS WEARER

1. Corneal ulcer

2. Allergy to contact lens solutions

3. Giant papillary conjunctivitis

4. Old lenses

5. Corneal abrasion

15. **The same woman returns 3 months later complaining that she awoke in the morning with severe pain, redness, and tearing in the left eye. It feels like the original scratch. She denies rubbing her eye or any other trauma. What may have happened?**
Patients who have had a corneal abrasion from a sharp object such as a paper edge or a fingernail may develop recurrent corneal erosions. Recurrent erosions also may be seen in patients who have corneal dystrophy, such as Meesmann's, map-dot-fingerprint, Reis-Buckler, lattice, macular, or granular dystrophy. Typically, patients awaken with severe pain and tearing, or symptoms develop after eye rubbing. On examination, an abrasion may be seen in the area of previous injury, or the epithelium may have healed the defect but appear irregular. Sometimes no abnormalities can be seen, and the diagnosis must be made from the history. Look carefully for any signs of dystrophy, especially in the other eye.
 Treatment consists of antibiotics, a cycloplegic, and a pressure patch for 24 hours when the defect is present. If the corneal epithelium is loose and heaped upon itself, debridement of the loose edges may be necessary first to allow the epithelial defect to heal. After healing, lubrication is crucial. If the eye is dry and the lid becomes stuck to the abnormal epithelium, the cycle will begin again. Artificial tears during the day and lubricating ointment at night will help. Some recommend a hypertonic solution of 5% sodium chloride, which theoretically draws out the water from the cornea and promotes epithelial adhesion to its basement membrane. If such treatment does not prevent further erosions, an extended-wear bandage soft contact lens worn for several months may help. Some patients require anterior stromal puncture, which causes small permanent corneal scars that prevent further erosions. Others have found excimer laser a promising treatment.

16. **A car mechanic complains of a painful red eye. He was fixing a muffler at the time of the onset of pain. What are your concerns?**
Most likely, he has a foreign body in his cornea or conjunctiva. It is important to find out what he was doing at the time of the injury. He states that he was hammering metal without safety glasses. This report increases your concern that he may have a ruptured globe. A metal piece that breaks off would travel at a high rate of speed.
 On exam, he has 20/20 vision in both eyes. You see no foreign bodies in the conjunctiva or the cornea. You evert the upper lid and find nothing. The intraocular pressure is 2 mmHg. The other eye has a pressure of 15 mmHg. A conjunctival defect with subconjunctival hemorrhage makes it impossible to determine whether a scleral laceration is present.

17. **What do you do now?**
First, put a shield over the eye to prevent further damage to the globe. It is best to examine and treat in the controlled setting of the operating room. The pupil should be dilated to determine

whether the foreign body can be seen with the indirect ophthalmoscope. The patient should have nothing else by mouth. A computed tomography (CT) scan of the orbits and brain (axial and coronal) is necessary to screen for foreign bodies in the eye, orbit, and brain. Always evaluate the patient systemically to make sure no other injuries are missed. Begin intravenous antibiotics such as cefazolin and ciprofloxacin. Give a tetanus toxoid booster.

18. **How do you proceed if, instead of a potential ruptured globe, you find a superficial metallic foreign body at 4:00 on the cornea?**
Document visual acuity. Sometimes an infiltrate may be found around the foreign body, especially if it is over 24 hours old. Usually, the infiltrate is sterile. Apply a topical anesthetic (proparacaine), and remove the foreign body with a 25-gauge needle or a foreign-body spud at the slit lamp. A rust ring may have formed, depending on how long the metal has been present. Often it can be removed with the same instruments. It is sometimes safer to leave a rust ring if it is deep or in the center of the visual axis. The rust ring will eventually migrate to the corneal surface, where it is easier and safer to remove. Dilate the pupil, and make sure that the vitreous and retina are normal. The history of hammering makes a dilated exam imperative.

Treatment consists of a cycloplegic, an antibiotic ointment or drug, and optional pressure patching. Large or central defects need follow-up to make sure that healing occurs without infection. An antibiotic such as erythromycin or trimethoprim/polymyxin is appropriate for the next 3–4 days.

19. **A lifeguard states that his eye has been red for a long time. He has a wing-shaped fold of fibrovascular tissue nasally in both eyes that extends onto the cornea. Should he be worried?**
The lesion is a pterygium (Fig. 7-5). A similar lesion called a pingueculum involves the conjunctiva but not the cornea. Both are usually bilateral. They are thought to result from damage due to chronic ultraviolet exposure or chronic irritation from wind and dust. They may be associated with dellen, an area of corneal thinning secondary to drying because the area adjacent to raised areas may not receive adequate lubrication. It is necessary to rule out conjunctival intraepithelial neoplasia, which is unilateral, often elevated, and not in a wing-shaped configuration.

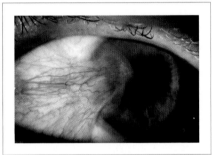

Figure 7-5. An early pterygium with triangular, fibrovascular growth from the conjunctiva (tail) onto the cornea (head). A deposit of iron in the corneal epithelium (Stocker line) may be seen anterior to the head. (From Kanski JJ: Clinical Ophthalmology: A Synopsis, 5th ed. New York, Butterworth Heinemann, 2004.)

Counsel the lifeguard to wear ultraviolet blocking sunglasses and to use artificial tears frequently, especially on sunny, windy days. Surgical removal of a pterygium is indicated if it interferes with contact lens wear, causes significant irritation, or involves the visual axis. Because the lesion may recur quite aggressively, surgery is deferred if possible. Antimetabolites such as mitomycin C are sometimes used to prevent recurrences.

20. **An unfortunate victim of domestic abuse had lye thrown in his face. What should you do?**
Even before you check vision, quickly check pH and then begin copious irrigation with saline or Ringer's lactated solution for at least 30 minutes. An eyelid speculum and a topical anesthetic will help. Make sure to irrigate the fornices. Stop irrigation only when pH of 7.0 is reached. If it is not reached after a significant time, check for particulate matter that may be trapping the chemical.

21. **What is his prognosis?**
Acids tend to have a better outcome than alkalis. Acids precipitate proteins, which limit penetration. Alkalis (lye, cement, plaster) penetrate more deeply. A mild burn may have only SPK or sloughing of part or all of the epithelium. No perilimbal ischemia is seen. Patients need a cycloplegic, antibiotic ointment, and pressure patching. Check intraocular pressure, which may be elevated by damage to the trabecular meshwork.

A moderate-to-severe burn has perilimbal blanching and corneal edema or opacification with a poor view of the anterior chamber. A significant anterior chamber reaction may be seen. The intraocular pressure may be elevated and the retina may be necrotic at the point where the alkali penetrated the sclera. The patient may need hospital admission to monitor intraocular pressure and corneal status. A topical antibiotic, cycloplegic, and pressure patching are used. Steroids may be used if the anterior chamber reaction or corneal inflammation is severe. However, they cannot be used for more than 7 days because they promote corneal melting. Collagenase inhibitors such as acetylcysteine (Mucomyst) may help in a melt. Cyanoacrylate tissue adhesive and an emergency patch graft or transplant may be necessary if perforation occurs. Patients require long-term care.

22. **A young boy presents with purulent discharge over the past few days. His mother thinks that he needs antibiotics. Do you agree?**
Yes. Purulent discharge signals bacterial conjunctivitis as opposed to the watery discharge of viral conjunctivitis. Patients usually have a conjunctival papillary reaction and no preauricular node. Gram stain and conjunctival swab for culture and sensitivities should be done if the conjunctivitis is severe.

23. **What are the common organisms responsible for bacterial conjunctivitis in children? How should you treat?**
Staphylococcus aureus, Streptococcus pneumoniae, and *Haemophilus influenzae* are common; *H. influenzae* is especially common in children. Topical antibiotics such as trimethoprim/polymyxin (Polytrim), ciprofloxacin, or erythromycin four times/day for 5–7 days is appropriate. *H. influenzae* should be treated with oral amoxicillin/clavulanate because of the possibility of systemic involvement, such as otitis media, pneumonia, or meningitis.

24. **A 27-year-old woman complains of red, irritated eyes with watery discharge over the past 6 weeks. A follicular conjunctivitis and palpable preauricular node are present. What is the differential diagnosis?**
Conjunctivitis lasting longer than 4 weeks is considered chronic (Fig. 7-6). The differential for chronic conjunctivitis includes chlamydial inclusion conjunctivitis, ocular toxicity, Parinaud's oculoglandular conjunctivitis, trachoma, molluscum contagiosum, and silent dacryocystitis.

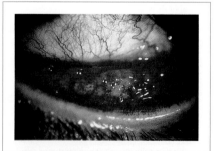

Figure 7-6. Chronic follicular conjunctivitis with large conjunctival follicles, most prominent in the inferior forniceal conjunctiva, and scant mucopurulent discharge. Lymphadenopathy is also present. (From Kanski JJ: Clinical Ophthalmology: A Synopsis, 5th ed. New York, Butterworth-Heinemann, 2004.)

25. **How do you proceed?**
History is important. On questioning, the patient reports a recent vaginal discharge. Chlamydial infection becomes high on the list. Such patients

also may have white peripheral subepithelial infiltrates and a superior corneal pannus. Stringy, mucous discharge is common. Obtain a chlamydial immunofluorescence test and/or a chlamydial culture of the conjunctiva. Giemsa stain will show basophilic intracytoplasmic inclusion bodies in epithelial cells as well as polymorphonuclear leukocytes. Tetracycline, doxycycline, or erythromycin should be taken orally for 3 weeks by the patient and her sexual partners. Topical ocular erythromycin, tetracycline, or sulfacetamide ointment is used at the same time. Counseling and evaluation for other sexually transmitted diseases should be done by the family physician.

26. **How do you diagnose the other causes of chronic conjunctivitis?**
    1. **Toxic conjunctivitis** is common with many drops (see question 2 for offending agents). These patients may also have allergic dermatitis around the eyes. Treat with preservative-free artificial tears.
    2. **Parinaud's oculoglandular conjunctivitis** presents with a mucopurulent discharge and foreign body sensation. Granulomatous nodules on the palpebral conjunctiva and swollen lymph nodes are necessary for the diagnosis. Fever and rash also may occur. The etiology includes cat-scratch disease (most common), tularemia (contact with rabbits or ticks), tuberculosis, and syphilis.
    3. **Trachoma** occurs in underprivileged countries with poor sanitation. It is also caused by chlamydial infection. Patients develop superior tarsal follicles and severe corneal pannus, which, if untreated, lead to significant dry eye, trichiasis, and scarring. Patients may become functionally blind. Diagnosis and treatment are the same as for chlamydial inclusion conjunctivitis.
    4. **Molluscum contagiosum** develops a chronic follicular conjunctivitis from a reaction to toxic viral products. On the lid or lid margin, multiple dome-shaped, umbilicated nodules are present. These lesions must be removed by excision, incision and curettage, or cryosurgery to resolve the conjunctivitis.
    5. **Dacryocystitis** is an inflammation of the lacrimal sac. Patients usually present with pain, erythema, and swelling over the inner aspect of the lower lid. They also may have a fever. However, a red eye may be the only sign. Pressure over the lacrimal sac may elicit discharge and a complaint of tenderness. Treatment is systemic antibiotics, warm compresses with massage over the inner canthus, and topical antibiotics. Watch patients closely because cellulitis can occasionally develop.

27. **A 40-year-old woman presents with a bright red eye that she noticed on awakening in the morning. On examination, she has a subconjunctival hemorrhage. What questions are important to ask?**
    You need to know whether this is her first episode. Does she have a history of easy bruising or poor clotting? Is she taking any medications or supplements that may increase bleeding time, such as warfarin, aspirin, vitamin E, or garlic? Has she been rubbing her eye or had any injury to her eye? Has she done any heavy lifting or straining? Has she been sneezing or vomiting—anything that may cause a Valsalva maneuver?

28. **She answers no to the above questions and states that this is her first episode. Should she be worried?**
    No. Reassure her that the symptoms will resolve within 2 weeks. Artificial tears will make her more comfortable. Tell her to return if she has further episodes.

29. **With further thought, she remembers two other hemorrhages in her left eye and reports that her menses have been much heavier recently. What now?**
    At this point, referral to an internist for a complete blood count with differential, blood pressure check, prothrombin time, partial thromboplastin time, and bleeding time is appropriate.

30. **A 60-year-old woman complains that her eyes have been red and burning over the past several weeks. She also has some tearing and photophobia. On exam, you notice mild conjunctival injection and a slightly low tear meniscus. Should you think of anything else?**

Make sure to elevate the upper eyelid. Superior limbic keratoconjunctivitis (Fig. 7-7) is a thickening and inflammation of the superior bulbar conjunctiva. Sometimes a superior corneal micropannus, superior palpebral papillae, and corneal filaments can be found. Fifty percent of patients have associated dysthyroid disease. Artificial tears and ointments are all that are necessary for mild disease. Silver nitrate solution (**not** cautery sticks) may be applied to the superior tarsal and bulbar conjunctiva; mechanical scraping, cryotherapy, cautery, or surgical resection or recession of the superior bulbar conjunctiva may be necessary for more severe disease.

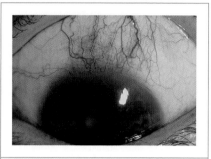

Figure 7-7. Superior limbic keratoconjunctivitis. Slit-lamp appearance of focal superior bulbar conjunctival injection is shown with rose bengal staining. (From Bouchard CS: Noninfectious keratitis. In Yanoff M, Duker JS [eds]: Ophthalmology, 2nd ed. St. Louis, Mosby, 2004.)

31. **A 22-year-old woman presents with mild redness in the temporal quadrant of her left eye for about 1 week. She notices no discomfort. On exam, she has normal vision. Large episcleral vessels beneath the conjunctiva are engorged in the area. They can be easily moved with a cotton swab, and no tenderness is present. The cornea and anterior chamber are clear. The sclera appears to be uninvolved. What is the diagnosis?**

You must distinguish between episcleritis (Fig. 7-8) and scleritis. A drop of 2.5% phenylephrine blanches the episcleral vessels but leaves any injected vessels of the sclera untouched. Look for any discharge or conjunctival follicles and papillae to rule out conjunctivitis.

Episcleritis is usually idiopathic. It may be diffuse or sectoral, unilateral or bilateral. Sometimes a nodule may be seen. Rarely, it is associated with collagen-vascular disease, gout, herpes zoster or simplex, syphilis, Lyme disease, rosacea, or atopy. Usually artificial tears and/or a topical vasoconstrictor/antihistamine drop, such as naphazoline/pheniramine, will suffice. If the patient is unresponsive, a mild steroid drop should help. Rarely, oral nonsteroidal anti-inflammatory drugs are necessary. Warn the patient that episcleritis may recur.

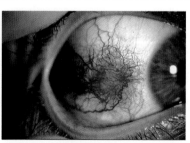

Figure 7-8. A slightly tender and mobile elevated nodule with epithelial injection is typical for nodular episcleritis. (From Kanski JJ: Clinical Ophthalmology: A Systematic Approach, 5th ed. New York, Butterworth-Heinemann, 2003.)

32. **The same patient returns 2 months later. Her left eye is still red, but it is now diffuse. She denies arthritis, rash, venereal disease, tick exposure, or other medical problems. She has been using a vasoconstrictor/antihistamine drop since her last visit. She began using it four times/day, then increased the frequency because her eye continued to be red unless she used it. She now applies drops every 1–2 hours. Does this make a difference?**
Counsel patients not to use a vasoconstrictor for longer than 2 weeks and no more than four times/day. Just as vasoconstrictor nose sprays produce dependence so that patients are congested unless they use them, so do eyedrops. She should stop the drop immediately. Her left eye will be very red for a time until dependence resolves.

33. **A 65-year-old woman with rheumatoid arthritis states that her left eye has been red and painful for a couple of weeks. The pain is severe and radiates to her forehead and jaw and has awakened her at night. It has worsened slowly. Her vision is decreasing. She thinks that she has had a similar condition before. On exam, the conjunctival, episcleral, and scleral vessels are injected temporally. The scleral vessels do not move, and the area is very tender. A scleral nodule is present. The sclera appears bluish in this area, adjacent to which is a peripheral keratitis with a mild anterior chamber reaction. The intraocular pressure is 24 mmHg in the affected eye and 16 mmHg in the unaffected eye. What may she have?**

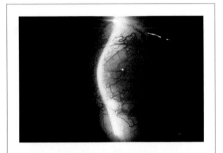

Figure 7-9. Nodular scleritis is painful with a nonmobile nodule associated with swelling of the episclera and sclera. (From Kanski JJ: Clinical Ophthalmology: A Systematic Approach, 5th ed. New York, Butterworth-Heinemann, 2003.)

Nodular anterior scleritis (Fig. 7-9). The inflamed blood vessels are much deeper than those seen in conjunctivitis or episcleritis and do not blanch with 2.5% phenylephrine. In addition, the cornea and anterior chamber are involved. The deep, boring pain is typical with scleritis.

34. **How else may scleritis present?**
- Diffuse anterior scleritis.
- Necrotizing anterior scleritis with inflammation. The pain is severe, and the choroid is visible through the transparent sclera. The mortality rate is high due to systemic disease.
- Necrotizing anterior scleritis without inflammation (scleromalacia perforans; Fig. 7-10). Such patients have almost a complete lack of symptoms, and most have rheumatoid arthritis.
- Posterior scleritis. It may mimic an amelanotic choroidal mass. An exudative retinal detachment, retinal

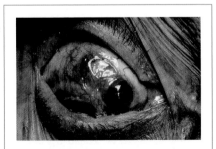

Figure 7-10. Scleromalacia perforans is a noninflammatory form of necrotizing scleritis. (From Kanski JJ: Clinical Ophthalmology: A Test Yourself Atlas. New York, Butterworth-Heinemann, 2002.)

hemorrhages, choroidal folds, and/or choroidal detachments may be seen. Restricted extraocular movements, proptosis, pain, and tenderness may also occur. Rarely is it related to a systemic disease.

35. **What percentage of patients with scleritis have systemic disease? What diseases are associated with scleritis?**
Fifty percent. The connective tissue diseases, such as rheumatoid arthritis, ankylosing spondylitis, systemic lupus erythematosus, polyarteritis nodosa, and Wegener's granulomatosis, are common associations. Herpes zoster ophthalmicus, syphilis, and gout also may cause scleritis. Less frequently, scleritis may be associated with tuberculosis, sarcoidosis, or a foreign body.

36. **What workup is appropriate for a patient with scleritis?**
Any avascular areas of the scleritis must be identified. The red-free filter on the slit lamp is helpful for this purpose. The severity of the disease is increased with more thinning. The risk of a melt is much higher. A dilated exam is necessary to check for posterior segment involvement. Patients should be referred to an internist or a rheumatologist for a complete physical exam, complete blood count, erythrocyte sedimentation rate (ESR), uric acid level, rapid plasmin reagin test (RPR), fluorescent treponemal antibody, absorbed test (FTA-ABS), rheumatoid factor, antinuclear antibody tests (ANA), fasting blood sugar, angiotensin-converting enzyme (ACE), CH50, complement 3, complement 4, and serum antineutrophilic cytoplasmic antibody (ANCA). If history or symptoms warrant, a purified protein derivative test (PPD) with anergy panel, a chest radiograph, sacroiliac radiograph, and/or B-scan ultrasonography to detect posterior scleritis should be ordered.

37. **How should you treat the patient?**
An oral NSAID, such as ibuprofen, 400–600 mg four times/day, or indomethacin, 25 mg three times/day, coupled with an antacid or H_2 blocker such as ranitidine is a good initial choice. If the patient is nonresponsive, oral steroids are the next step. In diseases such as systemic vasculitis, polyarteritis nodosa, and Wegener's granulomatosis, an immunosuppressive agent such as cyclophosphamide, methotrexate, cyclosporine, or azathioprine may be necessary. They may be used in combination. Decreased pain is an indication of successful treatment, although the clinical picture may not show a significant difference for a while.

Scleromalacia perforans does not have ocular treatment except for lubrication. Patch grafts are used if perforation is a significant risk. Immunosuppression for the underlying systemic disease may be necessary.

38. **What about topical steroids or a subconjunctival steroid injection?**
Topical steroids are not usually effective. Subconjunctival steroids are contraindicated because they may lead to scleral thinning and perforation.

39. **A 35-year-old man presents with severe photophobia, pain, and decreased vision in his right eye for two days. This condition has occurred several times before. He says that it is helped by using drops. On examination, his vision is 20/50 in the right eye and 20/20 in the left eye. His pupil is poorly reactive on the right and miotic. The left eye is normal, and no afferent pupillary defect is present. The right eye is diffusely injected, especially around the limbus. The anterior chamber is deep, but 2+ cell and flare are present with a few fine keratic precipitates. The left eye is clear. The right eye has an intraocular pressure of 5 mmHg; the left is 15 mmHg. Dilated exam is normal. What are the diagnosis and treatment?**
The diagnosis is acute, nongranulomatous anterior uveitis. A cycloplegic drop such as cyclopentolate, 1–2% three times/day, for mild inflammation, and scopolamine 0.25% or atropine 1% three times/day for more severe inflammation will relax the ciliary spasm, making

the patient more comfortable as well as preventing formation of synechiae in the angle and on the pupillary margin. Formation of synechiae increases the long-term risk of angle closure glaucoma. A steroid drop every 1–6 hours, depending on the severity of the anterior chamber inflammation, is started. If no response occurs, a sub-Tenon's injection or oral steroids may be necessary. Rarely, systemic immunosuppressive agents are necessary.

40. **A 68-year-old Asian American woman presents with an acutely painful red left eye that developed after a recent anxiety attack. She has blurred vision and sees halos around lights. She has vomited twice. On exam, she has a fixed, mid-dilated pupil and conjunctival injection. The cornea is cloudy. What are you concerned about?**

Angle-closure glaucoma. When the pressure rises quickly in the eye, severe pain and nausea with decreased vision develop. Asian Americans are at increased risk because of their shallow anterior chambers. Examination of the angle of the affected eye may be facilitated by glycerin to clear the corneal edema. If the shallow angle cannot be visualized, the other eye may reveal a narrow angle. For further information about diagnosis and treatment, see Chapter 17.

KEY POINTS: DISEASES THAT MAY MIMIC UVEITIS

1. Rhegmatogenous retinal detachment

2. Posterior segment tumors and lymphoma

3. Intraocular foreign body

4. Endophthalmitis

BIBLIOGRAPHY

1. Kunimoto DY, Kanitkar KD, Makar M: Wills Eye Manual: Office and Emergency Room Diagnosis and Treatment of Eye Disease, 4th ed. Philadelphia, Lippincott Williams & Wilkins, 2004.

2. Lin JC, Rapuano CJ, Laibson PR, et al: Corneal melting associated with use of topical nonsteroidal anti-inflammatory drugs after ocular surgery. Arch Ophthalmol 118:1129–1132, 2000.

3. Riordan-Eva P, Asbury T, Whitcher JP: Vaughn & Asbury's General Ophthalmology, 16th ed. Norwalk, CT, McGraw Hill/Appleton & Lange, 2003.

4. Tasman W, Jaeger EA: Wills Eye Hospital Atlas of Clinical Ophthalmology, 2nd ed. Philadelphia, Lippincott Williams & Wilkins, 2001.

CHAPTER 8

CORNEAL INFECTIONS

Sherman W. Reeves, MD, MPH, Elisabeth J. Cohen, MD, and Terry Kim, MD

1. **What is a corneal ulcer?**
   Infections of the cornea involve the epithelium and/or stroma. Some infections may occur strictly within the epithelium (i.e., herpes simplex epithelial keratitis), whereas others manifest as an infiltrate in the corneal stroma. The term "corneal ulcer" refers to the loss of stroma associated with an overlying epithelial defect (that stains with fluorescein) (Fig. 8-1). A corneal ulcer is usually considered infectious when accompanied by a stromal infiltrate, but may also be caused by noninfectious (or sterile) etiologies.

   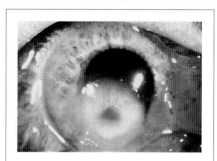

   Figure 8-1. Central pseudomonal corneal ulcer.

2. **What clinical features distinguish an infectious corneal ulcer?**
   Infectious corneal ulcers caused by bacterial, fungal, viral, and parasitic microorganisms elicit an inflammatory response that can manifest with conjunctival injection, a visible corneal infiltrate, and surrounding corneal edema. If the corneal inflammation is severe, anterior chamber cell and flare, keratic precipitates, and/or a hypopyon may also develop. Patients are usually symptomatic, with acute redness, pain, decreased vision, and/or photophobia (light sensitivity). Bacterial corneal ulcers may also be associated with a mucopurulent discharge.

3. **What clinical features distinguish a sterile corneal ulcer?**
   Sterile corneal ulcers are not due to infection with microorganisms. They may be caused by a large variety of etiologies including dry eye, exposure, neurotrophic keratopathy (e.g., from previous corneal herpetic infections), autoimmune disorders (e.g., rheumatoid arthritis), by a secondary immunologic response elicited by staphylococcal hypersensitivity or hypoxia (e.g., from contact lens wear). These ulcers often present with mild conjunctiva, minimal or absent corneal infiltrate, and/or epithelial defect, and a quiet anterior chamber (Fig. 8-2). Patients may notice decreased vision but often do not complain of significant redness, pain, or photophobia.

   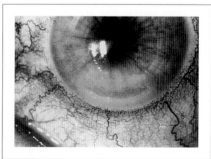

   Figure 8-2. Sterile corneal ulcer caused by rheumatoid arthritis.

4. **What conditions predispose to corneal infections?**
Any condition that disrupts the corneal epithelial integrity, including:
- Contact lens wear (number one risk factor!)
- Trauma (e.g., corneal abrasion)
- Structural eyelid abnormalities (e.g., ectropion/entropion, trichiasis)
- Dry eye
- Chronic epithelial disease (e.g., recurrent erosions, bullous keratopathy)
- Topical medication toxicity
- Local or systemic immunosuppression (e.g., steroids, diabetes, HIV)

5. **How can a contact lens wearer reduce the risk of infection?**
Contact lens wear is associated with at least 30% of microbial keratitis cases. The major risk factor identified for corneal infection with contact lens use is sleeping overnight in contact lenses, even if they are approved for extended wear. Patients need to know that disposable contact lenses are not any safer than conventional contact lenses and that lenses with higher oxygen permeability ("high DK" lenses) also increase risk. Proper contact lens cleaning and disinfection prior to reinsertion are also of crucial importance in reducing the incidence of contact lens-related corneal infections.

Cohen EJ, Fulton JC, Hoffman CJ, et al: Trends in contact lens-associated corneal ulcers. Cornea 24:51–58, 2005.

6. **Describe classic presentations and associations of various types of corneal infections (e.g., bacterial, viral, fungal).**
- **History of trauma with any vegetable matter:** Fungal keratitis
- **Oral and eyelid vesicles or repeated problems in only one eye:** Herpetic keratitis
- **Contact lens wear:** *Pseudomonas* or *Acanthamoeba* infection
- **Gram-positive organisms:** Focal, discrete infiltrate
- **Gram-negative organisms:** Spreading diffuse infiltrate
- ***Pseudomonas* infections:** Suppurative
- **Herpes simplex keratitis:** Epithelial dendrite
- ***Acanthamoeba* keratitis:** Ring infiltrate, pain out of proportion to exam
- **Fungal keratitis:** Feathery, irregular borders with satellite lesions (Fig. 8-3)

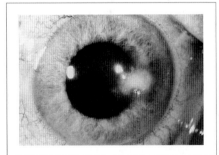

Figure 8-3. Infectious ulcer caused by filamentous fungus. Note the indistinct, feathery borders.

7. **When should smears and cultures be performed?**
Corneal scrapings for smears and cultures should be obtained on most corneal ulcers suspected to be infectious. Small, peripheral corneal infiltrates (less than 1 mm in diameter) do not necessarily have to undergo scraping prior to the initiation of intensive empiric broad-spectrum antibiotic therapy. Corneal infections that do not improve on therapy should undergo scraping or rescraping, and documentation of current antibiotic medication should be given to the laboratory.

McLeod SD, Kolahdouz-Isfahani A, Rostamian K, et al: The role of smears, cultures, and antibiotic sensitivity testing in the management of suspected infectious keratitis. Ophthalmology 103:23–38, 1996.

8. **How should smears and cultures be performed?**
   Corneal smears and cultures should be performed at the slit lamp after the patient has been given topical anesthetic drops. Corneal scrapings should be obtained using a sterile Kimura spatula, resterilized over a flame between each scraping, or with sterile calcium alginate swabs. Separate slides should be used for each smear (e.g., Gram's stain, potassium hydroxide [KOH]). Separate plates should be used for each culture and for Giemsa or calcfluor white stains.

9. **What smears and cultures should be obtained? What culture plates should be used?**
   See Table 8-1.

TABLE 8-1. SMEARS AND CULTURES FOR INFECTIOUS KERATITIS	
Routine Tests	**Tests for**
Gram stain (smear)	Bacteria
KOH or Giemsa stain (smear)	Fungi/yeasts
Sabaroud's dextrose agar culture plate (without cycloheximide)	Fungi
Chocolate agar culture plate	*Hemophilus* and *Neisseria* species
Thioglycolate culture broth	Aerobic and anaerobic bacteria
Optional Tests (as needed based on clinical suspicion)	**Tests for**
Gomori methenamine silver stain (smear)	*Acanthamoeba*, fungi
Acid fast stain (smear)	Mycobacteria
Calcoflour white stain (smear)	*Acanthamoeba*, fungi
Löwenstein-Jensen agar culture plate	Mycobacteria, *Nocardia* spp.
Non-nutrient agar culture plate with *E. coli* overlay	*Acanthamoeba*

10. **What is the diagnostic yield for smears and cultures performed prior to the initiation of therapy?**
    Although Gram's stain smears may provide early insight into the causative organism, they may be negative (with a highly variable positivity range of 0–57%). Smears must not be relied on too heavily because their correlation with culture results is low as a result of contamination by normal flora and improper staining/processing technique. On the other hand, cultures grow organisms in approximately 50–75% of suspected infectious ulcers. Though cultures performed prior to starting antibiotics have higher yield, clinical evidence suggests that the yield is not significantly diminished by antibiotic treatment if the infection is not responding.

11. **What is the recommended initial therapy for suspected infectious ulcers? How does one determine whether single-agent, broad-spectrum antibiotics or combination fortified antibiotics should be used?**
    In general, initial therapy for corneal ulcers must cover a broad range of gram-positive and gram-negative bacteria and be administered frequently (every 15–30 minutes). Previous multicenter studies have provided evidence that monotherapy with topical fluoroquinolones may be as effective as fortified antibiotics in many cases. It is our practice to treat small, peripheral ulcers with a single, fourth-generation fluoroquinolone antibiotic, such as gatifloxacin or

moxifloxacin, which has shown improved coverage of gram-positive organisms like streptococcal and staphylococcal species. We reserve combination fortified antibiotics for more severe, sight-threatening infections.

Kowalski RR, Dhaliwal DK, Karenchak LM, et al: Gatifloxacin and moxifloxacin: An in vitro susceptibility comparison to levofloxacin, ciprofloxacin, and ofloxacin using bacterial keratitis isolates. Am J Ophthalmol 136:500–505, 2003.

O'Brien TP, Maguire MG, Fink NE, et al: Efficacy of ofloxacin vs. cefazolin and tobramycin in the therapy of bacterial keratitis: Report from the Bacterial Keratitis Research Group. Arch Ophthalmol 113:1257–1265, 1995.

12. **How does the presence of a hypopyon affect the management of infectious keratitis?**
The presence of a hypopyon (Fig. 8-4) is indicative of corneal inflammation severe enough to cause a marked anterior chamber response. Therefore, the treatment should be intense, including hospitalization for frequent combined fortified antibiotics in most cases. For the most part, hypopyons associated with infectious corneal ulcers are sterile and do not require evaluation and treatment for endophthalmitis.

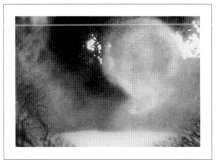

Figure 8-4. Hypopyon associated with infectious corneal ulcer.

13. **When should an anterior chamber and/or vitreous tap be performed?**
Whenever endophthalmitis is suspected. Endophthalmitis must be considered when there is severe inflammation after intraocular surgery or perforating trauma, especially when vitreous inflammatory cells are present. Once diagnosed, topical antibiotics are inadequate and intravenous antibiotics are unnecessary; antibiotics must be injected directly into the vitreous cavity after taking samples for culture (with vitrectomy indicated in severe cases). Endophthalmitis secondary to infectious keratitis in the absence of perforation is uncommon, and a sterile inflammatory response in the vitreous may be present that resolves with the clearing of the corneal infection.

14. **When should patients with corneal ulcers be hospitalized?**
   - If the patient lacks the ability or support to administer drops as frequently as every 30 minutes around-the-clock
   - If the patient lives too far away to be followed on a daily basis
   - Any condition requiring intravenous antibiotics or possible surgery (e.g., *Neisseria* infections involving the cornea and perforated corneal ulcers)

15. **When are systemic medications indicated?**
Systemic antibiotics are seldom indicated in bacterial corneal ulcers. However, oral antibiotics are used with impending or existing scleral involvement. Parenteral antibiotics play an important role in the treatment of aggressive infections from *Neisseria* and *Hemophilus* species with corneal involvement and impending perforation.

Systemic antifungal agents are used in some cases of fungal keratitis where the infiltrate involves deep corneal stroma or in cases that worsen on topical therapy alone. Oral acyclovir is the primary mode of therapy for patients with ocular herpes zoster and is also used by some physicians to treat primary herpes simplex infection.

16. **Other than antibiotics, what adjunctive therapy may be necessary in the treatment of corneal ulcers?**
Topical cycloplegic agents are often indicated to help relieve photophobia and pain from ciliary spasm and to help prevent posterior synechia.

   Severe anterior chamber inflammation may cause the intraocular pressure to increase, often necessitating the use of antiglaucoma medications. Pilocarpine should be avoided because of the phenomenon of blood-aqueous breakdown with subsequent increase in anterior chamber inflammation. In the case of impending or frank perforated corneal ulcer, cyanoacrylate tissue glue can be useful in temporarily and sometimes permanently sealing the open wound.

17. **How should the smear and culture results be used to modify treatment?**
Smears may provide a quick means of telling the clinician the general type of infection (e.g., bacterial, fungal, acanthamoeba) and can help start the appropriate empiric therapy. However, we recommend that broad-spectrum antibiotics be continued until culture results are available.

   Culture results identify the organism, help to target therapy, and eliminate extraneous medication. Sensitivities can be useful for guiding treatment, but must be interpreted with caution as they are based on drug levels attainable in the serum and not on drug concentrations in the cornea.

18. **What are the important immediate and delayed sequelae of corneal ulcers?**
The immediate concern with corneal ulcers is progressive thinning and perforation. Management and prognosis change considerably with perforation, and the concern for intraocular infection (i.e., endophthalmitis) rises dramatically. Perforated corneal ulcers can result in the loss of the eye. The delayed sequelae of corneal ulcers deal mainly with corneal scarring, which can severely limit visual acuity and function.

19. **How should impending and frank corneal perforations be managed?**
Any corneal infection associated with marked thinning or perforation (Fig. 8-5) should be protected with an eye shield without a patch. When the cornea becomes thinned to the point of imminent or existent corneal perforation, certain steps need to be taken. If the affected area is small, cyanoacrylate glue can be used to help seal the defect. However, most cases of perforation will eventually need patch grafting or corneal transplantation if the eye has visual potential.

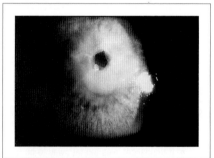

Figure 8-5. Perforated corneal ulcer.

20. **What steps should be taken when a corneal ulcer does not respond to empirical therapy?**
Reassess the situation. Is compliance a problem? Hospitalization eliminates this issue. If a culture has not been performed, this should be done so that therapy may be culture directed. If the empiric therapy is a fluoroquinolone, fortified antibiotics may be indicated. Consider toxicity from the antibiotics themselves, which may prevent the healing of an ulcer. Think also of the possibility of unusual organisms that would not be covered by broad-spectrum antibiotics: a fungal or mixed bacterial/fungal infection, a viral process with bacterial superinfection, or a protozoan such as *Acanthamoeba*.

21. **When should a corneal biopsy be considered?**
    Whenever an ulcer is failing intensive
    antibiotic therapy and the etiology
    remains unclear owing to negative
    cultures. *Acanthamoeba* (Fig. 8-6) is
    particularly difficult to grow in culture,
    and the infection may be deep in the
    cornea. If this organism is suspected, a
    corneal biopsy is the best opportunity to
    identify cysts (more commonly) or
    trophozoites in the tissue.
    A corneal biopsy may also be
    considered for deep corneal infiltrates
    that are not accessible with superficial
    scraping. Alternatively, a 6-0 or 7-0 silk
    suture can be passed through these
    stromal infiltrates and then placed in
    various culture media.

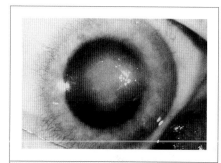

Figure 8-6. Central *Acanthamoeba* ulcer.

22. **What is the role of topical corticosteroids in the treatment of corneal ulcers?**
    The role of topical corticosteroids as an adjunctive therapy for corneal ulcers is controversial.
    Some advocate that corticosteroids help to reduce inflammation and decrease corneal scarring,
    whereas others fear that corticosteroids predispose to recrudescent infection and progressive
    thinning leading to perforation. Corticosteroids should not be used in the initial treatment of
    corneal ulcers and can be used in conjunction with antibiotics with extreme caution only after
    clinical improvement has been demonstrated with appropriate antibiotics.

23. **How are staphylococcal hypersensitivity infiltrates diagnosed and managed?**
    Corneal infiltrates due to staphylococcal
    hypersensitivity may be multiple, stain
    minimally or not at all with fluorescein,
    are located in the peripheral cornea
    separated from the limbus by a clear
    area (Fig. 8-7), and are not associated
    with anterior chamber inflammation.
    They accompany staphylococcal
    blepharitis and meibomitis and
    represent an immunologic reaction to
    staphylococcal antigens. Mild cases
    of staphylococcal hypersensitivity
    should be treated with lid hygiene and
    antibiotic ointment. In more severe
    cases, combined antibiotic-steroid
    drops or ointments can be added.
    If concerned about an infectious
    etiology, treat the infiltrate(s) initially
    with intensive antibiotics.

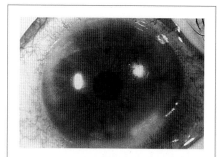

Figure 8-7. Staphylococcal hypersensitivity
infiltrate located in the inferior peripheral cornea.
Note its marginal location and clear separation from
the limbus.

24. **What is appropriate therapy for small peripheral infiltrates in a contact lens wearer?**
    Remember that small infiltrates in a contact lens wearer may be sterile or infectious. Sterile
    infiltrates are usually located in the peripheral subepithelium with an overlying intact epithelium
    and have minimal pain (Fig. 8-8). When in doubt, though, presume infection.

Patients with infiltrates should first stop all contact lens wear. One can forego scraping and treat presumed infectious infiltrates frequently (every 30–60 minutes) with a single broad-spectrum antibiotic (i.e., gatifloxacin or moxifloxacin) after a loading dose and then an antibiotic ointment (i.e., tobramycin) at bedtime. Patients should be followed closely and undergo scraping if the epithelial defect and infiltrate do not improve.

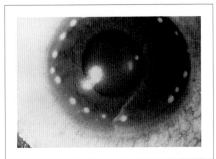

Figure 8-8. Small peripheral infiltrates caused by a sterile reaction to contact lens solution.

25. **When should a gonococcal infection be suspected? What additional workup and treatment should be initiated?**

A gonococcal infection should be suspected when an acute onset of marked conjunctival injection is associated with severe mucopurulent discharge, marked chemosis, and preauricular adenopathy (Fig. 8-9). Corneal infiltrates can progress rapidly and perforate within 48 hours. Workup should include conjunctival scrapings for immediate Gram's stain and culture using chocolate agar media. Treatment should include frequent irrigation with saline, a 1-gm intramuscular dose of ceftriaxone, and frequent topical fluoroquinolone drops. If the cornea is

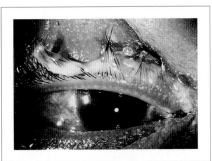

Figure 8-9. Gonococcal conjunctivitis with marked conjunctival injection and copious mucopurulent discharge on the eyelid margins.

involved or if compliance is problematic, the patient should be hospitalized for parenteral ceftriaxone therapy and close follow-up.

KEY POINTS: CORNEAL ULCERS

1. A corneal ulcer is infectious until proven otherwise.

2. You are never wrong to culture an ulcer.

3. Some small, peripheral ulcers can be treated empirically and closely followed.

4. Any ulcer not responding to therapy should be recultured.

26. **Why do herpetic infections occur?**

Herpes simplex keratitis (HSV) is usually caused by the type 1 virus, often spread by an oral "cold sore." The type 2 virus causes neonatal ocular infection after a newborn passes through an infected birth canal. Follicular conjunctivitis, corneal dendritic ulcers, cutaneous vesicles, and preauricular adenopathy may be seen.

Herpes zoster ophthalmicus (shingles of the eye) represents reactivation of the varicella zoster virus (VZV) in the first division of cranial nerve V (Fig. 8-10). Nerve damage in a dermatomal distribution may lead to severe and chronic pain. Associated keratitis, uveitis, and glaucoma may be severe, chronic, and difficult to treat.

27. **Why is herpes a recurrent disease?**
After primary contact with the herpes virus (HSV or VZV), the virus gains access to the central nervous system. The virus becomes latent in the trigeminal ganglia (HSV type 1 or VZV) or in the spinal ganglia (HSV type 2).

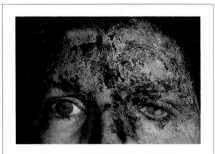

Figure 8-10. Herpes zoster ophthalmicus with crusting and ulceration of skin innervated by the first division of the trigeminal nerve. (From Kanski JJ: Clinical Ophthalmology: A Synopsis. New York, Butterworth-Heinemann, 2004.)

Recurrent attacks occur when the virus travels peripherally via sensory nerves to infect target tissues such as the eye. These attacks may be triggered by any of the following stressors: fever, ultraviolet light exposure, trauma, stress, menses, and immunosuppression. The most impressive example of this pathway of recrudescence is the dermatomal involvement of the zoster virus.

28. **Give some nonocular signs suggestive of a herpetic corneal infection.**
Some nonspecific signs of primary herpetic corneal infection include fever, malaise, and lymphadenopathy (especially preauricular adenopathy on the involved side). The vesicular skin rash of herpes zoster infections characteristically involves the dermatome of the first division of cranial nerve V on one side, does not cross the midline, and progresses to scarring. The presence of this rash on the tip of the nose (referred to as Hutchinson's sign) is a useful sign indicating probable ocular involvement, because both areas are innervated by the nasociliary nerve, a branch of cranial nerve (CN) V_1. Patients with herpes simplex can present with vesicular lesions in the perioral and periocular region that resolve without scarring.

29. **Are there differences between corneal infections caused by herpes simplex and herpes zoster viruses?**
Although corneal infections from herpes simplex and herpes zoster can present in a similar clinical fashion, there are subtle features that can help differentiate between the two. Herpes simplex keratitis is an episodic condition, whereas herpes zoster ophthalmicus results in chronic disease. The corneal dendrites of herpes simplex infections are epithelial ulcers whose edges stain brightly with fluorescein and have terminal bulbs (Fig. 8-11). Herpes zoster dendrites are raised lesions, do not have terminal bulbs, and do not stain well with fluorescein.

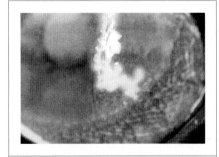

Figure 8-11. Classic herpes simplex dendrite staining brightly with fluorescein.

30. **What are the noninfectious manifestations of a herpetic keratitis?**
Some ophthalmic findings of herpetic keratitis are not directly caused by the viral infection itself but instead relate to the immunologic response to the infection. Examples of this phenomenon include chronic keratouveitis (where large keratic precipitates are associated with corneal edema) and disciform and necrotizing keratitis (in which stromal infiltration with leukocytes and neovascularization can occur with an intact epithelium).

Corneal scarring and neurotrophic ulcers are signs of previous herpetic keratitis that can be visually debilitating and potentially necessitate surgical intervention with penetrating keratoplasty or tarsorrhaphy.

31. **How should these infections be treated?**
Herpes simplex epithelial keratitis and conjunctivitis should be treated with frequent topical trifluorothymidine (Viroptic) drops. Zovirax ointment can be added for skin involvement but cannot be used in or near the eye. Disciform stromal keratitis should be managed with topical corticosteroids and prophylactic antiviral agents.

All herpes zoster infections, regardless of ocular involvement, are treated primarily with oral acyclovir (800 mg PO five times/day for 7–10 days). Skin lesions should receive antibiotic ointment and warm compresses. Topical medications should be added as needed according to other ocular involvement (e.g., conjunctivitis, uveitis, glaucoma).

32. **What is the role of topical corticosteroids in herpes simplex keratitis?**
Although topical corticosteroids are contraindicated in the presence of active epithelial disease, such as in dendritic keratitis, their use in treating herpes simplex stromal keratitis with an intact epithelium is beneficial. The Herpetic Eye Disease Study has documented that topical steroids and prophylactic antivirals are safe and effective in the treatment of stromal keratitis.

Wilhelmus KR, Gee L, Hauck WW, et al: Herpetic Eye Disease Study: A controlled trial of topical corticosteroids for herpes simplex stromal keratitis. Ophthalmology 101:1883–1895, 1994.

KEY POINTS: HERPETIC KERATITIS

1. Herpes simplex typically causes episodic keratitis.

2. Herpes zoster causes a dermatomal rash and chronic ulcers and pain.

3. Viroptic should be used for epithelial HSV keratitis.

4. Topical steroids are used for herpetic stromal keratitis.

5. All patients with VZV eye disease should receive oral acyclovir.

6. Oral acyclovir is beneficial only in certain types of HSV eye disease.

33. **When should oral acyclovir be used in herpes simplex keratitis?**
The Herpetic Eye Disease Study reported:
- Oral acyclovir (400 mg orally twice daily for 1 year) reduced the recurrence of ocular herpes simplex in patients who had one or more recurrent episodes.
- Oral acyclovir (400 mg orally five times/day for 10 weeks) may be helpful for treating herpes simplex iridocyclitis, but the results did not reach statistical significance.

- Oral acyclovir did not benefit patients with active stromal keratitis and did not prevent the development of stromal keratitis or uveitis in patients with active epithelial disease. Acyclovir is contraindicated during pregnancy and in patients with renal disease.

    Herpetic Eye Disease Study Group: Oral acyclovir for herpes simplex virus eye disease: Effect on prevention of epithelial keratitis and stromal keratitis: Arch Ophthalmol 118:1030–1036, 2000.

34. **Are corneal infections common after refractive surgical procedures such as laser in-situ keratomileusis (LASIK)?**
    Corneal infection is a potentially vision-threatening complication after LASIK but is fortunately uncommon. The incidence is estimated to be between 1 in 5,000 and 1 in 10,000. Although the epithelium is usually left intact in this procedure, the corneal flap created in LASIK produces a potential space in the corneal stroma for endogenous and exogenous flora to proliferate and result in an infection.

35. **What other conditions can be mistaken for a corneal infection after LASIK?**
    Although microbial infection should always be considered, the more common condition that manifests with an infiltrate under the flap is diffuse lamellar keratitis (DLK; Fig. 8-12). DLK is an inflammatory condition of unclear etiology that usually presents within 1–3 days after LASIK and has the appearance of sandy debris in the stromal interface (hence the term "sands of the Sahara syndrome").

    Smith RJ, Maloney RK: Diffuse lamellar keratitis: A new syndrome in lamellar refractive surgery. Ophthalmology 105:1721–1726, 1998.

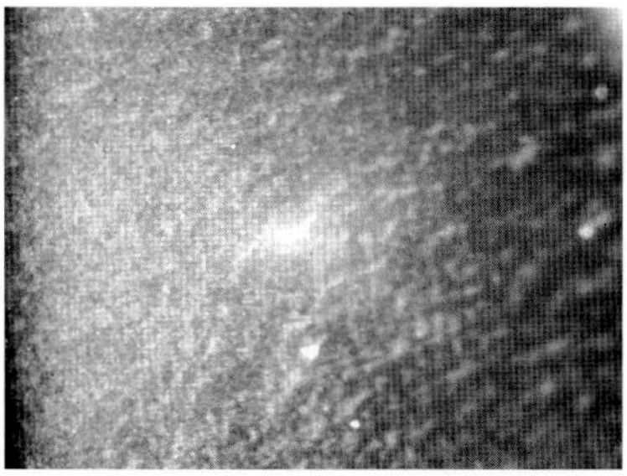

Figure 8-12. Advanced case of diffuse lamellar keratitis.

36. **Which clinical features help to distinguish DLK from an infectious process after LASIK?**
    DLK initially presents with a diffuse sandy infiltrate located in the periphery of the stromal interface. Patients are typically asymptomatic with a quiet eye. As the condition progresses, the infiltrate moves toward the center of the cornea and may begin to aggregate in clumps. Advanced cases of DLK can cause decreased vision and melting of the flap. Early treatment consists of frequent topical corticosteroids, and advanced cases may require systemic corticosteroids, lifting of the flap, and irrigation of the stromal interface. The lack of a distinct corneal infiltrate, conjunctival injection, cell and flare, and keratic precipitates favors the presence of DLK rather than infection.

KEY POINTS: LASIK INFECTIONS

1. Infections after LASIK are uncommon.

2. DLK is an inflammatory and not an infectious condition.

3. A suspicious infiltrate after LASIK should always be cultured.

37. **How should corneal infections after LASIK be prevented and managed?**
    Blepharitis should be treated preoperatively. Sterile technique, including hand scrubbing, sterile gloves, prepping solution (i.e., povidone iodine 10%), and draping of eyelashes, should be used. Postoperative treatment with a single-agent, broad-spectrum topical antibiotic also helps to reduce the incidence of infectious keratitis.

    Whenever an infection is suspected, the patient should be taken to an operating room where the flap can be lifted under a microscope for diagnostic smears and cultures. Depending on the severity of the infection, topical therapy with either a single-agent, broad-spectrum antibiotic or combination fortified antibiotics should be initiated.

OPHTHALMIA NEONATORUM

Janine G. Tabas, MD

1. **How does ophthalmia neonatorum typically present?**
   Inflammation of the conjunctiva within the first month of life is classified as ophthalmia neonatorum (neonatal conjunctivitis). A purulent or mucoid discharge is present from one or both eyes. Besides conjunctival injection, edema and erythema of the lids are often present.

2. **What is the usual means of transmission for neonatal conjunctivitis?**
   Conjunctivitis is usually transmitted to the newborn by passage through the mother's infected cervix at the time of delivery and reflects the sexually transmitted diseases prevalent in the community. It may be spread, however, by people handling the baby soon after birth.

3. **What is the most common cause of neonatal conjunctivitis in the United States?**
   Neonatal conjunctivitis is the most common ocular disease of newborns and is most often caused by *Chlamydia trachomatis* (6.2/1000 live births). One hundred years ago *Neisseria gonorrhoeae* was the leading cause of blindness in infants. Today gonococcal conjunctivitis is seen less in industrialized nations (3/1000 live births) because of neonatal ocular prophylaxis and better prenatal screening.

4. **List the common causes of ophthalmia neonatorum, their usual clinical presentations, and their approximate times of onset after birth.**
   See Table 9-1.

5. **Which type of neonatal conjunctivitis is associated with the most severe complications to the eye?**
   Neisseria gonorrhoeae has the ability to penetrate intact epithelial cells and divide within them. Its onset is rapid and can quickly lead to corneal perforation and endophthalmitis.

KEY POINTS: MOST COMMON CAUSES OF NEONATAL CONJUNCTIVITIS

1. Chemical

2. Chlamydial

3. Gonococcal

4. Bacterial

5. Herpetic

TABLE 9-1. COMMON CAUSES OF OPHTHALMIA NEONATORUM WITH TIME OF ONSET AND TYPICAL CHARACTERISTICS

Type	Time of Onset	Typical Characteristics
Chemical (e.g., silver nitrate drops)	Within hours of instillation	Self-limiting, mild, serous discharge (occasionally purulent) Lasts 24–36 hr
Chlamydia trachomatis	5–14 days	Mild-to-moderate, thick, purulent discharge (severity is variable) Erythematous conjunctiva, with palpebral more than bulbar involvement
Neisseria gonorrhoeae	24–48 hr	Hyperacute, copious, purulent discharge Lid swelling and chemosis common
Bacterial (nongonococcal)*	After 5 days	Variable presentation, depending on organism
Herpetic	Within 2 weeks	Conjunctiva only mildly injected Serosanguineous discharge Vesicular rash on lids sometimes seen Most have concomitant systemic herpetic disease

*Staphylococcus aureus, S. epidermidis, Streptococcus pneumoniae, S. viridans, Haemophilus influenzae, Escherichia coli, Pseudomonas aeruginosa.

6. **What other diagnostic tool is used to differentiate the various causes of neonatal conjunctivitis?**
   In most cases one cannot rely solely on clinical characteristics and time of onset for accurate diagnosis; therefore, initial therapy is also based on the results of Gram and Giemsa stains performed immediately on conjunctival swabs and scrapings. Their classic characteristics are listed in Table 9-2. Classic findings, however, are not seen in all cases. Specimens are also sent for culture and sensitivity testing and antigen detection tests. Treatment regimens are adjusted accordingly once the results are known, and clinical response is observed.

7. **Is a follicular reaction in the conjunctiva more indicative of a chlamydial or gonococcal infection?**
   Neither. Follicular reactions are not seen in the neonate because of the immaturity of the immune system.

8. **Why is Crede prophylaxis (2% silver nitrate drops) no longer the standard agent of choice for routine neonatal conjunctivitis prevention?**
   Crede prophylaxis is no longer the favored agent because of its high incidence of associated chemical conjunctivitis.

TABLE 9-2. GRAM AND GIEMSA STAIN FINDINGS WITH VARIOUS CAUSES OF NEONATAL CONJUNCTIVITIS

Cause	Stain	Findings
Chemical	Gram	Polymorphonuclear neutrophils (PMNs)
Chlamydial	Giemsa	Basophilic intracytoplasmic inclusion bodies in conjunctival epithelial cells
Gonococcal	Gram	Gram-negative intracellular diplococci in PMNs
Bacteria	Gram	Gram-positive or gram-negative organisms
Herpes simplex	Giemsa	Multinucleated giant cells, lymphocytes, plasma cells

9. **What is currently used for neonatal prophylaxis?**
   The American Academy of Pediatrics endorses the use of 1% tetracycline or 0.5% erythromycin ointment for neonatal prophylaxis. This is aimed primarily at preventing gonococcal conjunctivitis, which can have devastating ocular consequences. It is also effective for chlamydial infection.

10. **What is the differential diagnosis of neonatal conjunctivitis?**
    - **Birth trauma:** Usually evident by history.
    - **Foreign body/corneal abrasion:** Usually diagnosed by a combination of history and exam with fluorescein.
    - **Congenital glaucoma:** Accompanying early signs are tearing, photophobia, blepharospasm, and fussiness. Later signs include corneal edema and corneal enlargement. Intraocular pressure is elevated.
    - **Nasolacrimal duct obstruction:** Occurs in 6% of neonates and is usually associated with edema of the inner canthus and matting of the eyelids. Tearing is common, and the conjunctiva is usually not affected.
    - **Dacryocystitis:** Infection of the lacrimal sac, with erythema and swelling of the inner canthus and nasal conjunctival injection. Purulent drainage can often be expressed from the punctum.

11. **When is systemic treatment indicated for neonatal conjunctivitis? Why?**
    Systemic treatment is necessary for all cases of chlamydial, gonococcal, and herpetic conjunctivitis because of the potential for serious disseminated disease. A complete systemic examination is performed at the time of diagnosis to determine the extent of disease.

12. **List the potential ocular and systemic sequelae of untreated neonatal conjunctivitis.**
    See Table 9-3.

13. **What is the treatment for chlamydial conjunctivitis?**
    Oral erythromycin syrup is given for 2–3 weeks (50 mg/kg/day in four divided doses) along with erythromycin or sulfa ointment to the eye four times/day. The mother and her sexual partner also are treated with oral tetracycline, 250–500 mg four times/day, or doxycycline, 100 mg two times/day, for 7 days for presumed systemic disease, even if asymptomatic. Tetracycline cannot be used in children, pregnant women, or breast-feeding mothers because it will stain developing teeth.

TABLE 9-3. OCULAR AND SYSTEMIC SEQUELAE OF UNTREATED NEONATAL CONJUNCTIVITIS

Type	Ocular	Systemic
Chemical	None (a self-limited entity)	None
Chlamydial	Chronic infection may cause corneal scarring and symblepharon (adhesion of eyelid to eye)	Pneumonitis and otitis media
Gonococcal	Corneal ulceration, perforation, and endophthalmitis (may occur within 24 hr of onset)	Meningitis, arthritis, sepsis, and death
Bacterial	*Pseudomonas* sp. may cause corneal ulcer, perforation, and endophthalmitis	Usually none
Herpetic	Recurrences throughout life may cause corneal scarring and profound amblyopia. Chorioretinitis and cataracts also may develop.	Meningitis and disseminated CNS disease (mortality rate can be as high as 85%)

CNS = central nervous system.

KEY POINTS: POTENTIAL SYSTEMIC COMPLICATIONS OF NEONATAL CONJUNCTIVITIS

1. Pneumonitis

2. Meningitis

3. Otitis

4. Arthritis

5. Sepsis

14. **What is the treatment for gonococcal conjunctivitis?**
As a result of the high incidence of penicillin-resistant organisms, the Centers for Disease Control and Prevention recommends treatment with penicillinase-resistant antibiotics. Intravenous ceftriaxone (a third-generation cephalosporin) is started immediately and is given for 7 days at a dose of 25–50 mg/kg/day. The intravenous form can be changed to an oral equivalent, after significant improvement is noted, to complete a 7-day course. A single 125-mg intramuscular dose of ceftriaxone or a 100-mg/kg intramuscular dose of cefotaxime given immediately after diagnosis is an accepted alternative treatment.

Bacitracin ointment may be administered topically four times/day, and saline lavage is used hourly until the discharge is eliminated. Patients are generally hospitalized, and evaluated for evidence of dissemination.

Because of the high incidence of concomitant chlamydial infection in women who contract gonorrhea, the infant, mother, and her sexual partner are also treated systemically for chlamydia as outlined above. It is reasonable to test for other sexually transmitted diseases.

15. **What is the treatment for bacterial conjunctivitis?**
Erythromycin or gentamicin ointment applied four times/day for 2 weeks for gram-positive or gram-negative conjunctival swab results, respectively. Antibiotic choice may be altered later once culture and sensitivity results are known. In cases of corneal involvement, as seen with virulent organisms such as *Pseudomonas* sp., fortified topical antibiotics are administered and are often supplemented by systemic treatment.

KEY POINTS: POTENTIAL OCULAR COMPLICATIONS OF NEONATAL CONJUNCTIVITIS

1. Corneal scarring

2. Symblepharon

3. Corneal perforation

4. Endophthalmitis

16. **What is the treatment for herpes simplex viral conjunctivitis?**
Intravenous acyclovir, 10 mg/kg, is given every 8 hours for 10 days, along with vidarabine 3% ointment (Vira-A), five times/day, or trifluorothymidine 1% (Viroptic), every 2 hours, for 1 week.

17. **How can the incidence of ophthalmia neonatorum be reduced in future generations?**
The population most at risk for contracting neonatal conjunctivitis is infants born to mothers without adequate prenatal care or mothers involved with substance abuse. Because of its high association with serious systemic disease, neonatal conjunctivitis is still an important public health issue worldwide. Although not universally accepted, some countries (e.g., Sweden and England) have abandoned the use of routine prophylaxis after birth in favor of careful screening for sexually transmitted diseases and better prenatal care.

WEBSITE

1. www.emedicine.com/oph/topic/325.htm

BIBLIOGRAPHY

1. Albert DM, Jakobiec FA: Principles and Practice of Ophthalmology. Philadelphia, W.B. Saunders, 1994.

2. Chandler JW: Controversies in ocular prophylaxis of newborns. Arch Ophthalmol 107:814–815, 1989.

3. Cullom R, Chang B: The Wills Eye Manual—Office and Emergency Room Diagnosis and Treatment of Eye Disease. Philadelphia, J.B. Lippincott, 1994.

4. Hammerschlag M: Neonatal conjunctivitis. Pediatr Ann 22:346–351, 1993.

5. Laga M, Naamara W, Brunham R, et al: Single-dose therapy of gonococcal ophthalmia neonatorum with ceftriaxone. N Engl J Med 315:1382–1385, 1986.

6. O'Hara M: Ophthalmia neonatorum. Pediatr Clin North Am 40:715–725, 1993.

7. Weiss A: Chronic conjunctivitis in infants and children. Pediatr Ann 22:366–374, 1993.

CHAPTER 10

TOPICAL ANTIBIOTICS AND STEROIDS

Stephen Y. Lee, MD

1. **You are an antibiotic or steroid eyedrop just placed in the conjunctival fornix. Discuss the barriers to your journey into the eye.**

   Many eyedrop dispensers deliver a 50-µL eyedrop. However, only 20% of this volume is retained by the conjunctival cul-de-sac in most patients, and the excess immediately flows over the eyelids. Of the portion that remains, approximately 80% drains through the lacrimal system. In addition, because of the 15%/min tear turnover rate, almost all of the topically applied medication disappears from the conjunctival cul-de-sac in about 5 minutes. Irritating drugs produce reflex tearing and may be cleared more quickly.

   During this critical 5 minutes, the topically applied drug faces numerous tissue obstacles. Nonproductive absorption by the conjunctiva quickly disperses the medication systemically via the conjunctival vasculature. The small portion that penetrates the episclera faces the relative impermeability of the sclera and the tight junctions of the retinal pigment epithelium. The cornea poses three different barriers to entry. The corneal epithelium and the endothelium possess tight junctions that force the drugs to pass through the cellular membranes and limit passage of hydrophilic drugs. The corneal stroma is water-rich and limits movement of lipophilic drugs. Even after entry into the anterior chamber, the lens effectively limits most drug penetration, and very little enters the posterior segment of the eye through topical administration.

   Such formidable barriers seem insurmountable, but inflammation and infection render these barriers less effective, and modifications of the drug and/or its vehicle can facilitate entry into the eye. In addition, the desired site of action may be the ocular surface and not inside the eye.

2. **Given the above barriers, how would you increase delivery of topical antibiotics or steroids to the desired site of action?**

   The patient can perform punctal occlusion to decrease the amount of drainage through the lacrimal system by 65% and leave more drugs for intraocular absorption. Of course, frequent instillation also increases drug absorption, but the practical limit is probably every 5 minutes because the subsequent eyedrop can wash out the previous eyedrop before intraocular absorption.

   Changing the characteristics of the drug and/or its vehicle also improves delivery. Increasing the concentration of the drug may be limited by the solubility of the drug in the vehicle, and the high tonicity of higher concentrations triggers reflex tearing that quickly clears the drug from the ocular surface. Also, increasing lipid solubility of the drug appears to promote corneal passage despite the dual barrier characteristic of the cornea. In addition, adding surfactants that disturb the corneal epithelium dramatically increases drug entry.

3. **Name the three different formulations of topical medications and the advantages and the disadvantages of each.**
   - **Eyedrops** are easily instilled, but contact time is minimal, requiring frequent administration. In addition, the "pulse" nature of absorption invites transient overdose and toxicity.
   - **Suspensions** allow longer contact time, but the particulate nature of the preparation may be irritating and trigger reflex tearing. Suspensions settle to the bottom of the bottle

and need to be shaken before instilling the eyedrops. Patients also may complain of accumulation of the precipitates or forget to shake the bottle before administering the eyedrops.

- **Ointments** increase the contact time further, requiring the least frequent instillation, but leave a film over the eye that blurs vision. In addition, water-soluble drugs do not dissolve in the ointment vehicle and are present as crystals. Crystals are trapped in the ointment vehicle until the crystals on the surface of the ointment contact the ocular surface after the ointment vehicle melts with exposure to body temperature. This type of absorption allows entry of constant but low amounts of the drug.

Other methods of delivery include soft contact lenses, soluble ocular inserts, or implantable devices.

KEY POINTS: STRATEGIES TO INCREASE THE PENETRATION OF TOPICAL MEDICATIONS

1. Punctal occlusion.

2. Increase the frequency.

3. Increase the concentration of drug in the drop.

4. Increase the lipid solubility of the drug.

5. Use surfactants to disturb the corneal epithelium.

4. **A 60-year-old man complains of crusting of the eyelids in the morning and chronic foreign-body sensation. Examination reveals moderate blepharitis with numerous collarettes around the eyelashes. What would you recommend?**
Blepharitis often responds well to just warm compresses, but supplemental antibiotic ointments applied to the eyelash base or conjunctiva may be helpful, especially when numerous collarettes are seen around the eyelashes. Frequently used antibiotic ointments include erythromycin, bacitracin, and Polysporin. Erythromycin is a macrolide antibiotic that inhibits bacterial protein synthesis by binding to 50S ribosomal unit. It has a broad spectrum of coverage but suffers from poor intraocular absorption, and it is most appropriate for blepharitis and mild conjunctivitis. Bacitracin is composed of numerous polypeptides that inhibit bacterial cell wall synthesis. Polysporin combines bacitracin and polymyxin B, which are peptides that act like detergents to lyse bacterial cell membranes, and offers better coverage of gram-negative bacteria.

5. **A 30-year-old woman with "cold" symptoms presents with redness and mucous discharge in both eyes. The ocular symptoms began in the right eye 1 week ago but now involve both eyes despite treatment of the right eye with sulfacetamide 4 times/day, as prescribed by her family physician. Examination reveals bilateral follicular conjunctivitis with preauricular adenopathy. What would you recommend?**
History and examination are consistent with viral conjunctivitis. Artificial tears and cool compresses may provide comfort. Topical antibiotics are not required, but 1-week follow-up is advisable to look for potential membranous conjunctivitis, which may require topical steroids.

Sulfacetamide is a bacteriostatic structural analog of p-amino-benzoic acid and inhibits synthesis of folic acid. It has a broad spectrum of coverage and good corneal penetration and becomes more effective when combined with trimethoprim, which blocks a successive step in bacterial folate metabolism. It appears to be used often by nonophthalmologists for initial treatment of red eyes; it is fine for mild bacterial conjunctivitis but is not required for viral conjunctivitis.

6. **A 55-year-old woman complains of discharge and redness of her right eye for 4 weeks. Her family physician told her that she had "pink eye" and prescribed erythromycin ointment, then sulfacetamide, and then ciprofloxacin, but the symptoms have not improved. Examination reveals diffuse papillary conjunctivitis with purulent discharge. There is no preauricular adenopathy or previous history of "cold" symptoms. What should you do?**
   The patient has chronic bacterial conjunctivitis. Topical therapy usually brings prompt relief, and you should make sure that she uses the medications properly. Assuming that she is getting the medications into the eye in a proper dosing regimen, conjunctival cultures can be performed to look for resistant or unusual bacteria. Chronic dacryocystitis should be investigated by applying firm pressure below the medial canthal tendon in an attempt to produce a diagnostic purulent discharge through the lacrimal punctum. An abscess in the nasolacrimal sac may provide a source of bacteria resistant to topical antibiotics.

7. **A 25-year-old man holding a towel over his right eye complains of copious discharge that began in the morning. Examination reveals diffuse conjunctival hyperemia and chemosis with thick, purulent discharge. A prominent preauricular adenopathy is also present. What should you do?**
   Hyperacute bacterial conjunctivitis in sexually active patients should prompt a conjunctival smear and culture to look for gonococcal conjunctivitis. Although rare, gonococcal conjunctivitis requires immediate systemic antibiotics with topical antibiotics as an adjunctive treatment only.

8. **A 26-year-old physician in a general surgery residency with a doctorate in pharmacology presents with foreign-body sensation and photophobia in both eyes after sleeping with soft contact lenses during his call night. A midperipheral 2-mm corneal ulcer with surrounding corneal stromal edema is present with scant anterior chamber reaction. What should you do?**
   The chances of developing a corneal ulcer increase by a factor of ten when the patient sleeps with contact lenses. In addition, corneal cultures are recommended, although some ophthalmologists may manage small corneal ulcers without cultures (controversial).
   Initial therapy should cover a broad spectrum of bacteria. Traditionally, fortified cephalosporin and aminoglycoside have been used, but some believe that fluoroquinolones offer similar efficacy with less toxicity (controversial). In addition, fortified topical antibiotics are not universally available and need to be refrigerated.
   Fluoroquinolones inhibit bacterial DNA synthesis by binding to DNA gyrase and inhibiting the supercoiling of bacterial DNA. They offer a superb spectrum of coverage in in vitro studies, even against methicillin-resistant *Staphylococcus aureus*, if administered early in the course of infection. It appears to be highly effective for most corneal ulcers, especially contact lens-induced corneal ulcers, but large clinical series with attention to resistance and treatment failure have not been completed.
   Aminoglycosides bind to bacterial ribosomal subunits and interfere with protein synthesis. They offer a broad spectrum of coverage but require transport into the bacteria, which may be

reduced in anaerobic environments of an abscess. Coadministration of antibiotics that alter bacterial cell-wall structure improves aminoglycoside penetration into bacteria and produces a synergistic effect.

Cephalosporins are beta-lactam antibiotics synthesized or derived from compounds isolated from the fungus *Cephalosporium acremonium*. They inhibit bacterial transpeptidase, which is critical for bacterial cell-wall synthesis. In general, later generations provide broader coverage with better gram-negative but poorer gram-positive activity. Cephazolin is a first-generation cephalosporin that is traditionally combined with an aminoglycoside for the initial treatment of a corneal ulcer. It covers gram-positive and some gram-negative organisms but misses *Pseudomonas* sp. and, therefore, requires the addition of an aminoglycoside for initial broad-spectrum coverage.

9. **After corneal cultures are done, the patient is instructed to take ciprofloxacin every hour around the clock. Next day, he is in worse pain, and the corneal ulcer has enlarged to 3 mm with tenacious purulent discharge. What is your next step?**

   Make sure the eyedrops are getting into the eye. Ask the patient to demonstrate eyedrop administration. Several eyedrops fall on the floor, then on his cheeks, and finally he announces success when the eyedrops fall on his closed eyelids. Often, antibiotic failure is due to improper administration. Patients should be observed taking their eyedrops. A friend or family member may need to administer the eyedrops to be sure that the medications are getting to the source of infection, especially when frequent instillation is required. Indeed, some patients require hospitalization to receive intensive eyedrop administration.

   In addition, the patient should have taken the drug more often. The manufacturer's recommended dose of ciprofloxacin for corneal ulcers is two drops every 15 minutes for the first 6 hours, followed by two drops every half hour for the remainder of the first day. Then, two drops every hour for the second day, decreasing to two drops every 4 hours for days 3–14 are suggested. However, this regimen may be altered due to clinical exam and culture results. Frequent dosing of ciprofloxacin may produce a white precipitate over the ulcer, but this precipitate does not appear to impede the bactericidal activity and usually resolves when the dose is tapered.

   Ofloxacin is also used but has different manufacturer's recommendations:

   - **Days 1 and 2:** One to two drops every 30 minutes while awake
   - **Awaken at 4 and 6 hours after retiring:** Give one to two drops
   - **Days 3–7 or 9:** One to two drops hourly while awake
   - **Days 7–9 to completion:** One to two drops four times/day

   Fourth-generation fluoroquinolones, gatifloxacin and moxifloxacin, are also available with better gram-positive coverage and comparable gram-negative coverage.

10. **The patient now prefers a "proven" treatment regimen with a long history and requests topical fortified antibiotics. However, he recalls that minimal bactericidal concentration for most pathogenic bacteria is far below that provided by the fortified antibiotics and accuses you of wasting money and drugs. Is he right?**

    No. In vitro and in vivo results in other sites of the body may not be applicable to the eye. Indeed, in the vitreous, the dose-response relationship has been demonstrated up to 100 times the in vitro minimal bactericidal concentration.

11. **The patient reminds you that he is penicillin-allergic and does not enjoy anaphylaxis. What antibiotics should you choose? How do you begin therapy?**

    Penicillin is not often used in ophthalmology because of poor penetration into the blood ocular barrier and active transport out of the eye by the organic acid transport system of the ciliary body. However, inflammation improves ocular penetration. Penicillin inhibits bacterial transpeptidase and prevents bacterial cell-wall synthesis. Varieties of modification of the original compound have produced varying spectrums of activity. Penicillin G and V are still highly effective for many gram-positive and gram-negative bacteria, but many strains of *Staphylococcus aureus* and *epidermidis* are now resistant. Penicillinase-resistant penicillins such as methicillin are useful for penicillinase-producing staphylococci. Broad-spectrum penicillins, ampicillin, and amoxicillin, have better gram-negative coverage, and semisynthetic penicillins such as carbenicillin and ticarcillin extend coverage to *Pseudomonas, Enterobacter*, and *Proteus* spp.

    Immediate allergic response to penicillin, such as hives or anaphylaxis, is a strong contraindication for its use, and there is 10% cross-reactivity with cephalosporins. Therefore, for patients with penicillin allergy, cefazolin should be replaced with vancomycin. Vancomycin is a complex glycopeptide that inhibits bacterial cell-wall synthesis with principally gram-positive coverage, including methicillin-resistant *S. aureus* and *Streptococcus faecalis*, which is a frequent bacterial pathogen in infections of filtering blebs.

    As mentioned above, an aminoglycoside is synergistic with cell wall-inhibiting antibiotics, and the patient should be started on fortified vancomycin and tobramycin. Give the patient four doses—an alternating dose every 5 minutes—followed by alternation every half hour. Actual dosing may vary in different institutions.

12. **Next morning the ulcer looks worse with 4 mm corneal infiltrate and purulent material overlying the ulcer. The corneal culture confirms *Pseudomonas aeruginosa*. Why did the patient not improve?**

    Pseudomonas corneal ulcers sometimes require double coverage. Fortified ticarcillin should be added in a nonpenicillin-allergic patient. In this case, ciprofloxacin could be resumed.

13. **Next day, the ulcer looks stable, but the patient complains of persistent and perhaps worsening pain. Examination reveals diffuse punctate corneal epithelial defects, inferior conjunctival erythema, and swollen lower eyelids. What should you do?**

    Toxicity is often less severe with topical administration; indeed, some common topical antibiotics such as neomycin and polymyxin cannot be given intravenously because of systemic toxicity. However, intensive regimens of potent antibiotics often produce surface toxicity with prominent involvement of lower more than upper conjunctiva. Occasionally, only analgesics and cool compresses can be offered if the infection is not under control. Fortified vancomycin may be decreased because tobramycin and ciprofloxacin are more important for *Pseudomonas* ulcer, and the ulcer appears to be stabilizing.

14. **The patient slowly improves, but significant corneal scar remains. He would like binocular vision for his surgical career and asks you to get rid of his corneal scar. How do you respond?**

    Read on to learn about topical steroids. Often, inflammatory scars fade well with topical steroids. When, how much, and how long to use topical steroids is controversial, but a trial of topical steroids is certainly warranted before considering surgical options. The infection must be controlled first before applying any topical steroids.

KEY POINTS: CORNEAL ULCERS

1. Small, noncentral ulcers can be managed without cultures.

2. Fluoroquinolones every ½ to 1 hour initially may offer similar efficacy with less toxicity than fortified topical antibiotics.

3. *Pseudomonas* ulcers may require double coverage.

4. The use of topical steroids after the infection is controlled can decrease the size of the scar.

15. **Review the currently available topical antibiotics in generic and brand names.**
    See Table 10-1.

16. **How do topical steroids work?**
    The specific mechanisms of action of steroids are not completely understood. At a molecular level, inhibition of arachidonic acid release from phospholipids may be the most important effect. Arachidonic acid is converted to prostaglandins and related compounds that are potent mediators of inflammation. At a cellular level, steroids must be carried to the cytoplasm, where they bind to soluble receptors and then enter the nucleus to alter transcription of various proteins involved in immune regulation and inflammation. At the tissue level, steroids suppress the cardinal signs of inflammation such as edema, heat, pain, and redness through a variety of mechanisms. They cause vasoconstriction and decrease vascular permeability to inflammatory cells. Cellular and intracellular membranes are stabilized to inhibit release of inflammatory mediators such as histamine. Neutrophilic leucocytosis is inhibited, and macrophage recruitment and migration are also decreased. Overall, steroids are potent anti-inflammatory and immunosuppressive agents with wide-ranging ophthalmic applications, but their adverse effects as well as their benefits should be understood before use.

17. **Since steroids are not cures, what general categories of disorders warrant ophthalmic use of topical steroids?**
    Abelson and Butrus identify three broad categories of disorders that warrant steroid use: postsurgical, immune hyperreactivity, and combined immune and infectious processes. Remarkably, postoperative use of steroids has not been evaluated in a well-controlled, double-blinded study. Although their use in this setting is almost universal, some ophthalmologists report adequate control of postoperative inflammation with topical nonsteroidals for various ophthalmic procedures (controversial). The second category includes various uveitides, allergic and vernal conjunctivitis, corneal graft rejections, and other processes in which the immune system activity is harmful to the host tissue. The last category includes viral and bacterial corneal ulcers, especially herpes simplex and herpes zoster, in which control of infectious processes must be balanced with control of inflammation that may scar delicate ocular tissue.

18. **The physician with the residual corneal scar wants to minimize his corneal scar but is concerned about potential side effects of topical steroids. How do you advise him?**
    Exacerbation of the existing infection with reactivation of dormant organisms or inhibition of wound healing is the most immediate concern. Other well-known adverse effects include glaucoma and cataracts, but numerous other side effects have been observed, including blepharoptosis, eyelid skin or scleral atrophy, and mydriasis.
    Systemic absorption may be significant, and punctal occlusion should be encouraged. A 6-week regimen of topical 0.1% dexamethasone sodium phosphate has been shown to suppress the

TABLE 10-1. CURRENTLY AVAILABLE TOPICAL ANTIBIOTICS

Generic Name	Brand Name	Preparation
Gentamicin	Genoptic S.O.P.	0.3% ointment or solution
	Garamycin	
	Gentacidin	
	Gentak	
Tobramycin	Tobrex	0.3% ointment or solution
Bacitracin	AK-tracin	500 units/gm ointment
Chloramphenicol	Chloromycetin	0.5% ointment, 1.0% solution
	Ocu-chlor	
	Chloroptic	
Erythromycin	AK-mycin	0.5% ointment
	Ilotycin	
Fluoroquinolones		
Ciprofloxacin	Ciloxan	0.3% solution or ointment
Ofloxacin	Ocuflox	0.3% solution
Norfloxacin	Chibroxin	0.3% solution
Moxifloxacin	Vigamox	0.5% solution
Gatifloxacin	Zymar	0.3% solution
Levafloxacin	Quixin	0.5% solution
Bacitracin, neomycin, and polymyxin B	Neosporin	10,000 units, 3.5 mg, 400 units/gm ointment
Sulfisoxazole	Gantrisin	4% solution
Sulfacetamide	Bleph-10	10% solution or ointment
	AK-Sulf	10% solution or ointment
	Sodium Sulamyd	10% ointment or solution
Tetracycline	Achromycin	1% solution or ointment
Polymyxin and bacitracin	Polysporin	10,000 units/gm, 500 units/gm ointment
Trimethoprim and polymyxin B	Polytrim	0.1%/10,000 units/mL solution
Polymyxin B	Neomycin	10,000 units–1.75 mg–0.025 mg/mL solution
	Gramicidin (Neosporin)	

adrenal cortex, and some patients with systemic hay fever improve with topical ocular steroids. Of course, all of these effects are more frequent with intensive and chronic use of steroids.

19. **After a lengthy discussion, the patient agrees to try topical steroids. However, given his interest in pharmacology, he requests a brief discussion of the pharmacokinetics of a few of the available topical steroids.**
Topical steroids may be prepared as solutions, suspensions, or ointments. Phosphate preparations may be prepared as solutions because they are highly water-soluble in the aqueous

vehicles but penetrate less well into intact corneal epithelium than acetate or alcohol suspensions, which have biphasic solubility. Nevertheless, 1% prednisolone phosphate achieves a significant corneal level of 10 μg/gm within 30 minutes after instillation, which improves to 235 μg/gm when the corneal epithelium is removed. Dexamethasone phosphate enters the cornea and anterior chamber within 10 minutes, reaches a maximum in 30–60 minutes, and slowly disappears over the next few to 24 hours.

20. **The patient also requests that the most potent steroid be used with rapid taper so that the overall course may be shortened. Which steroid do you choose?**
Anti-inflammatory effects of topical steroids differ depending on the clinical setting and method of measurement. However, certain generalizations can be made:
- Higher concentrations and more frequent instillations, up to every 5 minutes, increase concentrations of steroids in the cornea and aqueous.
- With corneal epithelium intact, prednisolone acetate suspension > dexamethasone alcohol solution > prednisolone sodium phosphate solution > dexamethasone phosphate ointment.
- With corneal epithelial defects, prednisolone sodium phosphate solution > dexamethasone phosphate solution > prednisolone acetate suspension.

21. **The patient is started on 1% prednisolone acetate 4 times/day. His scar is beginning to recede, but he returns 2 days later with complaints of a white precipitate that forms in his conjunctiva and insists on a change of medication to prevent this annoying buildup. Which steroid do you choose now?**
Suspensions leave a milky precipitate that some patients find unpleasant. In addition, despite shaking the bottles before instillation, a variable amount of the suspension may be delivered if particles are not evenly distributed. Therefore, some ophthalmologists prefer phosphate solutions despite lower potency with intact epithelium. A change to 1% prednisolone phosphate is reasonable if patient compliance is improved.

22. **On day 10 of steroid therapy, the corneal scar is receding rapidly, but the patient complains of foreign-body sensation. Examination reveals large corneal epithelial dendrites. What should you do?**
Steroids do not cause herpetic keratitis but may promote herpetic keratitis when viral shedding is timed with the presence of steroids on the ocular surface. Often the dendrites are large and numerous in the presence of steroids, and steroids should be stopped or rapidly tapered. Of course, full dosing of trifluridine should be started.

23. **Fortunately, the dendrite heals rapidly and the previous corneal scar has faded significantly with return to 20/20 vision in that eye. Four years have passed, and the patient is now seeking employment. Opportunities are scarce, and his only job offer is from a large organized health company that hopes to use him as a pharmacist as well as a physician as a cost-saving measure. Understandably, he is stressed. Now he notices extreme photophobia and redness of his eye. Examination reveals corneal stromal edema and focal keratic precipitates consistent with herpes simplex keratouveitis. What should you do?**
Many stimuli, including stress, promote recurrence of herpetic keratitis. Other stimuli include menses, sun exposure, and fever. If the inflammation is severe or central vision is threatened, steroids should be given with trifluridine coverage to decrease corneal scarring and intraocular inflammation. One regimen may be trifluridine (Viroptic) and 1% prednisolone acetate, both four times/day. Other regimens may be acceptable, but an easily remembered regimen is to add trifluridine drop for drop with the topical steroids. Antiviral coverage is probably unnecessary below one drop/day of 1% prednisolone acetate. Vidarabine (Vira-A) ointment may be used instead of trifluridine.

24. **Two days later, only marginal improvement is noted, but intraocular pressure is 35 mmHg. What happened?**

   Significant steroid-induced rises in intraocular pressure have been demonstrated in up to 6% of patients after 6 weeks of topical dexamethasone, and patients with glaucoma or family history of glaucoma are particularly susceptible. The mechanism appears to be decreased aqueous outflow, perhaps as a result of deposition of mucopolysaccharides in the trabecular meshwork. The extent of intraocular pressure rise varies with type and dose of steroids. Usually, steroids with greater anti-inflammatory potency elicit greater elevation of intraocular pressure. For example, steroids with low intraocular bioavailability and potency, such as fluorometholone, cause lower rises in intraocular pressure after a greater duration of therapy than more potent steroids such as dexamethasone. Rimexolone claims to be the exception. It appears to have similar suppression of anterior chamber cell and flare as 1% prednisolone acetate with intraocular pressure elevation similar to fluorometholone. Regardless, the elevated intraocular pressure subsides, usually within 2 weeks, by decreasing or discontinuing steroid therapy, but topical aqueous suppressants may be needed in some patients.

   However, steroid-induced rises in intraocular pressure rarely occur in less than 2 weeks and certainly not after 2 days of steroid therapy. Patients with intraocular inflammations, especially in herpetic keratouveitis, may have increased intraocular pressure as a result of intraocular inflammation. Therefore, in the present patient, the topical steroids should be increased and not decreased.

25. **The frequency of prednisolone acetate administration was increased to every 3 hours while awake, and timolol, 2 times/day, was added. One week later intraocular pressure is normal, and intraocular inflammation has subsided. Prednisolone acetate is tapered to 2 times/day. The patient returns 2 days later with recurrence of pain and photophobia and return of intraocular inflammation. What happened?**

   You tapered the steroids too quickly. A useful rule is to decrease steroids by no more than half of the previous dose, especially in herpetic keratouveitis, in which rebound inflammation is frequent. Make sure that the patient is still taking the eyedrops. Sometimes patients abruptly stop the eyedrops when they feel better and then suffer rebound inflammation.

26. **Review the commonly available topical steroids and their generic and brand names.**

   See Table 10-2.

TABLE 10-2. COMMONLY AVAILABLE TOPICAL STEROIDS

Generic Name	Brand Name	Preparation
Dexamethasone sodium phosphate	AK-Dex, Decadron	0.05% ointment
	AK-Dex, Decadron	0.1% solution
Fluorometholone	FML forte	0.25% suspension
FML liquifilm, Fluor-op	0.1% suspension	
	FML S.O.P.	0.1% ointment
Fluorometholone acetate	Flarex	0.1% suspension
Prednisolone acetate	Predforte, Econopred plus	1% suspension
	Predmild, Econopred	0.125% suspension
Prednisolone sodium phosphate	Inflamase forte, AK-pred 1%	1% solution
	Inflamase mild, AK-pred 0.125%	0.125% solution
Rimexolone	Vexol	1% suspension
Loteprednol	Lotemax	0.5% suspension

BIBLIOGRAPHY

1. Abelson MB, Butrus S: Corticosteroids in ophthalmic practice. In Jakobiec FA, Albert D (eds): Principles and Practice of Ophthalmology, vol. 6. Philadelphia, W.B. Saunders, 1994, pp 1013–1022.

2. Axelrod J, Glew R, Barza M, et al: Antibacterials. In Jakobiec FA, Albert D (eds): Principles and Practice of Ophthalmology, vol. 6. Philadelphia, W.B. Saunders, 1994, pp 940–960.

3. Baum JL: Initial therapy of suspected microbial corneal ulcers. I: Broad antibiotic therapy based on prevalence of organisms. Surv Ophthalmol 24:97–105, 1979.

4. Callegan MC, Engel LS, Hill JM, et al: Ciprofloxacin versus tobramycin for the treatment of staphylococcal keratitis. Inv Ophthalmol Vis Sci 35:1033–1037, 1994.

5. Foster CS, Alter G, Debarge LR, et al: Efficacy and safety of rimexolone 1% ophthalmic suspension vs. 1% prednisolone acetate in the treatment of uveitis. Am J Ophthalmol 122:171–182, 1996.

6. Leibowitz HM, Bartlett JD, Rich R, et al: Intraocular pressure-raising potential of 1% rimexolone in patients responding to corticosteroids. Arch Ophthalmol 114:933–937, 1996.

7. Medical Economics Co. Inc.: PDR for Ophthalmic Medications 2001. Montvale, NJ, Medical Economics Co. Inc., 2000.

8. Stroman DW, Dajcs JJ, Cupp GA, et al: In vitro and in vivo potency of moxifloxacin and moxifloxacin ophthalmic solution 0.5%, a new topical fluoroquinolone. Surv Ophthalmol 50:S16–S31, 2005.

9. Tripathi RC, Tripathi BJ, Li J, et al: Ocular pharmacology. In Basic and Clinical Science Course, sect 2. San Francisco, American Academy of Ophthalmology, 1995, pp 312–354.

10. Ueno N, Refojo MF, Abelson M: Pharmacokinetics. In Jakobiec FA, Albert D (eds): Principles and Practice of Ophthalmology, vol. 6. Philadelphia, W.B. Saunders, 1994, pp 916–928.

CHAPTER 11

DRY EYES

Janice A. Gault, MD

1. **What is the definition of dry eye?**
   A dry eye or keratoconjuctivitis sicca (KCS) is a condition in which the tear film is abnormal and cannot lubricate the anterior surface of the cornea. The resulting changes in the ocular surface can cause ocular discomfort, scarring, and, in severe cases, loss of vision and perforation.

2. **Describe the normal tear film.**
   The normal tear film is a 0.1–0.5 mm convex band with a regular upper margin.

3. **What are the components of the tear film?**
   The normal tear film is made of three components. The outer layer is a thin lipid layer produced by the meibomian glands, which open along the upper and lower lid margins. The middle layer, the thickest, is composed of aqueous produced from the main and accessory lacrimal glands. The innermost layer is a mucin layer produced by conjunctival goblet cells.

4. **What is the function of the outer lipid layer?**
   It retards evaporation of the aqueous middle layer. If it is dysfunctional, evaporative dry eye will result.

5. **What causes dysfunction of the outer lipid layer?**
   Oil deficiencies as in meibomian gland dysfunction (i.e., blepharitis). Also, an abnormal lid contour as in ectropion or lid tumor, or poor blinking found in Bell's palsy.

6. **What is the function of the aqueous middle layer?**
   It supplies oxygen from the atmosphere to the corneal epithelium, washes away debris, and has antibacterial properties due to IgA, lysozyme, and lactoferrin present within it. If deficient, hyposecretive dry eye results, as found in Sjögren's syndrome.

7. **What is the function of the inner mucin layer?**
   It covers the villus surface of the corneal epithelium, converting it from a hydrophobic surface to a hydrophilic one thus allowing the aqueous layer to lubricate the cornea.

8. **What diseases of the conjunctiva can cause dry eye?**
   Conjunctival scarring can injure the goblet cells. Patients with cicatricial ocular pemphigoid, Stevens-Johnson syndrome, chemical burns (especially alkali), and graft-versus-host disease in bone marrow transplantation may have dry eye. Patients with other conjunctival disorders that accompany conditions such as aniridia may also have dry eyes. Vitamin A deficiency can result in the loss of goblet cells. This is becoming more common with the increase in gastric bypass procedures.

9. **What is necessary for the normal resurfacing of the tear film?**
   A normal blink reflex, normal lid anatomy and contour, and a normal corneal epithelium. Of course, a normal tear film makeup is essential.

10. **What are the types of dry eye?**
Basically, there are three main types:
- **Hyposecretive (i.e., Sjögrens or non-Sjögrens):** The aqueous component is decreased.
- **Evaporative:** This may be caused by eyelid abnormalities (i.e., Bell's palsy, ectropion) or corneal surface changes such as dellen.
- **Mixed:** This combines features of the other two.

11. **What are the symptoms of dry eye?**
Burning, irritation, foreign body sensation, light sensitivity, and blurred vision. Usually, the symptoms are worse in the afternoon and evening and better on awakening. A dry or dusty environment may cause more difficulties in patients with dry eye then others. Cigarette smoke can be extremely irritating. Symptoms are worse in low humidity environments, such as those with central air and in an airplane, during prolonged reading and driving with a decreased blink rate due to increased concentration, and windy conditions.

12. **What are the most common signs of dry eye?**
In the early stages, ocular symptoms may be more impressive than what is found on the examination. Signs of dry eye include a decreased tear meniscus, debris in the tear film, conjunctival injection, and superficial punctate keratitis and conjunctivitis. Abnormal fluorescein or rose bengal staining of the corneal and conjunctival epithelium in the exposed interpalpebral fissure (at 3 and 9 o'clock) of the lower third of the cornea is often present. The upper half of the cornea is usually spared. In more severe disease, filamentary keratitis can develop as well as corneal scarring. Blepharitis with a frothy tear film may be seen in tandem with dry eye.

13. **What is Sjögren's syndrome?**
Sjögren's syndrome is a triad of dry eye, dry mouth (xerostomia), and a collagen vascular disease. Rheumatoid arthritis is the most common, but systemic lupus erythematosus, Wegener's granulomatosis, scleroderma, systemic sclerosis, and primary biliary cirrhosis may also be associated. The lacrimal gland acini and ducts are damaged in the autoimmune disease.

14. **Who gets dry eye?**
Women are more likely to develop this than men, probably in relation to changes in hormone levels. It is also associated with birth control use. Contact lense wearers frequently have problems with dry eye.
  It may be seen in all age groups, but it is most common after 60 years of age. It can occur in patients in their 20s and 30s, but may be overlooked unless patients are specifically questioned about symptoms. LASIK and blepharoplasty can exacerbate underlying dry eye. Radiation treatments can also cause dry eye.

15. **What is the difference between fluorescein and rose bengal stains?**
Rose bengal stains mucin and epithelial cells that are dead or devitalized, but still in place. Fluorescein requires epithelial defects to stain. Thus, rose bengal will show earlier, more subtle abnormalities.

16. **How do you measure a tear break-up time (TBUT)?**
Instill fluorescein into the lower fornix. Ask the patient to blink several times and then stop. The TBUT is the time from the last blink to the development of a dry spot noted by black spots in the fluorescein film. Normal is 10 or more seconds. It decreases with age, but less than 5 seconds is good evidence for dry eye.

17. **What is Schirmer's test?**
    Schirmer's test filter strip is placed with the notched edge over the lid margin. The tear film in the lacrimal lake is absorbed over 5 minutes and measured. A normal Schirmer's test wets the strip 10 mm. Usually, it is done with topical anesthesia so as to not cause reflex tearing.

18. **What are the treatments for dry eye patients?**
    Patients should be treated based on symptoms. If a patient has a normal exam, but describes typical dry eye, treatment should still be instituted. Tear replacement therapy is the first choice. They can be used as needed depending on the patient's symptoms. Once or twice a day may be fine for some; others may need nearly every hour. Lacrisert is a solid form of artificial tear placed in the lower cul-de-sac that melts over a period of 12 hours. It is seldom used but can be very effective in a small number of patients. Lubricating ointments such as lacrilube can be used at night. It will blur vision, but may be necessary during the day if exposure is a significant problem, as in Bell's palsy.
    Patients should also be counseled to avoid conditions with low humidity such as central air heating, to prevent air from blowing into their eyes as from an air conditioner vent at home or in the car, and to use a humidifier while sleeping and at work if possible. Lubrication may need to be increased while flying, as airplane cabins have very low humidity, and while reading or studying, as the blink reflex is decreased.
    Newer contact lenses with a high-DK, high water content may be better tolerated by dry eye patients.

19. **What if the patient uses tears six to eight times a day and returns with red, painful eyes and more superficial punctate keratitis?**
    They may be sensitive to the preservatives in the tears. In these patients, preservative-free tears may be necessary.

20. **What if this is still not enough?**
    Punctal occlusion is an option. Patients who use tears every 2 hours or more may benefit from closing the lower puncta. Placement of a punctal plug can be easily done as an office procedure. Patients may notice local irritation for a short time, but this usually resolves. Occasionally, epiphora may result from overflow tearing and the plug can quickly be removed in the office. If the patient is comfortable with this, but the plug falls out, permanent closure can be done by using cautery. Between 10% and 20% of the tear film is drained through the upper puncta, and these may be closed subsequently if the lower lid punctal closure is not adequate to control symptoms. Lateral tarsorrhaphy is also available. Of course, any lid contour abnormalities should be addressed as well (e.g., ectropion, lid laxity).

KEY POINTS: SEVERE DRY EYE

1. Frequent tear use may make symptoms worse if the patient is sensitive to the preservatives.

2. Occlude the lower lid puncta first and then proceed to upper lid punctal occlusion.

3. Cyclosporine may increase tear production, but it may take months to see results.

21. **A patient with punctal occlusion returns with more irritation and burning since the procedure was done. The tear film meniscus is greatly improved. What happened?**
    If a patient has significant blepharitis, the symptoms can worsen after punctal occlusion. The debris is trapped and not drained and now has a higher concentration than before. Make sure blepharitis is treated adequately to prevent this.

22. **Is there any treatment to increase tear production?**
    Topical cyclosporine (Restasis) has been used recently as it decreases cell-mediated inflammation of the lacrimal tissue and ultimately can increase tear production. Patients need to use it twice a day for 1–3 months to get a response and then continue for up to 6 months or more. Some practitioners are using a mild steroid q.i.d. for the first 2 weeks to decrease inflammation and stinging until the cyclosporine begins to work.

23. **What is the role of acetylcysteine?**
    Acetylcysteine is a mucolytic agent used to break up mucous in patients that have filamentary keratitis and mucous plaques.

24. **What medications may be a cause of dry eye?**
    Topical eye drops such as those used in glaucoma can cause or worsen dry eye. The medication or the preservative may cause toxicity to the epithelial cells. Aminoglycoside antibiotics (i.e., Neosporin and gentamicin), β-blockers, and pilocarpine are common offenders.
    Systemic medications that can decrease tear production include antimuscarinics (scopolamine, Detrol), antihistamines, lithium, diuretics, estrogens (including birth control pills), antihypertensives (β-blockers, α-agonists), antidepressants, chemotherapy agents, antipsychotics, marijuana, and morphine.

BIBLIOGRAPHY

1. Chow CYC, Gibard JP: Tear film. In Krachmer JG, Mannis MJ, Holland EJ (eds): Cornea, vol. 1. St. Louis, Mosby, 1997, pp 49–60.
2. Fox FI: Systemic diseases associated with dry eye. Int Ophthalmol Clin 34:71–87, 1994.
3. Lemp MA: Report of the National Eye Institute/Industry Workshop on Clinical Trials in Dry Eyes. CLAO J 21:221–232, 1996.
4. Stevenson D, Tauber J, Reis BL: Efficacy and safety of cyclosporine A ophthalmic emulsion in the treatment of moderate-to-severe dry eye disease: A dose-ranging, randomized trial. The Cyclosporine A Phase 2 Study Group. Ophthalmology 107:967–974, 2000.
5. Tu EY, Rheinstrom S: Dry eye. In Yanoff M, Duker JS (eds): Ophthalmology, 2nd ed. St. Louis, Mosby, 2004, pp 520–526.
6. Kanski J: Clinical Ophthalmology: A Systematic Approach. Edinburgh, Butterworth-Heinemann, 2003.
7. Sall K, Stevenson OD, Mundorf TK, Reis BL: Two multicenter, randomized studies of the efficacy and safety of cyclospring ophthalmic emulsion in moderate to severe dry eye disease. CsA Phase 3 Study Group. Ophthalmology 107:1220, 2000.

CHAPTER 12

CORNEAL DYSTROPHIES

Sadeer B. Hannush, MD, and Lorena Riveroll, MD

1. **What are corneal dystrophies?**
   Corneal dystrophies are bilateral, inherited, noninflammatory, commonly progressive alterations of the cornea that are usually not associated with any other systemic condition. Most corneal dystrophies are autosomal dominant disorders occurring after birth. Because each dystrophy may exhibit a spectrum of clinical manifestations, examining multiple family members frequently aids in establishing the diagnosis.

2. **How do degenerations differ from dystrophies?**
   In contrast to dystrophies, degenerations are unilateral or bilateral aging changes that are not inherited. They are also not associated with systemic disease.

3. **Discuss the general anatomic classification of corneal dystrophies.**
   - **Anterior membrane dystrophies** include disorders affecting the corneal epithelium, epithelial basement membrane (Fig. 12-1), and Bowman's layer.
   - **Stromal dystrophies** occur anywhere in the stromal layer of the cornea between Bowman's layer and Descemet's membrane.
   - **Posterior membrane dystrophies** are primarily abnormalities of the endothelium and Descemet's membrane.

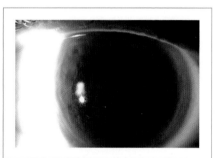

Figure 12-1. Typical mare's-tail sign in anterior basement membrane dystrophy.

KEY POINTS: DIFFERENCES BETWEEN CORNEAL DYSTROPHIES AND DEGENERATIONS

1. Corneal dystrophies are always bilateral.

2. They are inherited.

3. They may occur shortly after birth.

4. **Describe the inheritance patterns of anterior membrane dystrophies.**
   All anterior membrane dystrophies are autosomal dominant. Examples are Meesmann's juvenile epithelial dystrophy, epithelial basement membrane dystrophy, and corneal dystrophies of Bowman's layer.

5. **Which is the most common anterior membrane dystrophy? Which is strictly epithelial?**
Epithelial basement membrane dystrophy is by far the most common anterior membrane dystrophy. In fact, it has the highest prevalence of all of the corneal dystrophies. Areas of extra basement membrane result in maplike and/or fingerprint changes as well as intraepithelial microcysts. Five percent of otherwise normal corneas have been observed to have such changes.

Second in prevalence are the corneal dystrophies of Bowman's layer (CDBs): true Reis-Bücklers (CDB-1) and Thiel-Behnke honeycomb-shaped dystrophy (CDB-II). These disorders consist of gray reticular opacities beneath the epithelium.

Meesmann's dystrophy is the rarest of the three. This disorder, noted in the first few years of life, presents as a bilaterally symmetric pattern of microcysts or vesicles seen strictly in the epithelial layer of the cornea, usually in the interpalpebral fissure.

Küchle M, Green WR, Volcker HE, Barraquer J: Reevaluation of corneal dystrophies of Bowman's layer and the anterior stroma (Reis-Bücklers and Thiel-Behnke types): A light and electron microscopic study of eight corneas and review of the literature. Cornea 14:333–354, 1995.
Small KW, Mullen L, Barletta J, et al: Mapping of Reis-Bücklers' corneal dystrophy to chromosome 5q. Am J Ophthalmol 121:384–390, 1996.
Ridgway AE, Akhtar S, Munier FL, et al: Ultrastructural and molecular analysis of Bowman's layer corneal dystrophies: An epithelial origin. Invest Ophthalmol Vis Sci 41:3286–3292, 2000.

6. **What are the most common presenting symptoms of anterior membrane dystrophies?**
First are the symptoms associated with corneal erosions—pain, foreign body sensation, photophobia, and tearing, especially with opening of the lids during sleep or upon awakening in the morning. Erosions are most common in the setting of epithelial basement membrane dystrophy. The second symptom is blurred vision secondary to both corneal clouding and irregularity of the surface, most frequently seen in the dystrophies of Bowman's layer.

7. **Discuss treatment options for recurrent corneal erosions associated with anterior membrane dystrophies.**
The conservative approach includes the generous use of lubricating eyedrops during the day and ointments at night. Some physicians advocate the use of topical steroids to stabilize the basement membrane, and others advocate hypertonic saline, especially in ointment form at night to dehydrate the epithelium and aid in its attachment to the underlying layers. Patching, either conventional or with collagen or bandage contact lenses, hypothetically decreases the mechanical effect of lid movement on the already weakened corneal epithelium. Recalcitrant cases may require surgical intervention.

KEY POINTS: RECURRENT CORNEAL EROSIONS

1. Recurrent corneal erosions may be associated with anterior membrane and stromal dystrophies.
2. They have common symptoms: pain, blurred vision, and photophobia.
3. Recurrent corneal erosions are frequently amenable to medical therapy with lubrication and hyperosmotic agents.
4. They can be treated surgically with mechanical or laser keratectomy or stromal puncture.

8. **Discuss the role of surgery in the treatment of anterior membrane dystrophies.**
   In the setting of recalcitrant corneal erosions, mechanical debridement of the loose epithelium or anterior stromal puncture, together with the use of a bandage lens, may aid in re-epithelialization of the surface and adherence of the epithelium to the underlying layers. Mechanical debridement also may be used to remove an irregular epithelial basement membrane if an associated visual decline is noted. For the Bowman's layer dystrophies a more aggressive superficial or lamellar keratectomy may be required. Lamellar and penetrating keratoplasties also have been used.

9. **Do lasers have a role?**
   The yttrium-aluminum-garnet (YAG) laser has been used instead of a needle to accomplish anterior stromal puncture but does not offer a clear advantage. The excimer laser has been used for treatment of recurrent erosions associated with basement membrane dystrophies and for removal of deeper layers in conditions such as Reis-Bücklers and Thiel-Behnke dystrophies (phototherapeutic keratectomy [PTK]). Although in the first instance the excimer laser may not offer a clear advantage over debridement, in the second it has supplanted lamellar keratectomy as the treatment of choice.

10. **What controversy surrounds the dystrophies affecting Bowman's layer?**
    Until recently there has been some confusion over dystrophies affecting Bowman's layer because they present with two different sets of characteristics, but historically they have been lumped under Reis-Bücklers dystrophy. The first was described by Reis in 1917 and later by Bücklers in 1949, and the second by Thiel and Behnke in 1967. Küchle et al. recently divided the Bowman's membrane dystrophies into two classifications: corneal dystrophy of Bowman's layer type I and type II. Type I is synonymous with the original Reis-Bücklers dystrophy and equivalent to what also has been described as superficial variant of granular dystrophy. Type II is honeycomb-shaped and is also known as the Thiel-Behnke corneal dystrophy. The two dystrophies have slightly different characteristics on light microscopy. Transmission electron microscopy, on the other hand, differentiates them unequivocally.

11. **Describe the inheritance patterns of the stromal dystrophies.**
    - **Autosomal dominant:** Granular (Groenouw type I; Fig. 12-2), lattice, Avellino granular-lattice, Schnyder's crystalline, fleck, central cloudy of François, pre-Descemet, congenital hereditary (stromal), and posterior amorphous dystrophies
    - **Autosomal recessive:** Macular (Groenouw type II) and possibly gelatinous droplike dystrophies

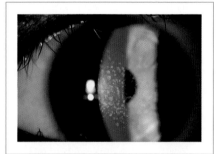

Figure 12-2. Slit-lamp appearance of granular dystrophy.

12. **Match the stromal dystrophy with the histochemical stain for the accumulated substance.**
    - **Granular:** Masson trichrome stains hyaline
    - **Lattice:** Congo red stains amyloid (amyloid deposits exhibit polarized light birefringence and dichroism)
    - **Macular:** Alcian blue stains mucopolysaccharides (glycosaminoglycans)
    - Lattice and macular dystrophies also stain with periodic acid-Schiff stain.

13. **Describe the clinical features of the three major stromal dystrophies.**
See Table 12-1.

TABLE 12-1. CLINICAL FEATURES OF THE THREE MAJOR STROMAL DYSTROPHIES			
Feature	Age of Onset		
	Granular dystrophy	Lattice dystrophy	Macular dystrophy
Deposits	First decade	First decade	First decade
Symptoms	Third decade or none	Second decade	First decade
Decreased vision	Fourth or fifth decade	Second or third decade	First or second decade
Erosions	Uncommon	Frequent	Common
Corneal thickness	Normal	Normal	Thinned
Opacities	Discrete with sharp borders and clear intervening stroma early but becoming hazy later, not extending to limbus	Refractile lines and subepithelial spots, diffuse central haze, not extending to limbus except in advanced cases	Indistinct margins with hazy stroma between, extending to limbus; central lesions more anterior and peripheral lesions more posterior

14. **Is lattice dystrophy associated with systemic amyloidosis?**
There are three types of lattice dystrophy. Only type II (Meretoja's syndrome or familial amyloid polyneuropathy type IV), which has less corneal involvement than types I or III, is associated with systemic findings, including blepharochalasis, bilateral facial nerve palsies, peripheral neuropathy, and systemic amyloidosis.

15. **What is the differential diagnosis of corneal stromal crystals? What systemic findings are associated with Schnyder's crystalline dystrophy?**
The differential diagnosis of corneal stromal crystals includes Bietti's peripheral crystalline dystrophy, cystinosis, and dysproteinemias, such as multiple myeloma, Waldenstrom's macroglobulinemia, and benign monoclonal gammopathy.

Schnyder's dystrophy (Fig. 12-3) is strongly associated with hypercholesterolemia with or without hypertriglyceridemia. There is no direct association with primary

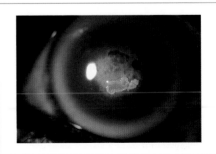

Figure 12-3. Schnyder's crystalline stromal dystrophy.

hyperlipidemias, and serum lipid levels do not correlate with the density of the corneal opacities. The dystrophy more likely represents a localized defect in cholesterol metabolism.

Of importance, not all patients with Schnyder's dystrophy have clinical evidence of corneal crystalline deposits.

Paparo LG, Rapuano CJ, Raber IM, et al: Phototherapeutic keratectomy for Schnyder's crystalline corneal dystrophy. Cornea 19:343–347, 2000.

16. **How does central cloudy dystrophy of François differ from posterior crocodile shagreen?**

Although some physicians have argued that location of the lesions differs in the two conditions, the lesions are clinically the same. It is generally accepted that the polygonal "cracked-ice" lesions of the central cloudy dystrophy of François are more central, deeper, and, by definition, bilateral with an inheritance pattern. On the other hand, posterior crocodile shagreen is more commonly peripheral and anterior stromal and is classified as degeneration. Of importance, both conditions are associated with normal corneal thickness and no recurrent erosions or significant visual compromise.

17. **What characterizes Avellino dystrophy?**

Avellino dystrophy also has been called granular-lattice dystrophy. The granular deposits occur in the anterior stroma early in the progression of the condition, followed later by lattice lesions in the mid to posterior stroma and finally by anterior stromal haze. More patients with Avellino dystrophy experience recurrent erosions than patients with typical granular dystrophy. Recently, the disease-causing genes of lattice dystrophy type I, granular dystrophy, Avellino dystrophy, and Reis-Bücklers dystrophy were mapped to chromosome 5q, suggesting one of the following possibilities:

1. A corneal gene family exists in this region.
2. These corneal dystrophies represent allelic heterogeneity (i.e., different mutations within the same gene manifest as different phenotypes).
3. They are the same disease.

18. **How are stromal dystrophies treated?**

To the extent that some dystrophies, such as lattice and Avellino, are associated with recurrent erosions, they are treated as discussed earlier. When the lesions obscure vision and are restricted to the anterior third of the stroma, they are usually amenable to surgical lamellar or phototherapeutic keratectomy (PTK) with the excimer laser. If the lesions are deeper, lamellar or penetrating keratoplasty is necessary.

19. **Is penetrating keratoplasty a definitive treatment?**

In most instances, penetrating keratoplasty for stromal dystrophies is associated with recurrence of the pathology in the graft as early as 1 year after surgery. The recurrent pathology is sometimes milder than in the original cornea but requires regrafting not infrequently (Fig. 12-4.)

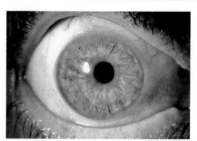

Figure 12-4. Appearance of eye after penetrating keratoplasty.

Dinh R, Rapuano CJ, Cohen EJ, Laibson PR: Recurrence of corneal dystrophy after excimer laser phototherapeutic keratectomy. Ophthalmology 106:1490–1497, 1999.

KEY POINTS: PENETRATING KERATOPLASTY ✓

1. Penetrating keratoplasty is the surgical procedure of choice for stromal and posterior membrane dystrophies.

2. The alternative for stromal dystrophies is deep anterior lamellar keratoplasty (DALK).

3. Penetrating keratoplasty does not prevent recurrence of stromal dystrophy in the donor graft.

4. The alternative for posterior membrane dystrophies is Descemet-stripping endothelial keratoplasty (DSEK).

20. **Name the three posterior membrane dystrophies.**
    - Posterior polymorphous dystrophy (PPMD)
    - Fuchs' endothelial dystrophy
    - Congenital hereditary endothelial dystrophy (CHED)

21. **What is their common clinical manifestation?**
    All three essentially share the pathway of corneal edema and increased thickness, resulting in visual compromise.

22. **Describe the inheritance patterns of the three posterior membrane dystrophies.**
    Posterior polymorphous and Fuchs' dystrophies have an autosomal dominant inheritance pattern. Two forms of congenital hereditary endothelial dystrophy exist. The autosomal dominant form presents in early childhood and is slowly progressive and frequently symptomatic. The autosomal recessive form presents at birth and is nonprogressive, but it is associated with significant visual compromise and nystagmus.

23. **Describe the main clinical characteristics of the three posterior membrane dystrophies.**
    See Table 12-2.

24. **How does Fuchs' dystrophy differ from cornea guttata?**
    Cornea guttata basically refers to a pattern of corneal guttae that are usually found on the central cornea. They sometimes coalesce, produce a beaten metal appearance, and are associated with increased pigmentation. This condition does not affect vision significantly. In 1910 Fuchs described a more severe form of the condition associated with stromal thickening and epithelial edema with secondary visual compromise (Fig. 12-5). This represents a different stage of the same dystrophy.

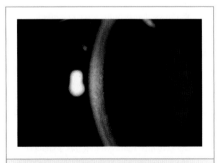

Figure 12-5. Fuchs' endothelial dystrophy.

Adamis AP, Filatov V, Tripathi BJ, Tripathi RC: Fuchs' endothelial dystrophy of the cornea. Surv Ophthalmol 38:149–168, 1993.

TABLE 12-2. MAIN CLINICAL CHARACTERISTICS OF THE THREE POSTERIOR MEMBRANE DYSTROPHIES

Feature	PPMD	Fuchs' Dystrophy	CHED
Onset	Second to third decades, rarely at birth	Fifth to sixth decades	Birth to first decade
Corneal findings	Vesicles, diffuse opacities, and corneal edema	Guttae, stromal thickening, epithelial edema, and subepithelial fibrosis	Endothelium rarely visible with marked corneal thickening and opacification
Other ocular abnormalities	Peripheral synechiae, iris atrophy/corectopia, and glaucoma	Narrow angles and glaucoma	None
Differential diagnosis	ICE syndrome, early-onset CHED	Pseudoguttae, Chandler's syndrome, herpes simplex keratitis, aphakic or pseudophakic bullous keratopathy, and other guttate conditions	Congenital glaucoma, metabolic opacification, Peters' anomaly, forceps injury, early-onset PPMD, and infectious etiologies

ICE = iridocorneal endothelial.

25. **Describe the workup of a patient with Fuchs' dystrophy.**
    - **History:** Ask about previous intraocular surgery
    - **Biomicroscopic examination:** Endothelial guttae, increased stromal thickness, and epithelial edema with possible subepithelial bullae
    - Intraocular pressure measurement
    - Ultrasound or optical pachymetry
    - Specular microscopy to evaluate number, size, and shape of endothelial cells

26. **What overlapping features are seen in PPMD and ICE syndromes?**
    Abnormal corneal endothelium, peripheral anterior synechiae, corectopia, and glaucoma.

27. **What is unique about the CHED cornea?**
    Markedly increased corneal thickness, unlike any other corneal dystrophy.

28. **Discuss management and prognosis of posterior membrane dystrophies.**
    Conservative management has a small role, especially in the earlier stages of Fuchs' dystrophy. Topical hypertonic saline solution, dehydration of the cornea with a blow-dryer, and reduction of intraocular pressure may decrease corneal edema and improve vision. Bandage contact lenses may be used in the setting of recurrent erosions or subepithelial bullae. However, when vision is significantly compromised by Fuchs' or other posterior membrane dystrophies, the definitive solution is penetrating keratoplasty. Penetrating keratoplasty has the best prognosis in Fuchs'

dystrophy, especially in the absence of glaucoma; a fairly good prognosis in PPMD in the absence of glaucoma; and a guarded prognosis in CHED, especially in the early pediatric age group. Currently, techniques of transplanting a posterior corneal lamella, including healthy donor endothelium to replace the affected recipient endothelium, are gaining popularity. Although more technically challenging, Descemet-stripping endothelial keratoplasty (DSEK) is emerging as the procedure of choice (Fig. 12-6).

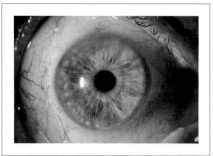

Figure 12-6. Appearance of eye 6 weeks after performance of Descemet-stripping endothelial keratoplasty (DSEK).

Price FW Jr, Price MO: Descemet's stripping with endothelial keratoplasty (DSEK) in 50 eyes: A refractive neutral corneal transplant. J Refract Surg 21:339–345, 2005.

29. **Can PPMD recur in the graft?**
Recurrence of PPMD has been reported.

30. **Discuss considerations for combined cataract extraction and corneal transplantation in patients with Fuchs' dystrophy.**
   - **First scenario: Visually significant cataract and borderline corneal function.** The decision whether to perform corneal transplantation at the time of cataract extraction may be based on a number of factors, including appearance of the corneal endothelium by specular microscopy, corneal thickness, visual variation throughout the day, and postoperative visual requirements of the patient. Patients with no evidence of frank stromal edema, including absence of morning blur and a stable central corneal thickness less than 620 μ, are likely to tolerate cataract extraction alone. The risk of corneal decompensation is outweighed by the advantage of rapid visual rehabilitation from cataract surgery alone. On the other hand, in patients with frank stromal edema, central corneal thickness greater than 650 μ, or an increase of more than 10% in corneal thickness in the morning compared with later in the day, the cornea is unlikely to tolerate routine cataract extraction. The patient will benefit from a triple procedure (i.e., cataract extraction with implant combined with penetrating keratoplasty or DSEK).
   - **Second scenario: Corneal edema requiring corneal transplantation and mild-to-moderate cataract.** One must weigh the added intraoperative risk of cataract surgery and the unpredictability of refractive error after a combined procedure against the risk of graft failure from secondary cataract extraction. Several retrospective studies indicate that most patients undergoing corneal transplantation alone eventually require cataract extraction. The incidence of corneal decompensation after secondary cataract surgery is small. To avoid increased costs and delay in visual rehabilitation, the triple procedure is recommended for patients with Fuchs' endothelial dystrophy and visually significant cataract over nonsimultaneous surgery.

   Note: With the development of DSEK and the associated rapid visual rehabilitation and predictability of refractive error when combined with cataract extraction with intraocular lens (IOL) implantation, more triple corneal procedures (DSEK + cataract extraction with IOL) are likely to be performed for combined moderate corneal endothelial disease and cataract.

Piñeros OE, Cohen EJ, Rapuano CJ, Laibson PR: Triple versus nonsimultaneous procedures in Fuchs' dystrophy and cataract. Arch Ophthalmol 114:525–528, 1996.

31. **List some interesting trivia about corneal dystrophy.**
    ■ The apostrophe in Fuchs' dystrophy is after the "s," not before.
    ■ In cornea guttata, guttata is the adjective describing the cornea. The actual excrescences of Descemet's membrane between the endothelial cells are corneal guttae, not corneal guttata.
    ■ Although keratoconus is usually bilateral and may have an inheritance pattern, it is considered an ectasia, not a dystrophy.

WEBSITES

1. www.corneasociety.com/links.cfm

2. www.nkcf.org

BIBLIOGRAPHY

1. Adamis AP, Filatov V, Tripathi BJ, Tripathi RC: Fuchs' endothelial dystrophy of the cornea. Surv Ophthalmol 38:149–168, 1993.
2. Arffa RC: Grayson's Diseases of the Cornea, 4th ed. St. Louis, Mosby, 1997.
3. Casey TA, Sharif KW: A Color Atlas of Corneal Dystrophies and Degenerations. London, Wolfe Publishing, 1991.
4. Coleman CM, Hannush S, Covello SP, et al: A novel mutation in the helix termination motif of keratin K12 in a U.S. family with Meesmann corneal dystrophy. Am J Ophthalmol 128:687–691, 1999.
5. Cullom RD, Chang B (eds): The Wills Eye Manual: Wills Eye Hospital Office and Emergency Room Diagnosis and Treatment of Eye Disease, 3rd ed. Philadelphia, J.B. Lippincott, 1999.
6. Dinh R, Rapuano CJ, Cohen EJ, Laibson PR: Recurrence of corneal dystrophy after excimer laser phototherapeutic keratectomy. Ophthalmology 106:1490–1497, 1999.
7. Klintworth GK: Advances in the molecular genetics of corneal dystrophies. Am J Ophthalmol 128:747–754, 1999.
8. Krachmer JH, Mannis MJ, Holland EJ: Cornea. St. Louis, Mosby, 1997.
9. Krachmer JH, Palay DA: Cornea Color Atlas. St. Louis, Mosby, 1997.
10. Küchle M, Green WR, Volcker HE, Barraquer J: Reevaluation of corneal dystrophies of Bowman's layer and the anterior stroma (Reis-Bücklers and Thiel-Behnke types): A light and electron microscopic study of eight corneas and review of the literature. Cornea 14:333–354, 1995.
11. Paparo LG, Rapuano CJ, Raber IM, et al: Phototherapeutic keratectomy for Schnyder's crystalline corneal dystrophy. Cornea 19:343–347, 2000.
12. Piñeros OE, Cohen EJ, Rapuano CJ, Laibson PR: Triple versus nonsimultaneous procedures in Fuchs' dystrophy and cataract. Arch Ophthalmol 114:525–528, 1996.
13. Price FW Jr, Price MO: Descemet's stripping with endothelial keratoplasty (DSEK) in 50 eyes: A refractive neutral corneal transplant. J Refract Surg. 21:339–345, 2005.
14. Price FW Jr, Price MO: Descemet's stripping with endothelial keratoplasty (DSEK) in 200 eyes: Early challenges and techniques to promote donor adherence. J Cataract Refract Surg 32:411–418, 2006.
15. Ridgway AE, Akhtar S, Munier FL, et al: Ultrastructural and molecular analysis of Bowman's layer corneal dystrophies: An epithelial origin. Invest Ophthalmol Vis Sci 41:3286–3292, 2000.
16. Small KW, Mullen L, Barletta J, et al: Mapping of Reis-Bücklers' corneal dystrophy to chromosome 5q. Am J Ophthalmol 121:384–390, 1996.
17. Stone EM: Three autosomal dominant corneal dystrophies mapped to chromosome 5q. Nature Genetics 6:47–51, 1994.
18. Waring GO, Rodriguez MM, Laibson RR: Corneal dystrophies. I: Dystrophies of epithelium, Bowman's layer and stroma. Surv Ophthalmol 23:71–122, 1978.
19. Waring GO, Rodriguez MM, Laibson RR: Corneal dystrophies. II: Endothelial dystrophies. Surv Ophthalmol 23:147–168, 1978.

CHAPTER 13

KERATOCONUS

Irving Raber, MD

1. **What is keratoconus?**
   Keratoconus is a noninflammatory ectatic disorder of the cornea that leads to variable visual impairment. The cornea becomes steepened and thinned, thereby inducing myopia and irregular astigmatism. In advanced stages the cornea assumes a conical shape; hence the term keratoconus. The condition is usually bilateral, although frequently asymmetric.

2. **Who gets keratoconus?**
   It is difficult to estimate the incidence of keratoconus because the diagnosis is easily overlooked, especially in the early stages. The reported incidence ranges from 400–600 per 100,000. There does not appear to be a gender predilection. Some studies report a female predominance, whereas other studies report a male predominance. There is no known racial predilection.

3. **What is the cause of keratoconus?**
   The cause of keratoconus is unknown. Various biochemical abnormalities have been documented in keratoconic corneas, including reduced collagen content, decreased or altered keratin sulfate molecules, reduced total protein and increased nonproteinaceous material, and increased collagenolytic and gelatinolytic activity associated with reduced matrix metalloproteinase inhibitor levels. Several studies have shown that the enzyme and proteinase inhibitor abnormalities are most prominent in the epithelial layer of the cornea, which suggests that the basic defect in keratoconus may reside in the epithelium and its interaction with the stroma. Recent evidence also suggests that abnormal processing of free radicals and superoxides within keratoconus corneas leads to buildup of destructive aldehydes and/or peroxynitrites. Eye rubbing has been implicated as a cause of keratoconus. When asked, patients with keratoconus will frequently admit to excessive eye rubbing.

4. **What is the relationship between contact lens wear and keratoconus?**
   The relationship between contact lens wear and keratoconus is controversial. Circumstantial evidence suggests that contact lens wear may lead to the development of keratoconus, especially long-term wearing of rigid contact lenses. Such patients tend to present at an older age and have a flatter corneal curvature than typical patients with keratoconus. In addition, the so-called contact lens-induced cones tend to be more centrally located in the cornea than the more characteristic cones, which are decentered inferiorly.

   In the syndrome known as contact lens warpage, contact lens wear induces irregular astigmatism without slit-lamp features of keratoconus. Discontinuing lens wear for weeks to months eliminates the irregular astigmatism and allows the cornea to resume its normal shape, whereas in the so-called contact lens-induced keratoconus the changes are permanent and do not resolve when contact lens wear is discontinued.

   Some contact lens practitioners are of the opinion that contact lenses can be used to flatten the cornea and reverse or at least retard further progression of keratoconus. However,

I believe that corneal flattening induced by contact lens wear in patients with keratoconus is temporary, and that the cornea reverts to its precontact lens shape once lens wear is discontinued.

5. **Is keratoconus hereditary?**
The role of heredity in keratoconus has not been clearly defined. The vast majority of cases occur sporadically with no familial history. However, some cases of keratoconus are transmitted within families. One study using corneal topography to diagnose subclinical cases of keratoconus documented evidence of familial transmission in 7 of 12 families (58.3%) of patients with keratoconus and no known family history of corneal or ocular disease. The authors postulate autosomal dominant inheritance with incomplete penetrance as the mode of transmission.

6. **What systemic conditions are associated with keratoconus?**
There is a definite relationship between atopy and keratoconus. The prevalence of atopic diseases such as asthma, eczema, atopic keratoconjunctivitis, and hay fever is higher in patients with keratoconus than in normal controls. Atopic patients are bothered by ocular itching, and excessive eye rubbing also may contribute to the development of keratoconus.

There is an association between Down syndrome and keratoconus. Approximately 5% of patients with Down syndrome manifest signs of keratoconus. The incidence of acute hydrops in patients with Down syndrome is definitely higher than in patients without Down syndrome. As in atopic subjects, patients with Down syndrome tend to be vigorous eye rubbers, which may explain, at least in part, the relationship with keratoconus.

Keratoconus is also associated with various connective tissue disorders, such as Ehlers-Danlos syndrome, osteogenesis imperfecta, and Marfan's syndrome. There are conflicting reports of an association between keratoconus, mitral valve prolapse, and joint hypermobility. One study has reported an association between keratoconus and false chordae tendineae in the left ventricle. The relationship between various connective tissue diseases and keratoconus suggests a common defect in the synthesis of connective tissue.

7. **What ocular conditions are associated with keratoconus?**
Keratoconus has been described in association with various ocular diseases, including retinitis pigmentosa, Leber's congenital amaurosis, vernal conjunctivitis, floppy eyelid syndrome, corneal endothelial dystrophy, and posterior polymorphous corneal dystrophy.

8. **What are the symptoms of keratoconus?**
The characteristic onset of keratoconus is in the late teens or early 20s. Symptoms usually begin as blurred vision with shadowing around images. Vision becomes progressively more blurred and distorted with associated glare, halos around lights, light sensitivity, and ocular irritation.

9. **How is the diagnosis of keratoconus made?**
Corneal topography can document the presence of keratoconus even before keratometric or slit-lamp findings become apparent. Placido rings of light are reflected off the cornea, and corneal curvature is derived from the distance between the rings and displayed as a color-coded map. Distortion of these rings may help in early diagnosis. In the early stages of keratoconus, the patient presents with myopic astigmatism. An irregular light reflex with scissoring on retinoscopy can be appreciated through the dilated pupil. As the disease progresses, the cornea steepens and thins with irregularity of the mires on keratometry and development of obvious keratoconus on slit-lamp examination.

KEY POINTS: DIAGNOSIS OF KERATOCONUS

1. Topographic mapping of the anterior corneal surface.

2. Elevation analysis of the anterior and posterior corneal surfaces.

3. Slit-lamp examination of the cornea.

4. Evaluation of the light reflex through a dilated pupil.

10. **What are the topographic signs of keratoconus?**
    The characteristic sign of keratoconus on topography is inferior midperipheral steepening (Fig. 13-1). Numerous studies have tried to develop quantitative topographic parameters to define keratoconus. In one recent study, central corneal power >47.20 diopters (D) combined with steepening of the inferior cornea compared with the superior cornea of >1.20 D detected 98% of patients with keratoconus. However, it may be difficult to make a definitive diagnosis of keratoconus based on topographic findings alone. This is of particular importance in patients seeking refractive surgery because the results of the surgery are poorly predictable in patients with keratoconus. Patients with apparently normal corneas may have inferior midperipheral steepening >1.20 D but normal central corneal powers in the range of 43–45 D. It is difficult to know whether such patients represent a forme fruste of keratoconus and, as such, should be dissuaded from considering refractive surgery. Each case must be analyzed on an individual basis.

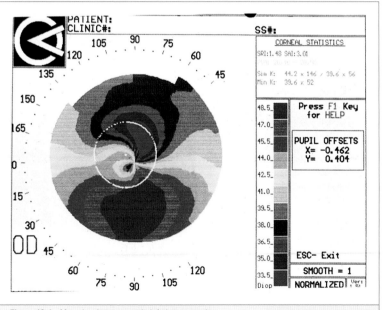

Figure 13-1. Map showing symmetric inferior steepening.

Newer scanning slit topographic units document elevation of the front and back corneal surfaces in relation to a computer-generated best-fit sphere. These instruments also present standard placido disc color maps as well as thickness measurements all across the cornea. The additional information can be helpful in differentiating between forme fruste or early keratoconus and asymmetric astigmatism in nonkeratoconic corneas.

11. **What are the slit-lamp findings of keratoconus?**

The earliest slit-lamp signs of keratoconus are apical thinning and steepening, usually located inferior to the center of the pupil. As the keratoconus progresses, the thinning and ectasia become more prominent with the development of apical scarring that begins in the anterior stroma and then appears in the deeper layers of the stroma (Figs. 13-2, 13-3, and 13–4). Fine linear striae become apparent in the deep stroma just anterior to Descemet's membrane, usually oriented vertically or obliquely. They are thought to represent stress lines in the posterior stroma and are known as Vogt's striae. They can be made to disappear when the intraocular pressure is transiently raised by applying external pressure to the globe. Moreover, in some mild cases of keratoconus, the pressure from rigid gas-permeable contact lens wear can induce the formation of such striae, which disappear when the lens is removed. A Fleischer ring is commonly seen outlining the base of the cone, the result of hemosiderin pigment deposition within the deeper layers of the corneal epithelium. A Fleischer ring may outline the cone only partially but, as the ectasia progresses, tends to become a complete circle with more dense accumulation of pigmentation that is best appreciated while viewing the cobalt blue filter on the slit lamp. Subepithelial fibrillary lines have been described in a concentric circular fashion just inside the Fleischer ring. The source of these fibrils is unknown but has been postulated as epithelial nerve filaments. Anterior clear spaces thought to represent breaks in Bowman's membrane are sometimes seen within the thin portion of the

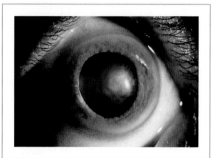

Figure 13-2. Apical scarring.

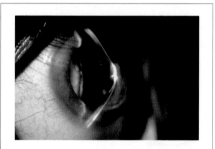

Figure 13-3. Apical thinning and scarring demonstrated in slit beam.

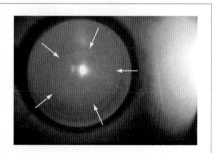

Figure 13-4. Cobalt blue illumination demonstrating Fleischer ring outlining the extent of the cone. *Arrows* point to margins of the ring.

conical protrusion. Prominent corneal nerves are reportedly more common in keratoconic corneas. In the more advanced stages, when the eye is rotated downward, the corneal ectasia causes protrusion of the lower lid, which is known as Munson's sign.

12. **How does keratoconus progress?**
The onset of keratoconus characteristically occurs in the mid to late teens, progressing slowly for several years before stabilizing. However, delayed onset or late progression of keratoconus is not uncommon. As the disease progresses, the corneal thinning and ectasia become more prominent with increasing apical scarring. Two types of cones have been described: (1) a small round or nipple-shaped cone that tends to be more central in location, and (2) an oval or sagging cone that is usually larger and displaced inferiorly, with the thinning extending close to the inferior limbus. Progression of keratoconus tends to manifest as increased thinning and protrusion, although enlargement of the cone also occurs with extension peripherally.

13. **What is acute hydrops?**
Acute hydrops (Fig. 13-5) occurs in the more advanced cases of keratoconus. Ruptures in Descemet's membrane allow aqueous to enter into the corneal stroma, resulting in marked thickening and opacification of the cornea that is usually restricted to the cone. The involved stroma becomes massively thickened with large, fluid-filled clefts, overlying epithelial edema, and bulla formation. Rarely, a fistulous tract may develop, with resultant leakage of aqueous through the fluid-filled stroma and epithelium on the corneal surface.

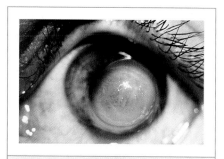

Figure 13-5. Acute hydrops.

The corneal edema gradually resolves over weeks to months as endothelial cells adjacent to the rupture in Descemet's membrane enlarge and migrate across the defect, laying down new Descemet's membrane. With healing, scarring tends to flatten the cornea, thereby facilitating the possibility of subsequent contact lens fitting. Some corneas with acute hydrops tend to develop stromal neovascularization that increases the potential risk of graft rejection if corneal transplantation becomes necessary. Acute hydrops is more common in patients with Down syndrome and vernal kerato-conjunctivitis, presumably related to the repeated trauma of eye rubbing in these patients.

Most cases of acute hydrops resolve spontaneously, requiring supportive treatment with topical hyperosmotic agents such as 5% sodium chloride drops and/or ointment to promote corneal deturgescence. Some patients with acute hydrops complain of severe photophobia and benefit from the use of topical steroids and/or cycloplegic agents. In addition, topical steroids should be instituted in patients with signs of corneal neovascularization. Once the hydrops has resolved, the patient can then try to resume contact lens wear if the central cornea has not become excessively scarred. Otherwise the only alternative is a corneal transplant.

14. **What is the histopathology of keratoconus?**
Most histopathologic studies of keratoconic corneas are performed on advanced cases that require penetrating keratoplasty. In addition, most patients were previous long-term contact lens wearers, which also may affect the histopathologic findings.

Changes have been described in every layer of the cornea. The stroma of the cone is thinner than the surrounding cornea. The apical epithelium tends to be flattened and thinned with scattered fragmentation and dehiscence of the epithelial basement membrane. Iron can be demonstrated in the epithelial cells outlining the cone, corresponding to the Fleischer ring.

Among the most characteristic histologic changes of keratoconus are breaks in Bowman's membrane that are sometimes filled with epithelium and/or stromal collagen. Ultimately, the anterior corneal stroma may become replaced with irregularly arranged connective tissue.

Descemet's membrane is normal unless acute hydrops has occurred. Depending on the stage of the reparative process, breaks in Descemet's membrane with curled edges subsequently become covered by adjacent endothelial cells that slide over and lay down new membrane. The corneal endothelial cells tend to be normal, although they may exhibit increased pleomorphism.

15. How is keratoconus treated?

Mild cases of keratoconus can be successfully managed with spectacles. However, as the keratoconus progresses and the amount of irregular astigmatism increases, patients become unable to obtain satisfactory vision with spectacle correction. Contact lenses can then be used to neutralize the irregular astigmatism, thereby offering significant visual improvement over spectacles. As the cornea becomes more distorted and ectatic, contact lens fitting becomes more difficult and vision deteriorates, ultimately necessitating surgical intervention.

16. What types of contact lenses are used to treat keratoconus?

Conventional spherical myopic soft contact lenses may be used successfully in mild cases of keratoconus with minimal manifest astigmatism. Toric soft contact lenses also may be used in some patients without excessive amounts of irregular astigmatism. The vast majority of patients with keratoconus are managed with rigid gas-permeable contact lenses. Fitting such lenses over a distorted ectatic cornea is difficult. Numerous lens designs are available for fitting patients with keratoconus, including varying diameters of spherical lenses, aspheric lenses, toric lenses, and lenses with multiple curvatures on the posterior surface, such as the Soper cone lens. The Soper cone lenses have a steeper central curve to vault the apex of the cone and a flatter peripheral curve to align with the more normal peripheral cornea. Computed topography is used by some contact lens practitioners to help fit these challenging patients.

Large gas-permeable scleral contact lenses are sometimes used to manage patients with prominent ectatic cones who cannot be fit with more conventional gas-permeable lenses and, for whatever reason, are not considered good candidates for corneal transplantation. A piggyback system is another option available for treating patients with keratoconus: A gas-permeable contact lens is fitted on top of a soft contact lens. This system is expensive and time-consuming for both practitioner and patient but can be helpful in managing select cases that have failed more conventional contact lens fitting. Another specialized lens design incorporates a rigid gas-permeable center with a soft peripheral skirt to reduce the edge awareness of conventional gas-permeable lenses. Moreover, such "saturn-style" lenses may actually center better and offer a more stable fit by virtue of their large diameter, which extends beyond the limbus.

17. What are the surgical options for treating keratoconus?

Surgical intervention is reserved for patients with keratoconus who cannot be successfully fit with contact lenses or who fail to obtain satisfactory vision with contact lenses. Atopic patients with keratoconus tend to come to surgery much more frequently than nonallergic patients because the allergic diathesis tends to interfere with contact lens tolerance.

- **Penetrating keratoplasty (full-thickness corneal transplantation)** is the most common surgical technique used to rehabilitate patients with keratoconus. The surgical procedure requires excision of the entire cone, frequently determined by the outline of the Fleischer ring.

If the cone extends close to the limbus (usually inferiorly), a large corneal graft is needed. Usually the grafted tissue is centered on the pupil, but when the cone is eccentric, an eccentric graft is used to encompass the entire cone, taking care to leave the optical zone free of sutures. Increasing graft size with proximity to the limbal blood vessel reduces the "immune privilege" of the usually avascular cornea, thereby increasing the risk of immunologic reaction.

- **Lamellar (partial-thickness) keratoplasty** may be used in patients with keratoconus, although the procedure is technically more difficult and in the hands of most surgeons achieves a slightly poorer visual outcome than a full-thickness procedure. However, a lamellar graft has the advantage of being an extraocular procedure that avoids the risk of endothelial rejection. Most cases of lamellar keratoplasty are performed as tectonic procedures for large cones in which the thinning extends out to the limbus. If a satisfactory visual result is not obtained, a smaller central full-thickness corneal transplant can subsequently be performed within the confines of the lamellar graft, thereby avoiding the increased risk of immunologic rejection with large full-thickness corneal transplants.

- **Intracorneal rings** are polymethylmethacrylate ring segments that are inserted into the midperipheral corneal stroma. They have recently been reported to be useful in treating mild keratoconus in patients who are contact lens-intolerant. The corneas included in the study were free of central scarring and no thinner than 400 microns. The rationale of the procedure is to reinforce the ectatic area of the cornea, thereby reducing corneal steepening and irregular astigmatism associated with keratoconus, with improvement in both uncorrected and best spectacle-corrected visual acuity. Further studies are needed to corroborate these findings and to determine if placement of these ring segments within keratoconus corneas will in fact slow or prevent progression of corneal ectasia.

- **Epikeratophakia** is a type of onlay lamellar procedure using a freeze-dried donor cornea that is sewn on top of a de-epithelialized host cornea. The purpose of this procedure is to flatten the cornea with the hope of offering improved spectacle-corrected visual acuity and/or better contact lens fitting. After initial enthusiasm in the late 1980s, the procedure has been abandoned by most surgeons because of complications and poor visual results. However, in select cases in which a full-thickness corneal transplant is contraindicated, such as patients with Down syndrome who may aggressively rub their eyes and dehisce a full-thickness wound or patients at high risk for immune rejection (e.g., multiple graft failures in the other eye), partial-thickness procedures such as lamellar grafts or epikeratophakia are worthy of consideration.

- **Thermokeratoplasty** is a technique in which heating the cornea to 90–120°C causes shrinkage of corneal collagen fibers with resulting flattening of the cornea. This procedure has been abandoned for the most part because of unpredictable results, induced scarring, and the potential for recurrent corneal erosions because of damage to the epithelial basement membrane complex. However, when the apex of the cone spares the visual axis, thermokeratoplasty may be used to flatten the cornea, thereby allowing more favorable spectacle-corrected visual acuity and/or contact lens fitting. In addition, thermokeratoplasty may be helpful in promoting resolution of acute hydrops.

Some patients with keratoconus develop an elevated subepithelial scar at the apex of the cone as the result of chronic apical irritation from contact lens wear. Corneal epithelial breakdown may develop over the scar, thereby interfering with contact lens wear. These scars can be removed manually with a blade or with the excimer laser, thereby allowing resumption of contact lens wear and sparing the patient an otherwise needed corneal transplant.

18. **What are the results of corneal transplant in patients with keratoconus?**
As mentioned previously, most corneal surgery for keratoconus involves penetrating keratoplasty. The results of such surgery are excellent with clear grafts in approximately 90% of patients, most of whom obtain visual acuity of 20/40 or better. The most frequent problem

arising in patients with keratoconus who undergo corneal transplantation is high postkeratoplasty astigmatism. However, the astigmatism following corneal transplant surgery tends to be regular as opposed to the irregular astigmatism of the original disorder. This difference allows most patients to achieve satisfactory visual results with spectacle correction, even if they have a large amount of astigmatism that most patients without keratoconus would not be able to tolerate in spectacles. Because keratoconus tends to be asymmetric, many patients undergoing corneal transplantation in one eye manage with a contact lens in the lesser involved eye and thus prefer to wear a contact lens in the operated eye as well. The contact lens tends to neutralize most of the astigmatism in the corneal transplant. A small percentage of patients may not be able to tolerate a large degree of astigmatism in spectacles. If they cannot be fit with a contact lens, they ultimately require keratorefractive surgery to reduce the astigmatic error.

It usually takes up to a full year or more for the corneal transplant wound to heal. If the patient is seeing well with the sutures in place, the sutures (most commonly 10–0 nylon) are left undisturbed and tend to disintegrate spontaneously over a few years. Sometimes disintegrating sutures erode through the corneal epithelium and cause a foreign body sensation. If they are not removed from the surface of the cornea, they may cause secondary infection. After sutures disintegrate and/or are removed, a significant change in the refractive error is frequently notable. All graft sutures should have disintegrated or be removed before keratorefractive surgery is contemplated.

Graft rejection occurs in approximately 25% of patients with keratoconus who undergo penetrating keratoplasty. Most rejections can be reversed with appropriate local steroid therapy if they are caught early. Irreversible rejection leads to permanent corneal clouding that requires repeat penetrating keratoplasty. A repeat graft has a reasonably good prognosis, although the success rate is lower than the primary graft and tends to diminish with each successive transplant if multiple graft failures occur.

WEBSITE

National Keratoconus Foundation
www.KNCF.org

BIBLIOGRAPHY

1. Bron AJ: Keratoconus. Cornea 7:163–169, 1988.
2. Colin J, Cochener B, Savary G, Malet F: Correcting keratoconus with intracorneal rings. J Cataract Refract Surg 26:1117–1122, 2000.
3. Kenney MC, Brown DJ, Rajeev B: The elusive causes of keratoconus: A working hypothesis. CLAO J 26:10–13, 2000.
4. Krachmer JH, Feder RS, Belin MW: Keratoconus and related noninflammatory thinning disorders. Surv Ophthalmol 28:293–322, 1984.
5. Lawless M, Coster DJ, Phillips AJ, Loane M: Keratoconus: Diagnosis and management. Aust NZ J Ophthalmol 17:33–60, 1989.
6. Macsai MS, Valery GA, Krackmer JH: Development of keratoconus after contact lens wear: Patient characteristics. Arch Ophthalmol 108:534–538, 1990.
7. Maeda N, Klyce SD, Smolek MD: Comparison of methods for detecting keratoconus using video keratography. Arch Ophthalmol 113:870–874, 1995.
8. Tuft SJ, Moodaley LC, Gregory WM, et al: Prognostic factors for the progression of keratoconus. Ophthalmology 101:439–447, 1994.

CHAPTER 14

REFRACTIVE SURGERY

Brandon D. Ayres, MD, and Christopher J. Rapuano, MD

1. **What are the refractive components of the eye?**
   The cornea and the lens refract incident light so that it is focused on the fovea, the center of the retina. The cornea contributes approximately 44 diopters (D) compared with only 18 D from the lens. In addition, anterior chamber depth and axial length of the eye contribute to refractive status.

2. **What are the different types of refractive errors?**
   - **Myopia,** or nearsightedness, exists when the refractive elements of the eye place the image in front of the retina.
   - **Hyperopia,** or farsightedness, exists when the image is focused behind the retina.
   - **Astigmatism** usually refers to corneal irregularity that requires unequal power in different meridians to place a single image on the fovea. Lenticular astigmatism (due to the lens) is less common than corneal astigmatism.
   - **Presbyopia** is the natural impairment in accommodation often noted around age 40 years. The power of the corrective "add" or bifocal segment to combat presbyopia increases with age.

3. **How is myopia related to age?**
   Myopia is common among premature infants, less common in full-term infants, and uncommon at 6 months of age, when mild hyperopia is the rule. Myopia becomes most prevalent in adolescence (approximately 25%), peaking by 20 years of age and subsequently leveling off. This information is important for determining the appropriate age to consider refractive surgery.

4. **What are the goals of refractive surgery?**
   Goals vary for each patient. Certain patients desire refractive surgery because of professional or lifestyle issues; examples include athletes and police, fire, and military personnel, who may find glasses or contact lenses hindering or even dangerous. Other patients, such as high myopes, may find spectacle correction inadequate because of image minification or may be intolerant of contact lenses. In general, the goals of refractive surgery are to reduce or eliminate the need for glasses or refractive lenses without altering the quality of vision or best-corrected vision.

5. **What features characterize a good candidate for refractive surgery? Are there any contraindications?**
   First, patients considering refractive surgery should be at least 18–21 years of age with a stable refraction. Patients with ocular conditions (severe dry eye or uveitis) or systemic diseases, and patients taking medications that impair wound healing are poor candidates. Keratoconus, a condition in which the cornea is irregularly cone-shaped, remains a contraindication for refractive surgery because results are unpredictable. Analysis of corneal curvature, often using computerized corneal topography, should be performed on all patients before surgery because early keratoconus has a prevalence of up to 13% in this population and may be missed by other diagnostic methods.

Second, patients' motivations and expectations should be explored thoroughly so that unrealistic hopes may be discovered preoperatively. For example, the patient who is constantly cleaning his or her glasses because of "excruciating glare" from dust on the lenses or who desires perfect uncorrected vision is not a good candidate for refractive surgery. A careful discussion of the risks and benefits of surgery is particularly important. Patients may want to try contact lenses before considering surgery. The concept of presbyopia must also be explained; many patients are prepresbyopic and have no understanding that achieving excellent uncorrected vision at distance will require correction for reading at near within a few years.

6. **How is corneal topography used in the evaluation of patients undergoing refractive surgery?**
   Corneal topography typically refers to the use of computer-based videokeratography to accurately evaluate corneal curvature. Most topographic systems use a video camera to detect reflected images of rings projected onto the cornea. A computer generates a topographic "map" of corneal curvature based on the measured distance between the rings reflected from the cornea (Fig. 14-1). Other topographic systems use slit beams, special photographic methods, or high-frequency ultrasound to evaluate corneal curvature and elevation. These systems can also estimate corneal thickness.

   Topography is extremely useful for evaluating patients undergoing refractive surgery because it generates precise images of corneal curvature that correspond to a large area of the cornea. Subtle corneal abnormalities, such as early keratoconus or contact lens-induced corneal warpage, may be detected by this method only. In addition, postoperative and preoperative topographic maps may be analyzed to generate "difference" maps that isolate the procedure-induced changes. Computerized corneal topography is also extremely useful for determining the cause of imperfect vision after refractive surgery, which is commonly due to irregular astigmatism.

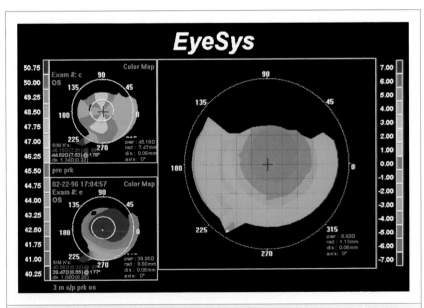

Figure 14-1. Corneal topography. Upper left shows preoperative myopic astigmatism. Lower left shows a central flattening 3 months after photorefractive keratectomy. On right, the difference map demonstrates treatment effect of the excimer laser.

7. **What are the major options for the surgical treatment of myopia?**
   - Radial keratotomy (RK)
   - Photorefractive keratectomy (PRK)
   - Laser in-situ keratomileusis (LASIK)
   - Intracorneal ring segments (Intacs)
   - Phakic intraocular lens (IOL) implants
   - Clear lens extraction

8. **How does RK reduce myopia?**
   Deep radial incisions created with a diamond blade cause steepening of the cornea peripherally, which results in secondary flattening of the central cornea. The number, length, and depth of incisions and the size of the clear, central optical zone along with the patient's age determine the refractive effect. Typically, four incisions are used for low myopia (Fig. 14-2) and eight incisions for moderate myopia. Optical zones <3 mm in diameter are associated with greater reduction of myopia but also greater risk of refractive instability and optical aberrations such as glare or starburst.

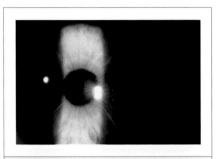

Figure 14-2. Three weeks after four-incision radial keratotomy.

   Sanders DR, Deitz MR, Gallagher D: Factors affecting predictability of radial keratotomy. Ophthalmology 92:1237–1243, 1985.
   Waring GO III: Refractive Keratectomy for Myopia. St. Louis, Mosby, 1992.

9. **What are the various RK techniques?**
   - The "American" technique involves making centrifugal incisions (from the center toward the limbus) with an angled diamond knife blade.
   - The "Russian" technique uses centripetal incisions (from the limbus toward the center) with a straight vertical diamond knife blade. The Russian technique gives deeper incisions and more refractive effect; however, there is greater danger of entering the optical zone.
   - A combined bidirectional technique uses an angled blade edge on one side for centrifugal incisions, which are performed first, combined with a vertical blade edge on the other side to perform a second centripetal incision. The vertical blade edge is sharp only at the tip so that the second incision stops at the optical zone. This technique allows the creation of a deep and square, rather than sloped, incision near the optical zone.

   Based on statistical analysis of previous cases, standardized nomograms are used to determine the number of incisions and optical zone size, depending on the patient's age and desired refractive change. Each ophthalmologist must monitor his or her own results to make surgeon-specific modifications in the nomograms.

10. **What results have been achieved with RK? What about complications?**
    Several major investigations have been performed, the most important of which is the Prospective Evaluation of Radial Keratotomy (PERK). This study showed that 60% of treated eyes were within 1 D of emmetropia up to 10 years postoperatively. After 10 years, 53% had at least 20/20 uncorrected vision, and 85% had at least 20/40 vision. However, 43% of eyes had a progressive shift toward hyperopia of at least 1 D after 10 years. This shift was noted to be worse for eyes with the smaller optical zone of 3 mm. Only 3% of patients lost two or more lines of best-corrected visual acuity, and all had 20/30 vision or better. Three of more than 400

patients complained of severe glare or starburst that made night driving impossible. Corneal perforations occurred in 2% of cases; none required a suture for closure. Overall, the best results were achieved in the low myopia group (−2.00 D to −3.00 D).

Waring et al. reported similar results in 615 eyes 1 year after RK using the Russian technique. Their data showed that 54% of eyes had 20/20 vision and 93% had 20/40 uncorrected vision 1 year postoperatively. One percent (six eyes) lost two to three lines of best-corrected vision, but all had 20/30 vision or better. Despite a significant increase in glare and fluctuation in vision from baseline, 90% of patients were satisfied with the outcome after RK. As with any invasive procedure, infection is a small but real risk (Fig. 14-3). With the tremendous advances in laser refractive surgery over the past decades, RK is rarely performed.

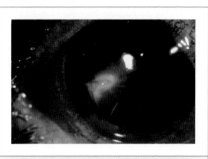

Figure 14-3. Infection at radial keratotomy incision.

Waring GO III, Casebeer JC, Dru RM: One-year results of a prospective multicenter study of the Casebeer system of refractive keratotomy. Casebeer Chiron Study Group. Ophthalmology 103:1337–1347, 1996.

Waring GO III, Lynn MJ, Gelender H, et al: Results of the prospective evaluation of radial keratotomy (PERK) study one year after surgery. Ophthalmology 92:177–198, 307, 1985.

Waring GO III, Lynn MJ, McDonnell PJ: Results of the prospective evaluation of radial keratotomy (PERK) study 10 years after surgery. Arch Ophthalmol 112:1298–1308, 1994.

11. **How does PRK reduce myopia?**
Unlike RK, which causes central corneal flattening indirectly through steepening of the corneal periphery, PRK involves direct laser treatment of the central corneal stroma. Specifically, the "**exci**ted di**mer**" (excimer) 193-nm UV laser causes flattening of the central cornea through a photoablative/photodecomposition process whereby more tissue is removed centrally than peripherally. Under topical anesthesia, the central corneal epithelium is removed either with a spatula or the laser. The laser is then used to ablate a precise quantity of stromal tissue with submicron accuracy to achieve the desired refractive effect.

12. **What results have been achieved with PRK? What about complications?**
In some respects, the results with excimer laser are comparable to those of RK for the same magnitude of myopia (−1.00 D to −6.00 D), as indicated by the Summit and VISX experience at 1 year:
- 68% were within 1 D of emmetropia (versus 60% for RK).
- 60% had at least 20/20 vision (versus 53% for RK).
- 90% had at least 20/40 vision without correction (versus 85% for RK).
- In the subgroup of patients with low-to-moderate myopia (1.5–2.9 D), 80% had at least 20/20 uncorrected vision.
- Refraction was generally stable by 6–9 months, depending on the amount of myopia treated. According to the United Kingdom excimer laser clinical trial, at 12 years:
- Postoperative refraction remained stable with no major change in mean spherical equivalent.
- 4% have residual corneal haze that did not reduce best-corrected visual acuity (Figs. 14-4 and 14-5).
- Nighttime halo was a significant problem (4-mm optical zone used in this study).

O'Brart DP, Corbett MC, Lohmann CP, et al: The effects of ablation diameter on the outcome of excimer laser photorefractive keratectomy. A prospective, randomized, double-blind study. Arch Ophthalmol 113:438–443, 1995.

Rajan MS, Jaycock P, O'Brart D, et al: A long-term study of photorefractive keratectomy; 12-year follow-up. Ophthalmology 111:1813–1824, 2004.

13. **Discuss the major advantages and disadvantages of PRK versus RK.**

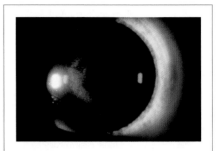

Figure 14-4. Mild stromal haze, 3 months after photorefractive keratectomy.

   - The cornea is weakened in RK but not in PRK because RK is an incisional technique. Permanent weakening of the globe may be important in patients who are at risk for blunt trauma (athletes, military personnel).
   - Unlike RK, PRK is associated with no diurnal variation in refraction.
   - It may be easier to resume soft lens wear after PRK than after RK (for the minority of patients who require contact lenses).
   - The "hyperopic shift" associated with RK is much less frequently experienced after PRK. The initial hyperopic phase after PRK, which precedes the return to emmetropia, may be prolonged in patients over the age of 40 because of decreased accommodative reserve.

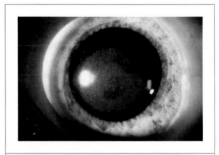

Figure 14-5. Moderate-to-severe stromal haze, 6 months after photorefractive keratectomy.

   - A significant advantage of RK is the relative speed of recovery. Patients undergoing RK may have excellent uncorrected vision on postoperative day 1. After PRK, healing of the epithelial defect may delay return of good vision and comfort for 1–2 weeks.
   - RK currently is less expensive than PRK.

14. **What is LASIK?**
    LASIK stands for laser in-situ keratomileusis. The procedure involves creating a corneal flap to ablate midstromal tissue directly with an excimer laser beam, ultimately flattening the cornea to treat myopia and steepening the cornea to treat hyperopia. Whereas earlier techniques of keratomileusis consisted of removing a corneal cap and resecting stromal tissue manually, technologic advancements have revolutionized this procedure into a highly automated process. Contemporary techniques use a suction ring with a blade guide, an automated microkeratome blade, and an excimer laser. After a lid speculum is placed and topical anesthetic is applied, the suction ring is centered on the cornea to apply a constant suction pressure >65 mmHg on the eye (as measured by an applanation tonometry device). The microkeratome blade is then placed on the guide of the suction ring and advanced to create a hinged flap with a depth approximately 15–25% of the corneal thickness. The blade stops approximately 0.5 mm short of a complete flap resection. The suction on the ring is shut off, and the flap is then lifted and moved to the side on its hinge, exposing a bed of bare stroma. Next,

the excimer laser is applied directly to the stromal tissue. Afterward, the corneal flap is replaced to its original position, typically without sutures, and allowed to heal.

Salah T, Waring GO III, el Maghraby A, et al: Excimer laser in situ keratomileusis under a corneal flap for myopia of 2 to 20 diopters. Am J Ophthalmol 121:143–155, 1996.

15. **How have advancements in the LASIK procedure helped to improve results?**
The use of a suction ring helps to maintain constant pressure on the eye so that the microkeratome blade makes a smooth and uniform cut through a single plane of corneal tissue. Automation of the microkeratome with a mechanically operated turbine drive on a blade guide also has contributed to producing a smooth, regular cut with the ability to leave a hinge (so that the corneal flap can be easily realigned to its original position). The excimer laser beam also allows for the controlled and monitored removal of stromal tissue, thereby adding greater precision, predictability, and reproducibility to the results.

Waring GO III, Carr JD, Stulting RD, et al: Prospective randomized comparison of simultaneous and sequential bilateral laser in situ keratomileusis for the correction of myopia. Ophthalmology 106:732–738, 1999.

16. **What is the range of myopia recommended for correction with LASIK?**
LASIK is generally recommended for myopia as low as 1 D and as high as 10–12 D, although it is FDA-approved for myopia up to 14 D.

17. **What are the advantages and disadvantages of LASIK versus RK and PRK?**
LASIK offers the advantage of minimal postoperative pain as well as earlier recovery of vision because the epithelium is left essentially intact. There is less chance of corneal scarring and haze than after RK and PRK. The disadvantages of LASIK include the brief intraoperative period of marked visual loss (due to high intraocular pressures generated by the suction ring), the risk of flap irregularities, subluxation or dislocation, and the expense of the procedure. Additional problems associated with LASIK include irregular astigmatism and the potential for epithelial ingrowth or infection under the flap.

LASIK offers several advantages to the surgeon. Because the technique involves making a flap in the anterior corneal stroma, the risk of corneal perforation associated with RK is virtually nonexistent. The creation of a uniform smooth flap with preservation of the central Bowman's layer also reduces the subepithelial scarring seen with PRK. The overall mechanization of the technique allows little room for surgeon error. However, its automated aspect also poses disadvantages. The surgeon has limited intraoperative control over creation of the flap and ablation of the stroma. The microkeratome also requires extensive care for proper performance. The suction ring device is cumbersome and can be difficult to place on a patient with narrow palpebral fissures or deep orbits. If the suction is released during the use of the microkeratome, the corneal flap may be damaged.

18. **How do the surgical results of LASIK compare with those of PRK?**
Several studies have compared the results of LASIK and PRK in both low-to-moderate and moderate-to-high myopia. Overall, the refractive and visual results are comparable after the first 1–3 months. LASIK definitely results in faster visual recovery. Pop and Payette compared the results of LASIK and PRK for the treatment of myopia between −1 and −9 D. They concluded that visual and refractive outcomes were similar at follow-up visits between 1 and 12 months, but LASIK patients were more likely to experience halos. In general, when refractive subgroups are analyzed, less predictable results are achieved in the higher myopia groups for both procedures. Nevertheless, LASIK may be the best corneal technique available for treating higher degrees of myopia. Long-term stability requires further study.

Pop M, Payette Y: Photorefractive keratectomy versus laser in situ keratomileusis: A control-matched study. Ophthalmology 107:251–257, 2000.

19. **What is "wavefront?" Are wavefront ablations any better than standard LASIK?**
In standard LASIK the spherical and cylindrical aberrations are measured using computerized corneal topography, and manifest and cycloplegic refraction. The excimer laser is then programmed based on this data. A wavefront measurement has the ability to measure many more aberrations than just sphere and cylinder. To measure a wavefront an aberrometer shines low-intensity laser light through the pupil. The laser light is then reflected off the retina, through the lens, pupil, and cornea, and is distorted by the refractive properties of the eye. This wavefront of light is then used to detect an infinite number of ocular aberrations (evaluated, for example, by Zernike polynomials or Fournier analysis).

In a wavefront ablation the data collected by the aberrometer is converted into a sphere and cylindrical equivalent (usually with room for a physician adjustment) and the customized ablation is carried out. Although the hope for wavefront-guided LASIK and PRK is high, clinical evidence that it is significantly better than carefully planned standard LASIK is lacking. Some studies have shown a reduction in higher order aberrations after wavefront-guided ablations, while others have shown an increase. As surgical technique and technology improve, perhaps the clinical results of wavefront LASIK will begin to outshine standard LASIK.

20. **Name the important potential complications of LASIK.**
Complications are uncommon and are not listed in order of frequency:
- Premature release of suction ring
- Intraoperative flap amputation
- Postoperative flap dislocation/subluxation (may require suturing of flap into place)
- Epithelialization of flap-bed interface (causes irregular astigmatism, light scattering, and possibly flap damage)
- Irregular astigmatism
- Infection
- Diffuse lamellar keratitis (DLK)
- Progressive corneal ectasia

Tham VM, Maloney RK: Microkeratome complications of laser in situ keratomileusis. Ophthalmology 107:920–924, 2000.

KEY POINTS: COMMON POTENTIAL CONTRAINDICATIONS TO LASIK

1. Thin cornea.
2. Irregular astigmatism.
3. Keratoconus.
4. Anterior basement membrane dystrophy.
5. Herpes simplex or zoster keratitis.

21. **What is diffuse lamellar keratitis (DLK)? How is it treated?**
DLK was originally termed "sands of the Sahara syndrome" because of the clinical appearance of a wavy inflammatory reaction in a LASIK flap interface. It generally appears 1–3 days after a primary LASIK procedure or an enhancement. The exact cause is unknown and is most likely multifactorial. Suspected etiologies include bacterial endotoxins, meibomian secretions, oils from the microkeratome, and excessive laser energy from the IntraLase femtosecond laser.

Treatment involves high-dose topical steroids. In severe cases, lifting the flap and irrigating the interface may be helpful.

Holland SP, Mathias RG, Morck DW, et al: Diffuse lamellar keratitis related to endotoxins released from sterilizer reservoir biofilms. Ophthalmology 107:1227–1234, 2000.

22. **What is Epi-LASIK? What are the potential advantages?**
Epi-LASIK is a modified surface ablation, which uses a keratome and an epithelial separator that creates a plane between the epithelial basement membrane and Bowman's membrane. As the "epitheliatome" passes over the eye it creates an epithelial flap on a hinge, very similar to a LASIK flap. The epithelial flap is then reflected, exposing the surface of Bowman's membrane. The excimer laser is then used to alter the shape of the cornea, after which the epithelial flap is repositioned. The advantage of Epi-LASIK is the safety of a surface procedure but with potentially faster visual recovery, less postoperative discomfort, and less haze than PRK. Preliminary clinical results suggest that Epi-LASIK is safe and effective for low myopia, but further studies need to be done before Epi-LASIK becomes fully established.

Pallikaris IG, Kalyvianaki MI, Katsanevaki VJ, Ginis HS: Epi-LASIK: Preliminary clinical results of an alternative surface ablation procedure. J Cataract Refract Surg 31:879–885, 2005.

23. **What is the femtosecond laser? What are its potential advantages?**
The femtosecond laser is a tool that uses ultrafast (15 kHz) pulses of energy to ablate tissue with extreme precision. The ultrashort pulses prevent heat buildup, thus allowing minimal to no damage to surrounding tissues. In refractive surgery this laser is used to cut a lamellar flap in the cornea. The potential advantages of using the femtosecond laser, or IntraLase, include greater safety, reproducibility of flap thickness, decreased flap complications, and decreased epithelial defects. Flap striae and interface deposits may also be reduced. Many physicians also feel the refractive outcome is improved especially in wavefront-guided procedures.

Binder PS: Flap dimensions created with the IntraLase FS laser. J Cataract Refract Surg 30:26–32, 2004.
Durrie DS, Kezirian GM: Femtosecond laser versus mechanical keratome flaps in wavefront-guided laser in situ keratomileusis: prospective contralateral eye study. J Cataract Refract Surg 31:120–126, 2005.
Touboul D, Salin F, Mortemousque B, et al: Advantages and disadvantages of the femtosecond laser microkeratome. J Fr Ophthalmol 28:535–546, 2005.

24. **What is progressive corneal ectasia?**
Corneal ectasia is progressive corneal thinning and steepening with irregular astigmatism that causes poor vision. It is thought to result mainly in eyes with "forme fruste" keratoconus, or from too thin a stromal bed after LASIK. Most surgeons believe that the stromal bed (calculated by taking the central corneal thickness minus the flap thickness minus the laser ablation) should be at least 250 μm to prevent corneal ectasia. However, other surgeons believe that the minimal stromal bed thickness should be greater. Long-term follow-up is required to determine the answer.

25. **What are intracorneal ring segments?**
Intracorneal ring segments (Intacs) are an FDA-approved procedure for the correction of low myopia, and more recently for mild to moderate keratoconus. This procedure involves the placement of two 150-degree arc segments of polymethylmethacrylate plastic at two-thirds depths in the peripheral cornea. This "tissue addition" results in flattening of the central cornea.

Rapuano CJ, Sugar A, Koch DD, et al: Intrastromal corneal ring segments for low myopia: A report by the American Academy of Ophthalmology. Ophthalmology 108:1922–1928, 2001.

26. **How much myopia do Intacs treat?**
Intacs are FDA-approved to treat between −1 and −3 D of nearsightedness in patients with no more than 1 D of astigmatism, and who are at least 21 years old.

27. **What are the refractive results of Intacs for myopia?**
   In the U.S. clinical trials at 1 year, 97% of patients had 20/40 vision or better, 74% had 20/20 vision or better, and 53% had 20/16 vision or better without correction.

28. **List the potential complications of Intacs.**
   Complications are not common and are not listed in order of frequency.
   - Induced astigmatism
   - Fluctuating vision
   - Anterior or posterior perforation of the cornea
   - Infection
   - White deposits along the ring segment
   - Extrusion of the ring segment

29. **Is the Intacs procedure reversible?**
   The Intacs can be removed, and most eyes return to their original refractions.

30. **What are phakic IOL implants?**
   These lens implants are placed in the eye without the removal of the patient's own crystalline lens. There are currently three main types: an anterior chamber lens clipped to the iris, an angle-supported anterior chamber lens, and a posterior chamber lens in the ciliary sulcus (just in front of the crystalline lens). Only the Artisan or Verisyse iris-clip anterior chamber lens is currently FDA-approved for −5 D to −20 D of myopia with up to 2.5 D of astigmatism.

   Alio JL, de la Hoz F, Perez-Santonja JJ, et al: Phakic anterior chamber lenses for the correction of myopia: A 7-year cumulative analysis of complications in 263 cases. Ophthalmology 106:458–466, 1999.

31. **What is the effect of the Verisyse phakic IOL implant on endothelial cell count?**
   The FDA found no significant loss in endothelial cell counts with the Verisyse iris-claw phakic IOL at 2 years after implantation. In a worst case scenario (by adjusting for measurement inaccuracy), 9% of eyes would have been at risk for 10% loss of endothelial cells at 12 months. Eyes at risk were found to have higher preoperative endothelial cell counts. Several authors have reported that the iris-claw lenses do accelerate endothelial cell loss.

   Benedetti S, Whomsley R, Baltes E, Tonner F: Correction of myopia of 7 to 24 diopters with the Artisan phakic intraocular lens: Two-year follow-up. J Refract Surg 21:116–126, 2005.
   Pop M, Payette Y: Initial results of endothelial cell counts after Artisan lens for phakic eyes: An evaluation of the United States Food and Drug Administration Ophtec Study. Ophthalmology 111:309–317, 2004.

32. **What are accommodative IOLs?**
   As opposed to the more common single-vision IOLs implanted after cataract surgery, which leave the eye with very little ability to focus, the accommodative IOLs allow the eye to move the implant by various mechanisms to allow a greater range of focus. The only FDA-approved accommodative IOL as of this date is the Crystalens by Eyeonics. The optic of the Crystalens is on hinges that allow for vitreous pressure to move the IOL anteriorly and posteriorly. This movement changes the refractive power of the IOL and allows patients greater reading ability. In the FDA 1-year trial, 98% of patients with bilateral implants were 20/25 at distance, 96% could read 20/20 at arms length, and 73% could read at near without any assistance from glasses or contact lenses.

33. **Are there any other surgical options for the treatment of myopia?**
   Because the crystalline lens adds about 18 D of power to the optical system, clear lens extraction may be used in patients with a comparable level of myopia. However, performing intraocular surgery for a purely refractive goal is controversial. In addition, highly myopic eyes carry a moderate risk of retinal detachment, which is increased after lens extraction.

34. **What are the treatment options for astigmatism?**
The correction of astigmatism is slightly more forgiving than the correction of myopia. A patient with 3.00 D of astigmatism is usually quite pleased with a postoperative residual of 1.25 D of cylinder correction because reasonably good vision results. Each of the procedures for myopia has adaptations to address astigmatism alone or simultaneously with myopia. Astigmatic keratotomy (AK) refers to making transverse (straight) or arcuate astigmatic cuts in the mid periphery of the steep corneal meridian. We have learned that crossing of transverse and radial incisions is problematic. Epithelial ingrowth into the stroma, healing difficulties, and significant scarring may result. Excimer laser photo-astigmatic refractive keratotomy (PARK) uses a cylindrical ablation pattern rather than spherical ablation to remove tissue in a chosen meridian (astigmatic correction). If compound myopic astigmatism is present, a combination of spherical and cylindrical patterns results in correction of both myopia and astigmatism. Similar astigmatic corrections have been achieved with LASIK. Whichever procedure is employed, the axis of the astigmatism should be marked with the patient seated, because it may shift when the patient reclines.

35. **What can be done about astigmatism after a corneal transplant?**
There are several options. First, selective removal of sutures in steep meridians may improve astigmatism. A rigid gas-permeable contact lens may be especially effective in alleviating irregular astigmatism. However, many patients do not tolerate or desire contact lenses after corneal transplant surgery. Once all sutures are out and the refraction is stable, arcuate relaxing incisions may be performed in the donor cornea along the steep meridian to reduce astigmatism. An alternative technique involves using a blade to open the wound partially and relax several clock hours of the graft-host junction as opposed to creating incisions in the donor tissue. As described above, the excimer laser also has been used to correct postcorneal transplant astigmatism. Relaxing incisions combined with compression sutures (across the graft-host interface) have been used successfully to correct astigmatism of 5–10 D by causing steepening of the cornea in the sutured median (Fig. 14-6). For astigmatism greater than 10 D, a wedge resection (of corneal tissue followed by sutured closure of the wound) may be performed in the flat meridian.

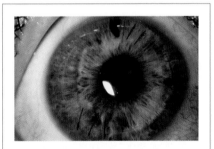

Figure 14-6. Treatment for postcorneal transplant astigmatism. Compression sutures were placed in the flat meridians (1:00–3:00 and 6:30–8:00), and relaxing incisions were performed in the graft wound 90 degrees away.

36. **A 40-year-old Olympic ski coach desires refractive surgery so that he may see distance clearly. His refraction is –3.00 × –2.00 at 180 in both eyes. The surgeon performs radial incisions for 3.00 D of myopia and transverse incisions to flatten the steep meridian by 2.00 D at 90 degrees. Is the patient happy?**
The patient is unhappy because of residual myopia. He now knows more about the "coupling effect" than his surgeon. When a transverse incision causes corneal flattening in one meridian, there is a compensatory steepening of the unincised corneal meridian 90 degrees away. In the case above, the coupling effect of the incised and unincised meridians (90 degrees apart) should have been anticipated. Radial incisions must be used to correct the 3.00 D of spherical myopia as well as the approximate 1.00 D of steepening

induced by the transverse incisions. In general, short incisions tend to cause less steepening of the unincised meridian than longer incisions.

37. **What about procedures for hyperopia?**
Of the available options, none is as effective or reliable as the procedures for myopia.

For low levels of hyperopia, **holmium laser thermokeratoplasty** has been used with some success. This procedure is FDA-approved for the "temporary reduction" of hyperopia in patients 40 years or older with between $+0.75$ D and $+2.50$ D of manifest spherical equivalent with -0.75 D of astigmatism. Eight (or 16) peripheral laser spots are placed in a ring (or two), each spot causing shrinkage of the stromal collagen and resulting in steepening of the central cornea. Problems to be resolved include regression of effect and induced astigmatism.

Conductive keratoplasty (CK) involves the use of low energy radiofrequency energy delivered to the cornea with a guarded needle in a ring pattern around the midperiphery of the cornea. The heat generated causes collagen shrinkage, allowing the central cornea to steepen. CK was FDA approved in 2002 for the treatment of hyperopia in patients 40 and older with a manifest refraction between $+0.75$ and $+3.25$ D. The procedure is effective for low to moderate hyperopia, but the trend is for regression over several years. CK has also recently been FDA approved to treat presbyopia in people over 40.

Hyperopic excimer laser PRK also has been approved by the FDA to treat hyperopia between $+1$ and $+6$ D. Treatment of hyperopic astigmatism also has been approved by the FDA in patients with $+0.5$–$+5.0$ D of sphere with refractive astigmatism of $+0.5$ to $+4.0$ D and a maximal manifest refraction spherical equivalent of $+6.0$ D at the spectacle plane. The laser is used to create a large, donut-shaped ablation that requires a generous epithelial defect (often 9 mm or more).

Hyperopic LASIK treatments are currently FDA approved to treat up to 6 D of hyperopia with up to 6 D of astigmatism. Performing the laser ablation under a corneal flap has the theoretical advantage of decreased haze (ablation performed deep to Bowman's layer) and faster healing response (no large epithelial defect).

Phakic intraocular lenses can treat hyperopia as well as myopia; however, they are not currently FDA approved to do so.

Clear lens extraction is a technique already familiar to most surgeons. Phacoemulsification is performed with implantation of one or two IOLs as required by the degree of hyperopia. However, accommodation is completely eliminated by the procedure. Moreover, the risks of intraocular surgery, including endophthalmitis, are difficult to justify in eyes without organic disease.

38. **What are the effects of refractive surgical procedures on corneal endothelial cells?**
Although endothelial cell loss was an early concern in RK, studies using specular microscopy have demonstrated only a small, nonprogressive loss of endothelial cells. After excimer laser treatment of myopia, studies in animals and humans suggest a small, insignificant loss of endothelial cells that diminishes over time. Certainly it is much more of a concern with intraocular surgery, especially phakic IOLs. Ongoing studies are important. As the treated population grows older, patients eventually will require cataract surgery. There are already case reports of a renewed hyperopic shift in post-RK patients undergoing cataract surgery. Is corneal decompensation in Fuchs' endothelial dystrophy accelerated by previous refractive surgery? Many questions remain unanswered. Effects of the laser itself, the inflammatory response, and toxicity of topically applied drugs may contribute to endothelial cell loss and require further study.

39. **What is the role of drugs in refractive surgery?**
The first issue is pain, which is important in all treatment modalities but most significant for PRK. After PRK, increased levels of prostaglandin E-2 have been found, which sensitize the pain

response of nerves. Topical nonsteroidal anti-inflammatory drugs (NSAIDs) such as ketorolac and diclofenac sodium have been shown to decrease pain by reducing prostaglandin E-2 levels. However, these agents also increase white blood cell response in the cornea and should be used concomitantly with a topical steroid. One study found increased sterile corneal infiltrates when topical NSAIDs were used alone.

Another issue is corneal haze after PRK. The cornea undergoes a wound-healing response to the excimer laser ablation. Activated keratocytes lay down new collagen and proteoglycan matrix (the haze). This is first apparent at 1 month postoperatively, peaks at 3 months, and then decreases as remodeling ensues. Several experimental and retrospective studies have shown that topical steroids reduce corneal haze after PRK. However, a prospective, double-masked study revealed no benefit from topical steroids versus placebos. Still, in a subgroup of patients steroids may be beneficial, and they are typically used postoperatively.

Topical steroids also have been studied in the modulation of corneal curvature. Despite controversy in the literature, topical steroids apparently help to prevent regression of myopic effect after PRK. In fact, cessation of steroids has been associated with myopic regression, which may be reversed on reinstituting therapy in certain patients.

Mitomycin C (MMC) is a cell cycle–nonspecific alkylating agent that targets rapidly dividing cells. MMC is being used by topical application during PRK for people with moderate to high myopia. The goal is to reduce the proliferation of keratocytes and fibroblasts, thus reducing the haze seen after moderate to deep ablations. MMC has shown great promise in refractive surgery and is felt to be safe for use on the cornea; however, the adverse reactions to MMC when used on the conjunctiva or sclera can be quite severe. Reported complications of MMC include corneal and scleral melts, cataract formation, and corneal edema.

GLAUCOMA

Mary Jude Cox, MD, and George L. Spaeth, MD

CHAPTER 15

1. **What is glaucoma?**
   Glaucoma is a highly heterogeneous group of conditions in which tissues of the eye become damaged. Usually the optic nerve is damaged, resulting in a characteristic optic neuropathy with associated visual-field loss. In conditions such as acute angle-closure glaucoma, the lens, cornea, and other structures may be affected as well. The etiology of glaucoma is multifactorial. Elevated intraocular pressure (IOP) is one of the factors responsible for the damage. The role of IOP in glaucoma damage is variable. Increased IOP is the sole cause for the damage in acute angle-closure glaucoma, whereas, in low-tension glaucoma (LTG), IOP may play less of a role in the disease process.

2. **How is glaucoma classified?**
   The broad classifications of glaucoma are somewhat artificial; they tend to blur as we learn more about the disease and its pathogenesis. Traditionally, glaucoma has been classified as open-angle or closed-angle based on the gonioscopic angle appearance. This differentiation plays an important role in treatment. Open- and closed-angle glaucoma have been further classified as primary or secondary. Open-angle glaucoma is classified as primary when no identifiable contributing factor for the increased IOP can be identified. Secondary glaucoma identifies an abnormality to which the pathogenesis of glaucoma can be ascribed. Examples include pseudoexfoliative, uveitic, angle recession, and pigmentary glaucoma.

3. **How prevalent is glaucoma?**
   Glaucoma is the second leading cause of irreversible blindness in the United States and the third leading cause of blindness worldwide. Primary open-angle glaucoma affects approximately 2.5 million Americans. Half are unaware that they have the disease. Population-based studies have shown prevalence among Caucasians 40 years of age and older ranging from 1.1% to 2.1%. The prevalence among African Americans is 3–4 times higher. Prevalence also increases with age. People over 70 have a prevalence 3–8 times higher than people in their forties.

   Tielsch JM, Sommer A, Katz J, et al: Racial variations in the prevalence of primary open-angle glaucoma. The Baltimore Eye Survey. JAMA 266:369–374, 1991.

4. **Name risk factors for the development of primary open-angle glaucoma (POAG).**
   Known risk factors include elevated intraocular pressure, age, race, and a positive family history of glaucoma. Decreased central corneal thickness also has been shown to contribute to the risk of developing glaucoma. Presumed risk factors for which evidence exists but sometimes appears conflicting include myopia and diabetes mellitus. Potential risk factors for which some association has been found include hypertension, cardiovascular abnormalities, and vasospastic conditions such as Raynaud's phenomenon or migraine. Disc hemorrhage, increased cup to disk ratio, and asymmetric cupping of the optic nerve may represent either risk factors or evidence of early disease.

   Caprioli J, Bateman J, Gaasterland D, et al: Primary Open-Angle Glaucoma: Preferred Practice Pattern. San Francisco, American Academy of Ophthalmology, 2003.

5. **Discuss the genetics of primary open-angle glaucoma (POAG).**
   POAG is most likely inherited as a multifactorial or complex trait. A combination of multiple genetic factors or a combination of genetic and environmental factors are required to develop

the disease. One specific gene, the TIGR/*myocilin* gene has been found to confer susceptibility to POAG. Family history is an important risk factor for the development of glaucoma. The Baltimore Eye Survey found the relative risk of having POAG is increased approximately 3.7 times for individuals having siblings with POAG.

Tielsch JM, Katz J, Sommer A, et al: Family history and risk of primary open-angle glaucoma. The Baltimore Eye Survey. Arch Ophthalmol 112:69–73, 1994.

Wolfs R, Klaver C, Ramrattan R, et al: Genetic risk of primary open-angle glaucoma: Population-based familial aggregation study. Arch Ophthalmol 116:1640–1645, 1998.

6. What is the pathogenesis of glaucoma?

The pathogenesis of glaucoma has been only partially elucidated. In some cases elevated intraocular pressure may cause optic nerve damage by mechanically deforming the optic nerve with posterior bowing of the lamina cribrosa. In other cases a decrease in perfusion of the optic nerve may cause damage. This may happen from a sudden drop in blood pressure in response to blood loss or medications. Anemia can also result in ischemia of the optic nerve. Focal vasospasm may contribute to decreased perfusion and ischemia in patients with the low-tension forms of glaucoma. In most patients, several different pathogenetic mechanisms probably operate simultaneously.

American Academy of Ophthalmology: Basic and Clinical Science Course, Section 10. San Francisco, American Academy of Ophthalmology, 2004.

7. What is the clinical presentation of primary open-angle glaucoma?

Primary open-angle glaucoma is slowly progressive and painless. It is usually bilateral but often asymmetric. Central visual acuity is relatively unaffected until late in the disease; therefore, patients are often asymptomatic. Advanced disease may be present before symptoms are noticed.

8. What is normal intraocular pressure (IOP)?

The line between normal and abnormal intraocular pressure is not clear. Mean intraocular pressure is around 16 mmHg, with a standard deviation of 3 mmHg. It is a non-Gaussian distribution skewed toward higher pressures. Elevated intraocular pressure has been shown to be a risk factor for glaucoma; however, only 5% of people with pressures above 21 mmHg eventually develop glaucoma. Conversely, patients with glaucoma damage may have intraocular pressures consistently in the normal range.

Colton T, Ederer F: The distribution of intraocular pressures in the general population. Surv Ophthalmol 25:123–129, 1980.

Dielemans I, Vingerling JR, Wolfs RC, et al: The prevalence of primary open-angle glaucoma in a population-based study in The Netherlands. The Rotterdam Study. Ophthalmology 101:1851–1855, 1994.

9. True or false: Loss of peripheral vision is a warning sign of early glaucoma.

False. Loss of temporal vision (side vision) is the last to be affected in most types of glaucoma. The first area to be damaged in most people with glaucoma is vision to the nasal side of central vision. This helps explain why patients do not notice loss of vision until the damage is marked. Both eyes provide vision to the nasal side so a blind spot is not noted with both eyes open until vision is lost in both eyes.

Caprioli J, Bateman J, Gaasterland D, et al: Primary Open-Angle Glaucoma: Preferred Practice Pattern. San Francisco, American Academy of Ophthalmology, 2003.

KEY POINTS: COMMON VISUAL-FIELD DEFECTS FOUND IN GLAUCOMA

1. Superior/inferior nasal step.

2. Superior/inferior arcuate defect.

3. Generalized depression.

4. Paracentral loss.

5. Temporal or central island with advanced disease.

10. **What is a glaucoma suspect?**
A glaucoma suspect is an adult who has an open angle on gonioscopy and one of the following findings in at least one eye:
- Optic nerve suspicious for glaucoma
- Visual-field defect consistent with glaucoma
- Elevated intraocular pressure consistently greater than 22 mmHg
If a patient has two or more of the above findings, then a diagnosis of glaucoma is more likely. The decision to treat a glaucoma suspect takes into account the above findings as well as additional risk factors and the general health of the patient.

   American Academy of Ophthalmology Basic and Clinical Science Course, Section 10. San Francisco, American Academy of Ophthalmology, 2004.

11. **In examination of the optic nerve, what findings could be consistent with a diagnosis of glaucoma or suspicion of glaucoma?**
Diffuse narrowing of the optic nerve rim, focal narrowing or notching of the optic nerve rim, vertical elongation of the optic cup, nerve fiber layer defects, nerve fiber layer hemorrhages, and asymmetric cupping of the optic nerves are all signs of glaucoma or suspicion of glaucoma. An acquired pit of the optic nerve is a pathognomonic sign of glaucoma.

   Coleman AL, Morrison JC, Callender O: Evaluation of the optic nerve head. In Higginbotham E, Lee D (eds): Clinical Guide to Glaucoma Management. Boston, Elsevier, 2004, pp 183–191.

KEY POINTS: COMMON OPTIC NERVE FINDINGS IN GLAUCOMA

1. Diffuse narrowing of the neuroretinal rim.

2. Focal narrowing or notching of the neuroretinal rim.

3. Nerve fiber layer defects.

4. Disc hemorrhages.

5. Asymmetry of optic nerve cupping.

12. A patient presents with optic nerve damage in one eye as pictured in Fig. 15-1. The other eye has lower pressures and a healthier optic nerve with a normal visual field. What is the prognosis for the healthier optic nerve?

The optic nerve in Fig. 15-1 shows complete loss of the inferotemporal rim. Optic nerve damage in one eye has been associated with a significant increased risk of future damage in the other eye. Twenty-nine percent of untreated fellow undamaged eyes will show visual-field loss in an average of 5 years.

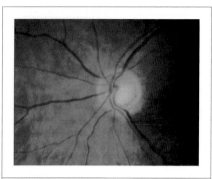

Figure 15-1. Complete loss of the neuroretinal rim is a sign of advanced glaucoma.

Kass MA, Kolker AE, Becker B: Prognostic factors in glaucomatous visual field loss. Arch Ophthalmol 94:1274–1276, 1976.

13. A 74-year-old African American female presents for a routine eye examination. She has not been to an ophthalmologist in 10 years. Her intraocular pressures are 26 mmHg in the right eye (OD) and 24 mmHg in the left eye (OS). Her optic nerves are as pictured in Fig. 15-2. What information is important to obtain from the patient?

The optic nerves in Fig. 15-2 show significant asymmetry with a narrower rim supertemporally in the right eye in comparison to the left eye. She has not been seen by an ophthalmologist for years. The history is a crucial part of the evaluation; it identifies possible secondary causes for glaucoma (e.g., trauma, steroid use) as well as risk factors such as family history, helps determine the visual demands and support system of the patient, and can give an idea of the patient's general health and life expectancy. All of these components combine to help formulate a treatment plan most likely to be agreeable to the patient, least likely to be damaging, and of an appropriate level of aggressiveness for each individual patient.

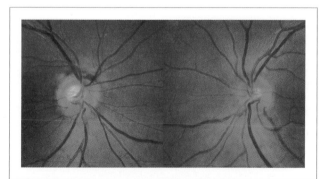

Figure 15-2. Asymmetry of the cup-to-disc ratio can be an early sign of glaucoma.

14.   If the patient in question 13 had been to another ophthalmologist several times a year and was presenting for the first time in your office, what information would be important to obtain?

Old records are valuable. Knowing about previous surgeries, lasers, and medicines (both those that worked and those that did not) helps formulate a current treatment plan. Previous intraocular pressure readings, former visual-field tests, and optic nerve evaluations can establish the rate of progression of the disease, a key piece of information in determining the level of aggressiveness needed in treatment.

15.   True or false: If the patient in question 13 had a normal visual field, she would be unlikely to have glaucoma.

False. Visual-field defects may not be apparent until as much as 50% of the optic nerve fiber layer has been lost.

16.   True or false: If the patient in question 13 had intraocular pressures of 19 mmHg OD and 18 mmHg OS, then she would be unlikely to have glaucoma.

False. A single intraocular pressure measurement in the normal range is not enough to eliminate the possibility of glaucoma. Several studies suggest that as many as 30–50% of individuals in the general population having glaucomatous optic nerve damage and visual-field defects have an initial IOP measurement of less than 22 mmHg. Diurnal IOP fluctuation and artificially low measurements due to decreased central corneal thickness or other factors may contribute to the normal IOP. In addition, patients with average pressure glaucoma have glaucomatous optic neuropathies without ever demonstrating elevated intraocular pressures.

Mitchell P, Smith W, Attebo K, et al: Prevalence of open-angle glaucoma in Australia. The Blue Mountains Study. Ophthalmology 103:1661–1669, 1996.

Sommer A, Tielsch JM, Katz J, et al: Relationship between intraocular pressure and primary open angle glaucoma among white and black Americans. The Baltimore Eye Survey. Arch Ophthalmol 109:1090–1095, 1991.

17.   How does intraocular pressure (IOP) fluctuate in glaucoma patients?

Individuals without glaucoma may have an IOP fluctuation of 2–6 mmHg over a 24-hour period. IOP in glaucoma patients may vary widely. Untreated glaucoma patients may vary by 15 mmHg or more. The majority of patients demonstrate the highest pressures in the morning with decrease throughout the day. Other patterns with peak pressures at night or midday as well as flat patterns without variation have been reported.

Zeimer RC: Circadian variations in intraocular pressure. In Ritch R, Shields MB, Krupin T (eds): The Glaucomas, 2nd ed. St. Louis, Mosby, 1996, pp 429–445.

18.   What role does central corneal thickness play in the evaluation of glaucoma?

Corneal thickness is important to consider for two reasons. First, corneal thickness affects the measurement of IOP so that the measured IOP may be inaccurate if the corneal thickness is not average. The actual average central corneal thickness is approximately 544 μ. IOP is about 5 mmHg lower than measured for each 100 μ that the cornea is thicker than normal. The IOP is actually higher than measured when the cornea is thinner than average. Second, a thin central cornea, in itself, is associated with more severe glaucoma. The Ocular Hypertension Treatment Study identified reduced central corneal thickness as a risk factor for glaucoma in patients with IOP between 24 mmHg and 32 mmHg.

Brandt JD, Beiser JA, Kass MA, et al: Central corneal thickness in the Ocular Hypertension Treatment Study. Ophthalmology 108:1779–1788, 2001.

Ehlers N, Bramsen T, Sperling S: Applanation tonometry and central corneal thickness. Acta Ophthalmol 53:34–43, 1975.

19. **Name factors that affect the measurement of intraocular pressure.**
    Intraocular pressure measurements can be overestimated and underestimated based on several factors (see Table 15-1).

TABLE 15-1. FACTORS INFLUENCING THE MEASUREMENT OF INTRAOCULAR PRESSURE
Overestimation of IOP
Pressing on the globe
Thick tear meniscus (too much fluorescein)
Thick central cornea
Valsalva (breath-holding or straining)
Thick neck/obese patients
Anxiety
Astigmatism
Orbital disease/restrictive ocular myopathy, as with Graves' disease
Corneal scarring and high corneal rigidity
Flat anterior chamber
Underestimation of IOP
Thin tear meniscus (too little fluorescein)
Thin central cornea
Corneal edema
Repeated IOP measurements/prolonged contact with cornea
Low corneal rigidity

20. **What is the primary goal of treatment of patients with glaucoma?**
    The primary goal in the treatment of glaucoma is enhancing the patient's health by improving or preserving his or her vision. One way of preserving vision is by lowering the intraocular pressure. It is important not to lose sight of the primary goal in treatment. All treatment options carry side effects and risks. The patient's general health and visual demands always need to be considered.

21. **Name different initial treatment options for primary open-angle glaucoma.**
    Options include observation or lowering intraocular pressure through eyedrops, laser trabeculoplasty, or surgery.

22. **What factors help determine which option to try?**
    When deciding on an initial treatment for a patient with glaucoma, several factors need to be considered. First, determine how aggressive the treatment needs to be. The level of aggressiveness takes into consideration the severity of the disease, the rapidity of progression, and the general health of the patient. Second, the toxicity and cost of the different treatment options need to be assessed. This will help predict compliance. For example, a 70-year-old healthy patient with advanced disease and an inability to tolerate medicines would most likely benefit from surgery. A healthy 45-year-old with mild-to-moderate disease may begin with medication or, if unable to be compliant or tolerate medicines, a laser trabeculoplasty. An elderly sick patient with mild-to-moderate disease may benefit from observation alone.

23. **Are eyedrops safer than oral medications?**

No. Eyedrops are directly absorbed into the blood through the nasal mucosa. This route bypasses the first-pass metabolism of drugs by the liver and can allow increased effects for a given amount of absorption.

24. **Are some optic nerves more resistant to intraocular pressure damage than others?**

Yes. Small nerves with no peripapillary atrophy but small central cups in which it is not possible to see laminar dots are less likely to become damaged than eyes with large optic nerves, large cups, peripapillary atrophy, and prominent laminar dots. A large cup does not necessarily correlate with glaucoma if the optic nerve itself is large. It is important to determine the optic nerve size when evaluating neuroretinal rim.

25. **A patient being treated for glaucoma presents for a follow-up examination with an optic nerve appearance as shown in Fig. 15-3. Discuss the findings.**

Figure 15-3 demonstrates an optic nerve with vertical elongation of the cup. Narrowing at the superior and inferior rim often occurs in glaucoma. A nerve fiber layer hemorrhage is present at the inferotemporal rim of the optic nerve. Disc hemorrhages are commonly found in glaucoma patients. They are important prognostic signs for the development or progression of visual-field loss.

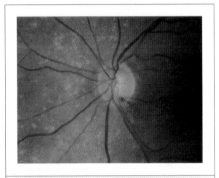

Figure 15-3. Elongation of the optic nerve cup can be an early finding in glaucoma. Splinter disc hemorrhages can be a prognostic indicator for progressive disease.

Diehl D, Quigley HA, Miller NR, et al: Prevalence and significance of optic disc hemorrhage in a longitudinal study of glaucoma. Arch Ophthalmol 108:545–550, 1990.

26. **Name five potential causes of disc hemorrhages.**

- Glaucoma
- Posterior vitreous detachments
- Diabetes mellitus
- Branch retinal vein occlusions
- Anticoagulation

27. **What is low-tension glaucoma (LTG)?**

Low-tension glaucoma is one of the traditional labels for a glaucomatous optic neuropathy that occurs without evidence of elevated intraocular pressure. Because "low" is a relative word, and because many people with "low-tension" have IOP above the mean, but in the average range, a better term is "average-pressure glaucoma" (APG). There is much controversy over whether APG is part of a spectrum of primary open-angle glaucoma with IOP that is not elevated above the average range, or its own disease entity. The optic nerve in patients with APG is susceptible to damage at normal IOP. Ischemia may contribute significantly to the progression of the disease. Studies suggest a higher prevalence of vasospastic disorders such as migraine or Raynaud's phenomenon, coagulopathies, cardiovascular disease, and autoimmune disease in patients with low-tension glaucoma. Nocturnal hypotension and anemia may also result in decreased optic nerve perfusion in patients with low-tension glaucoma.

28. **What disease entities can mimic LTG?**

Undetected "high-tension glaucoma" can mimic LTG. This could be the result of a missed elevation of IOP that occurs at times when the IOP was not measured, a thin central cornea, or an error in applanation. The patient could have suffered a previous episode of severe intraocular pressure elevation from a secondary glaucoma such as uveitic or steroid-induced glaucoma that had subsequently normalized. He or she could have suffered intermittent spikes from angle closure. The patient may have suffered an episode of optic nerve hypoperfusion due to blood loss from surgery or trauma. Compressive optic nerve lesions, ischemic optic neuropathy, congenital anomalies, and certain retinal disorders can also mimic APG (Table 15-2).

Kent AR: Low-tension glaucoma. In Higginbotham E, Lee D (eds): Clinical Guide to Glaucoma Management. Boston, Elsevier, 2004, pp 183–191.

TABLE 15-2. DIFFERENTIAL DIAGNOSIS OF GLAUCOMALIKE OPTIC DISCS AND VISUAL FIELDS

1. Missed elevated IOP
   - Diurnal variability
   - Incorrect measurement
   - Thin central cornea ($<500\ \mu$)
2. Previous IOP elevation, no longer present
3. Shock-induced optic neuropathy
4. Compressive optic neuropathy
5. Ischemic optic neuropathy
6. Giant cell arteritis (temporal arteritis)
7. Optic nerve anomalies (pituitary tumors, etc.)
8. Macular degeneration
9. Juxtapapillary choroiditis
10. Myopia
11. Demyelinating disease

29. **What tests should be considered in the workup of a patient with glaucomatous-appearing optic nerves and visual fields without elevated intraocular pressure?**
   Usually the diagnosis is clear on the basis of the appearance of the optic nerve, the visual field, and the asymmetry of IOP with the higher pressure in the eye with more damage. When not clear, a diurnal curve and central corneal thickness should be checked to be certain the condition is not a "high tension" glaucoma with low intraocular pressure readings. A computed tomography or magnetic resonance imaging scan to evaluate for compressive lesions of the optic nerve or chiasm may be indicated. If history or symptoms suggest, rapid plasma reagin/Venereal Disease Research Laboratory (RPR/VDRL), rheumatoid factor/antinuclear antibody (RF/ANA), or erythrocytic sedimentation rate (ESR) may be checked to look for syphilis, autoimmune diseases, or temporal arteritis (giant cell arteritis) as potential causes. If a patient is on blood pressure medicines or has a history of hypotension, a 24-hour Holter monitor to check for nocturnal hypotension may be indicated.

30. **How is average-pressure glaucoma treated?**
   The Collaborative Normal-Tension Glaucoma Study (CNTGS) found that by reducing the intraocular pressure by 30% the rate of visual-field progression was reduced from 35% to 12%. Lowering intraocular pressure is the mainstay of treatment for average-pressure glaucoma, as well as primary open-angle glaucoma.

Collaborative Normal-Tension Glaucoma Study Group: Comparison of glaucomatous progression between untreated patients with normal-tension glaucoma and patients with therapeutically reduced intraocular pressures. Am J Ophthalmol 126:487–497, 1998.

CHAPTER 16

ANGLE-CLOSURE GLAUCOMA

Anup K. Khatana, MD, and George L. Spaeth, MD

1. **What landmarks are seen in the anterior chamber (AC) angle?**
   The structures noted in anterior-to-posterior sequence are as follows (numbered list corresponds to number labels in Fig. 16-1):
   1. **Schwalbe's line:** The peripheral or posterior termination of Descemet's membrane, seen clinically as the apex or termination of the corneal light wedge. May be visible inferiorly as the most anterior nonwavy pigmented line
   2. **Anterior, nonpigmented, trabecular meshwork (TM):** Clear whitish band
   3. **Posterior, pigmented, trabecular meshwork (TM):** Variably pigmented band of homogeneous width. Usually most pigmented inferiorly (Fig 16-2)
   4. **Schlemm's canal:** Variably visible light grey band at the level of the posterior TM. Elevated episcleral venous pressure or pressure from the edge of the goniolens will cause blood to reflux, making it appear as a faint red band

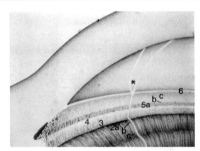

Figure 16-1. Diagram of anterior chamber anatomy.

   5. **Scleral spur:** Narrow, white band of sclera invaginating between the TM and ciliary body. Marks the insertion site of the longitudinal muscle fibers of the ciliary body to the sclera
   6. **Ciliary body (CB) band:** Pigmented band marking the anterior face of the ciliary body. Variably, iris processes may be seen as lacy projections crossing this band. By definition, iris processes do not cross the scleral spur. Projections that cross the scleral spur to the TM are peripheral anterior synechiae (PAS) and may be focal, pillar-like, or broad sheets
   7. **Iris**

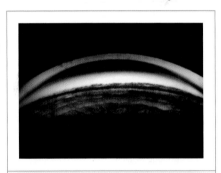

Figure 16-2. Inferior quadrant of heavily pigmented open angle.

2. **Why is a goniolens necessary to visualize the AC angle?**
   Light from the AC angle undergoes total internal reflection at the cornea-air interface, preventing direct visualization. A goniolens changes the refractive index at the interface, enabling visualization.

3. **What are the different kinds of goniolenses? How do they differ?**
   - **Direct gonioscopy** uses the **Koeppe** contact lens. This technique is cumbersome, requiring a supine patient; a clear, viscous liquid coupling medium such as methylcellulose; and a direct viewing system.
   - **Indirect gonioscopy** uses a mirrored contact lens, either the **Goldmann** three-mirror lens that also vaults the central cornea and requires a viscous coupling liquid, or the **Zeiss** (Fig. 16-3), **Posner**, or **Sussman** four-mirror lenses that directly contact the cornea and thus do not require a coupling agent beyond the patient's normal tear film.

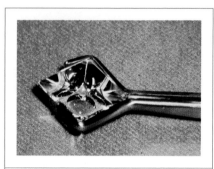

Figure 16-3. Zeiss goniolens.

4. **Which goniolens is preferred by most glaucoma specialists and why?**
   The Zeiss lens is preferred by a majority of glaucoma specialists for the following reasons:
   - Its speed and ease of use (it does not require a viscous coupling liquid, and, because of its four mirrors, it does not need to be rotated to see all 360 degrees of the angle).
   - The ability to perform indentation gonioscopy (which cannot be performed with the Goldmann lens because of its larger diameter), and its absence of suction effect on the eye (the suction effect of the Goldmann lens can sometimes artificially widen narrow angles). These two qualities can be critically important when evaluating eyes with narrow angles.
   - Elimination of the transient degradation of corneal clarity that is a consequence of the viscous liquid and Goldmann lens manipulation, which can make subsequent fundus examination difficult.

   Warning: When first mastering gonioscopy, the Zeiss lens can be more difficult than the Goldmann lens. In inexperienced hands, excessive indentation can easily occur that will make the angle appear wider than it really is. Zeiss gonioscopy demands a light touch. One way to make sure you are not pressing is for the contact to be so light that you occasionally lose part of the contact meniscus. If you see any corneal striae or if your view is not crystal clear, you are probably indenting.

5. **How is gonioscopy performed?**
   1. Topical anesthesia is essential for patient comfort and cooperation.
   2. Rest your elbow on the slit-lamp platform and your ring and/or small fingers on the side bar or on the patient's cheek to help stabilize your hand.
   3. Examination can be facilitated by asking the patient to stare straight ahead with the fellow eye without blinking.
   4. To facilitate viewing a particular quadrant of the angle with indirect gonioscopy, either tilt the mirror toward the quadrant or have the patient look toward that mirror. For example, when viewing the superior angle, either tilt the inferior mirror upward, toward the superior angle, or have the patient look down slightly, toward the inferior mirror.
   5. The superior-inferior relationships in the nasal and temporal mirrors and the nasal-temporal (right-left) relationships in the superior and inferior mirrors are preserved, not inverted as in indirect ophthalmoscopy. For example, when viewing the superior angle through the inferior mirror, an area of PAS seen at five o'clock in the mirror is actually at one o'clock, not eleven o'clock.

6. **How can I determine which patients may have narrow angles and need gonioscopy?**

The van Herick technique uses a thin slit beam focused at the limbus to approximate angle depth by comparing the peripheral AC depth to corneal thickness. A grade I has a peripheral AC depth less than one quarter of the corneal thickness; grade II is one quarter of the corneal thickness; a grade III is one half of the thickness; and a grade IV is one corneal thickness or more. Patients who are grade I or II certainly have narrow angles and should have gonioscopy. This technique, however, should never replace gonioscopy in eyes with clear media as part of a glaucoma evaluation. It falsely gives the appearance of an open angle in some eyes with plateau iris or anterior rotation of the ciliary body (see classification below).

7. **What are the different gonioscopic anterior chamber angle classification systems?**

Table 16-1 summarizes the **Scheie system**, which is rarely used, and the **Schaffer system**, which is the most commonly used.

The **Spaeth system**, however, is the most descriptive. The first element is a capital letter (A–E) for the level of iris insertion:

- **A** = Anterior to TM
- **B** = Behind Schwalbe's line, or at TM
- **C** = At scleral spur
- **D** = Deep angle, CB band visible
- **E** = Extremely deep

If during indentation gonioscopy, the true iris insertion is noted to be more posterior than originally apparent, the original impression is put in parentheses, followed by the true iris insertion outside parentheses.

The second element is a number that denotes the iridocorneal angle width in degrees at the level of the trabecular meshwork, usually from **5–45 degrees**.

The third element is a lower-case letter describing the peripheral iris configuration:

- **f** = Flat
- **b** = Bowed or convex
- **c** = Concave
- **p** = Plateau configuration

In addition, the pigmentation of the posterior TM is graded on a scale of 0 (none) to 4 (maximal). For example, (A)C10b, 2+PTM refers to an appositionally closed 10-degree angle that, with indentation, opened to the scleral spur and revealed moderate pigmentation of the posterior TM.

TABLE 16-1.	THE SCHEIE AND SCHAFFER CLASSIFICATION SYSTEMS				
	Grade 0	Grade I	Grade II	Grade III	Grade IV
Scheie		Wide open	Scleral spur visible, CB band not seen	Can only see to anterior TM	Closed
Schaffer*	Closed	10 degrees	20 degrees	30 degrees	40 degrees

*The angle is graded as a slit when it is between grades 0 and I.

8. How do I know if I can safely dilate a patient, with or without a slit lamp?

If no slit lamp is available, use a penlight and shine it from the temporal side perpendicular to the central visual axis. In an eye with a normal or "safe" anterior chamber depth, the entire nasal half of the iris will be illuminated as well as the temporal half. In an eye with a shallow or questionable anterior chamber depth, none or only part of the nasal half of the iris will be illuminated. This technique does not hold true in eyes with plateau iris.

If a slit lamp is available, angles that are less than or equal to 15 degrees are at risk for closure and probably should not be dilated. An eye with a 20-degree angle should be watched closely, as it may narrow further with time, and should be re-evaluated with tonometry and gonioscopy after dilation. An exception to these general guidelines is plateau iris (discussed later), in which the angle may be wider than 20 degrees and still at risk for closure. Thus, the peripheral iris configuration is also very important.

9. How is angle closure classified?

A. By clinical presentation
   I. Acute
   II. Subacute or intermittent
   III. Chronic

B. By mechanism
   I. Posterior pushing mechanism
      a. Pupillary block (can occur in phakic, pseudophakic, or aphakic eyes)
         1. Relative
            Idiopathic (i.e., primary angle closure)
            Miotic-induced
            Lens-induced
            Plateau iris
         2. Absolute or true: By posterior synechiae from any inflammatory etiology
      b. Lens-induced
         1. Phacomorphic (due to an intumescent cataractous lens or a swollen lens in a diabetic)
         2. Lens subluxation
            Trauma
            Pseudoexfoliation syndrome
            Hereditary/metabolic disorder (e.g., Marfan's syndrome, homocystinuria)
         3. Lens pushed forward
            Aqueous misdirection syndrome (malignant or ciliary-block glaucoma)
            Mass (e.g., tumor, retinopathy of prematurity [ROP], persistent hyperplastic primary vitreous [PHPV])
      c. Plateau iris
         1. True plateau iris
         2. Iris and ciliary body cysts
      d. Swelling/anterior rotation of the ciliary body (some overlap within this)
         1. Inflammatory (e.g., scleritis, uveitis, after panretinal photocoagulation)
         2. Congestive (e.g., after scleral buckling surgery, nanophthalmos)
         3. Choroidal effusion—secondary to medications (e.g., topiramate), hypotony after trauma or surgery, uveal effusion, etc.
         4. Suprachoroidal hemorrhage (SCH)—intraoperative or postoperative. Risk factors for SCH include previous intraocular pressure (IOP) elevation followed by hypotony, high myopia, advanced age, aphakia, previous vitrectomy, systemic hypertension or atherosclerotic vascular disease, and postoperative Valsalva maneuver
   II. Anterior pulling mechanism-synechial angle closure
      a. Chronic appositional closure from any of the above
      b. Intraocular inflammation (uveitis)
      c. Neovascular glaucoma

1. Central retinal vein occlusion (CRVO), accounts for one third of cases
2. Diabetes mellitus, accounts for another one third of cases
3. Carotid occlusive disease, comprises approximately 10% of cases
4. Miscellaneous (e.g., central retinal artery occlusion [CRAO], tumors, retinal detachment)

d. Iridocorneal endothelial (ICE) syndrome
   1. Progressive iris atrophy
   2. Chandler's syndrome
   3. Cogan-Reese syndrome

PRIMARY ANGLE CLOSURE (RELATIVE PUPILLARY BLOCK)

10. **What is the epidemiology of primary angle-closure glaucoma?**
    For **acute** angle closure, Eskimos (highest incidence) and Asians have a much higher incidence than Caucasians, who in turn have a higher incidence than black people. It is relatively more common in Northern European Caucasians than in Mediterranean Caucasians. The peak incidence is between the ages of 55 and 65. In Caucasians, women are three to four times more likely to develop angle closure than men. In black people, the incidence is equal between men and women. There is also a greater incidence in hyperopes. The inheritance appears to be polygenic.
    For **chronic** angle closure, black people have a higher incidence than Asians, who have a higher incidence than Caucasians. In addition, black people are more likely to develop chronic angle closure than acute angle closure.

11. **What are the symptoms of acute angle-closure glaucoma?**
    Patients may complain of ocular pain, redness, blurred or foggy vision, haloes around lights, nausea, and vomiting. The visual symptoms are partly caused by the corneal edema that occurs from the sudden severe rise in intraocular pressure (IOP). This, the most common presentation, is most often induced by stress, low ambient light levels, and occasionally by various medications. If the IOP exceeds the pressure in the ophthalmic or central retinal artery, visual loss occurs as a result of ischemia of the optic nerve or retina.

12. **Describe the signs or exam findings seen in primary acute angle-closure glaucoma.**
    - **Intraocular pressure (IOP):** Typically greater than 45 mmHg.
    - **Conjunctiva and episclera:** Dilated vessels.
    - **Cornea:** Epithelial and stromal edema.
    - **Anterior chamber:** Shallow; cells or flare variably present.
    - **Iris:** Dilated vessels (distinguish from neovascularization of the iris), mid-dilated nonreactive or sluggish pupil, and sector atrophy from ischemia (only if previous episodes have occurred).
    - **Lens:** Glaukomflecken (not seen acutely, but if present initially may indicate previous episodes of angle closure).
    - **Gonioscopy:** With narrow angle or closed angle, one may be unable to view structures owing to corneal edema (glycerin may be used to clear the cornea); superior angle is usually the narrowest and the first to develop peripheral anterior synechia (PAS).
    - **Optic nerve:** Occasional swelling and hyperemia from vascular congestion; may mimic papilledema.
    - **Retina:** May be normal or may show signs of vascular occlusion.
    - **Fellow eye:** Examination of the fellow eye is very important in making the diagnosis. It usually also has a shallow anterior chamber and narrow angle. If the fellow eye has a normal depth AC and a normal angle width, the diagnosis of primary angle closure should be seriously doubted, unless the involved eye is significantly more hyperopic.

KEY POINTS: COMMON SIGNS OF ACUTE PRIMARY ANGLE-CLOSURE GLAUCOMA

1. Dilated conjunctival and episcleral vessels.

2. Corneal edema.

3. Shallow anterior chamber with or without cells or flare.

4. Mid-dilated, sluggish, or unreactive pupil.

5. Lens glaukomflecken.

6. Shallow anterior chamber and narrow angle in fellow eye.

13. **How does subacute or intermittent angle closure present clinically?**
The symptoms are similar to an acute attack but usually less severe, tend to recur over days to weeks, and may be confused for headaches. They resolve on their own, often when the individual goes to sleep or enters a well-lit area (both induce miosis). These episodes can result in chronic angle closure. Between episodes, the IOP is normal and the ocular exam is usually normal, except for the presence of narrow angles and, sometimes, glaukomflecken, cataracts, and PAS on gonioscopy.

14. **How does chronic angle closure present clinically?**
It is usually asymptomatic, unless marked visual-field loss has occurred. Gradual closure of the angle, by simple apposition and/or PAS, leads to a more gradual rise in IOP. The IOP is more variable but tends to be somewhat lower than in acute angle closure. The cornea is usually clear, because the IOP rises gradually, resulting in a lack of pain, redness, decreased vision, or other symptoms. The most frequent exception to this is neovascular glaucoma, which is also caused by PAS but often presents with symptoms and signs similar to acute angle closure.

15. **What are the anatomic characteristics of eyes with primary angle closure?**
Short axial length, hyperopia, and anterior segment crowding.

16. **What is the pathophysiologic mechanism of relative pupillary block?**
The crystalline lens grows throughout life. In eyes that are predisposed, there is a gradually increasing apposition between the posterior iris surface and the anterior lens capsule. As the iridolenticular touch increases, the resistance to aqueous flow from the posterior to the anterior chamber increases, causing a gradual increase in the posterior chamber pressure. Under conditions in which the pupil is in a mid-dilated position (e.g., from stress, low ambient light levels, sympathomimetic or anticholinergic medications), the elevated posterior chamber pressure causes the lax or floppy iris to bow anteriorly and occlude the trabecular meshwork. In thinner or lighter-colored irides, this is more likely to cause an acute rise in IOP. Thicker irides are less likely to flop anteriorly, but rather are gradually pushed anteriorly, especially peripherally, leading to creeping chronic angle closure, with or without PAS, and a more gradual IOP rise (Fig. 16-4).

17. **What nonmedical maneuver may help to lower IOP even before medicating the patient?**
Even before starting medical treatment, indentation gonioscopy can sometimes help to lower IOP by pushing aqueous from the central AC peripherally, opening the angle if it is not sealed

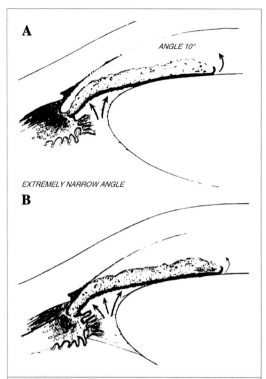

Figure 16-4. Mechanism of relative pupillary block closure. *A,* Extremely narrow angle with resistance to aqueous flow between the iris and lens, leading to increased posterior chamber pressure. *B,* Closed angle.

with PAS. This must be done carefully to avoid abrading the corneal epithelium, which is swollen and may abrade more easily than normal. However, this procedure rarely helps.

18. **How would you treat the involved eye medically?**
The "kitchen sink" approach is generally preferred, using some combination of the drugs listed below (Table 16-2). The use of miotics such as pilocarpine in narrow, potentially occludable, angles is a subject of some debate, even among glaucoma specialists. The rationale for miotic use is to pull the peripheral iris away from the TM, which opens the angle and prevents appositional closure. It may, however, make the angle narrower and potentially induce angle closure by causing the lens-iris diaphragm to move anteriorly with contraction of the ciliary muscle, which relaxes zonular tension and makes the pupillary block worse. If pilocarpine is used in such a patient, repeat gonioscopy should be performed 30–60 minutes after the initial drop. If the angle is not any wider, some would argue that a laser peripheral iridotomy (PI) should be performed right away. If this is not feasible, consider adding a beta blocker to decrease aqueous secretion until the PI is performed.
- **Topical inhibitors of aqueous secretion:** Beta blockers, carbonic anhydrase inhibitors (CAIs), and α2 adrenergic agonists.
- **Uveoscleral outflow enhancers:** The prostaglandin analogs, as well as the α2 agonist brimonidine, increase uveoscleral outflow. Their use in angle closure has not been studied as

TABLE 16-2. TREATMENT OF ANGLE-CLOSURE GLAUCOMA*

	IOP < 40 mmHg	IOP 40–60 mmHg	IOP > 60 mmHg or > 40 mmHg with cupping
First day of presentation	<ul><li>Topical pilocarpine 1%</li><li>Topical β blocker and α-agonist (possible topical carbonic anhydrase inhibitor)</li><li>Recheck at 1 hr</li></ul>	<ul><li>Topical pilocarpine 2%</li><li>Topical β blocker and α-agonist</li><li>Topical prednisolone 1%</li><li>IV acetazolamide 500 mg</li></ul>	<ul><li>Topical α-agonist and β blocker</li><li>IV acetazolamide 500 mg</li><li>Topical prednisolone 1%</li><li>Analgesics and antiemetics as needed</li></ul>
1 hr after presentation	IOP < IOP of other eye<ul><li>Topical β blocker and α-agonist 2 times/day</li><li>Topical prednisolone 1% as needed</li><li>Recheck at 1 hr</li></ul>	IOP reduced 50% but > IOP of other eye<ul><li>Topical pilocarpine 2%</li><li>Oral acetazolamide 500 mg</li><li>Recheck at 1 hr</li></ul>	IOP not reduced > 50%<ul><li>Topical pilocarpine 2%</li><li>Topical β blocker and α-agonist</li><li>Oral glycerol 50% 1 mg/kg (or mannitol if vomiting)</li><li>Recheck at 1 hr</li></ul>
2 hr after presentation	IOP < IOP of other eye<ul><li>Home on topical pilocarpine 1% 2 times/day and topical prednisolone 1% 4 times/day</li><li>Return next day</li></ul>	IOP reduced 50% but > IOP of other eye<ul><li>As per 6</li><li>Recheck at 1 hr</li></ul>	IOP still not reduced 50%<ul><li>Refer to specialist</li><li>Admit for IV mannitol</li><li>Maintain on oral acetazolamide 500 mg 2 times/day</li><li>Topical agents, α-agonists, β blockers 2 times/day</li><li>Keep NPO in preparation for surgery next day</li><li>If possible, have specialist see patient on same day</li><li>Do iridotomy or have specialist do iridoplasty (see "IOP elevated even after repeat mannitol[*]"). In unlikely event that cornea is clear, do iridotomy</li></ul>

TABLE 16-2. TREATMENT OF ANGLE-CLOSURE GLAUCOMA*—CONT'D

Second day	IOP < IOP of other eye	IOP elevated even after repeat manitol
	■ If eye uninflamed and cornea clear, do Nd:YAG peripheral iridotomy in affected eye	■ Clear cornea with glycerin
		■ Gonioscope again
	■ If eye inflamed and cornea not clear, defer peripheral iridotomy in affected eye *and* do peripheral iridotomy on fellow eye	■ Check disc
		■ If peripheral iridotomy not already done, try to do if able to see adequately
		■ If laser iridotomy already done and angle still closed, consider iridoplasty
		■ If IOP falls > 50% below presentation level, continue topical and oral medications and adjust therapy, depending on amount of cupping and future course of glaucoma
		■ If IOP does not fall > 50% below level at presentation, patient probably needs guarded filtration procedure
		■ If IOP falls > 50% below presentation level, continue topical and oral medications and adjust therapy, depending on amount of cupping and future course of IOP
Third day	■ Do Nd:YAG peripheral iridotomy on fellow eye if not already done	
	■ Arrange follow-up	
	■ Plan to do Nd:YAG laser iridotomy on affected eye as soon as cornea is clear and eye quiet	

*Glaucoma Service, Wills Eye Hospital/Jefferson Medical College.
Note: All topical medications apply to the afffected eye. No therapy in the form of drops is to be used in the unaffected eye unless that eye also has glaucoma or other ocular problems. Specifically, pilocarpine is *not* to be used in the unaffected eye.

extensively as some of the other agents, but they can also help lower the IOP. There is some theoretical concern that prostaglandin analogs could increase ocular inflammation. It should be remembered that miotics cause ciliary muscle contraction and decrease uveoscleral outflow.

- **Carbonic anhydrase inhibitors:** In patients who are not nauseated, an oral CAI is administered. If IV medications are available and the patient is unable to tolerate oral medications, IV acetazolamide is preferred as an adjunct to topical therapy because of its faster onset of action.
- **Hyperosmotic agents:** Hyperosmotic therapy reduces vitreous volume and can be a very powerful weapon in lowering IOP and breaking an attack. Glycerin and isosorbide can be given orally. Intravenous mannitol is the most potent agent for lowering IOP, but it also increases blood volume and should be used with caution.
- **Topical steroids:** Topical steroids (e.g., prednisolone 1% q.i.d.) are a useful adjunct to control the usually concurrent intraocular inflammation that may or may not be clinically apparent.
- **Miotics:** Pilocarpine helps to break the attack by pulling the peripheral iris away from the TM and increasing trabecular outflow. However, the pupillary sphincter (but not the ciliary muscle) usually becomes ischemic at IOPs above 40–50 mmHg and therefore unresponsive to miotics until the IOP is lowered with other medications. The duration of IOP elevation and sphincter ischemia ultimately determines whether or not the sphincter will respond to miotics even after the IOP is lowered. The usual concentration used is 1% or 2%. Pilocarpine should be used with caution, however, to avoid cholinergic toxicity. Also keep in mind that it may make some cases of angle closure worse. Some believe it should not be used in aphakic or pseudophakic pupillary block.
- **Topical glycerin:** Topical glycerin can be quite helpful to clear the cornea, which facilitates detailed examination of the eye and also laser treatment.
- **Others:** The α2 agonist, brimonidine, increases uveoscleral outflow, as do the prostaglandin analogs.

KEY POINTS: BASIC TREATMENT OF ACUTE PRIMARY ANGLE-CLOSURE GLAUCOMA

1. "Kitchen sink" approach of maximal medical topical therapy plus oral acetazolamide if patient not nauseated.

2. Oral hyperosmotics if above not effective and patient not nauseated, otherwise IV mannitol.

3. Laser peripheral iridotomy.

19. **How would you treat the involved eye with laser?**
Laser PI is the definitive first procedure of choice to relieve pupillary block (Fig. 16-5). Angle closure from any etiology other than pupillary block will not respond to iridotomy. The argon or Q switched YAG lasers may be used. The Nd:YAG laser is preferred because it is faster, easier, requires fewer bursts with less energy (causes less inflammation), is not dependent on iris color, and is less likely to cause complications such as posterior synechiae. The argon laser's thermal effect can help prevent bleeding and facilitate penetration of thick irides.

There is also some difference of opinion regarding the timing of the laser peripheral iridotomy in acute angle closure. If the IOP can not be reasonably controlled medically, then the PI must be performed immediately. If the pressure can be reasonably controlled medically, it may be better to defer the iridotomy for a few days for the following reasons:

- The corneal edema, from high pressure, and the Descemet's folds, from the abrupt lowering of pressure, can both make visualization and performing the iridotomy more difficult. In addition, because the anterior chamber is usually shallow, the corneal endothelium is closer to the point of laser energy focus and is more likely to be damaged from the concussion.
- The iris is usually also somewhat congested, edematous, and inflamed during an attack. This can make the iridotomy more difficult to perform; more power may be required to successfully penetrate the iris, and this can be more uncomfortable for the patient than when the eye is not inflamed.

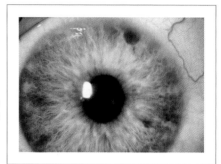

Figure 16-5. Patent laser peripheral iridotomy.

20. **What are the most common complications of laser PI?**
    The most troublesome problem is a ghost image resulting from light that has entered through the PI.
    - **Argon:** Posterior synechiae and localized cataracts. Argon laser PIs are more likely to close than are Nd:YAG PIs.
    - **Nd:YAG:** A hemorrhage may occur in up to 50% of eyes. It is usually small and localized to the area of the PI, but sometimes can form a significant hyphema. The bleeding may be controlled by applying gentle pressure on the eye with the contact lens. Even relatively large hyphemas are gone, or almost gone, the next day.
    Transient IOP spikes of more than 6 mmHg do occur in up to 40% of patients most often within the first 1–2 hours. Perioperative treatment with apraclonidine decreases the incidence and severity of post-laser IOP spikes. Beta blockers and CAIs have been used, but with less success. The incidence and severity of postoperative IOP elevation are similar with argon and Nd:YAG lasers.

21. **What are the indications for surgical intervention? What are the surgical options?**
    Surgery is indicated in an eye in which the combination of maximal tolerated medical and laser therapy has failed to control the IOP adequately. Evaluation of the disc and visual field, if possible, is essential.
    - **Clear corneal peripheral iridectomy:** In an eye with an ongoing or recent acute attack and if unable to successfully perform a laser iridotomy.
    - **Clear corneal peripheral iridectomy combined with goniosynechialysis:** If in the preceding scenario, peripheral anterior synechiae have already formed. This procedure involves breaking the synechiae in the angle to allow it to reopen.
    - **Guarded filtering procedure (GFP), or trabeculectomy:** In situations in which the preceding approach has failed or a patent laser PI has failed to resolve the attack.
    When operating on these eyes, it is important to remember that they already have shallower chambers and are more likely to develop flat chambers and aqueous misdirection (malignant or ciliary block glaucoma), both of which can complicate intra- and postoperative management. The use of miotics can also increase the chances of aqueous misdirection.

22. **When can you consider an attack to be completely "broken?"**
    When the intraocular pressure in the involved eye is the same as or lower than the IOP in the uninvolved eye at initial presentation, and the angle is open.

23. **What are the chances of the same thing happening to the fellow eye?**
There is a 40–80% chance of an acute attack in the fellow eye over the next 5–10 years.

24. **What would you recommend for the fellow eye?**
Prophylactic laser PI, when gonioscopic evaluation reveals a potentially occludable angle. It may be appropriate to treat the fellow eye first (if the angle is occludable), while waiting for the involved eye to quiet down and for the cornea to clear. The use of pilocarpine in the fellow eye to try to prevent angle closure by pulling the peripheral iris away from the TM until PI is performed is not without risk, as discussed in question 19.

25. **Describe the short- and long-term sequelae to the various structures of the eye after an acute angle-closure attack.**

   ■ **Cornea:** Shortly after lowering the IOP, the epithelial microcystic edema will resolve, and Descemet's folds may be seen from the acute reduction of IOP (Fig. 16-6). The stromal edema takes longer to resolve. In most cases, significant endothelial damage does occur. If the attack has caused enough endothelial injury, epithelial and stromal edema may persist. Endothelial pigment may result from the pigment released during iridotomy or from any ischemic atrophic regions of the iris.

   ■ **Anterior chamber:** Even after successful PI, the AC is usually still shallower than normal.

   ■ **Iris:** One may see a mid-dilated, nonreactive, or sluggish pupil, and sector atrophy and stromal necrosis from ischemia. Posterior synechiae may eventually develop long after a PI is performed owing to the alternate route available for aqueous humor flow. The pupil is often vertically oval.

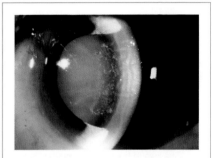

   Figure 16-6. Photograph of an eye after resolution of acute angle-closure attack. Note the corneal Descemet's folds, the PI at 12 o'clock at the upper edge of the photograph, and the lacy pattern of glaukomflecken under the anterior lens capsule.

   ■ **Lens:** Glaukomflecken (small whitish anterior subcapsular opacities representing areas of necrotic lens epithelium with adjacent subcapsular cortical degeneration; *see* Fig. 16-6) and development or progression of cataractous changes may be seen.

   ■ **Zonules:** Injury from an acute episode may not manifest itself until much later, when zonular weakness is noted during cataract extraction or from spontaneous subluxation or dislocation.

   ■ **Gonioscopy:** PAS.

   ■ **Optic nerve:** The disc congestion and swelling, if present, may take several days to resolve. Acute attacks typically produce more pallor than cupping; chronic angle closure usually produces more cupping than pallor, similar to open-angle glaucoma.

   ■ **Retina:** "Decompression retinopathy" may be seen after rapid lowering of IOP as scattered intraretinal hemorrhages concentrated more around the posterior pole and optic nerve. Peripapillary atrophy can also develop over time, along with focal nerve-fiber bundle defects, diffuse thinning of the retina, etc.

26. **What types of medications are contraindicated in narrow-angle glaucoma?**
Topical and systemic **sympathomimetic and anticholinergic medications,** such as those found in many over-the-counter antihistamine and cold remedies, as well as in antispasmodics for overactive bladder and some antiparkinsonian agents, should be avoided by people with eyes

that have narrow and potentially occludable angles until a prophylactic laser iridotomy is performed. These medications are not contraindicated in patients with eyes that have narrow but not occludable angles, or eyes with a patent iridotomy, or in patients with open-angle glaucoma.

Use **miotics** with caution in patients with narrow angles, regardless of occludability, because of the risk of causing further narrowing by anterior displacement of the lens-iris diaphragm. These patients should at least have repeat gonioscopy after commencing miotic therapy to rule out this possibility. If the angles do become significantly narrower, then one must consider discontinuation of miotic therapy or a prophylactic PI if there is a compelling reason for continuing miotic therapy.

KEY POINTS: LONG-TERM SEQUELAE OF ACUTE ANGLE-CLOSURE GLAUCOMA ATTACK

1. Corneal endothelial cell loss, endothelial pigment.

2. Permanently mid-dilated and unreactive pupil.

3. Iris sector atrophy, posterior synechiae.

4. Peripheral anterior synechiae in the angle.

5. Glaucomflecken, other cataractous changes.

6. Occasionally, lens zonular weakness.

7. Optic nerve pallor out of proportion to cupping.

27. **List some possible causes for persistent or recurrent IOP elevation after a successful PI.**
    - Peripheral anterior synechiae formation and/or undetected injury to the TM during the period of angle closure
    - Nonpupillary block angle closure (see question 9, classification, B.I.b.–d.)
    - Incomplete iridotomy will result in persistent IOP elevation. Occlusion of the iridotomy with debris or a membrane may cause a recurrent episode of pupillary block angle closure. Remember that transillumination does not equal patency.
    - Underlying or residual open-angle glaucoma component

PLATEAU IRIS

28. **Describe the epidemiology of plateau iris.**
    These patients are usually younger (typically fourth and fifth decades) and less hyperopic than patients with primary angle closure; they may even be myopic.

29. **How does it present clinically?**
    It may be noted on routine examination or present as an acute or chronic angle-closure glaucoma.

30. **What is plateau iris configuration (PIC)?**
    Anteriorly positioned (and sometimes larger than normal) ciliary processes push the peripheral iris more anteriorly than normal (Fig. 16-7). The central AC is usually slightly

shallow or normal depth, but the angle recess is narrower than the depth of the AC would suggest. The iris has a relatively flat contour, with a sharp peripheral drop-off at the angle approach. This finding is designated "p" in our gonioscopic system. A component of pupillary block is frequently present. With dilation, the peripheral iris folds into the angle and occludes the TM.

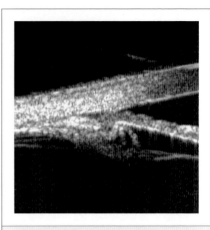

Figure 16-7. Ultrasound biomicroscope image of the anterior segment of an eye with plateau iris. Note the large ciliary processes causing anterior displacement of the peripheral iris and angle closure, while the central iris remains flat.

31. **How can plateau iris be distinguished from relative pupillary block (primary) angle closure on slit-lamp examination?**
    Primary angle closure normally presents with a shallow central AC and moderate to significant iris convexity, which is in contrast to the appearance of PIC noted above. With indentation gonioscopy, the angle is much harder to open and does not open as widely as a typical narrow angle. A "hills and valleys" profile may be seen when looking at the angle. In addition, indentation gonioscopy reveals the almost pathognomonic "double hump sign," characterized by posterior displacement of the midperipheral iris but a persistently anterior position of the peripheral iris. Persistence of the plateau iris appearance despite a patent iridotomy confirms the diagnosis clinically. High-resolution ultrasound biomicroscopy can also confirm the diagnosis.

32. **What is plateau iris syndrome?**
    Acute or chronic angle closure that develops with dilation, or even spontaneously, in an eye with plateau iris configuration and a patent PI.

33. **How is plateau iris treated?**
    The primary procedure of choice in an eye with (or at risk for) angle closure is **laser peripheral iridotomy,** to eliminate any component of pupillary block that may be present. In general, the older the patient, the more the pupillary block contributes, as a percentage, to the mechanism of angle closure. However, laser iridotomy is *not* adequate treatment in such cases; it is merely the necessary first step.

    Laser peripheral iridoplasty may be necessary in patients whose angle approach remains very narrow despite a patent PI. This technique uses the argon laser to apply burns circumferentially to the peripheral iris, which cause it to contract and pull away from the angle. Although the green wavelength is usually used, use of the yellow-green wavelength may improve absorption of laser energy in more lightly colored irides. One important potential complication that should always be discussed with the patient is the risk of a permanently larger pupil size postoperatively, and its attendant potential to increase problems with glare.

    Chronic miotic therapy can also be a useful alternative or adjunct to iridoplasty in eyes with a narrow approach despite a patent PI. With either method of therapy, the angle should be examined with gonioscopy after instillation of pilocarpine, and at regular 6- to 12-month intervals afterward, to document the effect on angle configuration.

AQUEOUS MISDIRECTION SYNDROME (MALIGNANT/CILIARY BLOCK GLAUCOMA)

34. What is aqueous misdirection syndrome?

Posterior misdirection of aqueous into the vitreous cavity causes an anterior displacement of the lens-iris diaphragm. It most commonly occurs after ocular (typically glaucoma-filtering) surgery, but can occur after laser procedures or, rarely, spontaneously. Miotic use and previous angle-closure glaucoma increase the risk of occurrence. It typically presents within the first postoperative week with a shallow to flat anterior chamber and a high IOP, but the IOP may be normal in an eye with a functioning filter. Serous choroidal effusion/detachment, pupillary block, and suprachoroidal hemorrhage should be ruled out.

35. How is aqueous misdirection treated medically?

- Cycloplegics relax the ciliary muscle, which increases zonular tension and pulls the lens-iris diaphragm posteriorly. Cycloplegics are also essential in the management of angle closure due to anterior rotation of the ciliary body. They may be required indefinitely.
- Aqueous suppressants.
- Hyperosmotic agents.
- Miotics are contraindicated.

36. How can aqueous misdirection be treated with laser if it is unresponsive to medication?

The goal of therapy is to reestablish aqueous flow from the posterior chamber to the anterior chamber, and to try to create a channel for aqueous flow from the posterior segment to the anterior segment.

- **Nd:YAG laser hyaloidotomy:** In pseudophakes and aphakes, using the Nd:YAG laser to disrupt the anterior vitreous face can be successful in resolving aqueous misdirection.
- **Argon laser treatment of ciliary processes:** Regardless of the lens status, this procedure can only be done if a surgical iridectomy or a relatively large laser iridotomy is present.

37. How can aqueous misdirection be treated surgically if refractory to medical therapy and/or laser?

The timing and mode of intervention depend on the following factors:

- Duration of misdirection without resolution.
- Degree and duration of shallowness or flatness of the anterior chamber. When there is contact between the corneal endothelium and the crystalline lens or an intraocular lens, surgical correction is urgent.
- IOP and optic nerve status.

The treatment options are as follows:

- **Anterior chamber reformation:** Occasionally can be performed at the slit lamp by injecting a small amount of air followed by viscoelastic through a peripheral corneal paracentesis wound. The initial air helps to confirm complete penetration of the needle through the cornea into the AC before injecting any viscoelastic. Because the IOP is almost always elevated with the aqueous misdirection syndrome, this is rarely an option.
- **Pars plana vitrectomy (PPV):** Aqueous misdirection can occasionally persist or recur even after PPV, especially in phakic eyes.
- **Lens extraction:** May be combined with vitrectomy. The posterior capsule and anterior hyaloid are usually incised to allow aqueous passage to the anterior chamber.

NEOVASCULAR GLAUCOMA

38. **What typically causes neovascular glaucoma (NVG)?**
Posterior segment (retinal) ischemia results in the production of angiogenic factors that stimulate the formation of a neovascular membrane on the iris (NVI). Vascular endothelial growth factor (VEGF) has been shown to be the primary angiogenic factor. As the membrane first grows into the angle and across the scleral spur to the TM, the angle appears anatomically open. Later, the membrane contracts, pulling the peripheral iris up to the TM and peripheral cornea, creating PAS. This latter process can occur over significant areas of the angle very quickly (often in a few days) producing an acute angle-closure glaucoma. Common causes of NVG are CRVO ($\frac{1}{3}$), proliferative diabetic retinopathy ($\frac{1}{3}$), and carotid occlusive disease (approximately 10%).

39. **How is neovascular glaucoma treated?**
    1. The underlying etiology of the neovascularization must be diagnosed and treated, usually with panretinal photocoagulation (PRP) or, if the lack of clear visualization of the retina precludes PRP, peripheral retinal cryotherapy for posterior segment ischemic processes. New anti-VEGF compounds injected into vitreous or AC can produce dramatic regression of NVI within 1–2 weeks.
    2. **Medical treatment.** The percent of angle that is closed with PAS as well as the outflow resistance of the TM still open will determine the potential for successfully treating the glaucoma medically. Even if the angle is completely closed, maximal tolerated aqueous suppressant and, if necessary, hyperosmotic therapy should be used in an attempt to temporize until surgery is performed. Miotics should not be used, because they decrease uveoscleral outflow and increase inflammation.
    3. **Surgical treatment.** One of the most important principles to remember when operating on these eyes, especially eyes with florid NVI, is to try to avoid rapid decompression of the eye; the fragile new vessels may rupture, creating a spontaneous hyphema that can significantly complicate subsequent management.
       - The **guarded filtering procedure (trabeculectomy)** has been used to control IOP in these eyes with poor results. The success rate is somewhat better if an adjunctive antimetabolite such as mitomycin C is used. The risk of filtration failure due to fibrosis is higher, presumably owing to the presence of angiogenic factors in the aqueous.
       - **Aqueous tube shunts** have become the procedure of choice for many glaucoma surgeons, but still have success rates of only approximately 70%, owing to the often poor prognosis of the underlying pathologic process.
    4. **Laser/cryo cyclodestruction.** This may be a viable option in eyes with minimal visual potential, as an attempt to control IOP for long-term comfort, and to prevent the need for enucleation for pain due to high IOP. Laser is highly preferred to cryo due to higher long-term success, much lower risk of phthisis bulbi, and much less postoperative pain and inflammation.

MISCELLANEOUS

40. **What are the different mechanisms of producing angle closure secondary to inflammation?**
    - PAS formation from any etiology
    - Complete pupillary block (secluded pupil) from posterior synechiae resulting in iris bombé
    - Uveal effusion causing anterior rotation of the ciliary body (uncommon)
    - Exudative retinal detachment pushing lens-iris diaphragm forward (rare)

41. **Describe nanophthalmos.**

A bilateral condition in which the globes are significantly shorter than normal, with an axial length less than 20 mm (mean 18.8 mm), with a corresponding hyperopia. In addition, the corneal diameter is smaller (mean 10.5 mm versus 12 mm for a normal adult) and the sclera is much thicker (often at least twice as thick) than normal. The unusually thick sclera creates an impediment to uveoscleral outflow that predisposes to choroidal effusions, either spontaneously or after surgery, and angle closure. Angle-closure glaucoma can also occur as a result of anterior-segment crowding without uveal effusions.

42. **List one systemic medication that can cause angle closure by producing ciliochoroidal effusions, and the principles for management of this type of angle closure.**

Topiramate, a sulfa-derived antiepileptic medication whose indications have expanded to include the treatment of migraine headaches and obesity, has been reported to cause idiosyncratic ciliochoroidal effusions with acute onset myopia and angle-closure glaucoma. Thus, a careful and thorough history can be crucial in making the diagnosis. These changes do gradually resolve with discontinuation of the medication. Pupillary block is usually not present and thus laser peripheral iridotomy is not helpful. Miotics will make the problem worse. The treatment includes topical and systemic aqueous suppressants, systemic hyperosmotics if necessary for IOP control, steroids, and cycloplegics to help pull the lens-iris diaphragm posteriorly.

WEBSITES

1. The Glaucoma Foundation:
   www.glaucomafoundation.org

2. Glaucoma Research Foundation:
   www.glaucoma.org

BIBLIOGRAPHY

1. Albert D, Jakobiec F: Principles and Practice of Ophthalmology, 2nd ed. Philadelphia, W.B. Saunders, 2000.
2. American Academy of Ophthalmology Basic and Clinical Science Course: Section 10, Glaucoma. 2005.
3. American Academy of Ophthalmology Preferred Practice Pattern: Primary Angle Closure Glaucoma. 2005.
4. Davidorf J, Baker N, Derick R: Treatment of the fellow eye in acute angle-closure glaucoma: A case report and survey of members of the American Glaucoma Society. J Glaucoma 5:228–232, 1996.
5. Rhee DJ, Goldberg MJ, Parrish RK: Bilateral angle-closure glaucoma and ciliary body swelling from topiramate. Arch Ophthalmol 119:1721–1723, 2001.
6. Ritch R: The pilocarpine paradox [editorial]. J Glaucoma 5:225–227, 1996.
7. Ritch R, Shields B, Krupin T: The Glaucomas, 2nd ed. St. Louis, Mosby, 1996.
8. Spaeth GL, Idowu O, Seligsohn A, et al: The effects of iridotomy size and position on symptoms following laser peripheral iridotomy. J Glaucoma 14:364–367, 2005.

CHAPTER 17

SECONDARY OPEN-ANGLE GLAUCOMA

Janice A. Gault, MD

1. **A 72-year-old man presents for a routine exam. He states that vision in the left eye is getting bad. On exam, he has vision of 20/30 in the right and counts fingers at 3 feet in the left. The intraocular pressure in the right eye is 25 mmHg; in the left eye, 42 mmHg. The optic nerve appears somewhat cupped on the right, severely so on the left. Visual fields reveal a significant nasal step in the right eye and a temporal island on the left. He does not have pseudoexfoliation syndrome or a Krukenberg spindle in either eye. His angles are deep. What do you suspect?**

   A history of trauma. The patient's prior occupation was boxing, and he was often hit in his left eye. Angle-recession glaucoma can be asymptomatic until many years later when visual loss occurs. On gonioscopy, the angle recession is determined by torn iris processes and posteriorly recessed iris, revealing a widened ciliary body band. Comparison with the other eye may help to identify this condition. Any patient with traumatic iritis or hyphema needs to be warned of this complication, which may occur many years later. Treatment is the same as with open-angle glaucoma except that miotic agents are ineffective and may even increase the intraocular pressure. Argon laser trabeculoplasty (ALT) is rarely effective.

2. **What should you look for to make a diagnosis of pseudoexfoliation glaucoma?**

   Fibrillar, "dandruff-like" material is deposited on the anterior lens capsule in a characteristic bull's eye pattern, most easily seen after pupillary dilation. This material is also seen clinically in the angle and on the iris. Gonioscopy reveals a heavily pigmented trabecular meshwork and a Sampolesi's line, which is pigment deposited anteriorly to Schwalbe's line (Fig. 17-1).

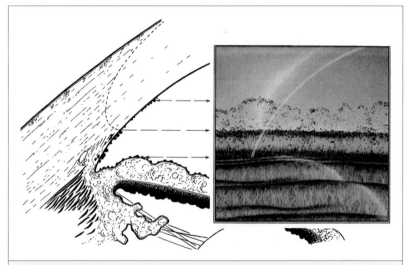

Figure 17-1. Sampolesi's line is a scalloped band of pigmentation anterior to Schwalbe's line. (From Alward WLM: Color Atlas of Gonioscopy. St. Louis, Mosby, 1994.)

Pseudoexfoliation syndrome is thought to be part of generalized basement membrane disorder, because it can be found histologically in other parts of the body. It may be unilateral or bilateral with asymmetry. Although pseudoexfoliation is infrequent in the United States, it accounts for more than 50% of open-angle glaucoma in Scandinavia. The condition is often more resistant to medical therapy than primary open-angle glaucoma and may require ALT, selective laser trabeculoplasty (SLT), or surgical therapy.

3. **Is the condition cured after cataract extraction?**
   No. The deposits continue, and cataract surgery has a higher risk in such patients. The zonules are weak, and synechiae are often present between the iris and anterior lens capsule. There is an increased risk of posterior capsular rupture.

4. **What is true exfoliative glaucoma?**
   Capsular delamination caused typically by exposure to intense heat, as seen in glassblowers.

KEY POINTS: PSEUDOEXFOLIATION GLAUCOMA

1. Bull's-eye deposits on anterior lens capsule.

2. Sampolesi's line on gonioscopy.

3. Less responsive to medical therapy.

4. Higher risk for complications in cataract surgery.

5. **A 24-year-old man with sarcoidosis presents with an intraocular pressure of 35 mmHg in the right eye and 32 mmHg in the left eye. He notes mild pain and some decreased vision but is otherwise asymptomatic. On examination, you notice 2+ cell and flare in both eyes as well as significant posterior synechiae and mutton-fat keratic precipitates. Gonioscopy reveals an open angle with no peripheral anterior synechiae. A dilated exam reveals no significant cupping of either optic nerve. What do you do?**
   Most likely, the inflammatory cells have clogged the trabecular meshwork. Intensive topical steroids and a cycloplegic should decrease the inflammatory load and break the synechiae to prevent angle closure from becoming an issue in the future. Antiglaucoma medications are also appropriate until the pressure decreases. However, miotics are contraindicated because they may cause further synechiae and precipitate angle closure. They also increase permeability of blood vessels and may contribute to an increase in inflammation. Prostaglandin agonists or analogues may also increase inflammation and should be avoided. The aggressiveness with which the pressure is lowered depends a great deal on optic nerve cupping.

6. **The same patient returns 14 days later with pressures of 40 mmHg and 45 mmHg in the right and left eye, respectively. Exam reveals minimal cell and flare in each eye as well as a significant decrease in the keratic precipitates. He has been using prednisolone acetate 1% every hour and atropine 1% three times/day. What should you do?**
   Gonioscopy. The differential of increased intraocular pressure in this situation includes:
   - Steroid response. Decreasing steroids lowers the pressure if this is the cause.
   - Cellular blockage of the trabecular meshwork from the inflammatory cells. Increasing the steroids lowers the pressure if this is the cause.

■ Synechiae formation causing an element of secondary angle closure or blocking of the meshwork. Gonioscopy determines whether the angle is open. Increased steroids may melt the synechiae.

Provided the angle is open and without neovascularization, the most likely cause is response to steroids. The increased intraocular pressure may occur anywhere from a few days to years after initiating therapy. The response has been noted in or around the eye after oral and intravenous administration of steroids and even with inhalers. Patients with Cushing's syndrome with excessive levels of endogenous steroids are also at risk. Optic nerve evaluation is crucial to determine the risks of damage. Decrease the steroid concentration or dosage, and start antiglaucoma therapy. A topical nonsteroidal agent may help decrease inflammation without increasing intraocular pressure. Fluorometholone and loteprednol (Alrex, Lotemax) are also less likely to increase intraocular pressure than other formulations of steroids; however, they have less potency in decreasing inflammation.

7. **What does a Krukenberg spindle look like? What does it mean?**
A Krukenberg spindle is a vertical pigment band on the corneal endothelium (Fig. 17-2). It is typically found in patients with pigmentary dispersion syndrome. The iris is often bowed posteriorly and rubs against the lens zonules. This process causes midperipheral spokelike iris transillumination defects. Gonioscopy reveals a densely pigmented trabecular meshwork for 360 degrees. The patient is often asymptomatic but may notice blurred vision, eye pain, and halos around lights after exercise or pupillary dilation. Pigmentary dispersion syndrome is more common in young adults and white, myopic males. It is usually bilateral.

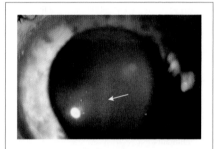

Figure 17-2. A Krukenberg spindle *(arrow)* is made of pigment deposited on the endothelium in pigmentary dispersion syndrome. (From Alward WLM: Color Atlas of Gonioscopy. St. Louis, Mosby, 1994.)

8. **How is pigmentary dispersion treated?**
If no optic disc damage is noted and the visual fields are normal, the patient may be observed. Treatment for intraocular pressure over 28 mmHg is usually indicated, although this point is controversial. Once damage is noted, miotics may be the first line of therapy because they minimize contact between the zonules and iris. However, miotics also cause myopic fluctuation and may not be practical in young patients, especially in myopes with lattice degeneration because of their increased risk of retinal detachment. Laser peripheral iridectomies (PI) have been recommended; they treat the posterior bowing of the iris and may theoretically cure the disorder. The pressures may still be elevated until the residual pigment in the trabecular meshwork is cleared. This treatment is controversial. Patients also respond well to ALT or SLT because of the increased pigment of the trabecular meshwork.

9. **A 95-year-old woman presents with a markedly red, painful right eye of 2 days' duration. Her vision is hand motions at 1 foot and 20/400 in the right and left eye, respectively. Exam of the right eye reveals a steamy cornea with a pressure of 60 mmHg and no view of the anterior chamber. The left eye has a brunescent cataract but appears to be deep and quiet with a pressure of 18 mmHg. With topical glycerin, the cornea clears in the right eye to reveal iridescent particles**

floating in the anterior chamber with a morgagnian cataract. **Gonioscopy reveals bilateral open angles. No view is obtained of either posterior chamber. What do you do now?**

The patient denies a history of uveitis. A B-scan of both eyes reveals only significant cataract without retinal detachment or intraocular tumor. The leakage of lens material through an intact lens capsule is obstructing the trabecular meshwork. If the diagnosis is in question, paracentesis may be done to examine the anterior chamber reaction microscopically. Macrophages are filled with lens cortical material (phacolytic glaucoma). Typically, the lens is hypermature, as in this patient. The intraocular pressure must be reduced and the inflammation controlled before surgical therapy is attempted. A steroid such as prednisolone acetate 1% every hour, a cycloplegic such as scopolamine 0.25%, three times/day, and antiglaucoma medications are started immediately. Cataract extraction is performed in the next day or two once the eye is less inflamed.

10. **A 64-year-old woman who had cataract surgery in the left eye 1 week ago presents to the emergency department complaining that the eye is red and painful with decreasing vision. What is your concern?**

    First, you must think of endophthalmitis. Any patient presenting after surgery with a red, painful eye with decreased vision must be presumed to have endophthalmitis until it is ruled out. The exam reveals vision of hand motions at 2 feet, a severely injected eye with corneal edema, 4+ cell and flare, and an intraocular pressure of 47 mmHg. The anterior chamber is filled with lens cortical material, and a rupture in the posterior capsule is seen. A large chunk of nuclear material is in the vitreous. The optic nerve is mildly cupped.

    Because the lens material is seen in the anterior chamber, treatment with steroids and antiglaucoma medications is appropriate, along with close observation. The diagnosis is most likely lens-particle glaucoma. The patient is started on prednisolone acetate 1% every 2 hours, scopolamine 0.25%, three times/day, latanoprost once daily, a beta blocker twice daily, apraclonidine twice daily, and acetazolamide sequels twice daily. In addition, because her pressure is so high, mannitol is given. When the pressure improves to 25 mmHg, she is sent home. The next day, she counts fingers at 5 feet, her intraocular inflammation is subsiding, and the pressure is 23 mmHg. Once her eye is less inflamed and the pressure well controlled, she is scheduled for removal of the remaining lens material. If the retained lens material is minimal, patients sometimes can be maintained on medical therapy until the eye clears without surgery.

11. **What other type of open-angle glaucoma can be caused by the lens?**

    Phacoanaphylactic glaucoma, which occurs after penetrating trauma or surgery. The patient is sensitized to the lens protein during a latent period and develops a granulomatous uveitis. This feature distinguishes it from lens particle glaucoma. Patients are treated medically and may need surgery to remove the lens if they do not respond adequately.

12. **What is Posner-Schlossman syndrome? Who gets it?**

    Patients are young to middle-aged. They notice unilateral attacks of mild pain, decreased vision, and halos around lights. Episodes tend to recur. Also known as glaucomatocyclitic crisis, this disorder is idiopathic. On exam, intraocular pressure is high, usually between 40 mmHg and 60 mmHg. The angle is open on gonioscopy without synechiae, and the eye is minimally injected. Anterior chamber reaction is minimal. The corneal epithelium may be edematous because of the acute rise in pressure. A few fine keratic precipitates may be present on the corneal endothelium, often inferiorly. Treatment includes steroids and antiglaucoma medications to reduce aqueous production. A cycloplegic agent is necessary only if the patient is symptomatic. The attacks usually resolve in a few hours to a few weeks. No therapy is needed between attacks. However, the risk of chronic open-angle glaucoma is increased in both eyes.

13. **What is the classic triad of Fuchs' heterochromic iridocyclitis?**

    Heterochromia, cataract, and low-grade iritis. The iritis is mild and does not cause synechiae. Characteristic stellate, colorless keratic precipitates are seen over the inferior endothelium. Fine new vessels may be seen in the angle but do not cause closure. The glaucoma is difficult to control and often does not correspond to the degree of inflammation. Steroids are not often helpful.

14. **A patient reports for postoperative check-up 1 day after cataract surgery. The pressure in the operated eye is 40 mmHg, and the patient complains of nausea. What is the most likely cause?**
Retained viscoelastic from surgery. The pressure usually increases 6 or 7 hours after surgery and normalizes within 24–48 hours, depending on the type of viscoelastic. Most eyes tolerate short-term pressures up to 30 mmHg; of course, tolerance depends on preexisting optic nerve status. Medical treatment and paracentesis to remove the viscoelastic are indicated to decrease pressure quickly and relieve nausea. Paracentesis is somewhat controversial because of the increased risk of endophthalmitis.

15. **What else can cause postoperative glaucoma?**
Hyphema, pigment dispersion, generalized inflammation, aphakic or pseudophakic pupillary block, malignant glaucoma (aqueous misdirection syndrome), and steroid-response glaucoma. In patients who have undergone an intracapsular cataract extraction, alpha-chymotrypsin is injected into the anterior chamber to dissolve the zonules. The zonular debris may block the trabecular meshwork postoperatively. Epithelial ingrowth may occur many months to years after surgery or trauma and block outflow.

16. **A patient had cataract surgery 1 year ago but continues to have episodes of anterior chamber cell and flare with increased intraocular pressure. Some of the cells are red blood cells. What is the diagnosis?**
Uveitis-glaucoma-hyphema (UGH) syndrome. The cells may layer out to produce a hyphema, usually as a result of irritation from an anterior chamber intraocular lens, although a posterior chamber lens may be involved. Gonioscopy may reveal where the irritation is occurring. Treatment consists of atropine, topical steroids, and antiglaucoma medications until the pressure is reduced. Argon laser of the bleeding site, if it can be identified, may be curative. However, exchange or removal of the intraocular lens may be necessary.

17. **How can raised episcleral venous pressure cause glaucoma?**
Aqueous drains from the anterior chamber through the trabecular meshwork, Schlemm's canal, and intrascleral channels to the episcleral and conjunctival veins. Normal drainage depends on an episcleral venous pressure that is lower than the pressure of the eye. Usually, it ranges from 8–12 mmHg. However, if it is higher than intraocular pressure, drainage does not occur. Blood will be seen in Schlemm's canal on gonioscopy. Drugs that reduce aqueous humor formation are obviously the most effective medical treatment.

KEY POINTS: CAUSES OF RAISED EPISCLERAL VENOUS PRESSURE

1. Thyroid ophthalmopathy.

2. Carotid and dural fistulas.

3. Superior vena cava syndrome.

4. Retrobulbar tumors.

5. Orbital varices.

6. Sturge-Weber syndrome.

18. **A patient with long-standing diabetes has had recurrent vitreous hemorrhage. While you are observing him waiting for the condition to clear, intraocular pressure increases to 35 mmHg. What should you suspect?**
When intraocular hemorrhages clear, hemolytic or ghost-cell glaucoma may develop. Hemolytic glaucoma occurs because macrophages full of hemoglobin block the trabecular meshwork. Reddish cells can be seen in the anterior chamber. In ghost-cell glaucoma, degenerating red blood cells block the aqueous outflow. Khaki cells in the anterior chamber may layer out to form a pseudohypopyon. Both conditions can be treated medically until the hemorrhage clears. However, because the intraocular pressure may become markedly raised, washout of the anterior chamber and/or vitrectomy often becomes necessary. In addition, the patient may be developing neovascular glaucoma; thus it is important to check the angles for new vessels and angle narrowing.

19. **What other conditions may cause open-angle glaucoma?**
    1. Intraocular tumor may cause secondary open-angle glaucoma by invasion of the chamber angle or blockage of the trabecular meshwork by tumor debris.
    2. Siderosis or chalcosis from a retained metallic foreign body.
    3. Chemical injuries from acid or alkali can shrink the scleral collagen or cause direct damage to the trabecular meshwork.
    4. Iridocorneal endothelial syndrome (ICE) is a spectrum of three entities that overlap considerably:
       - **Essential iris atrophy:** Iris thinning leads to iris holes and pupillary distortion
       - **Chandler's syndrome:** Mild iris thinning and distortion with hammered metal appearance of corneal endothelium
       - **Cogan-Reese syndrome:** Pigmented nodules on the iris surface with variable iris atrophy
       - Such patients are generally asymptomatic, middle-aged adults. Usually findings are unilateral with increased intraocular pressure and corneal edema. No treatment is necessary unless corneal edema and glaucoma are present.
    5. Posterior polymorphous dystrophy is a bilateral and autosomal dominant disease. Vesicles are seen at Descemet's membrane. Corneal edema occurs in severe cases. Iridocorneal adhesions may occur. Glaucoma is associated in 15%.

20. **What types of secondary open-angle glaucoma occur in children?**
    1. Glaucoma associated with mesenchymal dysgenesis is a spectrum of disease, but two main categories are recognized:
       - Axenfeld's anomaly consists of a prominent Schwalbe's ring with attached iris strands. Axenfeld's syndrome is the anomaly with coincident glaucoma and occurs in 50% of cases. It is autosomal dominant or sporadic.
       - Rieger's anomaly is Axenfeld's anomaly plus iris thinning and distorted pupils. Sixty percent of patients develop glaucoma; it is also autosomal dominant or sporadic. Rieger's syndrome is the anomaly associated with dental, craniofacial, and skeletal abnormalities.
    2. Aniridia is a bilateral, near-total absence of the iris. The strands may be seen only by gonioscopy. Glaucoma, foveal hypoplasia, and nystagmus may occur. The disorder may be autosomal dominant or sporadic. Patients with sporadic inheritance need to be evaluated for Wilms' tumor, which is associated in 25% of cases.
    3. Oculocerebrorenal syndrome (Lowe) is an X-linked recessive disease. Patients have aminoaciduria, hypotonia, acidemia, cataracts, and glaucoma.
    4. Congenital rubella may be associated with cataracts and pigmented retinal lesions. Cardiac, auditory, and central nervous abnormalities are often coexistent.
    5. Sturge-Weber syndrome.
    6. Neurofibromatosis.
    7. Glaucoma after cataract removal is a long-term risk for such patients.

BIBLIOGRAPHY

1. American Academy of Ophthalmology: Basic and Clinical Science Course, Section 10. San Francisco, American Academy of Ophthalmology, 1992.

2. Danyluk AW, Paton D: Diagnosis and management of glaucoma. Clin Symp 43:2–32, 1991.

3. Kunimoto DY, Kanitkar KD, Makar M: The Wills Eye Manual: Office and Emergency Room Diagnosis and Treatment of Eye Disease, 4th ed. Philadelphia, Lippincott Williams & Wilkins, 2004.

4. Shields MB: Textbook of Glaucoma, 4th ed. Baltimore, Williams & Wilkins, 1998.

CHAPTER 18

MEDICAL TREATMENT OF GLAUCOMA

Jeffrey D. Henderer, MD, and Richard P. Wilson, MD

1. **What classes of medications are used to treat glaucoma?**
   See Table 18-1.

2. **How do these medications work?**
   - **Miotics** constrict the longitudinal muscle of the ciliary body, which is attached to the scleral spur anteriorly and to the choroid posteriorly. When the longitudinal muscle constricts, it pulls the scleral spur posteriorly, pulling open the spaces between the trabecular beams and mechanically increasing the capacity for aqueous outflow.
   - The **adrenergic agonists** epinephrine and dipivefrin initially decrease aqueous production slightly, but their major action is to increase outflow through the trabecular meshwork. Apraclonidine and brimonidine decrease aqueous production. Brimonidine may have some increased uveoscleral outflow as well.
   - **β-blockers** and **carbonic anhydrase inhibitors** (CAIs) decrease aqueous production.
   - **Prostaglandin analogs** increase outflow through the uveoscleral outflow channels. Aqueous is absorbed into the face of the ciliary body or into the trabecular meshwork and then flows posteriorly around the longitudinal muscle fibers of the ciliary body posteriorly. It is absorbed into the choroid or passes out through the sclera.
   - **Hyperosmotic agents** increase the osmolarity of the blood, which in turn draws fluid from the posterior chamber into the blood vessels of the ciliary body.

3. **For patients in good health with primary open-angle glaucoma, what is the first drug to try?**
   The short answer is that any of the topical medications can be used. The choice is based on the desired amount of intraocular pressure (IOP) reduction, the possible side effects, and the relative costs of the medicines. The advantage of having four commonly used classes of medications (β-blockers, prostaglandin analogs, topical CAIs, and adrenergic agonists) is that therapy can be customized for each patient. Traditionally, most ophthalmologists have started with a β-blocker. However, the prostaglandin analogs have largely supplanted β-blockers as first-line therapy due to their ease of use, powerful hypotensive effect, and favorable side-effect profile. Latanoprost has replaced timolol as the most commonly prescribed glaucoma medication.

   If a patient would not be a good candidate for a prostaglandin, one of the other three classes of medicines can be used. Nonselective β-blockers are the most potent, and the cardioselective β-blocker (betaxolol), topical CAIs, and adrenergic agonists are all about equal in hypotensive effect. When used alone, topical CAIs and α-adrenergic agonists should be used 3 times/day to prevent possible IOP fluctuation (Fig. 18-1).

   Konstas AG, Stewart WC, Topouzis F, et al: Brimonidine 0.2% given two or three times daily versus timolol maleate 0.5% in primary open-angle glaucoma. Am J Ophthalmol 131:729–733, 2001.

4. **What medicine should be used as second-line therapy? Third-line therapy?**
   As in the case of first-line therapy, any of the medicine classes can be used as second- or third-line therapy. With several options available, the physician can attempt to tailor the choice to the patient's particular situation. If a prostaglandin has been used as first-line therapy, a β-blocker is often chosen as second-line therapy, and vice versa. As these medicines are the most

TABLE 18-1. COMMONLY USED AGENTS FOR GLAUCOMA MANAGEMENT

Chemical Name	Strength	Usual Dosage	Size
Miotics			
Pilocarpine hydrochloride	0.25, 0.5, 1, 2% 4, 6, 8, 10%	2–4 times/day	15, 30 mL
Pilocarpine-HS gel	4% gel	At bedtime	4-gm tube
Pilocarpine nitrate	1, 2, 4%	2–4 times/day	15 mL
Carbachol	0.75, 1.5, 2.25, 3%	2–3 times/day	15, 30 mL
Echothiophate iodide	0.03, 0.06%, 0.125, 0.25%	1–2 times/day	5 mL
Adrenergic agonists			
Dipivefrin hydrochloride	0.1%	1–2 times/day	5, 10, 15 mL
Epinephrine hydrochloride	0.5, 1, 2%	1–2 times/day	5, 10, 15 mL
Apraclonidine hydrochloride	0.5%	2–3 times/day	5 mL
Brimonidine tartrate	0.1, 0.15, 0.2%	2–3 times/day	5, 10, 15 mL
Prostaglandin analogs			
Latanoprost	0.005%	Daily	2.5 mL
Travoprost	0.004%	Daily	2.5, 5 mL
Bimatoprost	0.03%	Daily	2.5, 5 mL
Beta blockers			
Betaxolol hydrochloride suspension	0.25%	2 times/day	2.5, 5, 15 mL
Carteolol hydrochloride	1.0%	1–2 times/day	5, 10 mL
Levobunolol hydrochloride	0.25, 0.5%	1–2 times/day	5, 10 mL
Metipranolol	0.3%	1–2 times/day	5, 10 mL
Timolol maleate	0.25, 0.5%	1–2 times/day	2.5, 5, 10, 15 mL
Timolol hemihydrate	0.5%	1–2 times/day	5, 10, 15 mL
Timolol XE gel-forming solution	0.25, 0.5%	Daily	2.5, 5 mL
Carbonic anhydrase inhibitors			
Acetazolamide sodium	125, 250 mg	3–4 times/day	NA
Acetazolamide sequels	500 mg	2 times/day	NA
Methazolamide	25, 50, 100 mg	2–4 times/day	NA
Dorzolamide	2%	2–3 times/day	5, 10 mL
Brinzolamide	1%	2–3 times/day	5, 10 mL
Hyperosmotic agents			
Glycerin	50% solution	1–1.5 gm/kg (orally)	NA
Mannitol	20%, 50% solution	0.5–2 gm/kg (IV)	NA
Fixed combinations			
Timolol/dorzolamide	0.5%/2%	2 times/day	5, 10 mL

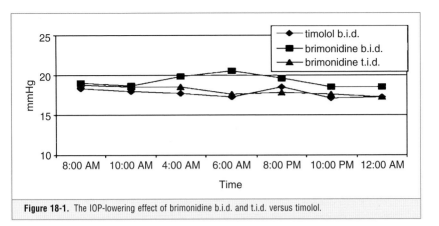

Figure 18-1. The IOP-lowering effect of brimonidine b.i.d. and t.i.d. versus timolol.

potent ones available and are both typically once-a-day medicines (β-blocker once per day in the morning and prostaglandin once per day in the evening), this regimen typically results in a very good hypotensive effect for the number of drops used. In addition, combination products may soon be released that will enable timolol/latanoprost or timolol/travoprost to be dispensed in a single drop, once a day. Additional product combinations are likely and fewer drops per day likely results in greater compliance.

The availability of the fixed combination of timolol/dorzolamide makes it easy to add dorzolamide as a second-line agent after timolol. This reduces the drop count from three or four to two per day.

Brimonidine can be an excellent choice for additive therapy. Brimonidine works much better than latanoprost when added to two or more medications. Epinephrine and dipivefrin are rarely used today. The next choice may be a topical CAI, if it has not been used previously.

Miotics are more difficult to use due to drop frequency and side effects but can be quite effective, especially in aphakic (no crystalline lens in the eye) patients. In phakic patients with little remaining accommodation and little cataract, pilocarpine is often well tolerated. It provides a pinhole effect that gives an increased depth of field for most patients. Many patients can read without reading glasses when taking pilocarpine, and no one needs trifocals if the pupils are adequately miotic.

Oral CAIs were once quite commonly used and are among the most potent of all hypotensive medications. Their side-effect profile and the availability of a variety of topical medicines limit their use today.

5. **Are there any hints for prescribing β-blockers?**
Nonselective β-blockers can often be used in the 0.25% dosage once daily for patients with light irides and the 0.5% dosage once daily for patients with dark irides. β-blockers block intrinsic β-1 and β-2 receptor tone; thus, when patients are asleep, β-blockers are ineffective because there is little tone. However, because aqueous production also declines at night, this fact is usually considered inconsequential. Thus, many ophthalmologists prescribe β-blockers once daily when patients awake in the morning. Brubaker's study, however, suggested that a nighttime dose might be the most effective. For patients with more advanced disease, a twice-daily regimen of 0.25% for lighter irides and 0.5% for darker irides is common. This regimen guards against going for a day without medication in patients who miss one prescribed drop. Betaxolol has far fewer systemic side effects than the nonselective β-blockers but is not as potent. Betaxolol results in a roughly 20% drop in intraocular pressure, while nonselective β-blockers achieve about a 25% reduction. β-blockers should be started as a one-eyed trial since 10% of patients show no effect

from topical nonselective β-blockers, and 10% of patients who had a significant effect from nonselective β-blockers have no effect from selective β-blockers.

In general, the side effects of this class of medications are identical to those of the oral β-blockers. Patients, and even physicians, often forget that eyedrops have systemic effects. Physicians must remember to ask about eyedrops when taking a complete medical history. β-blockers can exacerbate asthma or chronic obstructive pulmonary disease (COPD) and can cause bradycardia, lowered blood pressure, heart block, fatigue, exercise intolerance, impotence, and depression. In diabetics they may mask the symptoms of hypoglycemia. The selective β-blocker betaxolol is much less likely to trigger bronchospasm but still must be used with caution.

6. **How does one choose among the five nonselective β-blockers?**
In terms of effectiveness, there is little difference. However, there are subtle differences between them. Carteolol has intrinsic sympathomimetic activity that can reduce the chance of cardiovascular side effects. It also raises triglycerides and lowers high-density lipoproteins the least. It has the least allergenic potential and is the best tolerated in patients with dry eyes and extensive superficial punctate keratopathy. Levobunolol lasts the longest of the compounds that have been tested as once-daily drugs. Metipranolol is the least expensive and in once-daily dosage can fit many budgets. Timolol was the first β-blocker and is still considered the gold standard against which all other ocular hypotensive medications are judged. It has been formulated as both a nonviscous and viscous drop. The viscous formation (Timoptic XE from Merck, Timolol GFS from Falcon) remains in the tear film longer; consequently, intraocular absorption is greater and systemic absorption is reduced. This drug provides the best diurnal curve for pressure control with once-daily dosing and can reduce the possibility of systemic side effects.

7. **Any hints for prescribing prostaglandin analogs?**
The three prostaglandin analogs available today are all extremely effective at lowering intraocular pressure and are generally used as first-line therapy. They can be additive with any medicine, but tend not to work as well if added beyond second-line therapy. Latanoprost was released first and remains the most commonly used of the three medicines. It is an extremely powerful prostaglandin analog and in a 0.005% concentration it is 100 times more powerful than timolol or levobunolol. Travoprost is equally effective to latanoprost with greater conjunctival erythema but less effect on iris pigmentation. Bimatoprost appears to offer on average about 0.5 mm greater IOP reduction than the other prostaglandins, and in selected individuals, it may be significantly more powerful. The increased concentration of bimatoprost is accompanied by greater local ocular side effects.

Although there have been rare reports of systemic side effects, such as flulike symptoms, numerous ocular side effects can occur. The most common are conjunctival injection, increased pigmentation of the iris and eyelid skin, and growth of eyelashes. Increased iris pigmentation is the result of increased amount of melanin within iris melanocytes and seems to occur much more frequently in patients with hazel irides or who have iris nevi. While the other side effects are reversible, increased iris pigmentation is not. Ocular inflammation, including anterior uveitis and keratitis, has been rarely reported so in patients with a history of uveitis, it may not be the drug of choice. The drug has been associated with cystoid macular edema, especially in pseudophakes, although the eyes in which this occurs typically have other risk factors that may be responsible. Likewise, it can exacerbate or reactivate herpes keratitis. It also has been known to produce a herpes-like keratitis that clears when the drops are stopped.

8. **Any tips on prescribing adrenergic agonists?**
Adrenergic agonists may be classified into two groups. Epinephrine and dipivefrin, which is converted to epinephrine by the eye, make up the first group. They increase trabecular meshwork outflow. Apraclonidine and brimonidine make up the second group. They are α-2 selective agonists that reduce aqueous production. Brimonidine also may increase trabecular meshwork outflow.

The α-adrenergic compounds are characterized by a high allergic-reaction rate. Epinephrine is said to have an allergic rate of 50% by 5 years, and apraclonidine has an allergic rate of approximately 20% by 1 year. Because of its high allergy rate, apraclonidine is used almost exclusively for acute pressure control or to prevent pressure rise after laser procedures. Brimonidine is less likely to cause an allergy, but many patients develop one often months after starting the drug. Yet brimonidine can often be used successfully in patients that have had a previous allergic reaction to apraclonidine. The newer 0.15% and 0.1% formulation of brimonidine is packaged with a less-allergy-provoking preservative and has a reduced allergic rate.

Due to their high allergy rate and poor pressure lowering effect, epinephrine and dipivefrin are rarely used today. Brimonidine has become an important drug for treating glaucoma. It works as well as a nonselective β-blocker at peak effect, although less well at trough 6–12 hours later, and almost all patients have some reduction in pressure. Aside from allergy, it is well tolerated by the eye. Systemically, it can cause dry mouth and fatigue, which can be debilitating. Brimonidine is contraindicated in infants because it causes CNS depression and apnea. There is also some evidence from animal models of glaucoma that brimonidine may protect ganglion cells from death. There is no evidence of this property in humans, but this drug has sparked interest in treating glaucoma by mechanisms other than pressure reduction.

9. **Any tips on prescribing carbonic anhydrase inhibitors (CAIs)?**
Topical CAIs took more than 40 years to develop, and were particularly welcome as oral CAIs cause a myriad of side effects. The most common complaints with oral CAIs are lack of energy and lethargy, lack of appetite and weight loss, nausea and/or an upset stomach, and a metallic taste to foods. The most dangerous side effect is hypokalemia, especially when a CAI is combined with a potassium-reducing diuretic. This combination is dangerous in patients taking digitalis. Depression and aplastic anemia are other serious side effects. The same sort of side effects can be seen with the topical medications, but they are extremely rare. Because complaints are frequent with oral CAIs, most ophthalmologists rarely use them unless there is a need for acute pressure control, or if topical CAIs are not effective. There is no additional benefit to using topical CAIs concurrently with oral CAIs in the same patient. Dorzolamide allows IOP fluctuation when used twice daily. However, twice-daily usage gives an adequate response when combined with a topical β-blocker, which diminishes the wash-out effect of aqueous production. Brimonidine can often be used 2x/day when combined with another aqueous suppressant.

The two topical CAIs are equally effective, but brinzolamide might be a bit less irritating to the eye. Dorzolamide has been reported to augment blood flow to the optic nerve. This may help reduce the impact of free radicals that have been postulated to be a cause of glaucoma.

KEY POINTS: GLAUCOMA TOPICAL MEDICATIONS

1. Allow 5 minutes between drops to prevent one drug from washing the other out of the eye.

2. Punctal occlusion can dramatically reduce systemic side effects of glaucoma drugs.

3. A patient on glaucoma drugs with dry or irritated eyes may be developing a medication allergy. Check the conjunctiva of the lower lid for a follicular reaction.

4. Noncompliance is the most common cause of ineffective medication.

10. **How many eyedrops can be used?**

Most ophthalmologists believe that compliance becomes increasingly more difficult the more medicines are used. Most consider the combination of a prostaglandin analog, timolol/dorzolamide, and brimonidine to represent maximum medical therapy (5 drops/day). Surgical options are generally considered at this point, if not earlier. In selected cases additional medicines such as miotics or oral medication can be tried.

11. **What are the general rules for using eyedrops?**

1. Allow at least 5–10 minutes between applying any two topical eye medications.
2. Drops should be spaced at roughly stable intervals. Once-a-day medication should be used each evening or morning. Twice-a-day medicines should be used about 12 hours apart. It becomes harder to space three- and four-times-a-day medicines equally, but an effort should be made to try.
3. Topical medications all have systemic side effects. Punctal occlusion can reduce the systemic absorption to minimize these effects. The patient puts a finger adjacent to the nose where the two lids come together and pushes down on the bone. The drop is then instilled in the eye, and the lids are gently closed. This position is held for 3 minutes. This procedure dramatically reduces the amount of drug entering the system. Because a drug coming into contact with the nasal mucosa is absorbed rapidly and almost completely, it attains serum levels quite similar to those achieved by intravenous administration. Absorption through the nasal mucosa also prevents a first pass by hepatic enzymes, which gives the liver a chance to metabolize or detoxify the medication.
4. An important rule to remember is that topical medications should be initially prescribed as a one-eye therapeutic trial. This will help sort out a true drug effect from the patient's underlying diurnal intraocular pressure fluctuation. Although there can be some crossover effect (about 1–2 mmHg) in the fellow eye, the one-eyed therapeutic trial is the best way to determine the drug's effect. Unfortunately, the response in the first eye doesn't always correlate with the response in the fellow eye once the drug is used bilaterally. Still, most glaucoma specialists believe that a therapeutic trial provides critical evidence to justify the use of a medication.

Piltz J, Gross R, Shin DH, et al: Contralateral effect of topical β-adrenergic antagonists in initial one-eyed trials in the Ocular Hypertension Treatment Study. Am J Ophthalmol 130:441–453, 2000.

Realini T, Fechtner RD, Atreides SP, Gollance S: The uniocular drug trial and second-eye response to glaucoma medications. Ophthalmology 111:421–426, 2004.

12. **Pilocarpine is often used in the treatment of angle-closure glaucoma. What is its effect on the anterior chamber?**

Pilocarpine contracts the longitudinal muscle of the ciliary body, pulling on the scleral spur and mechanically opening the trabecular meshwork. However, it also pulls the lens-iris diaphragm forward, shallowing the anterior chamber. The contraction of the circular muscle of the ciliary body relaxes the stress on the zonules, allowing the lens to become more round, to float forward on a longer tether, and to act more like a natural cork in the pupil. This effect increases pupillary block and blows the peripheral iris closer to the trabecular meshwork. All of these effects tend to shallow the anterior chamber and narrow the anterior-chamber angle. Luckily, these effects are balanced by the miosis caused by the contraction of the sphincter muscle of the iris. Miosis pulls the peripheral iris away from the trabecular meshwork. Therefore, in most patients, although the anterior-chamber depth is decreased by pilocarpine, the peripheral angle is slightly widened. In some patients, however, shallowing of the peripheral angle may be more of a problem than angle crowding. In such patients, pilocarpine may cause angle closure. Therefore, one should gonioscope all patients with a narrow angle for whom a miotic is prescribed, both initially and periodically thereafter.

13. **If a patient does not show an expected response to a topical glaucoma medication, what should the ophthalmologist consider as the reason?**
   - **Ineffective medication:** Make sure that any medication is properly evaluated by a one-eyed trial.
   - **Noncompliance:** The most common cause for an ineffective medication is failure to take it. Kass et al. performed a study in which a microchip placed in the bottom of pilocarpine bottles recorded when the bottle was tipped upside down. The chip was camouflaged, and patients did not know that their drop use was being monitored. Overall, he found that 76% of the prescribed doses were taken. Six percent of patients took less than 25% of the drops, whereas 15% took only 50%. However, 97% of his patients reported that they were taking all of their medication. Not surprisingly, compliance was best on the day before the office visit. This behavior can explain why many patients have completely controlled intraocular pressures in the ophthalmologist's office but evidence progressive glaucoma damage.
   - **Inadequate interval between multiple drops:** Make sure that patients wait at least 5 minutes between drops, and that the drops are spread evenly over the course of the day.

   Kass MA, Meltzer DW, Gordon M, et al: Compliance with topical pilocarpine treatment. Am J Ophthalmol 101:515–523, 1986.

14. **Many patients taking topical medications complain of dry or irritated eyes. What should the treating ophthalmologist include as a routine part of the examination of all patients taking topical medication?**
   The treating ophthalmologist should examine the lower lid and observe the conjunctiva. If only papillae are present, the patient does not have a chronic allergy. If there is a significant follicular reaction, especially if follicles are present on the bulbar conjunctiva, the patient is more than likely allergic to the topical drops. Ocular allergies can appear immediately upon using the drop or months later. Brimonidine is well known for this but such a late reaction is commonly underappreciated and unrecognized. Pilocarpine is famous for causing symblepharon with chronic use. Among the topical nonselective β-blockers, carteolol seems to be the least irritating.

15. **In a patient with an ocular allergy secondary to topical medication, which is the most likely offender?**
   Among the medications now in use, apraclonidine has the highest incidence of allergic reaction, followed (in order) by epinephrine, dipivefrin, brimonidine (less with the 0.15% and 0.1% formulation), topical CAIs, prostaglandin analogs, β-blockers, and pilocarpine.
   Stopping the medicines in that order will usually help sort out which is the offender. Alternatively, have patients instill one drop in one eye and a different one in the fellow eye. Using carteolol and changing from pilocarpine to carbachol can be helpful too.

16. **Are any of the glaucoma medications safe for use in pregnant women? In children?**
   There are, in general, few data about the safety of glaucoma medicines in pregnancy. Most specialists would strongly consider stopping all glaucoma medicines during pregnancy and either forgoing treatment for the duration or considering a surgical option. Epinephrine compounds, although not very effective, can be considered. Because the fetal effects of most glaucoma drops have not been adequately tested, the use of an endogenous compound like epinephrine is reassuring.
   Dipivefrin and brimonidine are class B medications; all others are class C. In the postpartum period, topical CAIs and betaxolol may be useful, although both are secreted in breast milk and may affect the newborn. Topical CAIs in high doses have demonstrated harm to animal fetuses. Brimonidine is also secreted in breast milk, which is a serious problem. Because it causes

severe CNS depression in neonates, it cannot be used in nursing women. No study has determined whether dipivefrin is secreted in breast milk. Prostaglandin analogs are probably not a good choice in pregnancy.

Glaucoma in children is principally a surgical disease. Medications are typically used to lower the IOP until an exam under anesthesia can be performed and surgery done if needed. Topical or oral CAIs are a good choice in this group. Because of systemic side effects, β-blockers are used with caution in children. Brimonidine is a dangerous medication in neonates and infants. Its use has been associated with profound CNS depression and apnea. It is contraindicated in children under the age of 3 years and probably should not be used in children under the age of 8. Pilocarpine is useful after goniotomy or trabeculotomy but is not frequently used on a chronic basis. Prostaglandin analogs in theory would not be a good option because the uveoscleral outflow pathways may be compromised by the angle dysgenesis that is typical of infantile glaucoma. In juvenile glaucoma, however, their effect is highly variable, and they can be used after a successful therapeutic trial.

17. **Is there any evidence that current glaucoma medications are neuroprotective?**
There is only one proven neuroprotective treatment for glaucoma: to lower the intraocular pressure. Data from randomized, prospective controlled clinical trials such as the Collaborative Normal-Tension Glaucoma Study, the Advanced Glaucoma Intervention Study, the Ocular Hypertension Treatment Study, and the Early Manifest Glaucoma Study all indicate intraocular pressure reduction reduces the number of eyes that have continued glaucoma deterioration. Limited data suggest that the manner in which the pressure is reduced may be important. The Glaucoma Laser Trial found that patients initially treated with laser had less worsening of visual fields than patients who were initially treated with medication. This finding is probably due to the fact that the laser-first group had a 2-mm lower IOP on average, compared with the medicine-only group. On the other hand, the Collaborative Initial Glaucoma Treatment Study found no difference at 5 years of follow up between medicine and trabeculectomy with regards to the rate of glaucoma worsening. These more recent data seem to support the current general approach that, in theory, it makes no difference how you lower pressure as long as you lower it adequately. There is no consensus as to how much pressure lowering is adequate. This depends on several factors like the amount of disease, the rate of change of the glaucoma, the patient's wishes, and the life expectancy. Most glaucoma specialists would probably agree that, all things being equal, mild disease would require a 25–30% IOP reduction, moderate disease a 30–40% reduction, and advanced disease a 40–50% or more reduction.

There are reports that patients treated with betaxolol show less decline in visual function than patients treated with a nonselective β-blocker, despite the fact that these patients do not achieve the same degree of pressure reduction. Additional non-pressure-related optic nerve protection has been demonstrated for some medications in animal models of glaucoma and retinal ganglion cell death. The medications have been postulated to help upregulate neurotrophic growth factor (brimonidine), increase blood flow to help reduce free-radical damage (dorzolamide), and interfere with apoptotic cell death by acting as a calcium-channel blocker (betaxolol). At present, no human data indicate "neuroprotection" beyond pressure reduction for any other medicine.

Advanced Glaucoma Intervention Study (AGIS): 7. The relationship between control of intraocular pressure and visual field deterioration. Am J Ophthalmol 130:429–440, 2000.

Collaborative Normal-Tension Glaucoma Study Group: Comparison of glaucomatous progression between untreated patients with normal-tension glaucoma and patients with therapeutically reduced intraocular pressures. Am J Ophthalmol 126:487–497, 1998.

Heijl A, Leske MC, Bengtsson B, et al: Reduction of intraocular pressure and glaucoma progression: Results from the Early Manifest Glaucoma Trial. Arch Ophthalmol 120:1268–1279, 2002.

Kass MA, Heuer DK, Higginbotham EJ, et al: The Ocular Hypertension Treatment Study: A randomized trial determines that topical ocular hypotensive medication delays or prevents the onset of primary open-angle glaucoma. Arch Ophthalmol 120:701–713, 2002.

18. **Are there any glaucoma medications that are not designed to lower eye pressure?**

At present, no non-pressure-lowering medication has been conclusively demonstrated to be helpful in treating glaucoma. Many drugs are under investigation for this purpose. Some data from neurologic studies indicate that ginkgo biloba may be helpful. Memantine, an antiparkinsonian drug that blocks N-methyl-D-aspartate (NMDA)-receptor-induced glutamate toxicity, is currently being tested. Oral calcium-channel blockers have been demonstrated to have a limited effect on preserving visual function in some studies. An inhibitor of nitric oxide synthase was found to be helpful in a rat model of glaucoma. Other drugs that have been investigated for chronic neurologic disease are being evaluated for effectiveness in glaucoma. Agents that increase blood flow to the optic nerve and retina may also be useful. Neuroprotective vaccines have even been developed and tested in animal models. Retinal ganglion cell death in glaucoma occurs by apoptosis and in this way is similar to many chronic neurodegenerative diseases. Identifying the unique trigger in glaucoma and/or interfering with the mechanism of apoptotic cell death might yield multiple ways to treat glaucoma beyond IOP reduction. The trick will be to selectively target the tissue of concern and devise a drug delivery system that can bypass the blood-ocular barrier. It is likely that some type of "neuroprotective" agent will become an important adjunctive therapy for glaucoma in the future.

Neufeld A, Sawada A, Becker B: Inhibition of nitric-oxide synthase 2 by aminoguanidine provides neuroprotection of retinal ganglion cells in a rat model of chronic glaucoma. Proc Natl Acad Sci USA 96:9944–9948, 1999.

Schwartz M: Neurodegeneration and neuroprotection in glaucoma: development of a therapeutic neuroprotective vaccine: the Friedenwald lecture. Invest Ophthalmol Vis Sci 44:1407–1411, 2003.

Vorwerk CK, Lipton SA, Zurakowski D, et al: Chronic low-dose glutamate is toxic to retinal ganglion cells: Toxicity blocked by memantine. Invest Ophthalmol Vis Sci 37:1618–1624, 1996.

Wax MB, Tezel G, Edward D: Clinical and ocular histopathological findings in a patient with normal-pressure glaucoma. Arch Ophthalmol 116:993–1001, 1998.

KEY POINTS: COMMON SIDE EFFECTS OF TOPICAL GLAUCOMA MEDICATIONS

1. **Prostaglandin analogs:** Lash growth, iris and eyelid hyperpigmentation, allergic conjunctivitis, macular edema in pseudophakes, and flulike symptoms.

2. **β-blockers:** Bronchospasm, bradycardia, fatigue, poor exercise tolerance, depression, and decreased libido.

3. **Carbonic anhydrase inhibitors:** Stinging, metallic taste, and rash.

4. **Adrenergic agonists:** Dry mouth, allergic conjunctivitis, fatigue, and headache.

WEBSITE

Wills Glaucoma Service (medicine information)
www.wills-glaucoma.org/meds.htm

CHAPTER 19

TRABECULECTOMY SURGERY

Marlene R. Moster, MD, and Augusto Azuara-Blanco, MD, PhD

1. **What are the indications for trabeculectomy surgery?**
   Glaucoma surgery is indicated when neither medical nor laser therapy sufficiently controls glaucoma progression, and that progression is likely to diminish a patient's quality of life. Because visual needs and vision-related quality-of-life characteristics differ, patients should be assessed individually before physicians decide to perform surgery. Physicians should consider the likelihood of success and risk of complications from surgery prior to proceeding.

2. **What is the goal of glaucoma surgery?**
   The goal of glaucoma surgery is to lower the intraocular pressure (IOP) sufficiently to prevent further damage to the optic nerve and visual function while avoiding severe complications. As a guideline, an IOP reduction of 30% is generally satisfactory. However, the target reduction of IOP will depend on individual factors. In the Advanced Glaucoma Intervention Study (AGIS), patients with severe glaucoma with an average IOP of 12 mmHg after surgery had stable visual function after 5 years of follow-up. Because many patients with glaucoma do not have elevated IOP, the goal of glaucoma surgery is *not necessarily* to reduce IOP to less than 21 mmHg, but to tailor the pressure to the patient's needs.

   The Advanced Glaucoma Intervention Study (AGIS): 7. The relationship between control of intraocular pressure and visual field deterioration. Am J Ophthalmol 130:429–440, 2000.

3. **How do we inform patients about the risks of trabeculectomy surgery?**
   The risks and benefits of glaucoma surgery and alternative options must be carefully outlined to all patients in language that is easily understood. It is imperative to explain clearly the remote possibility of blindness or loss of the eye due to hemorrhage or infection. In addition, the possibility of sudden or permanent visual loss, failure to control IOP (which may be too high or too low), need for repeated surgery, droopy lid, discomfort, and significant blurring (common for the first 2 weeks) should be elaborated. Other risks include infection and endophthalmitis, deterioration of glaucoma, or cataract.

4. **Describe the factors associated with failure of glaucoma filtering surgery.**
   Unfavorable factors include previously failed glaucoma surgery, pigmented skin (nonwhite), neovascular changes, young age, intraocular inflammation, shallow anterior chamber, dislocated lens, vitreous in the anterior chamber, inability to use corticosteroids, previous retinal surgery, scarred or abnormal conjunctiva, and an inexperienced surgeon (Fig. 19-1).

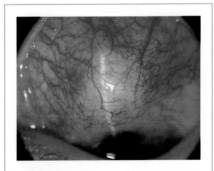

Figure 19-1. Failing filter with increased vascularization and inflammation surrounding the filtering bleb.

5. **Does a fornix versus a limbal–conjunctival approach affect outcome?**

   Fornix-based and limbal-based approaches produce similar results after trabeculectomy surgery. With a limbal-based approach the risk of a wound leak is much smaller. However, this incision appears to increase the likelihood of having a thin avascular and localized filtering bleb (Fig. 19-2). If a limbal-based flap is chosen, it should be made sufficiently posterior so that the closure is at least 10 mm or more from the limbus. If a fornix-based flap is chosen, it is imperative to assure the closure is watertight.

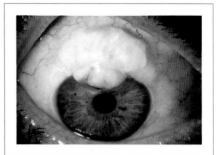

Figure 19-2. Corneal dissection of bleb following a limbal-based trabeculectomy causing discomfort and astigmatism.

6. **What medications should be stopped before filtration surgery?**

   Oral carbonic anhydrase inhibitors and miotics are stopped the night before surgery. Patients should continue their systemic medications. Coumadin or other blood thinners do not necessarily need to be stopped. However, it is convenient to confirm that the anticoagulation levels are within therapeutic range for the patient's condition. If the surgeon desires to stop the Coumadin prior to surgery, it is imperative to discuss this with the patient's internist as in some cases stopping may not be advisable.

7. **What are the choices of anesthesia?**

   General anesthesia is used in children and patients unable to cope with a local anesthetic procedure. There is a trend toward the use of sub-Tenon's or subconjunctival anesthesia. A facial nerve block is not necessary. A peribulbar block is preferred to retrobulbar techniques. A detailed description of our current technique ("blitz" anesthesia) follows:

   First, Xylocaine 1% jelly is placed in the operated eye in the preoperative room. Second, in the operating room, a paracentesis is made temporally and a small amount of aqueous is released from the anterior chamber, followed by an injection of 0.1 mL of 1% nonpreserved lidocaine (on a cannula). For a fornix-based conjunctival flap, an initial cut is made at the limbus, and 0.5 mL of anesthetic is injected with a cannula under the Tenon's layer both temporally and nasally. With a limbal-based flap, a 30-gauge needle is used to inject 0.5 mL, 10 mm posterior and parallel to the limbus, ballooning the Tenon's capsule and conjunctival space in both the nasal and temporal direction. When closing either a limbal- or fornix-based flap, additional lidocaine 1% is irrigated through the Tenon's capsule so that there is no sensation noted by the patient.

8. **Does a triangular versus a rectangular flap affect outcome?**

   The shape of the scleral flap is surgeon-dependent; there is probably no difference in clinical outcome with a triangular or rectangular flap. Although the shape of the flap is not important, its thickness may be. Thin flaps may offer better long-term filtration. However, very thin flaps should be avoided if mitomycin-C is used. Regardless of the shape of the scleral flap, sufficient sutures are necessary to prevent overfiltration.

9. **Does the size of the internal block affect outcome?**

   No. A 1-mm excision is sufficient, although some surgeons choose to create larger fistulas. Increased filtration results when one edge of the internal block coincides with one edge of the scleral flap. The more aggressive the surgery, the closer the internal block comes to one edge of the flap. The internal block can be removed with Vannas scissors or a punch.

10. Are iridectomy and paracentesis always necessary during filtration surgery?
Yes. An iridectomy is always performed to ensure that pupillary block does not occur. In addition, if the chamber shallows, the iris is less likely to occlude the ostium. A paracentesis can be made with either a sharp blade temporally or a 27-gauge needle on a syringe. A paracentesis is essential with each procedure because it allows reformation of the anterior chamber toward the end of surgery. By refilling the anterior chamber via the paracentesis, the surgeon has an appreciation of how much leakage is visible around the edges of the scleral flap.

11. How tight should I make the scleral flap?
The number of sutures and their tightness depend on the diagnosis, preoperative IOP, and how much leak is desired at the time of surgery. In general those patients at high risk for complications associated with hypotony should have tighter scleral flaps. For example, patients with inordinately high IOP, shallow anterior chamber, angle-closure glaucoma, aphakic glaucoma, or increased episcleral venous pressure are more likely to develop this.

With low-tension glaucoma, looser sutures with more flow may be indicated to ensure a lower initial postoperative intraocular pressure. The sutures can be lysed with an argon laser anywhere from day 1 through the first 2 weeks or longer if antimetabolites are used.

12. Are releasable sutures necessary?
Although releasable sutures are convenient, they are not necessary to achieve a good result. However, we tend to use additional releasable sutures tied into clear cornea because they allow tighter closure of the scleral flap, avoiding hypotony, and because of the ease with which they can be removed at the slit lamp (Fig. 19-3). The flap can be closed moderately tightly with permanent sutures, and the releasable sutures decrease the flow further. Selective removal between the first postoperative day and 1 month can easily be done at the slit lamp.

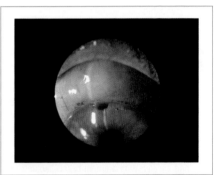

Figure 19-3. Low diffuse bleb with releasable suture still in place 1 week following a trabeculectomy.

13. Does it matter how far I dissect the scleral flap anteriorly?
In large myopic eyes, a perpendicular incision just anterior to the corneoscleral sulcus carries the flap well anterior to the trabecular meshwork. In removing the internal block, a satisfactory corneoscleral removal results. In contrast, in small hyperopic eyes and those with angle-closure glaucoma or peripheral anterior synechiae, an incision at the same point terminates just in front of the iris root. In these patients, an anterior dissection into the cornea is necessary both to ensure that the fistula will not be blocked by uveal tissue and to prevent bleeding (Fig. 19-4).

14. **Should atropine be used during the procedure?**
Only in patients with small eyes, shallow anterior chamber, or angle-closure glaucoma. Sterile 1% atropine drops are placed on the cornea to dilate the pupil maximally and to move the lens iris diaphragm posteriorly. This technique decreases the likelihood of a flat anterior chamber in the early postoperative period.

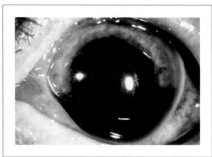

Figure 19-4. Spontaneous hyphema following a trabeculectomy in a 40-year-old woman with chronic angle closure and with no other risk factors.

15. **How often are steroids used in the postoperative period?**
It varies according to the surgeon's preference and the apparent inflammation, but at a minimum they should be used four times/day for one month (e.g., prednisolone acetate 1% or betamethasone 0.1%). In phakic eyes, topical steroids are tapered quickly after 4–6 weeks. In pseudophakic patients or eyes with signs of increased conjunctival or intraocular inflammation, the steroid treatment can be intensified. Some surgeons prefer the addition of a nonsteroidal anti-inflammatory drug (NSAID) two to four times/day in conjunction with the steroids over a 1–2 month period.

16. **How can you avoid a flat anterior chamber after trabeculectomy?**
The amount of leakage underneath the scleral flap ultimately determines the postoperative pressure. To minimize the chance of a flat anterior chamber (Fig. 19-5), additional 10–0 nylon sutures, with or without releasable sutures, should be used to minimize the flow at the end of the procedure. Laser suture lysis may then be used to increase selectively the flow under the scleral flap and improve control. If the sutures are cut too aggressively, a flat anterior chamber may result.

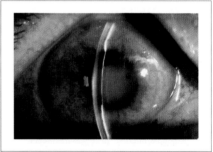

Figure 19-5. Flat anterior chamber, grade II (contact between peripheral and central iris and cornea), and resultant cataract following a trabeculectomy.

17. **What do you do when a wound leak occurs in the immediate postoperative period?**
Unless the leak is very brisk, it usually heals within the first few days. If antimetabolites have been used, healing may take longer. If the leak is near the limbus, either a collagen shield or a bandage contact lens may help. If a leak is very brisk or associated with a flat filtering bleb or with a shallow anterior chamber, surgical closure is necessary. If the leak is located at the wound, restitching is indicated. If there is a buttonhole, a purse-string knot with a rounded-body 11–0 nylon is very helpful.

KEY POINTS: HOW TO AVOID COMPLICATIONS OF TRABECULECTOMY

1. Identify high-risk conditions (e.g., angle-closure, elevated episcleral venous pressure, previous conjunctival surgery).

2. Avoid hypotony with proper suture technique of the scleral flap (with or without releasable sutures).

3. Use paracentesis to evaluate amount of filtration under the scleral flap and decide whether more or fewer sutures are required.

4. After closing the conjunctiva, inject balanced salt solution (BSS) into the anterior chamber to raise the bleb and confirm absence of leaks.

18. **What do you do if there is vitreous loss at the time of the trabeculectomy?**
A "dry" vitrectomy (without balanced salt solution [BSS] infusion) with viscoelastic is very helpful. It can be done through the scleral flap and peripheral iridectomy. If an inordinate amount of vitreous is present, it is probably best to proceed with a full anterior vitrectomy. Vitreous loss is rare in phakic eyes that have no history of trauma, prior iridectomy, or other predilection toward lens dislocation. Vitreous loss is more frequent in eyes that are aphakic or pseudophakic in the presence of zonular weakening (see next question).

19. **Which ocular conditions may predispose to vitreous loss during trabeculectomy surgery?**
Preoperative conditions such as ocular trauma, Marfan's syndrome, pseudoexfoliation, homocystinuria, and high myopia may predispose to vitreous loss during trabeculectomy surgery.

20. **Describe the indications of antimetabolites in trabeculectomy surgery.**
The most important innovation in glaucoma-filtering surgery in the recent past is undoubtedly the use of 5-fluorouracil and mitomycin C, which inhibit normal wound healing and facilitate the formation of highly functioning filtering blebs (Fig. 19-6). Although current antifibrotic agents have improved surgical outcomes, their associated complications should be considered. The indications for antimetabolite use with trabeculectomy include cases with scarring of the superior conjunctiva, previously failed filters, younger than 50 years, pseudophakia, aphakia, ocular inflammation, or advanced optic nerve and visual field injury with desired postoperative pressure less than 14 mmHg.

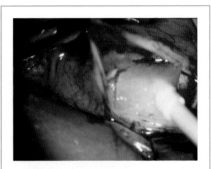

Figure 19-6. Sponge soaked with mitomycin C placed under the conjunctiva and Tenon's capsule prior to making the scleral flap.

Wilkins M, Indar A, Wormald R: Intra-operative mitomycin-C for glaucoma surgery. Cochrane Database Syst Rev; CD002987, 2001.

21. **How does 5-fluorouracil differ from mitomycin C?**
Mitomycin C (MMC, 0.1–0.5 mg/mL) is 100 times more potent than 5-fluorouracil (5-FU, 25–50 mg/mL). Whereas 5-FU affects primarily the S-phase of the cell cycle, MMC inhibits fibroblastic proliferation regardless of the phase of the cell cycle. Intraoperative application is done with several Weck-cell sponges on the sclera under the conjunctiva and Tenon's capsule, treating a large area of the superior globe. The sponges are left in place for 3–5 minutes if 5-fluorouracil has been chosen, and 1–5 minutes if MMC has been applied, depending on the risk for failure.

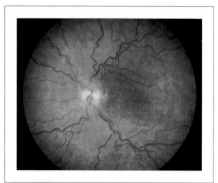

Figure 19-7. Hypotony with chorioretinal folds at the macula. IOP was 4 mmHg.

22. **Are antimetabolites indicated in primary filtering procedures?**
It depends on the surgeon's choice. Although MMC and intraoperative 5-FU increase the success rate of trabeculectomy, postoperative complications of hypotony (Fig. 19-7), suprachoroidal hemorrhage (Fig. 19-8), choroidal detachment, flat anterior chambers, bleb leaks (Fig. 19-9), and late endophthalmitis (Fig. 19-10) may be more common. A prudent approach would be to use no antimetabolites or only 5-fluorouracil on primary surgeries in patients with few risk factors for failure and without severe disease.

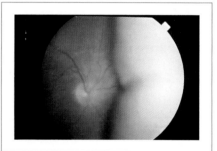

Figure 19-8. Suprachoroidal hemorrhage 1 week after filtering surgery in a patient with known heart disease, valve replacement on blood thinners.

23. **What do you do when the iris blocks the trabeculectomy site in the immediate postoperative period?**
One option is to place Miochol via the paracentesis into the anterior chamber in an attempt to constrict the pupil and dislodge it from the trabeculectomy site. A viscoelastic agent is then injected, and either a cannula or 30-gauge needle can be used to remove the iris carefully from the trabeculectomy site. On occasion, the iris does not occlude the ostium completely, and good filtration may occur around it.

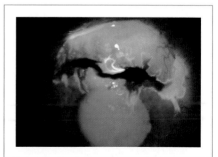

Figure 19-9. Leaking bleb following a mitomycin C trabeculectomy 6 months after surgery.

24. **What if the ciliary processes roll anteriorly and block the trabeculectomy site during surgery?**

    Ciliary processes commonly block the trabeculectomy site in small hyperopic eyes, chronic angle closure, and nanophthalmos. After the trabeculectomy specimen is removed, the ciliary processes may roll into the filtering site. In most cases, closure of the scleral flap, reforming the anterior chamber, and reestablishing normal anatomy allow the ciliary processes to revert to their normal positions. If, after deepening the anterior chamber, the ciliary processes continue to block the trabeculectomy opening, they can be cauterized and cut away. Care must be taken not to disturb the vitreous face.

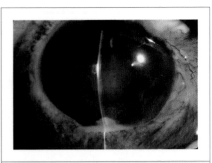

Figure 19-10. Endophthalmitis following a trabeculectomy resulting in poor vision.

25. **When is it necessary to give postoperative 5-FU injections?**

    Supplementary 5-FU injections, 0.1 mL (5 mg), may be given in the early postoperative period if the bleb is thickened, red, and vascularized. This option is left to the surgeon's discretion. This treatment appears to be effective to decrease the chances of bleb scarring and failure. When repeated injections are used, corneal epithelial toxicity may appear and should be monitored. If there are signs of keratopathy, 5-FU injections should be delayed (Fig. 19-11).

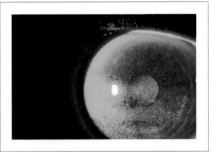

Figure 19-11. Superficial punctuate keratopathy following repeated injections of 5-FU in a failing filter.

The Fluorouracil Filtering Surgery Study Group: Five-year follow-up of the fluorouracil filtering study. Am J Ophthamol 121:349–366, 1996.

26. **What do you do if the bleb starts to fail?**

    If the bleb is red, thick, and injected, an increase of topical steroid regimen and 5-fluorouracil injections is indicated. Digital massage in the early postoperative period increases the outflow, but it is not effective in the long term to maintain the bleb function. Aggressive suture lysis should be considered. Sometimes, regardless of all efforts, the bleb fails and may have to be repeated in another location, using antifibrotic agents. Alternatively, bleb needling can be tried (see next question).

KEY POINTS: HOW TO IMPROVE YOUR SUCCESS RATE

1. Use intraoperative mitomycin C in high-risk cases.

2. Use postoperative 5-fluorouracil when the bleb has early signs of scarring and failure.

3. Cut or release sutures when function of filtering bleb is suboptimal.

4. Consider needling with 5-fluorouracil or mitomycin C when the bleb has failed.

27. **What is the technique of bleb needling?**

Needling can be done in the operating room or at the slit lamp. A sterile technique is required, including the use of topical diluted Betadine. Subconjunctival injection of 1% nonpreserved lidocaine is used. A 27-gauge needle is introduced into the subconjunctival space 8–10 mm away from the scleral flap, is directed toward the bleb, and if possible, under the scleral flap to ensure an outpouring of aqueous. Needling could be supplemented with 5-FU. Some surgeons use 0.1 mL of 0.4mg/mL MMC diluted with 0.1 mL of 1% nonpreserved lidocaine injected on a 30-gauge needle under the conjunctiva and Tenon's capsule 5–10 minutes prior to needling the bleb. The MMC/lidocaine mixture should be completely dissipated prior to the procedure. The point of needle entry into the conjunctiva is cauterized with a disposable hand-held unit. Post-operative topical antibiotics and steroids are used.

Shetty RK, Warluft L, Moster MR. Slit-lamp needle revision of failed filtering blebs using high-dose mitomycin-C. J Glaucoma 14:52–56, 2005.

28. **What is the differential diagnosis for a flat anterior chamber?**

The most common cause of a flat chamber after glaucoma surgery is excessive filtration. Other possibilities include serous choroidal detachment, hemorrhagic choroidal detachment, pupillary block, and malignant glaucoma (Table 19-1). With excessive filtration and serous choroidal detachment, the IOP is low. With a hemorrhagic choroidal detachment, the IOP may be low, normal, or high and usually is associated with pain. With both pupillary block and malignant glaucoma, the IOP is typically elevated, and the cornea often edematous.

TABLE 19-1.   PREVENTION OF MALIGNANT GLAUCOMA (AQUEOUS MISDIRECTION)

1. Detect high-risk cases (angle closure glaucoma, small, hyperopic eyes).
2. Minimize intraoperative shallowing of anterior chamber.
3. Perform a large peripheral iridectomy.
4. Avoid overfiltration.
5. Cautious suture lysis.
6. Use cycloplegics. Taper cycloplegics slowly.

---

29. **How urgent is the management of a flat anterior chamber?**

Grade I (contact between the peripheral iris and the cornea) commonly occurs in the presence of excessive filtration. Treatment includes use of cycloplegics and mydriatics and careful observation. Improvement is usually spontaneous. A grade I may worsen and become a grade II (contact between the peripheral iris and cornea up to the pupil). This progression may be a poor prognostic sign, especially if the pressure is falling and the bleb is flattening. Grade II may recover spontaneously or progress to grade III (contact between the corneal endothelium and lens). Grade III is a surgical emergency and must be corrected promptly or the cornea will decompensate.

30. **What are the indications to drain a choroidal detachment?**

Whenever the pressure consistently falls, the bleb flattens, and the chamber shallows despite reformation with viscoelastic material, drainage of the associated choroidal detachment is indicated. Appositional "kissing" choroidal effusions that do not improve after a few days should also be drained (Fig. 19-12). A full-thickness scleral incision is made in one of the inferior quadrants to reach the suprachoroidal space. Reformation of the anterior chamber is done simultaneously with BSS through the paracentesis tract.

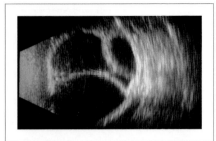

Figure 19-12. Ultrasound of kissing choroidals following a filtering procedure in an eye with chronic angle closure.

TRAUMATIC GLAUCOMA AND HYPHEMA

Douglas J. Rhee, MD

CHAPTER 20

1. **What is a hyphema?**
   A hyphema is blood in the anterior chamber. The appearance of a hyphema may range from microscopic, seen only at the slit lamp as erythrocytes circulating in the aqueous, to a total hyphema that fills the entire anterior chamber.

2. **List the causes of a hyphema.**
   There are three major causes: trauma to the globe, intraocular surgery, or spontaneous anterior segment hemorrhage in association with ocular or systemic conditions, such as neovascularization of the iris or anterior chamber angle, intraocular tumors, or clotting disorders (Table 20-1).

3. **What is the most common cause of a traumatic hyphema?**
   Blunt anterior segment trauma.

4. **Describe the pathophysiology of a traumatic hyphema.**
   Blunt ocular trauma results in ocular indentation, which causes a sudden expansion of ocular tissues and an immediate rise in the intraocular pressure. The sudden forceful displacement of the cornea and limbus posteriorly and peripherally may result in splitting or tearing of these tissues. As the tissues tear, blood vessels in the vicinity may rupture, resulting in a hyphema.

5. **List the anterior segment structures that may split or tear in response to blunt ocular injury.**
   - **Central iris:** Sphincter tear
   - **Peripheral iris:** Iridodialysis
   - **Anterior ciliary body:** Angle recession
   - **Separation of ciliary body from the scleral spur:** Cyclodialysis
   - **Trabecular meshwork:** Trabecular meshwork tear
   - **Zonules/lens:** Zonular tears with possible lens subluxation
   - **Separation of the retina from the ora serrata:** Retinal dialysis

6. **When a patient presents with a hyphema due to blunt ocular trauma, which anterior segment structure is the most likely source of the hemorrhage?**
   Hyphema as a result of blunt ocular trauma most commonly occurs as a result of angle recession, a tear in the anterior face of the ciliary body between the longitudinal and circular ciliary body muscles. Rupture of the blood vessels in the vicinity of the tear results in a hyphema. The most frequently ruptured blood vessels include the major arterial circle of the iris, arterial branches to the ciliary body, and the recurrent choroidal arteries and vein crossing between the ciliary body and episcleral venus plexus.

7. **What ocular injuries may be associated with a traumatic hyphema?**
   - **Ocular wall:** Ruptured globe at the cornea, limbus, and/or sclera
   - **Cornea/conjunctiva:** Epithelial abrasion, laceration, subconjunctival hemorrhage
   - **Iris:** Sphincter tears, iris dialysis, mydriasis (long-term)

TABLE 20-1. HYPHEMA CLASSIFICATION BY ETIOLOGY

I. Trauma

  A. Blunt—rupture of iris or ciliary body blood vessels

  B. Penetrating—direct severing of blood vessels

II. Intraocular surgery

  A. Intraoperative bleeding

    1. Ciliary body or iris injury—most common when performing cyclodialysis, peripheral iridectomy, guarded filtration procedure, and cataract extraction

    2. Laser peripheral iridectomy—bleeding is more common with the YAG laser than with the argon laser

    3. Argon laser trabeculoplasty—rarely

    4. Selective laser trabeculoplasty—extremely rare

    5. Cyclodestructive procedures—common, depending on the mechanism of elevated intraocular pressure (e.g., neovascular glaucoma)

  B. Early postoperative bleeding

    1. Dilation of a traumatized uveal vessel that was previously in spasm

    2. Conjunctival bleeding that enters the anterior chamber through a corneoscleral wound or a sclerostomy

  C. Late postoperative bleeding

    1. Disruption of new vessels growing across the corneoscleral wound

    2. Reopening of a uveal wound

    3. Chronic iris erosion from an intraocular lens causing fibrovascular tissue growth

III. Spontaneous

  A. Neovascularization of the iris

    1. Retinal detachment

    2. Central retinal vein occlusion, central retinal artery occlusion, carotid occlusive disease

    3. Proliferative diabetic retinopathy

    4. Chronic uveitis

    5. Fuchs' heterochromic iridocyclitis

  B. Intraocular tumors

    1. Malignant melanoma

    2. Juvenile xanthogranuloma

    3. Retinoblastoma

    4. Metastatic tumors

  C. Iris microhemangiomas—may be associated with diabetes mellitus and myotonic dystrophy

  D. Clotting factors

    1. Leukemia

    2. Hemophilia

    3. Anemias

    4. Aspirin

    5. Coumadin

    6. Ethanol

    7. Nonsteroidal anti-inflammatory drugs (NSAIDs)

    8. Vitamin C/gingko

IV. Indirect: spillover from vitreous hemorrhage

Adapted from Gottsch JD: Hyphema: Diagnosis and management. Retina 10:S65–S71, 1990.

- **Angle:** Angle recession, iris dialysis, cyclodialysis cleft
- **Lens:** Traumatic cataract (acute: capsular rupture, chronic: direct injury)
- **Vitreous:** Vitreous detachment, vitreous prolapse
- **Retina:** Retinal tear, detachment, and/or dialysis (vessel rupture, vascular occlusion)
- **Retinal pigment epithelium and choroids:** Choroidal rupture
- **Optic nerve:** Avulsion, optic nerve crush (chronic: glaucoma)

8. **Describe an appropriate approach toward the workup of a patient with a hyphema.**

   The primary responsibility is to search for ruptured globe and ocular foreign body in all patients who present with a traumatic hyphema. The color, character, extent of the hyphema, and associated ocular injuries, including corneal blood-staining status, should be documented. Gonioscopy is usually best deferred, but, if necessary, it may be performed gently, taking care to avoid a rebleed. Before a possible rebleed obscures the view, a dilated lens and fundus examination should be performed without scleral depression.

   Past medical and ocular history may identify risk factors for the bleeding episode and the chance of future complications. Sickle cell test and Hgb electrophoresis are suggested for all black and Hispanic patients and anyone with a positive family history. Establishing the exact nature of the trauma helps to estimate the likelihood of a possible ocular or orbital foreign body and/or ruptured globe. The exact timing of the injury is crucial in enabling one to predict when a patient will be at greatest risk for a rebleed, and to help determine the expected time of clearing and the length of necessary treatment.

   Four to six weeks after the injury, careful gonioscopy of the recovered eye may reveal an angle recession. At this time, one may also perform a dilated fundus examination with scleral depression to rule out peripheral retinal injury, such as described in the Table 20-1.

KEY POINTS: TRAUMATIC HYPHEMA

1. All patients should be evaluated for systemic injuries (e.g., computed tomographic [CT] scans, x-rays).

2. All patients should be evaluated for intraocular foreign bodies and ruptured globes as well as other ocular injuries.

3. Recurrent hemorrhages occur in 0.4–35% of patients, usually 2–5 days after trauma.

4. Corneal blood staining occurs in 5%.

9. **What are pertinent questions to ask a patient who presents with a traumatic hyphema? Why?**
   1. **When did your injury occur?** Establishing the exact time of the injury is important because there is an increased rate of rebleed in patients who present more than 24 hours after trauma, and it will help to determine how soon a patient will be at greatest risk for a rebleed.
   2. **What type of injury did you sustain?** The type and severity of an injury is important to help assess the likelihood of associated systemic injuries, an ocular or intraorbital foreign body, and the possibility of a ruptured globe.
   3. **Do you or any of your family members have a medical history of bleeding disorders or sickle cell disease?** The answer to this question may help to establish a possible etiology for the hyphema and to determine what type and how aggressive the treatment should be.

4. **What types of medications do you take (including alcohol intake)?** Antiplatelet or anticoagulant effects of aspirin, NSAIDs, Coumadin, and alcohol may predispose a patient to developing a hyphema or a rebleed after trauma and should be discontinued if possible.

10. **How are hyphemas managed?**
There is no consensus regarding the appropriate treatment for hyphema. Traditionally, most patients with a hyphema were admitted to the hospital for bed rest and sedation and were given a monocular or binocular patch for approximately 5 days. Today, compliant patients with a microhyphema and a low risk for rebleed are often followed as outpatients. It still appears prudent to hospitalize those patients who have a layered hyphema (Fig. 20-1), who are at increased risk for rebleed, have sickle cell disease, or are not compliant.

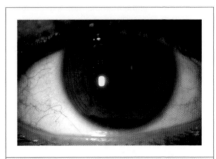

Figure 20-1. Layered hyphema.

Patients are given a protective shield over the affected eye to decrease any inadvertent trauma. The head is elevated (to allow the blood to layer inferiorly and thus assist with visual rehabilitation and prevent clot formation in the papillary aperture), and systemic blood pressure is controlled in an attempt to decrease the hydrostatic pressure in the traumatized blood vessels to minimize the risk of recurrent hemorrhage. Patients should be examined gently once or twice a day.

The medical management of hyphema includes the following:
1. Discontinuation of antiplatelet and anticoagulant medications
2. Treatment with cycloplegic drops, oral or topical steroids, antiemetics, and antifibrinolytics
3. Intraocular pressure control as necessary
   - β-blockers
   - α-agonists
   - Carbonic anhydrase inhibitors and hyperosmotics (except in sickle cell disease or trait because of the risk of increased sickling with these medications)
   - Avoid miotics and prostaglandin analogs, which may increase inflammation.

11. **Explain the rationale for the use of antifibrinolytic agents in the treatment of hyphema.**
Antifibrinolytic agents are used in an effort to reduce the chance of recurrent hemorrhage. Their use is controversial, especially in populations with a low risk of rebleeding. Fibrinolysis of a clot that seals a recently ruptured blood vessel may result in a repeat hemorrhage from that site. Tranexamic acid and aminocaproic acid decrease the rate of clot hemolysis by initiating the conversion of plasminogen to plasmin, which results in stabilization of the clot that seals the ruptured blood vessel. The injured vessel now has more time to heal permanently prior to fibrinolysis of the clot, thus reducing the risk of recurrent hemorrhage.

12. **Name the most common adverse effects associated with aminocaproic acid treatment.**
Nausea, vomiting, and postural hypotension are frequently encountered side effects of aminocaproic acid. It is therefore recommended that patients who receive aminocaproic acid be transported via wheelchair, particularly during the first 24 hours, to prevent possible complications from postural hypotension. Antiemetics may be used as necessary.

13. **In what setting is aminocaproic acid contraindicated?**
Aminocaproic acid use is contraindicated in the presence of the following:
- Active intravascular clotting disorders, including cancer
- Hepatic disease
- Renal disease
- Pregnancy

Cautious use is recommended in patients at risk for myocardial infarction, pulmonary embolus, and cerebrovascular disease.

14. **Why are patients with sickle cell disease or sickle cell trait at a particularly high risk for developing complications from a hyphema?**
Once pliable biconcave erythrocytes transform into elongated ridged sickle cells, they are unable to pass through the trabecular meshwork easily. The trabecular meshwork becomes obstructed with these cells, leading to a marked rise in intraocular pressure, even in the setting of a relatively small hyphema. Factors that encourage sickling include acidosis, hypoxia, and hemoconcentration. Patients with sickle cell are also predisposed to infarction of the optic nerve, retina, and anterior segment at minimally elevated intraocular pressures. This predisposition is thought to occur because of vascular sludging by sickled cells, which leads to ischemia and microvascular infarction. Therefore, vigorous and aggressive therapy for intraocular pressure control is suggested for patients with sickle cell disease.

Many glaucoma medications (except β-blockers and prostaglandin analogs) are generally avoided because they may increase sickling:
1. Carbonic anhydrase inhibitors, particularly acetazolamide, may increase the concentration of ascorbic acid in the aqueous, which decreases the pH and leads to increased sickling in the anterior chamber.
2. Epinephrine compounds and α-agonists may cause vasoconstriction with subsequent deoxygenation and increased intravascular and intracameral sickling.
3. Hyperosmotics may cause hemoconcentration, which may lead to vascular sludging and sickling, which increases the risk of infarction in the eye as well as other organs.
4. Surgical interventions are used earlier and at lower intraocular pressures than in people who do not have sickle cell trait or disease (see question 15).

KEY POINTS: TRAUMATIC HYPHEMA AND SICKLE CELL DISEASE

1. More aggressive management is required to prevent optic nerve damage and central retinal artery occlusion.
2. Beta blockers and prostaglandin analogs should be used for intraocular pressure control.
3. Carbonic anhydrase inhibitors, epinephrine compounds, α-agonists, and hyperosmotics may increase sickling and are therefore contraindicated.

15. **What level of intraocular pressure is considered medically uncontrolled?**
An intraocular pressure that is considered uncontrolled depends upon the patient in question. (Some guidelines are included in subsequent discussions.) Surgery is generally not indicated in a patient with a healthy optic nerve unless, despite medical therapy, the intraocular pressure is around 50 mmHg for 5 days, or greater than 35 mmHg for a more prolonged period of time. In the patient with previous glaucomatous optic nerve damage, however, the threshold for surgical intervention is lower and depends upon the level at which the intraocular pressure

is considered to be likely to cause further optic nerve damage. In such patients, surgery may be appropriate within hours or days of the initial trauma. As previously discussed, aggressive therapy is required for patients with sickle cell disease, as these patients are predisposed to optic nerve damage and central retinal artery occlusion at minimally elevated intraocular pressures. Surgery is generally indicated in a patient with sickle cell disease if the intraocular pressure exceeds 24 mmHg for more than 24 hours despite medical therapy.

16. **List the indications for surgical intervention in the management of a hyphema.**
    As a rule, patients with true eight-ball hyphemas require prompt surgical intervention (see question 26); in contrast, approximately 5% of all traumatic hyphemas demand surgical management. Indications for surgical intervention include the following:
    - A large hyphema that persists for more than 10 days
    - A total hyphema that persists for more than 5 days (after which time peripheral anterior synechiae are more likely to develop)
    - Early corneal blood staining
    - An intraocular pressure that cannot be controlled medically and threatens to damage the optic nerve or cornea or result in retinal vascular occlusion, particularly in patients with sickle cell trait or disease.

17. **Name the major complications associated with a hyphema.**
    - Corneal blood staining
    - Recurrent hemorrhage
    - Secondary glaucoma
    In addition to the preceding complications, patients with sickle cell anemia or sickle cell trait have a predisposition to central retinal artery occlusion and optic nerve damage at only minimally elevated intraocular pressure owing to vascular sludging of the sickled cells, which leads to ischemia and vaso-occlusion.

18. **What is corneal blood staining?**
    Endothelial cell decompensation results in passage of erythrocyte breakdown products (particularly iron from hemoglobin and lipid from cell membranes) into the stroma, creating a yellowish-brown discoloration of the posterior stroma. Corneal blood staining may resolve over months or years, first peripherally and then posteriorly.

19. **What percent of patients with a hyphema develop corneal blood staining?**
    Five percent.

20. **In which setting is corneal blood staining most likely to occur?**
    - Recurrent hemorrhage
    - Compromised endothelial cell function
    - Larger hyphemas that are prolonged in duration
    - Usually, but not always, in association with an elevated intraocular pressure

21. **What is the differential diagnosis of the appearance of bright red blood in the anterior chamber within the first 5 days after a patient has suffered a traumatic hyphema?**
    - Recurrent hemorrhage
    - Fibrinolysis and hemolysis of a clotted hyphema
    Recurrent hemorrhage must be differentiated from hemolysis that occurs as a clotted hyphema resorbs, particularly if the patient has been treated with aminocaproic acid. A rise in intraocular pressure associated with accelerated hemolysis can mimic a rebleed and may occur 24–96 hours after use of aminocaproic acid has been discontinued.

A patient who has been treated with aminocaproic acid should continue to have his or her intraocular pressure monitored several days after discontinuation of therapy in the event that there is a spike in intraocular pressure associated with accelerated hemolysis.

22. **In the setting of a traumatic hyphema, when is a patient at greatest risk for developing a recurrent hemorrhage?**
Between 2 and 5 days following blunt ocular trauma, perhaps due to clot fibrinolysis and retraction.

23. **How common is a recurrent hemorrhage?**
A recurrent hemorrhage generally occurs in 0.4–35% of patients who suffer a traumatic hyphema.

24. **What is the significance of a recurrent hemorrhage? Why is it important to try to prevent it?**
A recurrent hemorrhage carries a poorer prognosis than the initial hyphema. Most rebleeds are larger than the initial hyphema and carry an increased risk of developing a secondary glaucoma and corneal blood staining; visual outcome is worse, and there is a more frequent need for surgical intervention.

25. **List the risk factors that may be associated with an increased risk of developing a recurrent hemorrhage.**
   - Antiplatelet or anticoagulant ingestion
   - Black and Hispanic race
   - Hypotony
   - Younger age
   - Larger initial hyphema

26. **What is an eight-ball hyphema?**
An eight-ball or black-ball hyphema is a hyphema that has clotted and taken on a black or purple color (Fig. 20-2). The black or purple appearance of an eight-ball hyphema is due to impaired aqueous circulation, which leads to a subsequent decrease in the oxygenation of the intracameral blood and results in the characteristic black- or purple-colored clot. It is believed that impaired aqueous circulation occurs as a result of either pupillary block from the clot or direct tamponade effect by the clot at the level of the trabecular meshwork. The impairment in aqueous circulation prevents the clotted black-ball hyphema from being reabsorbed. These hyphemas carry a graver prognosis with respect to developing secondary glaucoma.

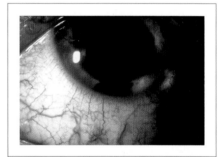

Figure 20-2. Clotted hyphema.

27. **How is an eight-ball hyphema different from a total or 100% hyphema?**
An eight-ball hyphema describes blood in the anterior chamber that has clotted and taken on a black or purple appearance. A total, or 100%, hyphema is one in which the blood filling the anterior chamber appears bright red. A hyphema that consists of bright red blood indicates that there is continuous aqueous circulation within the anterior chamber, which results in a significantly more favorable prognosis than an eight-ball hyphema.

28. **What is the prognosis for an eight-ball hyphema?**
Patients who develop an eight-ball hyphema carry a poor prognosis with respect to developing secondary glaucoma. Most, if not all, patients develop an elevated intraocular pressure that is usually severe and frequently difficult to control with medical therapy. Surgical intervention to evacuate the clot and/or decrease the intraocular pressure is generally required for most patients with an eight-ball hyphema.

29. **When is the optimal time to remove a clotted or eight-ball hyphema? Why?**
It is thought that the optimal time for evacuation of a clotted hyphema is 4–7 days after the hemorrhage, because it is at this time that there is maximal consolidation and retraction of a clot from adjacent structures and thus a decreased risk of causing new bleeding. However, extremely high intraocular pressures, with which vascular infarcts are a significant risk, are seen more commonly with eight-ball hyphema.

30. **What types of surgical techniques can be used to evacuate a hyphema?**
Surgical techniques in managing a hyphema include:
- Paracentesis and anterior-chamber washout alone or in association with a guarded filtration procedure (i.e., trabeculectomy).
- Clot expression with limbal delivery.
- Automated clot removal with a vitrectomy instrument. (Take care to avoid lens and cornea; vasodilators can help maintain the chamber during removal of the clot. Keep the iris between the vitrectomy instrument and lens to minimize the risk of iatrogenic cataract.)
- Peripheral iridectomy with or without a guarded filtration procedure to relieve pupillary block, which may be associated with an eight-ball hyphema.

Figure 20-3 provides an algorithm for the workup and management of a patient who presents with a hyphema.

31. **List the types of secondary glaucoma associated with a traumatic hyphema.**
An acute rise of intraocular pressure is generally due to obstruction of the trabecular meshwork by erythrocytes or their breakdown products. The intraocular pressure at which medical or surgical therapy is initiated should be individualized and depends upon the presence of previous glaucomatous optic nerve damage, corneal endothelial dysfunction, or sickle cell disease.

Late secondary glaucoma may develop weeks to years after a hyphema. Causes of late secondary glaucoma are listed in Table 20-2.

32. **Is the chance of developing secondary glaucoma related to the size of the hyphema?**
Although there are conflicting reports, the chance of developing a secondary glaucoma may be related to the size of the hyphema. Secondary glaucoma occurred in 13.5% of those eyes in which blood filled half of the anterior chamber, in 27% of those eyes in which blood filled greater than half of the anterior chamber, and in 52% of those eyes in which there was a total hyphema. However, the amount of blood may simply be an indirect marker of the degree of trauma.

Recurrent hemorrhages are often larger than the initial hyphema and carry a greater risk for developing secondary glaucoma. Patients with eight-ball hyphemas develop glaucoma virtually 100% of the time.

33. **Why and when is it important to perform gonioscopy on patients who have suffered a hyphema?**
The gonioscopic appearance of angle recession may change with time. Immediately following blunt eye trauma, a hyphema may obscure adequate visualization of the angle. Thorough gonioscopic evaluation with indentation is recommended approximately 6 weeks after trauma, at which time the eye has recovered, the hyphema has resolved, and the risk of further injury has been minimized. Clues that may help the ophthalmologist diagnose an old angle recession

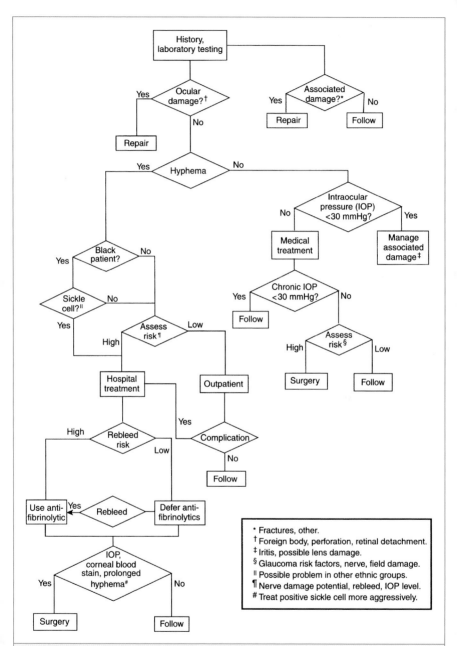

Figure 20-3. Treatment algorithm for ocular trauma and glaucoma. (From Higginbottom EJ, Lee DA: Clinical Guide to Glaucoma Management. Woburn, MA, Butterworth-Heinemann, 2004.)

TABLE 20-2.   SECONDARY GLAUCOMAS ASSOCIATED WITH TRAUMATIC HYPHEMA

A. Early

1. Trabecular meshwork obstruction with fresh red blood cells and fibrin, resulting in secondary open-angle glaucoma
2. Pupillary block by the blood clot, resulting in secondary angle-closure glaucoma
3. Hemolytic glaucoma
4. Steroid-induced glaucoma from treatment

B. Late

1. Angle-recession glaucoma
2. Ghost-cell glaucoma
3. Peripheral anterior synechiae formation, resulting in secondary angle-closure glaucoma
4. Posterior synechiae formation with iris bombé, resulting in secondary angle-closure glaucoma
5. Hemosiderotic or hemolytic glaucoma

include the presence of torn iris processes, depression or tears of the trabecular meshwork, and increased whitening of the scleral spur.

Up to 10% of patients with greater than 180 degrees of angle recession will eventually develop a chronic traumatic glaucoma. The term **angle-recession glaucoma** may also be used to describe the chronic traumatic glaucoma that occurs in association with an angle recession.

34. **Given a history of ocular trauma, how can one make the diagnosis of angle recession on gonioscopic examination?**
    Angle recession can be diagnosed by careful gonioscopic examination of the injured eye and by comparing it with the fellow, nontraumatized eye. Gonioscopy may reveal an irregular widening of the ciliary body, indicating a tear between the longitudinal and circular muscles of the ciliary body. A normal, nonrecessed ciliary body band is usually not as wide as the trabecular meshwork and should be roughly even in width throughout its entire circumference. Angle recession is found in 60–90% of patients with a traumatic hyphema (Fig. 20-4).

35. **Explain the difference between a cyclodialysis and an angle recession.**
    Although not as common as angle recession, cyclodialysis can occur secondary to blunt compressive trauma. Traumatic cyclodialysis occurs when the ciliary body is torn from its attachment at the scleral spur. A cyclodialysis differs from an angle recession in the following manner: An angle recession is a tear within the ciliary body itself, whereas a cyclodialysis is a tear between the ciliary body and the scleral spur. Disinsertion of the uvea from the sclera allows free passage of the anterior chamber aqueous fluid to the suprachoroidal space, thus permitting direct access to the uveoscleral outflow pathway. Temporary or permanent hypotony is usual. A cyclodialysis cleft should be suspected and carefully searched for when the intraocular pressure remains low after ocular trauma. Other causes for a low intraocular pressure following trauma are retial detachment and an inflammatory-mediated decrease in ciliary body production.

36. **Once a cyclodialysis cleft is suspected, how can it be diagnosed?**
    A traumatic cyclodialysis cleft can be diagnosed by careful gonioscopic examination. Although the wall of the cyclodialysis cleft is white (i.e., sclera), it appears shaded, owing to the fact that one is looking down into a hole. This is opposed to the gonioscopic appearance

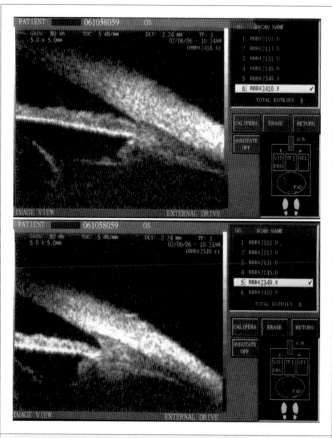

Figure 20-4. Angle recession ultrasound biomicroscopy (UBM). ***Top,*** Normal angle. ***Bottom,*** Angle recession.

of angle recession, which appears simply as an enlarged ciliary body band secondary to a tear in the ciliary body itself. Treatment for a cyclodialysis cleft includes atropine, laser, and surgical repair. Ultrasound biomicroscopy (UBM) provides high resolution (up to 50-μ) images of the anterior chamber angle, which can be particularly helpful if the cleft is small or as part of the preoperative evaluation to map the extent of a large cleft (see Fig. 20-4).

37. **How long after a traumatic hyphema is a patient at risk for developing angle-recession glaucoma?**
Angle-recession glaucoma may develop weeks to many years following blunt ocular trauma. Patients who develop traumatic or subsequent angle-recession glaucoma may have an underlying predisposition to primary open-angle glaucoma (POAG). It is believed that the infliction of trauma to a meshwork that is already predisposed to reduced aqueous outflow (POAG) may be just enough to push an already compromised trabecular meshwork over the edge, resulting in an angle-recession glaucoma. Evidence to support this underlying predisposition to reduced aqueous outflow includes the unusually high incidence of POAG in the nontraumatized fellow eye and an increased tendency for the intraocular pressure to be increased by topical

corticosteroids. Therefore, management of patients with angle recession includes long-term follow up of both the injured and uninjured eyes.

38. Explain the pathophysiology of angle-recession glaucoma. Is it a direct result of injury to the ciliary body?

No. Angle recession is merely a marker for anterior segment contusion injury, specifically injury to the trabecular meshwork. Angle-recession glaucoma is thought not to be due to the angle recession itself (i.e., a tear in the ciliary body) but rather due to (1) direct trabecular meshwork damage from the blunt trauma or (2) an extension of a Descemet's-like membrane covering the trabecular meshwork.

39. Describe treatment for angle-recession glaucoma.

Eyes with secondary traumatic glaucoma have reduced conventional outflow owing to trabecular meshwork injury, and may therefore shift over to primarily uveoscleral outflow. Miotics may actually paradoxically increase the intraocular pressure, possibly by decreasing uveoscleral outflow. Laser trabeculoplasty does not have a high rate of success in this setting. Prostaglandin analogs, β-blockers, carbonic anhydrase inhibitors, cycloplegics, and filtration surgery are the most effective treatments for angle recession glaucoma.

BIBLIOGRAPHY

1. Berrios RR, Dreyer EB: Traumatic hyphema. Ophthalmol Clin 35:93–103, 1995.
2. Caprioli J, Sears ML: The histopathology of black-ball hyphema: A report of two cases. Ophthalmic Surg 15:491–495, 1984.
3. Chi TS, Netland PA: Angle recession of glaucoma. Int Ophthalmol Clin 35:117–126, 1995.
4. Coles WH: Traumatic hyphema: An analysis of 235 cases. South Med J 61:813, 1968.
5. Crouch ER, Frenkel M: Aminocaproic acid in the treatment of traumatic hyphema. Am J Ophthalmol 81:355–360, 1976.
6. Dietse MC, Hersh PS, Kylstra JA, et al: Intraocular pressure increase associated with epsilon aminocaproic acid therapy or traumatic hyphema. Am J Ophthalmol 106:383–390, 1988.
7. Goldberg MF: Antifibrinolytic agents in the management of traumatic hyphema. Arch Ophthalmol 101:1029–1030, 1983.
8. Gottsch JD: Hyphema: Diagnosis and management. Retina 10:S65–S71, 1990.
9. Herschler J: Trabecular damage due to blunt anterior segment injury and its relationship to traumatic glaucoma. Trans Am Ophthalmol Otolaryngol 83:239–248, 1977.
10. Kennedy RH, Brubaker RF: Traumatic hyphema in a defined population. Am J Ophthalmol 106:123–130, 1988.
11. Kutner B, Fourman S, Brein K, et al: Aminocaproic acid reduces the risk of secondary hemorrhage in patients with traumatic hyphema. Arch Ophthalmol 105:206–208, 1987.
12. McGetrick JJ, Jampol LM, Goldberg MF, et al: Aminocaproic acid decreases secondary hemorrhage after traumatic hyphema. Arch Ophthalmol 101:1031–1033, 1983.
13. Parrish R, Bernardino V: Iridectomy in the surgical management of eight-ball hyphema. Arch Ophthalmol 100:435–437, 1982.
14. Ritch R, Shields MB, Krupin T: The Glaucomas, 2nd ed. St. Louis, Mosby, 1996.
15. Sears ML: Surgical management of black-ball hyphema. Trans Am Acad Ophthalmol Otolaryngol 74:820–827, 1970.
16. Shields MB: Textbook of Glaucoma, 4th ed. Baltimore, Williams & Wilkins, 1998.
17. Shingleton BJ, Hersh PS, Kenyon KR: Eye Trauma. St. Louis, Mosby, 1991.
18. Spaeth GL, Levy PM: Traumatic hyphema: Its clinical characteristics and failure of estrogens to alter its course. A double-blind study. Am J Ophthalmol 62:1098–1106, 1966.
19. Tesluk GC, Spaeth GL: The occurrence of primary open-angle glaucoma in the fellow eye of patients with unilateral angle-cleavage glaucoma. Ophthalmology 92:904–912, 1985.

20. Volpe NJ, Larrison WI, Hersh PS, et al: Secondary hemorrhage in traumatic hyphema. Am J Ophthalmol 112:507–513, 1991.

21. Wilson FM: Traumatic hyphema pathogenesis and management. Ophthalmology 87:910–919, 1980.

22. Wilson TW, Jeffers JB, Nelson LB: Aminocaproic acid prophylaxis in traumatic hyphema. Ophthalmic Surg 21:807–809, 1990.

23. Wolff SM, Zimmerman LE: Chronic secondary glaucoma. Am J Ophthalmol 54:547–562, 1962.

CATARACTS

Richard Tipperman, MD

CHAPTER 21

1. **Explain the derivation of the word *cataract*.**
   Cataract comes from the Greek word *cataractos,* which describes rapidly running water. Rapidly running water turns white, as do mature cataracts.

2. **What is the leading cause of blindness worldwide?**
   Believe it or not, cataracts, which are treatable, remain one of the leading causes of blindness worldwide.

3. **What is a nuclear sclerotic cataract?**
   A nuclear sclerotic cataract describes the sclerosis or darkening that is seen in the central portion of the lens nucleus. This type of cataract is typically seen in older patients. As the equatorial epithelial cells of the lens continue to divide, they produce compaction of the more central fibers and sclerosis.

4. **What produces the brown color seen in cataracts?**
   The brown color comes from urochrome pigment.

5. **What is "second sight?" How is it associated with nuclear sclerotic cataracts?**
   As patients develop nuclear sclerotic cataracts, the increased density of the lens causes the patient to become increasingly nearsighted. As a result of their nearsightedness, many patients who required spectacles to help them read find that they are able to read small print up close without glasses. In the past, this phenomenon was termed "second sight." Of interest, patients erroneously believe that their eyes are getting stronger or better, whereas the opposite is the case. Second sight indicates progression of the cataract.

6. **What are the typical symptoms of nuclear sclerotic cataracts?**
   In general, all types of cataracts cause decreased vision. Nuclear sclerotic cataracts tend to cause problems with distance vision but preserve reading vision because of the above-mentioned nearsightedness.

7. **What are posterior subcapsular cataracts?**
   Posterior subcapsular cataracts are granular opacities seen mainly in the central posterior cortex just under the posterior capsule. They have a hyaline type of appearance.

8. **What are the symptoms of posterior subcapsular cataracts?**
   Unlike patients with nuclear sclerotic cataracts, patients with posterior subcapsular cataracts often have good distance vision but typically have blurred near vision. In addition, patients with posterior subcapsular cataracts often have extreme difficulty with glare so that in dim illumination they function well, whereas with bright illumination their vision decreases significantly.

9. **What are the associated systemic findings in patients with cataracts?**
   In general, **nuclear sclerotic cataracts** are seen in elderly patients, although they may occur in young patients as well. In younger patients, they are often associated with high myopia.

Posterior subcapsular cataracts are common in patients with diabetes, patients who have taken steroids, and patients with a history of intraocular inflammation, such as uveitis.

10. **What are the major potential causes of cataracts in infants?**
Common causes of congenital cataracts include familial inheritance, intrauterine infection (e.g., rubella), metabolic diseases (e.g., galactosemia), and chromosomal abnormalities. Complete evaluation by a pediatrician is mandatory for any infant with a congenital cataract.

11. **What is a morgagnian cataract?**
A morgagnian cataract is a mature cataract in which the cortex liquefies and the mature central nucleus can be seen within the liquefied cortex.

12. **What is phacolytic glaucoma?**
Phacolytic glaucoma may occur with morgagnian and mature cataracts. Liquefied cortex traverses the capsular membrane and enters the posterior chamber, producing an inflammatory response that clogs the trabecular meshwork and results in elevated intraocular pressure.

13. **What is phacomorphic glaucoma?**
As the cataract matures, the lens becomes enlarged (intumescent). As the lens enlarges, it pushes the iris root and ciliary body forward, narrowing the angle between the iris and peripheral cornea in the region of the trabecular meshwork. If the angle becomes narrow enough, the pressure may become elevated because of angle closure. Treatment involves removal of the cataract.

14. **What is pseudoexfoliation? What is its relationship to cataracts?**
Pseudoexfoliation is a condition in which basement membrane material from the zonules and lens capsule is liberated onto the anterior lens capsule and anterior chamber. Patients with pseudoexfoliation have a predisposition for the development of glaucoma, presumably because of clogging of the trabecular meshwork by the exfoliated material. Patients with pseudoexfoliation often present a challenge for the cataract surgeon because their pupils tend to dilate poorly, and they often have weak or loose zonules that cause intraoperative complications with disinsertion of the zonules. Because of their propensity for developing glaucoma, patients often have postoperative pressure elevations.

15. **A patient underwent successful and uncomplicated cataract surgery and years after their surgery, the IOL completely dislocated. What associated ophthalmic condition would the patient be likely to have?**
Pseudoexfoliation.

16. **What is true exfoliation syndrome as opposed to pseudoexfoliation syndrome?**
True exfoliation is found in glassblowers who stand in front of hot furnaces throughout the day. Large sheets of material come off the anterior lens capsule. Such cataracts are termed **glassblower's cataracts**. With modern techniques of processing glass, they are no longer seen. Because the type of material produced in pseudoexfoliation seemed similar to the material produced in a glassblower's cataract, it was termed pseudoexfoliation to distinguish it from the exfoliative material produced by heat exposure.

17. **What systemic syndromes should be considered in a patient with a spontaneously dislocated natural lens?**
In these patients, the zonular support system has been disrupted. Spontaneous dislocation of the lens is most common in Marfan's syndrome and homocystinuria. Typical patients with Marfan's syndrome are tall, thin, and lanky and exhibit arachnodactyly. The lenses in Marfan's syndrome tend to dislocate superiorly. In homocystinuria, the lenses tend to dislocate inferiorly.

Trauma also should be considered in all patients with a dislocated lens. Rarely, pseudoexfoliation can be a cause.

KEY POINTS: DISLOCATED AND SUBLUXATED LENSES

1. Patients with a natural lens that is dislocated should be evaluated for trauma.

2. Marfan's syndrome most often causes lenses to dislocate superiorly. Patients need evaluation for possible cardiac and aortic abnormalities and retinal detachments.

3. Homocystinuria most often causes lenses to dislocate inferiorly. Patients have a high risk of thromboembolic events.

18. **What other clinical findings are common in patients with a traumatic cataract?**
Blunt trauma may produce a cataract. Patients often have associated sphincter tears and may even have iridodialysis or angle recession. If the trauma has been severe, some or all of the zonules may be broken, causing the lens to be mobile within the eye. This phenomenon is called **phacodonesis.** Retinal detachment and optic neuropathy also may be present and cause decreased vision.

19. **What are the indications for cataract surgery?**
The basic indication for cataract surgery is reduced visual function that interferes with activities of daily living. This indication obviously varies, depending on the patient's age and degree of activity. For instance, a 40-year-old accountant with an early posterior subcapsular cataract may be much more symptomatic than an 85-year-old who no longer reads or drives. Cases in which cataract surgery is medically necessary (e.g., phacomorphic and phacolytic glaucoma) are extremely uncommon. Patients with cataracts should be informed that cataract surgery is almost always an elective procedure and that leaving the cataract alone will not hurt or damage the eye. However, it is important to be aware of state standards of Snellen visual acuity and visual field for driving vision and to inform patients accordingly. They can be found in the Physicians' Desk Reference (PDR) for ophthalmic medicines.

20. **Does a cataract need to be "ripe"?**
Many years ago, when cataract surgery was performed by removing the entire lens and leaving the patient aphakic, the cataract needed to be dense enough to remove in a single entire piece and to be causing sufficiently poor vision that the patient would benefit from cataract surgery.
  Currently "ripeness" of the cataract is no longer a consideration. The indications for cataract surgery in general are functional visual difficulties secondary to the cataract, which are interfering with the patients day-to-day activities or overall quality of life. Typically if the patient has a Snellen visual acuity (or glare disability) that reduces their vision to 20/50 or worse, they may be considered candidates for cataract surgery.

21. **What is aphakia? What are aphakic spectacles? What is pseudophakia?**
Aphakia is the condition in which the patient's natural lens *(phakos)* has been removed surgically, leaving the patient without a lens. This is the result of intracapsular surgery. **Aphakic spectacles** describe the heavy "coke bottle" glasses patients had to wear to achieve the needed focusing power of the eye with the natural lens missing. **Pseudophakia** or "artificial lens" is the term used to describe an eye with an intraocular lens (IOL).

22. **How is the IOL power determined? What is the most commonly used IOL power?**
The appropriate IOL power for a patient is determined by measuring the curvature of the patients cornea (keratometry values) as well as the length of the eye (axial length measurement). These

two measurements are then utilized by multivariable "IOL power equations" to help determine the most appropriate lens for the individual patient.

The most commonly used IOL power is 18D.

23. **What are multifocal IOLs? How do multifocal IOLs work?**
With standard cataract surgery and conventional intraocular lens (IOL) there is only one fixed focal distance. Therefore, if a patient achieves good uncorrected distance vision following cataract surgery, they will not be able to see at near without correction because the artificial lens cannot accommodate to adjust its focal length the way a natural phakic lens can.

New technology multifocal IOLs now allow patients the ability to see both in the distance and up close. In the United States there are three Food and Drug Administration (FDA)-approved IOLs that achieve these results with different technologies: The crystal lens utilizes a thin small optic lens that is designed to flex and produce a degree of accommodation; the ReZoom lens uses differing radii of curvature to create a zonal refractive lens to achieve its multifocality; and the ReSTOR lens uses a combination of refractive and diffractive optics to create multifocal images.

24. **What is IFIS? What is a flomax pupil?**
IFIS is an acronym for intraoperative floppy iris syndrome. This condition occurs in patients who are taking tamsulosin (Flomax) for benign prostatic hypertrophy. Tamsulosin is a systemic sympathetic α_1-A receptor blocker, which improves lower urinary tract flow by relaxing the neck of the bladder neck and prostatic smooth muscle.

Patients taking tamsulosin who undergo cataract surgery manifest pupillary abnormalities that include a flaccid iris, which undulates and billows in response to intraocular fluid currents. There is also a tendency for the iris to prolapse through both the phaco incision and paracentesis. Last, there is typically a progressive intraoperative pupillary constriction despite apparent adequate pharmacologic dilation at the initiation of surgery. These iris abnormalities are believed to occur because the smooth muscle in the iris also has α_1-adrenoreceptors that are affected by tamsulosin.

Because cataract surgery is more difficult in patients with poorly dilating pupils and abnormalities as noted above, cataract surgery on patients taking tamsulosin can be more difficult as well. Interestingly, even if patients discontinue their tamsulosin for up to 4 weeks prior to cataract surgery, the pupil abnormalities persist. Surgical strategies for dealing with this situation include utilizing a highly cohesive viscoelastic agent and iris retractors.

www.ascrs.org

25. **What is the difference between an anterior chamber lens and a posterior chamber lens? What is "the capsular bag"?**
A posterior chamber lens is typically utilized in routine cataract surgery. During surgery a circular opening termed a capsulorrhexis is made in the capsule that surrounds the cataractous lens. The cataract is removed and then the new lens is placed into "the capsular bag," which is the membrane that is left behind once the cataract is removed. This region of the eye is termed the posterior chamber, hence the IOL that resides there is termed a posterior chamber lens.

At times it is not possible to place a posterior chamber lens either because of inherent weakness in the capsular bag or an intraoperative complication that disrupts its integrity. In these cases one of the options is to place a lens in the front (or anterior) portion of the eye; hence the term anterior chamber lens. Anterior chamber lenses fixate in the eye by resting on the scleral spur. If not positioned correctly, these IOLs have the potential to chafe the sensitive uveal tissue in the iris and create complications.

26. **What is posterior capsular opacification? What is a secondary membrane? Can a cataract grow back?**
The new IOL replaces the cataractous lens by resting inside the capsular bag. Slowly, over time, residual epithelial cells in the capsular bag can grow across the posterior portion of the capsule

and cause it to become hazy or cloudy. Over time, the capsule can become so cloudy it may seem as if the cataract has "come back." The cataract can never come back, but the secondary membrane can become cloudy.

27. **What is a YAG capsulotomy?**
    When the reduced vision becomes clinically significant, the patient may undergo a Nd:YAG capsulotomy. The initials are an acronym for **n**eo**d**ymium, **y**ttrium, **a**luminum, and **g**arnet, which are the materials utilized to allow the laser to function properly and open the membrane.

28. **What is the origin of the term laser?**
    Laser is actually an acronym for **l**ight **a**mplification by **s**timulated **e**mission of **r**adiation.

29. **What is the difference between an "intracap" and an "extracap?"**
    An **intracap** describes intracapsular cataract extraction. This is the "old" type of cataract surgery back in the days when patients had a very large incision made at the corneoscleral limbus and the entire lens surrounded by the lens capsule was removed (usually with the aid of a freezing probe termed a *cryoprobe*). In these cases no lens was replaced and the patient was left aphakic.

    In an **extracap** or extracapsular surgery, the capsule surrounding the lens is opened and the cataractous lens removed. The capsule, however, remains in the eye to support and hold the new posterior chamber IOL.

30. **What is couching?**
    Couching describes an ancient technique for cataract surgery where a needle was inserted into the eye and used to push the opaque cataract back into the vitreous cavity. Although the complication rate of this is extremely high and the visual result limited, in antiquity it would allow patients with mature light perception cataracts to be able to regain a limited degree of vision.

BIBLIOGRAPHY

1. Datilles M: Clinical evaluation of cataracts. In Tasman W, Jaeger E (eds): Duane's Clinical Ophthalmology, vol. 1. Philadelphia, Lippincott-Raven, 1996, pp 1–15.
2. Datilles M, Kinoshita J: Pathogenesis of cataracts. In Tasman W, Jaeger E (eds): Duane's Clinical Ophthalmology, vol. 1. Philadelphia, Lippincott-Raven, 1996, pp 1–9.
3. Datilles M, Magno B: Cataract: Clinical types. In Tasman W, Jaeger E (eds): Duane's Clinical Ophthalmology, vol. 1. Phildelphia, Lippincott-Raven, 1996, pp 1–25.

CHAPTER 22

TECHNIQUES OF CATARACT SURGERY

Sydney Tyson, MD, MPH

1. **What are the indications for cataract surgery?**
   In general, the decision to have cataract surgery is elective. It is based on a patient's personal needs and the physician's judgment as to the probability of visual improvement. For some people, even a slight loss of vision is unacceptable. Others may choose to delay surgery because their cataracts do not seriously interfere with their lives. The key question is whether the patient perceives the cataract as interfering with his or her quality of life. Of course, the physician must be aware of state visual acuity requirements for driving.

2. **What are two nonsurgical methods of managing a cataract?**
   - **Refraction:** Patients with a cataract may experience a myopic (near-sighted) shift or so-called second sight. Occasionally, glasses can compensate for such shifts. However, if the shift is large and unilateral, binocular vision may be compromised by image size differences between the two eyes. This anisometropia may push patients to have surgery.
   - **Pupillary dilation:** An expanded pupil allows light rays to enter around a central cataract (such as a posterior subcapsular cataract) rather than be blocked by light rays that attempt to pass through a hazy cataract.

3. **What preoperative tests are used to gauge visual impairment?**
   No single test adequately describes the effect of cataracts on a patient's visual functioning, but the most widely used tests are:
   - Snellen visual acuity (i.e., 20/20).
   - Potential acuity testing. This test estimates postoperative visual acuity by projecting a Snellen acuity chart through the patient's cataract. It is most often used to determine whether a patient's visual symptoms are due more to cataract or retinal disease.
   - Glare/contrast sensitivity testing. This test simulates lighting conditions outdoors and determines a patient's vision when functioning in more normal conditions. The high-contrast situation in a Snellen test can overestimate a patient's abilities. A patient may have 20/40 acuity in a dark room but may have 20/100 with glare testing, which could significantly impair driving.

KEY POINTS: TESTS OF VISUAL IMPAIRMENT

1. Snellen visual acuity

2. Contrast sensitivity

3. Glare testing

4. Potential acuity meters

4. **What are the basic steps in removing a cataract?**
   1. The pupil is dilated.
   2. The eye and eyelids are disinfected with an antiseptic, usually iodine based.
   3. The eye and eyelids are anesthetized, and a speculum is placed to open the eyelids.
   4. An incision is made into the anterior chamber (AC).
   5. A viscoelastic (viscous, protective gel) is injected into the AC.
   6. The anterior capsule is opened with a capsulotomy or capsulorrhexis to gain access to the lens mass.
   7. The nucleus is removed manually or by phacoemulsification.
   8. The residual cortex is removed.
   9. An intraocular lens (IOL) is inserted.
   10. The wound is closed.

5. **How is the eye anesthetized for surgery?**
   Most surgeons prefer local rather than general anesthesia for adult cataract surgery. Facial akinesia with a short-acting agent such as lidocaine or hyaluronidase (a diffusion enhancer) may be used to prevent squeezing of the eyelids during surgery. There are three types of local anesthesia:

   - **Retrobulbar:** Anesthetic (usually a combination of a short- and long-acting agent with hyaluronidase) is injected inside the muscle cone to achieve akinesia and anesthesia of the globe (Fig. 22-1).
   - **Peribulbar:** Anesthetic is injected outside the muscle cone. Although this block takes longer to take effect (12–25 minutes), there are fewer potential complications because a shorter needle is used.
   - **Topical:** Advances in technology have allowed skilled surgeons to perform the cataract procedure in 10–15 minutes. With such short operative times, prolonged anesthesia and akinesia become less critical. Topical drops of short-acting agents such as lidocaine or tetracaine may be used to anesthetize the eye sufficiently to complete the procedure. The advantage to the patient is instantaneous binocular vision postoperatively without the risk of injection-related, potentially sight-threatening complications.

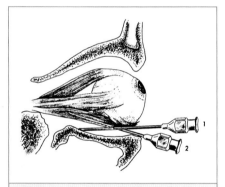

Figure 22-1. Retrobulbar injection. If the tip of the needle strikes the floor of orbit as it is inserted, it is withdrawn slightly and directed more superiorly. (From Jaffe NS, Jaffe MS, Jaffe GF: Cataract Surgery and Its Complications. St. Louis, Mosby, 1990.)

6. **What are the disadvantages of topical anesthesia for cataract surgery?**
   - Because there is no akinesia, the eye can move during surgery.
   - Patient selection is crucial. Patients need to follow the commands of the surgeon.

7. **What is couching?**
   Couching is one of the most ancient surgical procedures. It was the first known technique of cataract removal and was first described by the Indian physician Susruta circa 800 BC. Popular in the United States until the 1850s, couching involves piercing the eye with a needle, then dislocating the entire lens backward and downward into the posterior chamber. Although it may seem crude by modern surgical standards and prone to myriad complications, it is still performed in the Third World, where advanced technology is not available.

8. **What are the two most common ways to remove a cataract?**
   - **Intracapsular surgery** was the procedure of choice from its discovery by Jacques Daviel in 1752 until the early 1970s. It is accomplished with a cryoprobe, an instrument that freezes the tissue. Intracapsular surgery is rarely performed in the United States today except in cases of dislocated lenses.
   - **Extracapsular cataract extraction (ECCE)** is the most popular technique. There are two types—manual extraction and phacoemulsification. Both methods require the use of an operating microscope that permits magnification. In extracapsular surgery the anterior capsule of the lens is removed, the hard nucleus is expressed, and the remaining soft cortical fragments are removed with either an automated or a manual device (Fig. 22-2). The advantage of extracapsular surgery is preservation of the posterior capsule, which permits a pocket for an intraocular lens. This method also minimizes the complications associated with vitreous loss.

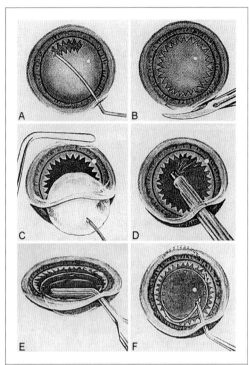

Figure 22-2. Extracapsular extraction. *A*, Multiple small cuts are made in the anterior capsule. *B*, Full-thickness incision is completed with scissors. *C*, Nucleus is removed. *D*, Cortex is aspirated. *E*, Inferior haptic is inserted through incision and passed under the iris. *F*, Tip of the superior haptic is grasped with a forceps and advanced into the anterior chamber; as the superior pole is clearing the edge of the pupil, the arm is pronated to ensure that when the haptic is released, it will spring open under the iris and not out of the incision. (From Kanski JJ: Clinical Ophthalmology: A Systematic Approach, 2nd ed. Boston, Butterworth-Heinemann, 1989.)

9. **What is phacoemulsification?**
   Invented by the late Dr. Charles Kellman in 1967, phacoemulsification is a sophisticated form of extracapsular surgery that permits mechanical removal of a cataract through a 3.0-mm incision (Fig. 22-3). This reduction in incision size results in faster visual recovery and fewer complications, making phacoemulsification still one of the most significant advances in cataract surgery. Conventional extracapsular surgery requires a wound size of 150 degrees (approximately 10 mm).

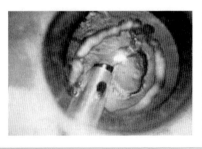

Figure 22-3. The removal of nuclear material by phacoemulsification. (From Koch PS, Davidson JA: Textbook of Advanced Phacoemulsification Techniques. Thorofare, NJ, Slack, 1991.)

10. **How does the phacoemulsification machine work?**
Although the machine is complex, its functions are simple: irrigation, aspiration, and ultrasonic vibration via a handpiece. The phacoemulsification handpiece consists of a hollow 1-mm titanium needle that fragments a cataract by vibrating at 40,000 times per second. The fragmented pieces are then aspirated through the tip of the needle and into a drainage bag. An irrigation solution flows from a bottle suspended above the machine and into the eye through the needle. This fluid serves to cool the needle and to maintain proper anterior chamber depth.

11. **What are the advantages and disadvantages of phacoemulsification?**
   - **Advantages** are a small incision, fewer wound problems, less astigmatism, more rapid physical rehabilitation, and less risk of expulsive hemorrhage.
   - **Disadvantages** are machine dependency, a longer learning period, complications while learning, expensive equipment, difficulty with a hard nucleus, and good pupil dilation is needed.

12. **How is a capsulotomy performed?**
There are two types of capsulotomies: a can-opener capsulotomy and a continuous-curve capsulorrhexis (CCC). The can-opener capsulotomy is a series of jagged punctures performed with a bent needle. Although it is simple to perform, it is prone to peripheral extension of its jagged edges. The CCC is made by tearing the capsule so that the edges remain sharp, well demarcated, and strong. Forces are distributed more evenly and prevent an anterior capsule extension from becoming a posterior capsular tear. This approach permits safe utilization of phaco techniques that use shearing or rotational forces. Implants are held more securely and center better (Fig. 22-4).

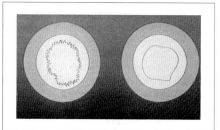

Figure 22-4. *Left,* Can-opener capsulotomy. *Right,* Continuous-curve capsulorrhexis. (From Koch PS, Davidson JA: Textbook of Advanced Phacoemulsification Techniques. Thorofare, NJ, Slack, 1991.)

   Location. The nucleus can be disassembled in the anterior chamber or in the capsular bag. Anterior chamber removal is less popular because of the higher risk of corneal endothelial damage. However, in cases with capsular rupture, this method of removal can prevent nuclear pieces from moving posteriorly into the vitreous.
   Nucleus handling. The nucleus can be disassembled as a whole (sculpting) or by first splitting it (nucleofractis) into pieces. Harder nuclei are more readily and safely removed with a splitting technique within the capsular bag. However, a capsulorrhexis is mandatory because the forces exerted during splitting may cause peripheral extension of a can-opener capsulotomy with possible posterior capsular rupture.
   The type of capsulotomy and anticipated method of cataract extraction are closely interrelated. The planned location and technique of nucleus emulsification are affected by such variables as nucleus consistency (hard or soft lens), pupil size, zonular (lens ligament) integrity, and the presence of intraoperative complications.

13. **Are lasers used to remove cataracts?**
Traditionally, the answer would be no, but in June 2002 the Food and Drug Administration (FDA) approved the Dodick PhotoLysis System for cataract removal. The system uses an indirectly pulsed neodymium:yttrium-aluminum-garnet laser (Nd:YAG) to generate shock

waves that emulsify the cataract. Currently, the only advantage for laser machines is their name. Patients love lasers. Otherwise, the newer, more energy efficient forms of ultrasound perform equally well or better in all other parameters. The future will tell which type of system prevails.

14. **Once a cataract is removed (aphakia), what are the options to restore vision?**
    - **Thick aphakic glasses** are rarely used today because they create visually annoying magnification (approximately 25%) and distortion.
    - **Contact lenses** are a better alternative to visual restoration (magnify only 7%), but many elderly patients do not possess the manual dexterity necessary to handle them. Long-term extended-wear lenses can help in this regard.
    - **Intraocular lenses** are the best and most common alternative to restoration of normal vision after cataract surgery, because they almost duplicate the aphakic eye. Magnification is minimal, and peripheral vision is normal.

15. **Who invented intraocular lenses?**
    In 1949, Sir Harold Ridley was the first person to insert an implant into the posterior chamber. Most authorities agree that this was one of the most significant advances in cataract surgery.

16. **Of what are implants made?**
    During World War I it was noted that British Spitfire fighter pilots who had Plexiglas (polymethylmethacrylate [PMMA]) embedded in their eyes from shattered canopies tolerated the material well. PMMA lenses became the gold standard. Advances in technology led to the creation of soft or foldable materials made from silicone and acrylic materials. These materials have come into favor mainly because they can be inserted through much smaller incisions.

17. **Describe the most common design and shape of IOLs.**
    Implants are composed of an optical portion called the "optic" and a nonoptical portion called the "haptic," which is used for fixating the IOL.
    Most optic designs are unifocal (distance only). Multifocal designs, which reduce or eliminate the need for reading glasses, are now available. Toric IOLs, which can correct preexisting astigmatism, are also available. Optics can be round or oval, with or without positioning holes, and range in size from 5 to 7 mm. Lens haptics can be looped or plate style (mostly seen in foldable implants) and made of the same or different material as their optics. Anterior chamber lenses are designed with special haptics that allow proper fixation in the delicate anterior chamber angle.

18. **What are the most common positions of IOLs?**
    Capsular bag, ciliary sulcus, and anterior chamber. Capsular bag fixation is preferred because it affords excellent lens stability far away from the corneal endothelium.

19. **Is an implant indicated in every aphakic patient?**
    No. Implants are generally not used in children or in eyes with severe anterior segment disease or inflammation. However, implants to treat children who are aphakic are becoming more common.

20. **How is the power of an IOL determined?**
    The most common method of determining IOL power (P) uses a regression formula called SRK. The formula is $P = A - 2.5\, L - 0.9\, K$. The components of this formula include axial length (length of the eye) measurement (L), which is determined by A-scan ultrasonography; average corneal curvature (K), which is determined by keratometry; and an A constant (A), which is specific for each lens type. The closer the implant is to the retina, the greater the

A constant. Therefore the A constant is larger for posterior chamber implants than for anterior chamber implants. Newer IOL calculation formulas have been gaining in popularity. These third- and fourth-generation formulas, such as the SRK/T and Holladay II formulas, have offered surgeons the ability to predict IOL powers with uncanny accuracy. These next-generation formulas are especially important in determining IOL power in extremely short or long eyes.

21. **How is the surgical wound closed?**
The need for wound closure is directly related to wound size and construction. Larger ECCE incisions can be reapproximated with 10-0 nylon sutures, in a radial, running, or combination technique. The major consideration with these closure techniques is postoperative astigmatism. The tighter sutures are tied, the greater the astigmatism and the more distorted the early postoperative vision. Phaco incisions are smaller and valvelike in construction. This makes them essentially self-sealing and astigmatism free, although some surgeons sleep better at night if at least one suture is placed.

22. **How should patients be managed postoperatively?**
The postoperative patient is seen within the first 48 hours of surgery—preferably within 24 hours. Intraocular pressure, wound integrity, anterior chamber inflammation, and IOL positioning are assessed. Typical postoperative medications include (1) antibiotic solutions for infection control and (2) steroids and/or nonsteroidal anti-inflammatory drugs for controlling the inflammation. Patients are then seen at 1-week, 1-month, and 3- to 6-month intervals. In advanced small-incision surgeries, refractions are usually stable by 1 month. Eyeglasses may be given at this visit.

23. **What are the most significant trends in cataract surgery?**
  - Topical versus retrobulbar anesthesia for cataract surgery
  - Clear corneal versus scleral incisions
  - Conversion to phacoemulsification from ECCE
  - Foldable IOLs versus rigid PMMA lenses
  - Multifocal versus monofocal implants
  - Sutureless wound closure

24. **What does the future hold for cataract surgery?**
Improvements and advances in the way that cataracts are removed will continue. Important hardware and software advances in ultrasound technology will include new phaco needles, improved fluidics, and improved instrumentation, which will allow safer, more efficient removal of cataracts.

   In addition, nonultrasound methods for cataract removal will reduce incision size even further, including the mechanical approach (Catarex, which is in preclinical development, uses a rotating blade and whorl-like fluidics to remove lens material through a 1-mm capsulorrhexis; AquaLase, now available, uses fluid micropulses to emulsify the lens) and the laser approach, as previously discussed. Both nonultrasound methods are expected to eliminate the risk of thermal injury to the wound site.

   Breakthroughs in IOL design and function also will continue. Different IOL materials, such as Collamer and hydrogel, promise improved biocompatibility and reduced postoperative inflammatory response. These lenses are ideal for patients with iritis, glaucoma, or diabetes. IOL design will more closely mimic the natural lens. The FDA recently approved the Crystalens accommodating IOL. This IOL restores accommodation by closely approximating the function of original lenses, thereby reducing or eliminating the need for reading glasses postoperatively. IOL designs are available to correct for the eye's optical aberrations. The Tecnis Z9000 is the first IOL designed to reduce these aberrations and improve the quality of vision by enhancing contrast sensitivity. Finally, a light-adjustable IOL by Calhoun vision is an experimental IOL design made of a light-absorbing polymer that allows precise and noninvasive postoperative modification of the lens power by applying light to the IOL. The era of spectacle-free postoperative vision is on the horizon.

BIBLIOGRAPHY

1. American Academy of Ophthalmology: Cataract in the Otherwise Healthy Adult Eye (Preferred Practice Patterns). San Francisco, American Academy of Ophthalmology, 1989.

2. Boyd B: The Art and Science of Cataract Surgery. Coral Gables, FL, Highlights of Ophthalmology, 2001.

3. Buratto L: Phacoemulsification: Principles and Techniques. Thorofare, NJ, Slack, 1998.

4. Gills J: Cataract Surgery: The State of the Art. Thorofare, NJ, Slack, 1998.

5. Jaffe N, Horowitz J: Lens and cataract. In Podos S, Yanoff M (eds): Textbook of Ophthalmology, vol. 3. New York, Gower Medical Publishing, 1992.

6. Johnson S: Phacoemulsification. In Focal Points (Clinical Modules for Ophthalmologists), vol. XII. San Francisco, American Academy of Ophthalmology, 1994.

7. Kratz R, Shammas H: Color Atlas of Ophthalmology: Cataracts. Philadelphia, Lippincott Williams and Wilkins, 1991.

8. Maloney W, Grindle L: Textbook of Phacoemulsification. Fallbrook, CA, Lasenda Publishers, 1988.

9. Stein H, Slatt B, Stein R: The Ophthalmic Assistant, 6th ed. St. Louis, Mosby, 1994.

10. Steinert R: Cataract Surgery: Technique, Complications, and Management. Philadelphia, W.B. Saunders, 1995.

CHAPTER 23

COMPLICATIONS OF CATARACT SURGERY

John D. Dugan, Jr., MD, and Robert S. Bailey, Jr., MD

1. **What complications may result from local anesthesia for cataract surgery?**
   - **Retrobulbar hemorrhage** is the most common complication from retrobulbar injection. Blood collects in the retrobulbar space, often causing proptosis of the involved eye and a tense orbit. If not treated, it may lead to severe, irreversible optic nerve ischemia.
   - **Ocular perforation** may occur if the needle perforates the globe. The risk of this complication is greatest in highly myopic eyes with long axial lengths.
   - **Optic nerve sheath hemorrhage** may occur if the needle penetrates the optic nerve. It may result in a secondary central retinal vein and/or central retinal artery occlusion.
   Peribulbar injections given with a shorter needle have become more popular recently, as has topical anesthesia for cataract surgery.

2. **How do you treat a retrobulbar hemorrhage?**
   Blood collecting in the retrobulbar space may cause a secondary increase in intraocular pressure from the pressure of the blood on the globe. When a retrobulbar hemorrhage occurs, intermittent pressure is applied initially to the globe to tamponade the bleeding. The intraocular pressure should be measured. If it is significantly elevated, a lateral canthotomy should be performed. This technique is often successful in relieving the pressure on the globe. Surgery is usually cancelled when a retrobulbar hemorrhage occurs.

KEY POINTS: MOST COMMON INTRAOPERATIVE COMPLICATIONS OF CATARACT SURGERY

1. Posterior capsule rupture

2. Dislocated lens fragment

3. Iris trauma

4. Thermal corneal injury

5. Descemet tear/detachment

6. Poor intraocular lens (IOL) placement

7. Choroidal/expulsive hemorrhage

3. **What are the common complications related to the cataract wound?**
   - **Wound leak or dehiscence:** Occurs when apposition of the cataract wound is inadequate. Aqueous humor can be seen leaking from the involved area of the wound.
   - **Wound burn:** Transfer of heat from the vibrating needle of the phacoemulsification instrument can induce an incision burn, which often adversely affects wound apposition.

- **Hypotony:** If a wound leak is present, a low intraocular pressure is usually found.
- **Flat anterior chamber:** If the wound leak is large enough, the anterior chamber becomes shallow and may become flat with the iris contacting the cornea.

  Most wound leaks require repair in the operating room with additional sutures to achieve a watertight closure.

4. **What is iris prolapse? How is it treated?**
   If a wound leak is present, the iris often becomes incarcerated in the wound and may prolapse through the wound, which leads to increased inflammation and increased risk of infection. Prolapse requires repair to be performed in an operating room. If the iris is viable, it can be reposited in the eye; if not, it can be excised. Additional sutures are then applied to the area of the wound dehiscence.

5. **What types of intraocular hemorrhage may occur during or after cataract surgery?**
   - **Hyphema or blood in the anterior chamber** can be seen as a layering or meniscus of blood in the anterior chamber. Blood vessels in the base of the cataract wound or possibly from the iris are usually the source of the blood. Most often the blood clears spontaneously, and no treatment is required. The intraocular pressure needs to be monitored closely because secondary elevation may occur.
   - **Expulsive choroidal hemorrhage** is the most feared complication of cataract surgery and is caused by rupture of choroidal vessels, most often during surgery. The rupture causes a rapid rise in intraocular pressure with loss of the anterior chamber, iris prolapse, and possible prolapse of the entire intraocular contents if not recognized and treated promptly. Fortunately, it has an occurrence rate of 0.2%.

6. **What is the incidence of posterior capsule rupture for an experienced surgeon during cataract surgery?**
   Most studies report between 1% and 3%.

7. **What are the possible consequences of posterior capsule rupture?**
   Posterior capsule rupture often is associated with vitreous loss.
   It may also result in loss of lens material into the vitreous cavity (Fig. 23-1). It also increases the risk of endophthalmitis and retinal detachment.

8. **What are some of the risk factors for expulsive choroidal hemorrhage? How are they treated?**
   Patients with advanced age, systemic hypertension, arteriosclerosis, glaucoma, and long axial-length eyes are at greater risk. The most important factor in treatment is time. The wound must be closed as quickly as possible; the surgeon may tamponade the wound with his or her thumb until a suture is ready. Sutures should be rapidly placed and the patient's eye closed. Some surgeons advocate performing posterior sclerotomies to release accumulated blood. The prognosis for visual outcome is usually quite poor.

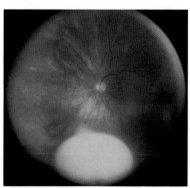

Figure 23-1. Posterior capsule rupture may lead to loss of nuclear fragments into the vitreous. In this case nearly the entire lens "dropped" following a circumferential extension of a radial tear during capsulorrhexis.

KEY POINTS: POSTOPERATIVE CATARACT SURGERY COMPLICATIONS

1. Corneal edema

2. Cystoid macular edema

3. Inflammation/uveitis

4. Wrong IOL power

5. Secondary membrane

6. Glaucoma/elevated intraocular pressure (IOP)

7. Wound leak

8. Retinal detachment

9. Diplopia

10. Ischemic optic neuropathy

9. **What are the causes of postoperative inflammation?**
   - **Operative trauma.** All eyes show some postoperative uveitis, characterized by cell and flare reaction in the anterior chamber. Despite individual variation, the degree of inflammation is usually proportionate to the degree of trauma induced by the surgical procedure. Procedures with longer surgical times and/or additional procedures (i.e., vitrectomy or iris manipulation) show greater amounts of inflammation.
   - **Retained lens material.** Fragments of lens material—either nucleus or cortical remnants—may cause inflammation. In almost all cases cortical remnants resorb and require no additional treatment. Nuclear fragments may become a source of chronic inflammation that leads to macular edema. Most nuclear remnants require surgical removal.
   - **Foreign body reaction to intraocular implants** may occur. This is more common when implants are poorly positioned and specifically when they are in contact with uveal tissue. Some patients, particularly those with a history of uveitis, may react to the intraocular lens (IOL) material.

10. **How does infectious endophthalmitis present? When does it usually occur?**
    The classic presentation includes severe ocular pain, decreased vision, eyelid swelling, conjunctival chemosis, and hypopyon. Corneal edema and diminution or loss of the red reflex often occur. This condition must be suspected in any patient who presents with more inflammation than expected postoperatively. On average, patients developed signs and symptoms 6 days after surgery. More than three-fourths of patients developed signs and symptoms within 2 weeks (Fig. 23-2).

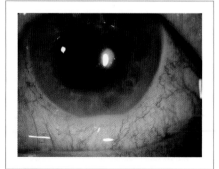

Figure 23-2. A layered hypopyon is seen in this case of postoperative endophthalmitis.

11. **What are the common organisms cultured from the vitreous of endophthalmitis patients?**
In the Endophthalmitis Vitrectomy Study the most common causative pathogens were gram-positive, coagulase-negative organisms (e.g., *Staphylococcus epidermidis*), followed by other gram-positive organisms, such as streptococci and *Staphylococcus aureus*.
http://www.nei.nih.gov/neitrials/viewStudyWeb.aspx?id=29

KEY POINTS: FINDING OF ENDOPHTHALMITIS VITRECTOMY STUDY

1. Systemic antibiotics provide *no* benefit in treating endophthalmitis
2. Intravitreal antibiotics for *all* endophthalmitis patients
3. If vision is *better* than hand movements: intravitreal tap and biopsy
4. If vision is *worse* than hand movements: full three-port pars plana vitrectomy

12. **What are the causes of corneal edema after cataract surgery?**
Corneal edema frequently occurs adjacent to the cataract wound and usually resolves spontaneously. Surgical trauma, preexisting endothelial corneal dystrophy, and elevated intraocular pressure may cause central corneal edema. Treatment of elevated intraocular pressure and topical steroids, as necessary for inflammation, are important. Often, central edema resolves. Corneal or epithelial transplantation may be necessary for patients when corneal edema persists (Fig. 23-3).

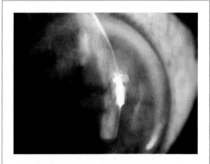

Figure 23-3. Corneal edema such as this is characterized by thickening of the cornea with Descemet's folds and, frequently, microcystic epithelial changes. It is more commonly seen in patients with preexisting endothelial cell loss (Fuchs' dystrophy) or dysfunction.

13. **What are the causes of vitreous loss during cataract surgery? Why is vitreous loss important?**
Vitreous loss may result from rupture of the posterior lens capsule or weakness or dehiscence of lens zonular apparatus. Vitreous loss increases risk of retinal detachment, cystoid macular edema, and endophthalmitis. The additional surgical trauma also may lead to an increase in corneal trauma and secondary central corneal edema.

14. **What is the incidence of retinal detachment after cataract surgery? Which patients are at greater risk?**
Retinal detachment occurs in 1–2% of patients in most reported series. Patients predisposed to retinal detachment because of high myopia, lattice degeneration, and a history of retinal detachment in the fellow eye are at greatest risk. Vitreous loss at the time of surgery also raises the risk of retinal detachment. The risk of retinal detachment after cataract surgery has decreased with the advent of extracapsular cataract extraction, which has replaced intracapsular extraction.

15. **What is cystoid macular edema?**
Cystoid macular edema (CME) occurs when fluid accumulates in the cells in and around the center of the macula, known as the fovea. Fluid may leak from the capillaries surrounding the fovea. CME typically presents 4–8 weeks after cataract surgery with a decrease in central visual acuity (Fig. 23-4).

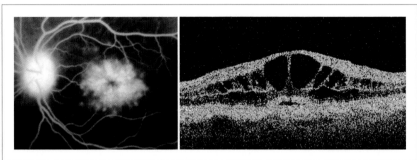

Figure 23-4. Cystoid macular edema after cataract surgery (Irvine-Gass Syndrome) has historically been documented with fluorescein angiography *(left)*, where it has a classic petaloid appearance in late frames of the angiogram. More recently, optical coherence tomography is increasingly being used to diagnose and follow macular edema *(right)*.

16. **What patients are likely to suffer from CME? How is it treated?**
Cystoid macular edema is more common after intracapsular than extracapsular cataract extraction. It is also more common when vitreous loss occurs, especially if vitreous or iris becomes incarcerated in the wound. It may occur in uncomplicated cases.
    Treatment of CME is controversial because a significant percentage of cases resolve spontaneously. Initial treatment often includes topical steroids or nonsteroidal anti-inflammatory medications (Acular). Acetazolamide (Diamox) has been shown to reduce edema in some cases and is often used as an oral medication. More recently, intravitreal triamcinolone has been shown to help cystoid macular edema, although the improvement may be transient. When vitreous or iris is adherent to the wound, lysis of vitreous strands with surgery, neodymium: yttrium-aluminum-garnet (Nd:YAG) laser, or wound revision may be beneficial. Pars plana vitrectomy has been used with success in some patients who suffer from chronic CME.

17. **What is a secondary membrane?**
A secondary or "after-cataract" membrane develops after extracapsular cataract surgery. The posterior capsule opacifies when persistent lens fibers adhere to the capsule, or the remaining lens fibers undergo metaplasia. Patients typically present with progressive decrease in vision or problems with glare after surgery.

18. **When does a secondary membrane develop? How frequently does it occur?**
Usually, secondary membrane begins to develop several months after surgery, although in many cases the membrane may take 1 year or more to become visually significant. The opacification rate varies from 8% to 50% in various series. Recently, squared posterior optic edge designs have lowered this rate, particularly with acrylic material optics.

19. **How is a secondary membrane treated? What complications may occur?**
A physician can perform a capsulotomy as a primary or secondary surgical procedure by cutting open the posterior capsule with a needle knife. This technique has been largely replaced by use

of the Nd:YAG laser. Complications of laser capsulotomy include transient intraocular pressure rise, retinal detachment, and CME.

20. **What are the most common complications related to IOLs?**
   - Implantation of the wrong power IOL may result in unacceptable refraction.
   - Decentration or dislocation of the IOL may produce unwanted optical images, including monocular double vision.
   - Mechanical chafing of the IOL against the iris or ciliary body may cause chronic inflammation. Chronic uveitis and secondary glaucoma, CME, or corneal decompensation may develop. Patients with these complications may require IOL repositioning or exchange.

21. **Why are patients with diabetes at greater risk when undergoing cataract surgery?**
   Diabetic retinopathy may accelerate dramatically after cataract surgery. This risk is greatest if the posterior capsule ruptures.

   Jaffe GJ, Burton TC, Kuhn E, et al: Progression of nonproliferative diabetic retinopathy and visual outcome after extracapsular cataract extraction and intraocular lens implantation. Am J Ophthalmol 114:448–459, 1992.

22. **What are the major problems in managing patients with preexisting glaucoma and cataracts?**
   - Many patients have been on glaucoma therapy, including miotics that constrict the pupil. Such therapy may make cataract surgery more difficult and often requires surgical maneuvers to enlarge the pupil.
   - Postoperative pressure may rise because of retained viscoelastic material and inflammation. This elevation in pressure is often more severe and prolonged in patients with glaucoma. Elevation of pressure may cause additional optic nerve damage and visual field loss and result in loss of central vision in patients with advanced glaucoma. A glaucoma procedure may be combined with cataract surgery in patients with advanced or poorly controlled glaucoma.
   - Patients with glaucoma who have had previous filtration surgery and develop cataracts may require a different approach to cataract surgery. A shift in the location of the incision to avoid damage to the filtration site is often necessary. Inflammation from the surgical procedure may cause failure of a previously functioning filter postoperatively.

23. **What medication is associated with intraoperative floppy iris syndrome?**
   Tamsulosin (Flomax) is a systemic α-1 antagonist medication used to treat prostatic hypertrophy. This drug relaxes the smooth muscle in the bladder neck and prostate. It has been postulated that the same receptor is present in the iris dilator smooth muscle resulting in loss of normal iris muscle tone.

24. **What are the indications for capsular tension rings?**
   Capsular tension rings may be used in a variety of patients. Most frequently they are used in patients with zonular laxity or instability. Most often this is in patients with pseudoexfoliation syndrome. It may also be a useful management tool in trauma cases or in patients who develop zonular dialysis as a result of the surgical procedure.

AMBLYOPIA

Steven E. Brooks, MD

CHAPTER 24

1. **What is amblyopia?**
   Amblyopia may be defined as a potentially reversible loss in visual function (e.g., acuity, contrast sensitivity, motion perception, binocularity), in one or both eyes, that results from inadequate or abnormal stimulation of the visual system during a critical period of early visual development.

   Brooks SE: Amblyopia. Ophthalmol Clin North Am 9:171–184,1996.
   von Noorden GK: Binocular Vision and Ocular Motility, 5th ed. St. Louis, Mosby, 1996.

2. **Explain the concept of the "critical" or "sensitive" period.**
   This period is central to the concept of amblyopia. It refers to a developmental time frame early in life during which there is robust plasticity within the visual system, particularly the visual cortex. Although not precisely defined, this period extends from birth to approximately 8–10 years of age. During this period the visual system is profoundly affected by the quality of visual stimulation it receives. Abnormal visual experience can lead to developmental abnormalities at both the structural and functional levels. Amblyopia occurs, and it should be detected and treated, during the critical period.

   Harwerth RS, Smith EL III, Duncan GC, et al: Multiple critical periods in the development of the primate visual system. Science 232:235–238, 1986.

3. **How is amblyopia generally classified?**
   Amblyopia is classified according to the underlying mechanism: strabismic, optical defocus, pattern or form deprivation, and organic.

   Optical defocus encompasses anisometropia as well as bilateral severe ametropia. Pattern or form deprivation amblyopia is caused by lesions that physically obstruct the visual axis, such as a congenital cataract, corneal opacity, vitreous hemorrhage, or ptosis. Organic amblyopia occurs secondary to a defined lesion of the visual pathways, such as a macular scar or coloboma. It is fundamentally different from the other types, because some or all of the vision loss is irreversible, and not simply a secondary effect on receptive fields in the lateral geniculate nuclei and visual cortex.

4. **How does strabismus cause amblyopia?**
   Manifest strabismus disrupts sensory fusion. As a result, the vision from one eye must be suppressed in order to avoid diplopia and visual confusion. If a child with strabismus develops a strong preference for the use of one eye over the other, the nondominant eye may become amblyopic because of chronic suppression.

5. **How prevalent is amblyopia?**
   In the United States it is estimated to be 2–5%.

6. **What factors place children at increased risk for amblyopia?**
   - Developmental delay
   - Positive family history of amblyopia
   - Prematurity

   These factors lead to a twofold to sixfold increase in a child's chance of developing amblyopia.

7. **What anatomic changes have been shown to occur in amblyopia?**
Although few human data are available, extensive animal studies have shown several neuroanatomic alterations in amblyopia. The primary abnormality appears to be the atrophy of cells in the layers of the lateral geniculate nucleus and visual cortex serving the amblyopic eye. These changes can be partially or wholly reversed if the amblyopia is successfully treated.

Crawford ML, Harwerth RS: Ocular dominance column width and contrast sensitivity in monkeys reared with strabismus or anisometropia. Invest Ophthalmol Vis Sci 45:3036–3042, 2004.
Wiesel TN, Hubel DH: Single-cell responses in striate cortex of kittens deprived of vision in one eye. J Neurophysiol 26:1003–1007, 1963.

8. **How early should children be screened for amblyopia?**
The American Academy of Ophthalmology recommends the following time points for routine screening of vision in children:
- Newborn to 3 months
- 6 months to 1 year
- 3 years
- 5 years

The optimal time to diagnose and treat amblyopia is as soon as it occurs, but it is critical to do so before the close of the critical period (ideally before the child is 5 years of age).

American Academy of Ophthalmology: Comprehensive Pediatric Eye Evaluation, Preferred Practice Pattern. San Francisco, American Academy of Ophthalmology, 1992.

9. **What are some clinical techniques to check for amblyopia in nonverbal children?**
Fixation preference testing is especially useful (Fig. 24-1). A lack of spontaneous alternation in visual fixation between the two eyes suggests amblyopia in the nonpreferred eye. Similarly, a child who consistently objects to occlusion of one eye but not the other can be assumed to have decreased vision in the eye that he or she will allow to be covered. Visual evoked potentials and preferential looking (e.g., Teller acuity cards) tests can be used to measure visual acuity. The Bruckner test, comparing the quality and symmetry of the red reflex between the two eyes by using a direct ophthalmoscope, can help detect small-angle strabismus or anisometropia.

Fischer N, Brooks SE: Effect of fixation target on fixation preference testing. Am Orthoptic J 49:105–110, 1999.
Tongue AC, Cibis GW: Bruckner test. Ophthalmology 88:1041–1044, 1981.
Wright KW, Walonker F, Edelman P: 10-Diopter fixation test for amblyopia. Arch Ophthalmol 99:1242–1246, 1981.

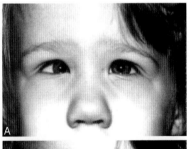
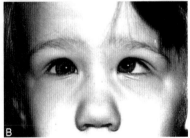

Figure 24-1. Child with esotropia showing spontaneous alternation in fixation. *A,* The left eye is used for fixation. *B,* The right eye is used for fixation. Alternating fixation is good evidence against the presence of amblyopia in children with strabismus.

10. **What is the usual presenting complaint of a child with anisometropic amblyopia and at what age?**
Similar to other forms of amblyopia, anisometropic amblyopia is generally asymptomatic. Detection in children depends on effective screening programs. Because of the lack of an overt external sign, such as strabismus or ptosis, the average age at presentation for anisometropic amblyopia is approximately 5–6 years, when school-initiated screening programs begin.

11. **Besides visual acuity, what other aspects of visual function may be affected in amblyopia?**
   - Binocular vision and stereoacuity
   - Contrast sensitivity
   - Motion perception and processing
   - Spatial localization

12. **How does anisometropia cause amblyopia?**
In anisometropia the retinal image in one eye is always defocused. If fixation is not alternated, the chronically defocused eye becomes incapable of processing high-resolution images.
In addition, the binocular rivalry between the blurred image in one eye and the clear image in the other eye leads to foveal suppression of the blurred image as a way to avoid visual confusion. In the absence of strabismus, the suppression affects the foveal region, where high-grade visual acuity is processed and binocular rivalry is poorly tolerated. As a result, such patients often display peripheral sensory fusion and gross stereopsis (monofixation syndrome), and maintain good ocular alignment.

   Brooks SE, Johnson D, Fischer N: Anisometropia and binocularity. Ophthalmology 103:1139–1143, 1996.
   Townsend AM, Holmes JM, Evans LS: Depth of anisometropic amblyopia and difference in refraction. Am J Ophthalmol 116:431–436, 1993.

13. **Which is more likely to produce amblyopia—unilateral or bilateral ptosis? Why?**
Unilateral ocular abnormalities are much more likely to lead to amblyopia than binocular ones. If one eye has a competitive advantage over the other, its afferent connections become stronger and more numerous while those of the other eye atrophy and retract. This competition also forms the basis for treating amblyopia. The amblyopic eye, by one means or another, must be given a temporary competitive advantage over the dominant eye.

KEY POINTS: AMBLYOPIA FUNDAMENTALS

1. Amblyopia is a potentially reversible loss of vision caused by abnormal visual stimulation during early visual development.

2. The critical period for amblyopia extends from birth to ages 8–10 years.

3. Testing vision with isolated optotypes may overestimate acuity in amblyopia because the effects of crowding are eliminated.

4. Amblyopia is characterized by functional and structural changes in the visual cortex and lateral geniculate nuclei.

14. **What steps should be taken before patching or penalization?**
The first step is to identify and treat any organic causes for vision loss. The second step is to ensure a clear visual axis. For example, this may require removal of a congenital cataract or

vitreous hemorrhage. Significant refractive errors should also be corrected. It may be helpful, during the course of treatment, to correct even relatively low degrees of hyperopia or astigmatism in the amblyopic eye, because the accommodative effort of an amblyopic eye is often reduced.

15. **What are some of the risks associated with full-time patching?**
The complete absence of any binocular interaction during the patching period may cause a phoria to decompensate into a tropia. Unfortunately, once present, the tropia may not resolve once patching is discontinued and may require corrective surgery. Amblyopia can also be induced in the eye being patched. Children can safely receive full-time occlusion of the sound eye for up to 1 week per year of life before the next follow-up visit without significant risk of inducing occlusion amblyopia in the sound eye.

16. **What are some alternative treatments to patching?**
Penalization refers to the intentional degradation of visual acuity in the sound eye by either optical or pharmacologic means. For example, the sound eye might be effectively blurred by intentional undercorrection of its refractive error, using atropine drops to prevent accommodation, or both. Translucent filters can be placed over the spectacle lens of the sound eye to degrade the vision. Penalization techniques are best suited for patients with a high degree of hyperopic refractive error in the sound eye and in whom the amblyopia is mild to moderate (20/100 or better).

Pediatric Eye Disease Investigator Group: A comparison of atropine and patching treatments for moderate amblyopia by patient age, cause of amblyopia, depth of amblyopia, and other factors. Ophthalmology 110:1632–1637, 2003.

Pediatric Eye Disease Investigator Group: The course of moderate amblyopia treated with atropine in children: experience of the amblyopia treatment study. Am J Ophthalmol 136:630–639, 2003.

Repka MX, Cotter SA, Beck RW, et al: A randomized trial of atropine regimens for treatment of moderate amblyopia in children. Ophthalmology 111:2076–2085, 2004.

17. **At what point can amblyopia treatment be discontinued?**
When the acuity in the treated eye is equal to that of the sound eye. The decision is less clear when there is some persistent deficit in visual acuity. If poor compliance can be ruled out, many practitioners continue to patch until no further improvement is noted after three consecutive treatment intervals (3–4 weeks each per interval). The eye examination and refraction should also be repeated to detect uncorrected refractive error or structural lesions. These guidelines may be modified, especially if there is a component of organic amblyopia. Once treatment is discontinued, children should be periodically rechecked to detect recurrences.

18. **What are some of the factors affecting the success of amblyopia treatment?**
   - Age of onset
   - Compliance with treatment regimen
   - Depth of amblyopia
   - Presence of associated ocular anomalies or injuries

19. **Can the vision of an amblyopic eye ever improve in adulthood?**
Although the critical period has passed, significant improvements in adulthood have been reported in cases in which the sound eye was lost to enucleation. The presence of central fixation in the amblyopic eye before the loss of the sound eye seemed to be the single most important predictor of the extent of visual improvement.

Studies looking at the potential use of pharmacologic agents such as levodopa to recover vision from amblyopic eyes in visually mature patients have demonstrated only small and temporary improvements. Such agents are not used in routine clinical practice.

El Mallah MK, Chakravarthy U, Hart PM: Amblyopia: Is visual loss permanent? Br J Ophthalmol 84:952–956, 2000.

Harwerth RS, Smith EL III, Duncan GC, et al: Effects of enucleation of the fixing eye on strabismic amblyopia in monkeys. Invest Ophthalmol Vis Sci 27:246–254, 1986.

Leguire LE, Komaromy KL, Nairus TM, Rogers GL: Long-term follow-up of L-dopa treatment in children with amblyopia. J Pediatr Ophthalmol Strabismus 39:326–330, 2002.

Leguire LE, Walson PD, Rogers GL, et al: Levodopa/carbidopa treatment for amblyopia in older children. J Pediatr Ophthalmol Strabismus 32:143–151, 1995.

Vereecken EP, Brabant P: Prognosis for vision in amblyopia after loss of the good eye. Arch Ophthalmol 102:220–224, 1984.

20. **Is color vision affected in amblyopia?**
    Generally speaking, color vision is not affected by amblyopia, although some investigators have found mild abnormalities in color perception. Eyes with severe amblyopia, particularly those with loss of foveal fixation, tend to demonstrate such abnormalities more consistently than eyes with milder degrees of amblyopia.

21. **Does amblyopia cause a relative afferent pupillary defect?**
    Generally speaking, amblyopia does not cause an afferent pupillary defect (APD), because the pathologic changes in amblyopia are located in the posterior visual pathways, not in the retina or optic nerve. If an eye suspected of having amblyopia is found to have a relative APD, it is imperative that a retinal or optic nerve lesion is ruled out.

    Greenwald MJ, Folk ER: Afferent pupillary defects in amblyopia. J Pediatr Ophthalmol Strabismus 20:63–67, 1983.

22. **In which of the following conditions is amblyopia most likely to occur: Congenital esotropia, Accommodative esotropia, Intermittent exotropia, or Constant exotropia?**
    Accommodative esotropia. Patients with this condition, particularly if there is significant anisometropia, are less likely to alternate fixation than patients with congenital esotropia or exotropia. Patients with intermittent exotropia are unlikely to develop amblyopia, because they spend a fair amount of time being bifoveal.

23. **What is the effect of neutral density filters on the vision of an amblyopic eye compared with a normal eye?**
    The visual acuity of a normal eye is progressively reduced by neutral density filters, whereas that of an amblyopic eye may remain unchanged or even improve slightly. This finding has led investigators to postulate that the vision in an amblyopic eye more closely resembles that normally occurring under scotopic conditions (i.e., rod mediated).

24. **What is the crowding phenomenon? What is its significance in amblyopia?**
    The crowding phenomenon refers to a loss of spatial acuity when optotypes are presented in close proximity, or surrounded by other visual details, rather than in isolation. The crowding phenomenon is seen in both normal and amblyopic eyes but tends to be much more pronounced in amblyopia. Because of this, measurement of acuity by isolated optotypes may overestimate acuity in amblyopia.

25. **What is eccentric fixation?**
    Eccentric fixation is seen in severe amblyopia as well as other conditions in which foveal fixation is severely compromised. It refers to use of nonfoveal areas of the retina for visual fixation. The fixation in such eyes is generally unsteady and poorly maintained. It appears as though the eye is looking elsewhere when, in fact, it is simply attempting to fixate using a nonfoveal area of the retina.

26. **Can refractive surgery be used to treat anisometropic amblyopia in children?**
    Currently, refractive surgery is not considered a good treatment option. Although investigators have reported successfully performing laser-assisted in-situ keratomileusis (LASIK) and photorefractive keratectomy (PRK) in pediatric patients, the surgical risks, lack of data on

long-term safety and predictability, and continued need for occlusion or penalization treatment render this form of treatment highly investigative at the present time.

Nucci P, Drack A: Refractive surgery for unilateral high myopia in children. JAAPOS 5:348–351, 2001.

Paysee EA, Hamill MB, Hussein MA, Koch DD: Photorefractive keratectomy for pediatric anisometropia: safety and impact on refractive error, visual acuity, and stereopsis. Am J Ophthalmol 138:70–78, 2004.

KEY POINTS: AMBLYOPIA TREATMENT GUIDELINES

1. Part-time occlusion therapy can be as effective as full-time occlusion if compliance is good.

2. Atropine penalization is most effective if the sound eye is at least moderately hyperopic.

3. Amblyopia treatment can be successful, with good compliance, up to 10 years of age.

4. Refractive errors in the amblyopic eye should be fully corrected during treatment.

27. **What is the upper age limit for treatment of amblyopia?**
Generally speaking, for optimal outcome, amblyopia should be detected and treated before age 6 years. However, there are several reports of successful treatment in older children (e.g., 7–14 years), if excellent compliance with treatment is maintained. This is particularly true for anisometropic amblyopia, and less so for strabismic and pattern deprivation amblyopia.

Mintz-Hittner HA, Fernandez KM: Successful amblyopia therapy initiated after age 7 years: Compliance cures. Arch Ophthalmol 118:1535–1541, 2000.

Park KH, Hwang JM, Ahn JK: Efficacy of amblyopia therapy initiated after 9 years of age. Eye 18:571–574, 2004.

Pediatric Eye Disease Investigator Group: A prospective, pilot study of treatment of amblyopia in children 10 to <18 years old. Am J Ophthalmol 137:581–583, 2004.

28. **Should anisometropia be corrected if amblyopia is not present?**
Several studies have found a positive relationship between the degree of anisometropia and incidence of amblyopia, whereas others have failed to find such a relationship. The American Academy of Ophthalmology's current preferred practice guidelines regarding amblyopia suggest that anisometropia in excess of 3 diopters (D) of myopia, 1.5 D of hyperopia, and 1.5 D of astigmatism be considered for empirical correction in young children in an attempt to minimize the risk of amblyopia. Experimental data in adults suggest that even lower levels of anisometropia can significantly affect high-grade binocular interactions.

American Academy of Ophthalmology: Amblyopia, Preferred Practice Pattern. San Francisco, American Academy of Ophthalmology, 1992.

Brooks SE, Johnson D, Fischer N: Anisometropia and binocularity. Ophthalmology 103:1139–1143, 1996.

29. **When should strabismus surgery be performed in a patient with amblyopia?**
Traditional teaching dictates that amblyopia should be fully treated before strabismus surgery. More recent studies suggest that surgery may be performed during the course of amblyopia treatment if the physician believes that recovery of binocular vision may be improved, or treatment of the amblyopia facilitated. It is likely that the management of any given case will need to be determined individually, and that both practice patterns can be effectively used.

Lam GC, Repka MX, Guyton DL: Timing of amblyopia therapy relative to strabismus surgery. Ophthalmology 100:1751–1756, 1993.

CHAPTER 25

ESODEVIATIONS

Scott E. Olitsky, MD, and Leonard B. Nelson, MD

1. **What is an esodeviation?**
    A convergent deviation, noted by crossing or in-turning of the eyes, is designated by the prefix *eso-*.

2. **What are the different types of esodeviations?**
    - **Esophoria** is a latent tendency for the eyes to cross. This latent deviation is normally controlled by fusional mechanisms that provide binocular vision or avoid diplopia. The eye deviates only under certain conditions, such as fatigue, illness, stress, or tests that interfere with the maintenance of normal fusional abilities (e.g., covering one eye).
    - **Esotropia** is a manifest misalignment of the eyes. The condition may be alternating or unilateral, depending on the vision. In alternating strabismus, either eye may be used for definitive seeing while the fellow eye deviates. In cases of unilateral esotropia, the deviating eye is noted in the description of the misalignment (left esotropia).

3. **How common is strabismus in infants?**
    Infants are rarely born with straight eyes. Alignment may vary intermittently from esotropia to orthotropia to exotropia during the first few months of life. Forty percent of newborn infants seem to have straight eyes, 33% may display exotropia, and approximately 3% may be esotropic. Many infants have variable alignment and cannot easily be classified in any single category.

    Archer SM, Sondhi N, Helveston EM: Strabismus in infancy. Ophthalmology 96:133–137, 1989.

4. **What is pseudoesotropia?**
    Pseudoesotropia is characterized by the false appearance of esotropia when the visual axes are actually aligned. Pseudoesotropia may be caused by a flat, broad nasal bridge; prominent epicanthal folds; or a narrow interpupillary distance that causes the observer to see less sclera nasally than expected, which creates the impression that the eye is turned in toward the nose.

5. **What is congenital esotropia?**
    Congenital esotropia describes a condition in which a child develops a convergent strabismus, with no identifiable cause, before the age of 6 months.

6. **What are the characteristics of congenital esotropia?**
    - **Large deviation:** The characteristic angle of congenital esotropia is considerably larger than angles of esotropia acquired later in life (Fig. 25-1). Average deviations in most series reported in the literature

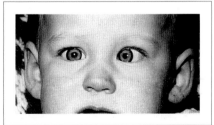

Figure 25-1. A child with congenital esotropia. Note the characteristic large angle of crossing.

are between 40 and 60 prism diopters. The diagnosis of congenital esotropia should be reconsidered in a child with a relatively small deviation.

- **Normal refractive error:** Children with congenital esotropia tend to have cycloplegic refractions similar to those of normal children of the same age.

7. **What is cross-fixation?**

Children with equal vision and a large esotropia have no need to abduct either eye. They use the adducted, or crossed, eye to look to the opposite field of gaze. This is called cross-fixation.

8. **Why do some children with congenital esotropia appear to have an abduction deficit?**

In children with good vision in both eyes, and who demonstrate cross-fixation, neither eye will appear to abduct. If amblyopia is present, only the eye that sees better will cross-fixate, making the amblyopic eye appear to have an abduction weakness.

9. **How can a pseudoabduction deficit be distinguished from a true abduction deficit?**

- Rotating the infant's head, either with the infant sitting upright in a moveable chair or by using a doll's head maneuver
- Patching one eye for a short period

10. **What is the differential diagnosis of an infant with esotropia?**

- Pseudoesotropia
- Congenital sixth nerve palsy
- Duane's retraction syndrome
- Early-onset accommodative esotropia
- Möbius' syndrome
- Sensory esotropia
- Nystagmus blockage syndrome
- Esotropia in the neurologically impaired

11. **How is vision evaluated in a child with congenital esotropia?**

The following observations can be made in order to look for equal vision in a child with a large-angle esotropia:

- Spontaneously alternates fixation
- Holds fixation with either eye when one eye is covered and then uncovered
- Cross-fixation present in both eyes

12. **How common is amblyopia in congenital esotropia?**

Amblyopia may occur in as many as 40–72% of infants with congenital esotropia.

13. **What are the goals in the treatment of congenital esotropia?**

- Development of normal sight in each eye
- Reduction of distant and near deviation as close to orthotropia (straight eyes) as possible
- Development of at least a rudimentary form of binocular vision

14. **What level of binocular vision can develop in children with congenital esotropia?**

- Classically, it has been taught that patients with congenital esotropia do not develop bifoveal fixation (perfect binocular vision) regardless of their age at treatment.
- Alignment within 10 prism diopters of orthotropia early in life is often associated with the attainment of some degree of binocular vision and stereopsis.

- Some surgeons have suggested that surgery performed on a patient at a very early age can lead to the development of bifoveal fixation.

15. **When is congenital esotropia treated?**
    - Most surgeons attempt to operate on children with congenital esotropia between 6 and 12 months of age, usually with bilateral medial ictus incisions.
    - Some surgeons operate on patients who are younger than 6 months of age in hopes of providing higher levels of binocular vision.

    Birch E, Stager D, Wright K, Beck R: The natural history of infantile esotropia during the first six months of life. J AAPOS 2:326–328, 1998.

    Ing M, Costenbader FD, Parks MM, Albert DG: Early surgery for congenital esotropia. Trans Am Ophthalmol 62:1419–1427, 1966.

16. **Why is it important to treat amblyopia before surgical correction of congenital esotropia?**
    - Detecting reduced vision in an infant is easier in the presence of a large esotropia.
    - Judgment about fixation preference is difficult in a preverbal child with straight eyes.
    - Occlusion therapy in children at a young age generally requires only a small amount of time to equalize vision.
    - If the vision is not equal after surgery, the chance of developing binocular vision and maintaining ocular alignment is lowered.
    - Parental incentive to comply with the often-arduous task of occlusion therapy is greatly diminished once the child's eyes are straight.

17. **What other motility disorders are often associated with congenital esotropia?**
    - **Inferior oblique overaction:** Elevation of the eye during adduction (Fig. 25-2); occurs in 78% of cases; most common in second or third year of life; may require surgery.
    - **Dissociated vertical deviation:** Slow upward deviation; occurs in 46–90% of cases; onset greatest in second year of life; may require surgery.
    - **Nystagmus:** Latent or rotary possible; occurs in 50% of cases; usually diminishes with time.

    Hiles DA, Watson A, Biglan AW: Characteristics of infantile esotropia following early bimedial rectus recession. Arch Ophthalmol 98:697–703, 1980.

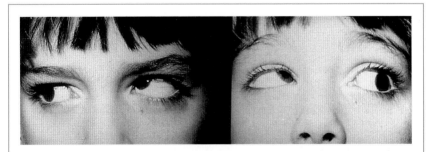

Figure 25-2. Inferior oblique overaction. As the eye adducts (moves toward the nose), it elevates.

18. **What is accommodative esotropia?**
    A convergent deviation of the eyes associated with activation of the accommodative reflex (Fig. 25-3).

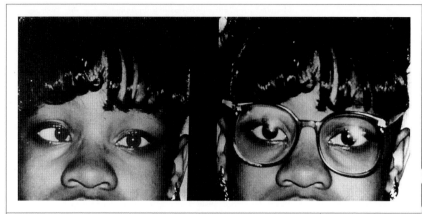

Figure 25-3. Accommodative esotropia. As the child attempts to accommodate (focus), the eyes cross *(left)*. With glasses that eliminate the need to accommodate, the eyes are straight *(right)*.

19. **At what age does accommodative esotropia develop?**
   Accommodative esotropia usually occurs in a child between 2 and 3 years of age. Occasionally, children who are 1 year of age or younger present with all of the clinical features of accomodative esotropia.

   Coats DK, Avilla CW, Paysse EA, et al: Early-onset refractive accommodative esotropia. J AAPOS 2:275–278, 1998.

20. **What are the three types of accommodative esotropia?**
   - Refractive
   - Nonrefractive
   - Partial or decompensated

21. **What three factors influence the development of refractive accommodative esotropia?**
   - Uncorrected hyperopia
   - Accommodative convergence
   - Insufficient fusional divergence

   Raab EL: Etiologic factors in accommodative esodeviation. Trans Am Ophthalmol Soc 80:657–694, 1982.

22. **How do the aforementioned three factors lead to accommodative esotropia?**
   A hyperopic person must exert excessive accommodation to clear a blurred retinal image. This, in turn, stimulates excessive convergence. If the amplitude of fusional divergence is sufficient to correct the excessive convergence, no esotropia results. However, if the fusional divergence amplitudes are inadequate, or if motor fusion is altered by some sensory obstacle, esotropia results.

23. **What is the AC:A ratio?**
   The accommodative convergence:accommodation (AC:A) ratio describes how many prism diopters a person's eyes converge for each diopter that they accommodate. The normal AC:A ratio is approximately 3–5 prism diopters of convergence per diopter of accommodation.

24. **How can the AC:A ratio be measured?**
   - Heterophoria method. A strabismic deviation is recorded in prism diopters for a distance of 6 meters *(D)* and near at one-third meter *(N)*. After measuring the patient's interpupillary distance in centimeters (PD), the AC:A ratio can then be calculated as follows:

$$AC:A = (PD) + N - D$$

Near measurement distance (in diopters)
- The gradient method. A strabismic deviation is measured at distance with any refractive error fully corrected. The deviation is then remeasured at distance through a convex or concave lens. The AC:A ratio is then calculated as:

$$AC:A = \text{deviation without lens} - \text{deviation with lens}$$

Dioptric power of lens
- Distance–near comparison. Most physicians prefer to assess the ratio using the distance–near comparison. This method is easier and quicker because it uses conventional examination techniques and requires no calculations. The AC:A relationship is derived simply by comparing the distance and near deviation. If the near measurement in an esotropic patient is >10 prism diopters, the AC:A ratio is considered to be abnormally high.

25. **How can refractive accommodative esotropia be treated?**
    - Spectacles correct the hyperopic refractive error.
    - Miotics are anticholinesterase inhibitors that alter the AC:A ratio so that a given amount of accommodation leads to a smaller amount of accommodative convergence.

26. **Why are spectacles a better option than miotics in the treatment of refractive accommodative esotropia?**
    - Spectacles control accommodation more reliably than glasses.
    - Miotics may cause pupillary cysts and, in adults, retinal detachments and cataracts.
    - Miotics may result in prolonged apnea after anesthesia if succinylcholine is used.

27. **What is the relationship between accommodative esotropia and congenital esotropia?**
    Recurrent esotropia may occur in approximately 25% of patients who have been successfully treated for congenital esotropia. Most of these patients (80%) respond to correction of hyperopia, even if the level of hyperopia is small.

KEY POINTS: ESOTROPIA

1. Amblyopia is best treated before surgery for congenital esotropia.

2. The diagnosis of congenital esotropia should be reconsidered in the presence of a small-angle deviation.

3. A complete exam is required to rule out other disorders in all patients who present with early-onset esodeviation.

4. Refractive accommodative esotropia is best treated with spectacles.

5. A neurologic work-up should be considered for patients who present with an acute esotropia and normal levels of hyperopia.

28. **What is nonrefractive accommodative esotropia?**
    Nonrefractive accommodative esotropia is associated with a high AC:A ratio. The effort to accommodate elicits an abnormally high accommodative convergence response. The amount of

esotropia is greater at near deviation than at distance because of the additional accommodation required to maintain a clear image at near.

29. **How can nonrefractive accommodative esotropia be treated?**
    - Bifocals eliminate the additional accommodative effort required at near and therefore reduce the near esotropia.
    - Miotics may be used to reduce the AC:A ratio but have the potential side effects mentioned in question 26.
    - Surgery may be performed to eliminate the esotropia at near and to correct the AC:A ratio permanently.
    - Observation. Some ophthalmologists choose simply to observe patients as long as the patients' eyes remain straight at distance. The esotropia at near may resolve on its own as the AC:A ratio normalizes during childhood.

30. **What is partial or decompensated accommodative esotropia?**
    Refractive or nonrefractive accommodative esotropias do not always occur in their "pure" forms. Glasses may reduce the esodeviation significantly. Sometimes the esotropia initially may be eliminated with glasses, but a nonaccommodative portion slowly becomes evident despite the maximal amount of hyperopic correction consistent with good vision. The residual esodeviation that persists is called the deteriorated or nonaccommodative portion. This condition commonly occurs with a delay of months between onset of accommodative esotropia and antiaccommodative treatment.

31. **How is partial or decompensated accommodative esotropia treated?**
    - Surgery may be indicated if the deviation is larger than an amount that allows development of binocular vision.
    - Surgery is generally performed for the nonaccommodative portion of the esotropia only, not for the full deviation that is present without glasses in place.

32. **What are the characteristics of the nystagmus blockage syndrome?**
    - It begins in early infancy and is associated with esotropia.
    - The nystagmus is reduced or absent with the fixating eye in adduction.
    - As the fixating eye follows a target moving laterally toward the primary position and then into abduction, the nystagmus increases and the esotropia decreases.

33. **What is cyclic esotropia?**
    - A rare disorder that classically describes a large-angle esotropia alternating with orthophoria or a small-angle esodeviation on a 48-hour cycle.
    - It may result from an aberration in the biologic clock or a combination of defects in the clock, oculomotor nuclei, superior colliculi, or other nuclei.
    - Unpredictable response to various forms of therapy with the exception of surgery, which is usually curative.

34. **What are the characteristics of acute acquired comitant esotropia (AACE)?**
    - Rare condition that occurs in older children and adults
    - Dramatic onset of a large angle of esotropia with diplopia
    - Normal levels of hyperopia
    - Has been reported after periods of interruption of fusion, such as occlusion therapy for amblyopia

35. **How should patients with AACE be managed?**
    - A careful motility analysis to rule out a paretic deviation.
    - Consider further work-up, including computed tomography or magnetic resonance imaging.

MISCELLANEOUS OCULAR DEVIATIONS

Janice A. Gault, MD

CHAPTER 26

1. **What is the differential diagnosis of exotropia?**
   - Congenital exotropia
   - Sensory exotropia
   - Third-nerve palsy
   - Duane's syndrome
   - Craniofacial abnormalities with divergent orbit (e.g., Apert's syndrome or Crouzon syndrome)
   - Myasthenia gravis
   - Thyroid disorder
   - Medial wall fracture
   - Slipped medial rectus muscle or excessively resected lateral rectus
   - Orbital inflammatory pseudotumor
   - Convergence insufficiency
   - Internuclear ophthalmoplegia

2. **A mother notices that her 4-month-old infant seems to be "wall-eyed." What is your concern as a physician?**
   First, check whether deviation or pseudostrabismus is present. A wide interpupillary distance or temporal dragging of the macula from retinopathy of prematurity or toxocariasis may cause pseudoexotropia. The light reflex test or cover testing elucidates this point. Also, make sure that the eyes move normally. Have the patient follow a light or a brightly colored toy to exclude paralysis or muscle restriction. If this test is normal and you notice true strabismus, quantify it at near and far. Check the cycloplegic refraction, and do a complete dilated exam. Anisometropic amblyopia may cause an eye to deviate, but it usually presents as esotropia in the younger age group. Also, a corneal lesion, cataract, glaucoma, or retinal lesion such as a toxoplasmosis scar or retinoblastoma may cause the deviation. These conditions must be ruled out.

   Once you have determined that the remainder of the exam is normal, you realize that the infant has an alternating exotropia of 40 prism diopters. Congenital exotropia is much rarer than congenital esotropia, but they have much in common. Both have a large angle of deviation and rarely develop amblyopia because of alternating fixation. The refractive error is normal. Early surgery is recommended to allow development of stereoacuity.

3. **A mother notices that her 2-year-old boy has a left eye that deviates outward when he is tired or has a fever. What is your concern as a physician?**
   Intermittent exotropia, which is the most common type of exotropia. The onset varies from infancy to 4 years of age. It may progress through the following three phases:
   - **Phase one:** Exophoria at distance and orthophoria at near occur when the patient is fatigued or daydreaming. He has diplopia and often closes one eye. When aware of the deviation, he is easily able to straighten his eyes, often after a blink.
   - **Phase two:** Exotropia at distance and exophoria at near. When the exotropia becomes more constant, suppression develops and the diplopia becomes less frequent. The exotropia remains after a blink.

- **Phase three:** The exotropia is constant at distance and near. There is no diplopia because of suppression.

  Vision must be equalized by correcting any significant refractive error and patching the nondeviating eye. Surgery should be done when the patient progresses beyond phase one, but preferably before phase three.

4. **An 18-year-old patient complains of blurred near vision and headaches while reading. Do you believe her, or is she just trying to get out of doing her homework?**

   Check her ocular deviations at near and far. She may be experiencing convergence insufficiency, which is common in teenagers and young adults. It is often idiopathic but may be exacerbated by fatigue, drugs, uveitis, or an Adie's tonic pupil. Exodeviation is greater at near than at distance and causes asthenopia. Exophoria at near may be all that is seen. The near point of convergence is more distant than normal (>3–6 cm for patients younger than age 20; >12 cm for patients older than age 40), and the amplitude of accommodation is reduced.

   Because she is symptomatic, treat her with base-in prisms for reading to help convergence. Near point exercises or "pencil push-ups" can improve fusional amplitudes. These exercises are performed by having the patient slowly move a pencil from arm's length toward the face while focusing on the eraser. Have the patient concentrate on maintaining one image of the eraser. Repeat 10 times several times a day. Once this is mastered, pencil push-ups can be done while holding a 6-diopter base-out prism over one eye. Rarely, medial rectus resection may be necessary.

5. **What if the fusional capacities are normal and there is no exodeviation?**

   The problem may be accommodative insufficiency, which has similar symptoms in the same age group. However, accommodation is reduced. First check the manifest and cycloplegic refraction. The patient may be underplussed and need a stronger hyperopic refraction. If refraction is normal, plus lens reading glasses will help. A 4-diopter base-in prism will cause blurring during reading, whereas patients with convergence insufficiency will note that print becomes clearer.

6. **Some patients have the opposite problem: esotropia that is worse at distance than near. What is this condition called?**

   Divergence insufficiency. Fusional divergence is reduced. Treatment is with base-out prisms and, rarely, lateral rectus resections. However, divergence insufficiency is a diagnosis of exclusion, and divergence paralysis must be ruled out because it may be associated with pontine tumors, head trauma, and other neurologic abnormalities. Neuro-ophthalmic evaluation is necessary.

7. **What is Duane's syndrome? What are the different types of this disorder?**

   Duane's syndrome is a congenital motility disorder characterized by limited abduction, limited adduction, or both. The globe retracts, and the palpebral fissure narrows on attempted adduction. A "leash effect" may cause upward deviation at the same time. There are three types of the syndrome:

   - Type 1—limited abduction (most common) (Fig. 26-1)
   - Type 2—limited adduction
   - Type 3—both limited abduction and limited adduction (rarest type)

   There are three females to every two males afflicted with Duane's syndrome. The left eye is involved in 60% of cases; in 18% of cases, both eyes are involved. Sixty percent of patients also have an associated esotropia, 15% have exotropia, and 25% are orthophoric. A and V patterns are common. Amblyopia, attributable to anisometropia, occurs in approximately one-third of cases. Surgery is done to correct a head turn, but resection should not be performed because it exacerbates the narrowing of the fissure and globe retraction.

8. **What is the cause of Duane's syndrome?**
   The cause is unclear, but it appears that the lateral rectus muscle is innervated by the third nerve, causing co-contraction of the medial and lateral rectus muscles. This theory explains the globe retraction and fissure narrowing.

9. **What other features may be associated with Duane's syndrome?**
   Goldenhar's syndrome, deafness, crocodile tears, and uveal colobomas.

10. **What is the differential diagnosis of hypertropia?**
    - Myasthenia gravis
    - Thyroid eye disease
    - Orbital inflammatory pseudotumor
    - Orbital trauma (may cause inferior rectus entrapment)
    - Fourth cranial nerve palsy
    - Pseudohypertropia
    - Skew deviation—see Chapter 30

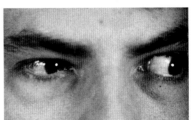
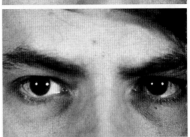
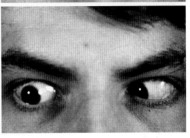

Figure 26-1. Duane's syndrome affecting the right eye. In primary position *(middle)*, the eyes are aligned. There is reduction in the right palpebral fissure height on left gaze *(top)* and right upper eyelid retraction as well as an abduction deficit on right gaze *(bottom)*. (From Burde RM, Savino PJ, Trobe JD: Clinical Decisions in Neuro-Ophthalmology, 3rd ed. St. Louis, Mosby.)

KEY POINTS: BROWN'S SYNDROME

1. Inability to elevate affected eye when adducted.

2. Hypertropia may be present in primary gaze.

3. Patient may turn head away from affected eye with chin-up position.

4. Ten percent of cases are bilateral.

5. Forced adduction reveals superior oblique muscle restriction.

11. **What is the cause of Brown's syndrome?**

Brown's syndrome (Fig. 26-2) may be congenital or acquired. The cause may be related to mechanical restriction of the superior oblique tendon. Examples include trauma, surgery, or inflammation in the region near the trochlea.

12. **How is Brown's syndrome treated?**

Acquired cases may be observed because they may improve spontaneously. Some improve with steroid injections near the trochlea. If no improvement is seen by 6 months, the superior oblique muscle may be weakened with a tenotomy. Some surgeons recess the ipsilateral inferior oblique at the same time to prevent an inferior oblique overaction postoperatively. Patients need to be aware that they will never be able to elevate the affected eye normally in adduction.

13. **What is the differential diagnosis of Brown's syndrome?**
   - **Inferior oblique palsy:** The three-step test reveals a superior oblique overaction that is not present in Brown's syndrome. In patients with diplopia, vertical deviations in primary gaze, or an abnormal head position, a superior oblique tenotomy or recession of the contralateral superior rectus is done. Forced ductions reveal no restriction.
   - **Double elevator palsy:** Patients cannot elevate the affected eye in any field of gaze (Fig. 26-3). Ptosis or pseudoptosis may be seen. A chin-up position helps to maintain fusion if a hypotropia is present in primary gaze. If no chin-up position is seen with hypotropia, amblyopia is present. Treatment for a large vertical deviation or an abnormal head position is inferior rectus recession if the inferior rectus is restricted or transposition of the medial and lateral rectus toward the superior rectus (Knapp procedure) if no restriction is present.
   - **Blowout fracture with entrapment of the inferior rectus muscle:** History elucidates this injury, and forced ductions show restriction. Confirm with an orbital computed tomographic (CT) scan.
   - **Thyroid disease:** Restriction is found on forced ductions, the strabismus is acquired and incomitant, lid retraction also may be noted. A CT scan reveals enlarged extraocular muscles.

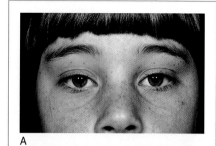

A

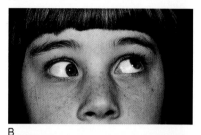

B

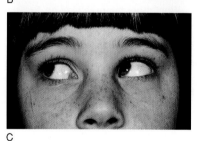

C

Figure 26-2. Brown's syndrome affecting the right eye. *A,* Usually straight in the primary position. *B,* Limited right elevation in adduction and occasionally also in the midline. *C,* Usually normal right elevation in abduction. (From Kanski JJ: Clinical Ophthalmology: A Systematic Approach, 5th ed. New York, Butterworth-Heinemann, 2003.)

14. **What is Möbius' syndrome?**
    A congenital syndrome with varying abnormalities of the fifth through twelfth cranial nerves. Patients may have a unilateral or bilateral esotropia with inability to abduct the eyes even on doll's head maneuvers. Patients also may exhibit limb, chest, and tongue defects and may have significant feeding difficulties.

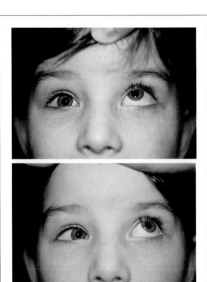

15. **A 48-year-old man undergoes medial rectus resection and lateral rectus recession for a sensory exotropia of 35 prism diopters in the left eye. He presents the next day with an exotropia of 60 prism diopters in primary position and an inability to abduct the eye. What is your diagnosis?**
    A slipped or lost medial rectus muscle. It is important to double-lock the suture through the tendon and muscle when reattaching the rectus muscle to the globe to prevent this complication. Reoperation is necessary to find the muscle and reattach it in the appropriate position. If you cannot locate the muscle, a transposition of the superior and inferior rectus muscles helps to correct the exotropia.

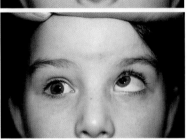

Figure 26-3. Right monoelevation deficit showing defective elevation in all positions. (From Kanski JJ: Clinical Ophthalmology: A Systematic Approach, 5th ed. New York, Butterworth-Heinemann, 2003.)

16. **A patient complains that her right eye is hypertropic. The light reflex test and covering test show her to be orthophoric. What may be going on?**
    Pseudohypertropia. She may have a vertically displaced macula from retinopathy of prematurity or toxocariasis. Eyelid retraction of the right eye may cause the right eye to appear hypertropic. Vertical displacement of the globe superiorly by a mass, such as a mucocele, may cause a similar appearance.

17. **A young boy has developed chin-up position and seems to move his head rather than his eyes to locate objects. On examination, he has poor ductions and versions in all fields of gaze as well as bilateral ptosis. Forced ductions reveal restrictions in all extraocular muscles. What is your diagnosis?**
    Congenital fibrosis syndrome. The normal muscle tissue is replaced by fibrous tissue to varying degrees. It may be unilateral or bilateral. The eyes may exhibit little-to-no vertical or horizontal movements, depending on the number of muscles involved, as well as esotropia

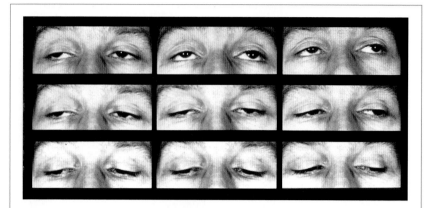

Figure 26-4. Chronic progressive external ophthalmoplegia. (From Kanski JJ: Clinical Ophthalmology: A Test Yourself Atlas, 2nd ed. New York, Butterworth-Heinemann, 2002.)

or exotropia. Amblyopia is common. Ptosis with chin elevation is a frequent manifestation. The cause is unknown. The goal of surgery is to restore orthophoria in primary gaze.

18. **A 20-year-old man with no history of strabismus complains that he cannot open his eyes well. You notice that ductions and versions are severely reduced and that he has bilateral ptosis. There is no restriction on forced ductions. What is your diagnosis?**
   Chronic progressive external ophthalmoplegia (CPEO). This condition begins in childhood with ptosis and progresses slowly to total paresis of the eyelids and extraocular muscles (Fig. 26-4). It may be sporadic or familial. Patients usually do not have diplopia. A frontalis sling procedure may be necessary to elevate the eyelids.

19. **What other evaluations are important?**
   Check for retinal pigmentations, and order an electrocardiogram to check for heart block. The triad of CPEO, retinal pigmentary changes, and cardiomyopathy is known as Kearns-Sayre syndrome (Fig. 26-5). Patients may require pacemakers to prevent sudden death. Inheritance is by maternal mitochondrial DNA.

20. **What other diseases may be associated with CPEO?**
   - **Abetalipoproteinemia (Bassen-Kornzweig syndrome):** Patients have retinal pigmentary changes similar to retinitis pigmentosa (RP), diarrhea, ataxia, and other neurologic signs.
   - **Refsum's disease:** Patients have an RP-like syndrome with an increased phytanic acid level. They also may have neurologic signs.

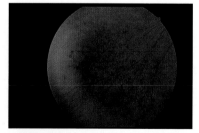

Figure 26-5. Kearns-Sayre syndrome. (From Kanski JJ: Clinical Ophthalmology: A Test Yourself Atlas, 2nd ed. New York, Butterworth-Heinemann, 2002.)

- **Ocular pharyngeal dystrophy:** Patients have difficulty with swallowing. The condition may be autosomal dominant.

21. **What is congenital ocular motor apraxia?**
In this rare disorder patients are unable to generate normal voluntary horizontal saccades. To change horizontal fixation, a head thrust that overshoots the target is made. The head is then rotated back in the opposite direction once fixation is established. Vertical saccades are normal, but vestibular and optokinetic nystagmus are impaired. Strabismus may be associated.

22. **A patient complains of diplopia. On examination, he has paresis of the third, fourth, and fifth cranial nerves on the right side. What can cause multiple ocular motor nerve palsies?**
Anything that damages the cavernous sinus and/or superior orbital fissure, including the following:
- Arteriovenous fistula—carotid-cavernous (C-C) sinus dural shunts
- Cavernous sinus thrombosis
- Tumors metastatic to cavernous sinus
- Skin malignancy with perineural spread to cavernous sinus
- Pituitary apoplexy—patients often have extreme headache with bilateral signs and decreased vision; need emergent intravenous steroids and neurosurgical consultation
- Intracavernous aneurysm
- Mucormycosis—more likely in diabetics, especially in ketoacidosis, and any debilitated or immunocompromised patient; look for an eschar in the nose and palate; emergent consultation with otolaryngology for débridement imperative
- Herpes zoster
- Tolosa-Hunt syndrome—acute idiopathic inflammation of the superior orbital fissure or anterior cavernous sinus (diagnosis of exclusion)
- Mucocele
- Meningioma
- Nasopharyngeal carcinoma
  Multiple cranial nerve palsies also may occur with brain stem lesions and carcinomatous meningitis. Other entities that can mimic multiple cranial nerve palsies include:
- Myasthenia gravis
- CPEO
- Orbital lesions such as thyroid disease, pseudotumor, or tumor
- Progressive supranuclear palsy
- Guillain-Barré syndrome

23. **What is Parinaud's syndrome?**
Also known as dorsal midbrain syndrome, Parinaud's syndrome is characterized by a supranuclear gaze paresis with nuclear oculomotor paresis and pupillary abnormalities. Active upward gaze is diminished, but elevation is seen with doll's head maneuver. Attempts at upward gaze cause retraction-convergence nystagmus and palpebral fissure widening (Collier's sign). Pupils are mid-dilated and do not react to light but react normally to accommodation.

24. **What is the cause of Parinaud's syndrome?**
In children, pinealoma and aqueductal stenosis are the most common causes. In adults, demyelination, infarct, and tumor are most common.

25. **Describe the presentation of a patient with internuclear ophthalmoplegia.**
A young woman with a history of optic neuritis complains of double vision when looking to one side. She is unable to adduct on attempted contralateral gaze and exhibits horizontal

nystagmus in the abducting eye. Adduction on convergence is normal. The condition may be unilateral or bilateral. Exotropia may be present if the condition is bilateral.

26. **Where is the causative lesion?**
In the medial longitudinal fasciculus. Causes include multiple sclerosis, ischemic vascular disease, brain stem tumor, and trauma.

BIBLIOGRAPHY

1. American Academy of Ophthalmology: Pediatric Ophthalmology and Strabismus, San Francisco, 2000.
2. Kunimoto DY, Kanitkar KD, Makar M: The Wills Eye Manual: Office and Emergency Room Diagnosis and Treatment of Eye Disease, 4th ed. Philadelphia, Lippincott Williams & Wilkins, 2004.
3. Nelson LB, Catalano RA: Atlas of Ocular Motility. Philadelphia, W.B. Saunders, 1989.

CHAPTER 27

STRABISMUS SURGERY

Bruce M. Schnall, MD

1. **How are forced ductions performed?**
   Before beginning surgery, place an eyelid speculum in both eyes. Using one- or two-toothed forceps, grasp the conjunctiva at the limbus. Move the eye horizontally and vertically. The resistance encountered in moving the eye is compared with what normally would be expected, as well as with the resistance encountered in performing the same forced duction on the other eye.

2. **Why perform forced ductions?**
   Forced ductions are performed to detect "tight muscles" or restrictions in eye movement. If the forced ductions indicate that a muscle is restricted, the affected muscle should be recessed. For example, if a patient has a vertical deviation, the superior rectus on the hypertropic side or the inferior rectus on the fellow eye may be recessed. If forced ductions show resistance to elevating the fellow eye, the preferred surgery is recession of the inferior rectus.

3. **When correcting a horizontal or vertical strabismus, how do you decide how many muscles to recess or resect?**
   The angle of the deviation determines the number of muscles to recess or resect. Whereas a small-angle strabismus (<20 diopters) may be corrected by operating on one muscle only, a large deviation may require surgery on three or four rectus muscles. Most major texts contain tables that provide a guide as to how much surgery should be performed for the angle (measured in prism diopters) of strabismus. The tables indicate how many muscles should be operated on and the amount of recession or resection.

4. **When doing a recess-resect procedure, should you first perform the recession or the resection?**
   The recession is performed first. In a resection the muscle is shortened and then brought forward to the insertion. This procedure creates tension on the resected muscle, making it difficult to bring the resected muscle to the insertion site. Initial recession of the antagonist muscle decreases the tension pulling the globe away from the resected muscle and makes it easier to bring the resected muscle to the insertion site and to tie the sutures on the resected muscle.

5. **When performing surgery on an oblique muscle and rectus muscle of the same eye, on which muscle do you operate first?**
   The oblique muscles are more difficult to identify and isolate on the muscle hook than the recti. Strabismus surgery creates swelling of Tenon's capsule and bleeding, which can obscure the view and make identification of the oblique muscles difficult. Therefore, it is preferable to operate on the oblique muscles first, when Tenon's capsule and the tissues surrounding the oblique muscles are the least swollen and distorted. The recti are more easily hooked and identified. There should be no difficulty in isolating the correct rectus muscle, even in the presence of significant bleeding and swelling of Tenon's capsule associated with oblique muscle surgery.

6. **What type of needle is used to suture the muscle to the sclera?**
A spatulated needle, which has cutting surfaces on the side, decreases the risk of perforating the globe. The sclera is thinnest just posterior to the insertion of the rectus muscles (0.3 mm).

7. **What is an adjustable suture?**
Various techniques of placing and tying scleral sutures allow the muscle to be moved forward or backward during the immediate postoperative period. If a patient has an immediate overcorrection or undercorrection, the muscle can be moved to improve the alignment. This suture adjustment is performed within 24 hours of the initial surgery.

8. **When should an adjustable suture be used?**
The use of an adjustable suture is at the discretion of the surgeon. Some surgeons do not perform adjustable suture surgery, citing the fact that the correction seen immediately after strabismus surgery is variable and may not be indicative of the long-term result. Others use adjustable sutures in cases in which the results of strabismus surgery are difficult to predict, such as reoperations and restrictive or paralytic strabismus. Often, adjustable sutures are used in patients with thyroid disease.

9. **What is a transposition procedure?**
A transposition procedure usually involves the placement of either part or the entire tendon of the adjacent recti muscles to the insertion of the palsied or underacting muscle. For instance, in double-elevator palsy the tendon of the lateral and medial recti may be sutured to the nasal and temporal borders of the superior rectus insertion.

Plager DA, Neely DE: Transposition procedures. In Tasman W, Jaeger EA (eds): Duane's Clinical Ophthalmology, vol. 6. Philadelphia, Lippincott-Raven, 2004, pp 1–12.

10. **When is a transposition procedure performed?**
A transposition procedure is the procedure of choice when the function of one or more recti muscles is severely limited, as with third-nerve, sixth-nerve, or double-elevator palsy.

11. **How are A and V patterns of strabismus treated?**
In cases of oblique muscle overaction, the appropriate oblique muscle should be weakened. Weakening of the inferior oblique muscles corrects a V pattern, whereas weakening of the superior oblique muscles corrects an A pattern (Fig. 27-1). In patients with no oblique muscle dysfunction, the horizontal recti are supraplaced or infraplaced. The medial recti are displaced toward the point of the A or V pattern, whereas the lateral recti are moved in the opposite direction. A useful acronym is **MALE**, which stands for **M**edial recti to the **A**pex, **L**ateral recti to

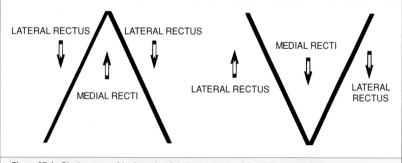

Figure 27-1. Displacement of horizontal arch in the treatment of A and V pattern strabismus.

the Empty space. For example, to treat a V pattern esotropia without oblique muscle overaction, the medial recti are recessed and infraplaced (moved inferiorly) by half of the tendon width.

12. **What surgery can be done for Brown's syndrome?**
In Brown's syndrome, a congenitally short or tight superior oblique tendon creates a mechanical restriction of elevation when the eye is in adduction, as confirmed at surgery with forced duction testing. Brown's syndrome is treated surgically by superior oblique tenotomy, recession, or a tendon expander.

13. **What are the indications for surgery in Brown's syndrome?**
Hypertropia in primary gaze or abnormal head position (face-turn or chin-up position).

14. **In strabismus surgery in patients with Duane's syndrome, is it better to recess or resect?**
Resection would increase the globe retraction; therefore, resections are avoided. Recessions or, less commonly, transposition procedures, are performed.

KEY POINTS: MOST COMMON COMPLICATIONS OF STRABISMUS SURGERY

1. Overcorrection or undercorrection
2. Anterior segment ischemia
3. Infection
4. Adherence syndrome
5. Diplopia
6. Scleral perforation
7. Slipped or lost muscle
8. Operating on the wrong muscle

15. **What are the signs of infection after strabismus surgery?**
Infection may take the form of cellulitis, subconjunctival abscess, or endophthalmitis. Cellulitis is most common with an estimated incidence between 1 case in 1000 and 1 case in 1900 surgeries. It typically occurs 2–3 days after surgery. The most common symptoms are marked swelling and pain. Suspected cellulitis requires prompt treatment with systemic antibiotics as well as careful examination to make certain that the patient does not develop endophthalmitis.

Kivlin JD, Wilson ME, and the Periocular Infection Study Group: Periocular infection after strabismus surgery. J Pediatr Ophthalmol Strabismus 32:42–49, 1995.

16. **What are the signs and symptoms of endophthalmitis after pediatric strabismus surgery?**
The signs of endophthalmitis typically appear 1–4 days after surgery and include lethargy, asymmetric eye redness, eyelid swelling, and fever. Patients who develop endophthalmitis experience an increase in eyelid swelling and redness during the postoperative period rather than a decrease, as expected during a normal postoperative course. On examination, the patient

has a decreased red reflex and signs of vitreal inflammation. If endophthalmitis is suspected, prompt evaluation and treatment are required.

Recchia FM, Baumal CR, Sivalingam A, et al: Endophthalmitis after pediatric strabismus surgery. Arch Ophthalmol 118:939–944, 2000.

17. **What should you do if you suspect that you perforated the globe when passing the scleral suture?**
If a scleral perforation is suspected, indirect ophthalmoscopy should be performed in the operating room at completion of the strabismus surgery. If a retinal perforation is seen on ophthalmoscopy, retinal consultation or repeat examinations with the indirect ophthalmoscope are indicated. Treatment is controversial. Whereas some surgeons advocate treatment with cryotherapy or indirect laser, others simply observe the patient. The incidence of retinal detachment after scleral perforation is believed to be low. At the same time, cryotherapy may increase the incidence of retinal detachment by stimulating vitreous changes. In patients predisposed to retinal detachment (for example, high myopes), however, serious consideration should be given to treatment of a retinal perforation at the time of strabismus surgery. Some strabismus surgeons believe that scleral perforation increases the risk of endophthalmitis and therefore recommend sub-Tenon's injection of prophylactic antibiotics if the globe is perforated.

Awad AH, Mullaney PB, Al-Hazmi A, et al: Recognized globe perforation during strabismus surgery: Incidence, risk factors, and sequelae. J AAPOS 4:150–153, 2000.
Sprunger DT, Klapper SR, Bonnis JM, Minturn JT: Management of experimental globe perforation during strabismus surgery. J Pediatr Ophthalmol Strabismus 33:140–143, 1996.

18. **What is a slipped muscle?**
The muscle is contained within a capsule. While operating on a rectus muscle it is possible to mistakenly engage only the capsule on the suture. After the muscle is reattached to the eye, it may slip back within its capsule, which results in further weakening of the muscle and consecutive deviation. For instance, if a slipped muscle occurred in recessing a medial rectus muscle for esotropia, exotropia and limited adduction will develop in the involved eye over time.

19. **How is a slipped muscle prevented?**
In placing the suture through the muscle, make locking bites on either end of the muscle. Locking bites should be made by placing the suture through the muscle perpendicular to its insertion, engaging the tendon, rather than tangentially. Tangential placement may engage only the capsule.

Parks MM, Bloom JN: The "slipped muscle." Ophthalmology 86:1389–1396, 1979.

20. **What is the adherence syndrome?**
The orbital fat is separated from the globe by Tenon's capsule. If an accidental opening is made in the portion of Tenon's capsule that separates the orbital fat from sclera, orbital fat may be pressed through the opening and adhere to the globe. This adherence often results in limited eye moments. It is best treated by prevention. The orbital fat comes forward around the equator of the globe to within 10 mm of the limbus. Care should be taken not to cut Tenon's capsule more than 10 mm from the limbus.

21. **How can strabismus surgery cause anterior segment ischemia?**
The anterior ciliary arteries accompany the recti muscles. They penetrate the sclera at the muscle's insertion site, contributing significantly to the blood supply of the anterior segment. In standard strabismus surgery the anterior ciliary vessels are cut when the rectus muscle is disinserted.

Rubin SE, Nelson LB: Complications of strabismus surgery. Ophthalmol Clin North Am 5:157–164, 1992.

22. **How is anterior segment ischemia avoided?**

By not operating on more than two recti muscles in one eye at the same time. It is also possible to dissect the anterior ciliary vessels from the rectus muscle and preserve them. Surgery to preserve the anterior ciliary vessels is performed only when the risk of anterior segment ischemia is high, such as in older patients with cardiovascular disease or patients with a history of previous rectus muscle surgery.

McKeown CA, Shore JW, Lambert HM: Preservation of the anterior ciliary vessels during extraocular muscle surgery. Ophthalmology 96:498–506, 1989.

CHAPTER 28

NYSTAGMUS

Robert D. Reinecke, MD

1. **What is nystagmus?**
   The eyes oscillate repetitively and typically symmetrically as well, in a to-and-fro horizontal direction with a fast jerk in a consistent direction in respect to orbital coordinates. Often the nystagmus is exclusively vertical, other cases are purely torsional, and occasional cases are a mixture of all three. The term *nystagmus* seems to have arisen from the sleepy head jerk. As the head of a drowsy student slowly falls to one side, often a head jerk brings the head back to an upright position. That head movement resembles the eyes' movements of nystagmus.

2. **Why don't all patients see the visual scene bobbing?**
   Oscillopsia occurs when the efferent copied nerve impulses do not match the motor nerve impulses or if there is a nonadaptive change. In general, nystagmus and/or strabismus occur before the age of 6 years when adaptation is easier.

3. **Is there any other means of adaptation to prevent oscillopsia when the eyes' movements and the eyes' relative positions to each other are not matched?**
   Yes. Each eye can sample independently, such that only a small time frame is used, rather like a stroboscopic presentation.

4. **Are patients with well-adapted nystagmus (i.e., no oscillopsia or diplopia) able to see their own eyes move when they look in a mirror?**
   No, they cannot see their own eyes move in a mirror. To show a patient what he or she looks like to others, you must make a movie of the eye movements and show them the movie.

5. **Why don't many nystagmus patients see well?**
   Usually something else is going on, such as hypoplasia of the fovea and macula, albinism, and, of course, the nystagmus itself may not allow quite enough fixation time to see the object.

6. **List the major types of nystagmus.**
   - **Vestibular nystagmus,** which is caused by pathology of the vestibular system. The hallmark is the similarity of nystagmus in all fields of gaze and a slow component that is linear.
   - **Latent nystagmus,** which is an inherited form of nystagmus that becomes manifest only when binocularity is lost or thought by the patient to be lost. The slow phase has decreasing velocity and the fast phase beats toward the fixing eye. When binocular vision is lost, the nystagmus is called **manifest latent nystagmus**.
   - **Amaurotic nystagmus** is not a true repetitive nystagmus but, rather, a roving of the eyes as if the patient is searching for something.
   - **Idiopathic infantile nystagmus** (IIN) is the type most commonly seen. Often, clinicians refer to this as motor nystagmus. It is frequently associated with ocular and systemic albinism, high astigmatism, and various retinal problems. The typical natural history helps in the diagnosis.

7. **What is the natural history of IIN?**
   At approximately 3 months of age the patient develops wide-swinging eye movements and, not uncommonly, is thought to be blind. At approximately 8 months to 1 year of age, small pendular

eye movements are substituted, and some control of fixation is reported. Then, at approximately 18 months to 2 years of age the jerk nystagmus of adulthood is developed with its null zone.

8. **What is the null zone of IIN?**
    The null zone is the direction of gaze in respect to orbital coordinates that minimize the amplitude and frequency of nystagmus. Because a position of gaze that minimizes the nystagmus allows better vision, it is common for patients to seek out the null zone with an ensuing habitual head positioning.

9. **Is the null zone the same for each eye?**
    Yes, but there is an exception. If the patient finds that he or she can converge the eyes, causing an esotropia (the nystagmus blockage syndrome), the patient may cross-fixate and appear to have the null zone of each eye in the adducted position. Such patients are typically not stable after strabismus surgery. Overcorrections and undercorrections are common.

10. **What are the subtypes of IIN?**
    The principal and most common subtype is periodic alternating nystagmus, in which the null zone drifts back and forth horizontally with a cycle lasting 30 seconds to 6 minutes (see questions 25 and 26).

11. **Do patients with poor vision also have the same natural history of the nystagmus waveform evolution?**
    Unfortunately, yes. Care must be taken to look for albinism, achromatopsia, Leber's congenital amaurosis, hypoplasia of the optic disc, and delayed visual development.

12. **Is a distinctive nystagmus associated with specific ocular pathology?**
    To date, only the unique nystagmus of achromatopsia seems somewhat distinctive as it evolves to an oblique direction from a horizontal pendular direction.

13. **Does IIN ever disappear spontaneously?**
    Rarely, yes. More commonly the patient has spasmus nutans, which is not recognized and, of course, by its very definition the spasmus nutans disappears after a year or so.

14. **What is the hallmark of spasmus nutans?**
    Asymmetry of the nystagmus. For example, if the jerk of one eye is horizontal and the other eye is vertical, the presumed diagnosis is spasmus nutans. Magnetic resonance imaging (MRI) would be a suitable consideration in search of midbrain pathology.

15. **Does nystagmus mean that the patient is blind?**
    No, to the contrary. You must have or have had some vision to develop nystagmus.

16. **Are some types of nystagmus present at birth?**
    Yes, bidirectional jerk nystagmus is the most common type and portends good vision.

17. **You often hear of nystagmus associated with untreated congenital cataracts. Is it distinctive?**
    The answer is uncertain. Often the nystagmus typical IIN and the course of the natural history just described is observed. If the patient develops roving eye movements, bad vision should be suspected.

18. **Does a patient need vision to have nystagmus?**
    Yes, but the vision may be poor. The retinal or systemic conditions may worsen or cause blindness, and the typical IIN persists.

19. **If one sees what seems to be the natural history of IIN, should an MRI be obtained?**
No. However, if the nystagmus is not symmetrical, the diagnosis of spasmus nutans should be entertained. Spasmus nutans consists of the following triad: (1) nystagmus that is unilateral or bilateral and asymmetric; (2) head nodding; and (3) torticollis. Patients develop spasmus nutans at 4–12 months of age and symptoms usually disappear within 2 years of onset. The etiology is unknown, but patients often are neurologically normal. However, because a chiasmal glioma may mimic spasmus nutans nystagmus, an MRI is warranted.

20. **If the nystagmus is vertical, will the patient develop a preferred chin-up or chin-down head position?**
Yes. Patients develop a head position in relationship to the null zone in the same fashion as patients with horizontal nystagmus. The null zone is in the direction of the slow phase of the nystagmus. Therefore, if the patient has obvious downbeat nystagmus, it will be worse on up gaze and the null zone will be downward, with a preferred chin-up head position.

21. **Do patients with torsional IIN exhibit a head tilt in respect to torsion?**
Occasionally. The physician needs to examine the infant carefully with the slit lamp in order to look for torsional nystagmus.

22. **How can torsional IIN be observed and diagnosed?**
Slit lamp observation of the iris is the most sensitive test.

23. **Is the pivot of the torsion always on the visual axis?**
No, and exceptions may cause some difficulty in diagnosis. If the pivot is on the visual axes, the eye rotates clockwise and counterclockwise about the visual axis—the object of fixation (visual axis)—and vision is only modestly degraded. In fact, the nystagmus often is not noted unless an examiner studies the iris or disc. If, however, the pivot is to the left (e.g., on the left brow), the patient will have a component of horizontal and vertical nystagmus. This combination results in a "windshield wiper" nystagmus in which the radii of each eye varies much like an automobile windshield wiper when the pivot of rotation is located asymmetrically.

24. **Do patients develop torsional nystagmus late in childhood or later in life?**
Both. If the nystagmus is asymmetric, it is most likely caused by midbrain pathology. More commonly, the torsional nystagmus was present all along, but not observed.

25. **What is alternating in periodic alternating nystagmus?**
The null zone. As you watch the patient read his or her best acuity line, the patient will change head position to maximize acuity by pointing the head in such a manner to allow the visual axis to remain in the null zone.

26. **What is the time cycle of period alternating nystagmus?**
Approximately 90 seconds is most common, but the cycle may be as short as 30 seconds or as long as 6 minutes.

27. **Is congenital periodic alternating nystagmus commonly associated with any other ocular problem?**
Yes. Albinism is the most common association—and most commonly overlooked. Look for it carefully.

28. **Does acquired periodic alternating nystagmus imply central nervous system pathology?**
Yes, but be careful. Often the nystagmus is overlooked if the patient compensates well by changing head position. If it is truly acquired, midbrain pathology is common.

29. **Does acquired periodic alternating nystagmus respond to pharmacologic treatment?**
   Yes. Baclofen often works.

30. **Does *congenital* periodic alternating nystagmus respond to any drug?**
   None has been reported to date.

KEY POINTS: GLASSES FOR NYSTAGMUS

To get the best visual acuity in a patient with nystagmus:

1. Use careful refraction.

2. Use dry retinoscopy.

3. Correct all astigmatism.

4. Use top line of full projector screen.

5. Watch for latent nystagmus—add plus 4.00 to nonfixating eye rather than occluding.

---

31. **What is the danger of missing the diagnosis of periodic alternating nystagmus?**
   If a Kestenbaum or Anderson procedure is done (e.g., for a head turn accompanying an eccentric null zone of IIN), a more severe head turn in the opposite direction will result.

32. **What is the surgical treatment of periodic alternating nystagmus?**
   The best procedure seems to be recession of all four recti muscles by a large amount with slightly more recession of the lateral as opposed to the medial muscles.

33. **Most patients with IIN have vision that is better at near than at distance. Why?**
   Most patients have an accommodative convergence:accommodation (AC:A) ratio that results in exophoria at near. The patient uses fusional convergence to overcome the exophoria. Fusional convergence dampens the nystagmus amplitude and frequency and in so doing improves the vision.

34. **Because convergence improves vision, should minus lenses be used to stimulate accommodative convergence?**
   No. Only fusional convergence (i.e., overcoming exophoria) dampens nystagmus. Accommodative convergence does not dampen nystagmus and even works against the patient by increasing accommodative demands and may cause the near point to recede with reduced visual acuity at near.

35. **Are bifocals helpful to a teenage patient with IIN?**
   Often, yes. If the accommodation cannot provide a near point that is close to the patient (with accompanying magnification and increased exophoria), bifocals can be a great help.

36. **Is photophobia common with IIN?**
   No. If photophobia is present with nystagmus, look for achromatopsia.

37. **Do patients with albinism have photophobia?**
   For the most part, no. However, some albinos do not like excessive light, and dark tints are occasionally helpful.

38. **You may have heard that contact lenses lessen nystagmus. Do they help?**
For the most part, no. Remember, however, that many patients with nystagmus have considerable astigmatism. Those that do may well be helped with toric contact lenses, particularly if the null zone is eccentric at points where spectacles distort the images. Usually, contact lenses seem to help for a brief period, then patients adapt to them and are back to where they were.

39. **Many patients with nystagmus have vision of approximately 20/50 and want to pass the magic barrier of 20/40 to obtain a driver's license. What can you do to help?**
For the most part, such patients are safe drivers as far as vision is concerned. If you project the full screen of letters and ask them to read the top line as you reduce the print size, you will find that many read two lines or so better. Hence, you can endorse their improved vision as adequate for driving.

40. **Aside from using a full screen of letters, what should one do when checking the visual acuity of a nystagmus patient with unexpected poor vision?**
Be sure to measure binocular visual acuity. If binocular vision is better, try occluding the nonfixing eye with a plus 4.00 lens and ask the patient to read with the opposite eye. In other words, look for latent nystagmus.

41. **Clinically, how do you distinguish manifest latent nystagmus (MLN) from IIN?**
As you occlude each eye, with MLN the direction of the jerk changes toward the fixing eye. With IIN the direction of the nystagmus remains constant on covering either eye, but the direction of the nystagmus fast phase changes when you cross to the other side of the null zone.

BIBLIOGRAPHY

1. Abadi RV, Whittle JP, Worfolk R: Oscillopsia and tolerance to retinal image movement in congenital nystagmus. Invest Ophthalmol Vest Sci 40:339–345, 1999.
2. Gottlob I: Nystagmus. Curr Opin Ophthalmol 9:V32–V38, 1998.
3. Gottlob I: Eye movement abnormalities in carriers of the blue cone monochromatism. Invest Ophthalmol Vest Sci 35:3556–3560, 1994.
4. Gradstein L, Reinecke RD, Wizov SS, Goldstein HP: Congenital periodic alternating nystagmus. Ophthalmology 104:918–929, 1997.
5. Jacobson L: Visual dysfunction and ocular signs associated with periventricular leukomalacia in children born preterm. Acta Ophthalmol Scand 77:365–366, 1999.
6. Kerrison J, Koenekoop RK, Arnould VJ, et al: Clinical features of autosomal dominant congenital nystagmus linked to chromosome 6p12. Am J Ophthalmol 125:64–70, 1998.
7. Kerrison J, Vagefi MR, Barmada MM, Maumenee IH: Congenital motor nystagmus linked to Xq26–q27. Am J Human Genet 64:600–607, 1999.
8. Mellott ML, Brown J Jr, Fingert JH, et al: Clinical characterization and linkage analysis of a family with congenital x-linked nystagmus and deuteranomaly. Arch Ophthalmol 117:1630–1633, 1999.
9. Reinecke RD: Idiopathic infantile nystagmus: Diagnosis and treatment. AAPOS 1:67–82, 1997.
10. Stahl J, Averbuch-Heller L, Leigh RJL: Acquired nystagmus. Arch Ophthalmol 118:544–549, 2000.
11. Sprunger DT, Wasserman BN, Stidham DB: The relationship between nystagmus and survival outcome in congenital esotropia. J AAPOS 4:21–24, 2000.

VI. NEURO-OPHTHALMOLOGY

THE PUPIL

Barry Schanzer, MD, and Peter J. Savino, MD

CHAPTER 29

1. **What muscles control the size of the pupil? Describe their innervation.**
   The iris sphincter muscle causes pupillary constriction and is innervated by the parasympathetic nervous system. The iris dilator muscle causes pupillary dilation and is innervated by the sympathetic nervous system. Thus, when sympathetic tone is increased, the pupil is larger, and when parasympathetic tone is increased, the pupil is smaller.

2. **Trace the pathway of the parasympathetic innervation of the pupil.**
   Parasympathetic fibers begin in the Edinger-Westphal nucleus in the oculomotor nuclear complex. With cranial nerve (CN) III they exit the midbrain and travel in the subarachnoid space and cavernous sinus. They follow the inferior division of CN III into the orbit, where they synapse at the ciliary ganglion. Postganglionic fibers are then distributed to the iris sphincter and ciliary body via short ciliary nerves.

3. **Trace the pathway of the sympathetic innervation of the pupil.**
   The first-order neuron begins in the posterior hypothalamus. The fibers travel caudally to terminate in the intermedial lateral cell column of the spinal cord at levels C8-T1, otherwise known as the ciliospinal center of Budge. Pupillomotor fibers exit from the spinal cord and ascend with the sympathetic chain to synapse in the superior cervical ganglion, constituting the second-order neuron. The third-order neuron begins with postganglionic fibers of the superior cervical ganglion. These fibers travel with the internal carotid artery to enter the cranial vault. In the cavernous sinus the fibers leave the carotid artery to join the ophthalmic division of CN V and enter the orbit through the superior orbital fissure. The sympathetic fibers reach the ciliary body and dilator of the iris by passing through the nasociliary nerve and long posterior ciliary nerves.

4. **Trace the pathway of the pupillary light reflex.**
   The pupillary light response begins with the rods and cones of the retina. Afferent pupillomotor fibers travel through the optic nerves and semidecussate at the optic chiasm. They then follow the optic tracts and exit before the lateral geniculate body to enter the brain stem via the brachium of the superior colliculus. Pupillomotor fibers synapse in the pretectal nuclei, which then project equally to the ipsilateral and contralateral Edinger-Westphal nuclei. The pupillary fibers travel with CN III to innervate the iris sphincter and cause pupillary constriction, as described in question 2.

5. **What is an afferent pupillary defect? How should you examine for it?**
   The swinging flashlight test is used to elicit a relative afferent pupillary defect (RAPD). If you shine a light into one eye of a normal subject, both pupils constrict to the same degree. If you swing the light over to the other eye, the pupil stays the same size or constricts minimally. In patients with RAPD the affected eye behaves as if it perceives a dimmer light than the normal eye; therefore, both pupils constrict to a lesser degree when the light is shone in the affected eye. Thus, if you shine the light in the right eye of a patient with left RAPD, both pupils constrict. If you swing the light to the left eye, it is perceived as dimmer and the pupils dilate. Note that this is a *relative* APD and signifies a difference in the pupillary response between the two eyes. However, if both eyes are equally abnormal, there may be no RAPD (Fig. 29-1).

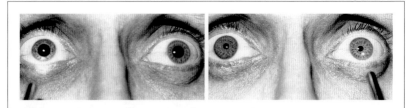

Figure 29-1. Demonstration of a large afferent defect in the right eye. This is best demonstrated when the light is alternated from eye to eye at a steady rate. The light is kept just below the visual axis and 1–2 inches (3–5 cm) from each eye. Each eye is illuminated for approximately 1 second, then the light is switched quickly to the other eye. This technique allows comparison of the initial direct pupil contraction with light in each eye. (From Kardon RH: The pupil. In Yanoff M, Duker JS [eds]: Ophthalmology, 2nd ed. St. Louis, Mosby, 2004, pp 1360–1369.)

6. **A lesion in which anatomic areas may cause an afferent pupillary defect?**
   A lesion anywhere in the afferent pupillary pathway may cause an RAPD—that is, retina, optic nerve, optic chiasm, optic tract, or along the course of pupillary fibers from the optic tract to pretectal nuclei. Pupillary fibers leave the optic tract prior to the lateral geniculate body. Therefore, any lesion from the lateral geniculate body posteriorly does not cause an RAPD. A retinal lesion causes an RAPD only if it is rather large. An optic nerve lesion causes an RAPD in the ipsilateral eye. A lesion in the optic chiasm may cause an RAPD if one optic nerve is affected more than the other. An optic tract lesion causes an RAPD in the eye with the most visual field loss. Typically, in patients with a mass lesion of the optic tract, an RAPD is produced in the ipsilateral eye because of apulateral optic nerve compression, but an ischemic lesion causes an RAPD in the contralateral eye. A lesion in the brain stem in the area of the pretectal nuclei may cause an RAPD without visual defects.

7. **What is anisocoria? How should one examine a patient with anisocoria?**
   Anisocoria is a difference in the size between the two pupils. In anyone who has anisocoria, the pupil size should be measured in both bright and dim light. If the anisocoria is greater in bright light, the larger pupil is abnormal and constricts poorly, which is usually caused by a defect in parasympathetic innervation. If the anisocoria is greater in dim light, the smaller pupil is abnormal because it dilates poorly, usually because of a defect in pupillary sympathetic innervation. If the difference in the size of the two pupils remains the same in bright and dim light, the anisocoria is physiologic and not pathologic.

8. **What is the differential diagnosis of a unilateral dilated, poorly reactive pupil?**
   - Third-nerve palsy
   - Pharmacologic paralysis (an anticholinergic medication such as atropine)
   - Adie's tonic pupil
   - Iris damage (e.g., sphincter tears secondary to trauma or posterior synechiae)

9. **What are the clinical findings in a third-nerve palsy?**
   CN III innervates the superior, medial, and inferior recti and inferior oblique and levator palpebrae muscles. Therefore, in a complete CN III palsy, ptosis is complete and the eye is in the down-and-out position; it does not move up, down, or medially. The parasympathetic nerves that innervate the pupillary sphincter travel with CN III; therefore, if those fibers are affected, the pupil will be dilated and nonreactive.

10. **What are some possible causes of third-nerve palsy?**
    In adults the most common causes are microvascular ischemia in the nerve, aneurysm (usually of the posterior communicating artery), trauma, and neoplasm. In children, aneurysm is rare, and consideration must be given to ophthalmoplegic migraine.

11. **What is the significance of pupil involvement or pupil sparing in third-nerve palsy?**

    Pupil involvement in third-nerve palsy suggests a compressive lesion such as aneurysm or tumor. Pupil sparing is suggestive of microvascular ischemia. The parasympathetic fibers are on the outer portion of CN III and are more susceptible to external compression and less susceptible to ischemia, which is usually axial in the nerve.

12. **What is the appropriate work-up for an isolated third-nerve palsy with pupillary sparing?**

    In patients in the vasculopathic age group, the most likely cause is microvascular ischemia. Patients may simply be followed with the expectation that the ocular misalignment will improve. Certainly a medical work-up for hypertension or diabetes is appropriate. If there is no improvement in 3–6 months, neuroimaging should be performed. Patients too young for the vasculopathic age group should have a magnetic resonance imaging (MRI) scan. If the scan is negative, other hematologic investigations and lumbar puncture should be considered.

13. **What is the appropriate work-up for an isolated third-nerve palsy with pupillary involvement?**

    The first step is to perform an emergent MRI and magnetic resonance angiography (MRA) or CT angiography scan. This important MRA or CTA must be done before catheter arteriography. If the scan is negative, a catheter arteriogram must be performed to rule out an aneurysm. If the scan is negative in children younger than age 10, an arteriogram is not necessary because the likelihood of an aneurysm is very low. Ten years is an arbitrary age based on the principle that aneurysms rarely occur in young children.

KEY POINTS: MANAGEMENT OF THIRD-NERVE PALSY

1. Pupil involvement in third-nerve palsy suggests a compressive lesion.

2. Pupil involving third-nerve palsy requires immediate MRI and MRA. If negative, conventional catheter angiography should be performed to rule out aneurysm.

3. Pupil-sparing third-nerve palsy in a patient in the vasculopathic age group may be observed with the presumption that the palsy is caused by microvascular ischemia.

4. Pupil-sparing third-nerve palsy in a patient not in the vasculopathic age group warrants an MRI and an MRA.

14. **What is an Adie's tonic pupil? What is its natural history?**

    Adie's tonic pupil is a postganglionic defect in the parasympathetic innervation to the pupil. The clinical finding is a dilated pupil that is usually slightly irregular and shows segmental iris constriction at the slit lamp. There also may be light/near dissociation, with characteristically slow and tonic constriction and redilation phases. This condition is benign and most commonly affects women in their second to fourth decades.

15. **How do you test for an Adie's pupil?**

    An Adie's tonic pupil constricts to dilute pilocarpine 0.1–0.12%, whereas a normal pupil does not. This is a result of denervation hypersensitivity.

16. **What is Horner's syndrome?**

    Horner's syndrome is a clinical syndrome characterized by ptosis, miosis, and occasionally anhidrosis (Fig. 29-2). Any lesion in the sympathetic innervation to the eye can cause this syndrome.

17. **What is the cause of ptosis in Horner's syndrome?**
    Ptosis in Horner's syndrome is caused by decreased sympathetic tone in Mueller's muscle. Mueller's muscle is responsible for approximately 2 mm of elevation of the upper eyelid. Thus the ptosis in Horner's syndrome is mild (only approximately 2 mm).

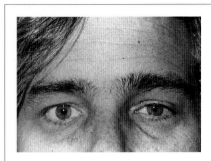

Figure 29-2. Horner's syndrome with ptosis and miosis on the left. Note that the left lower eyelid is higher than the right lower eyelid. This inverse ptosis is a result of interruption of sympathetic innervation to the analog of Mueller's muscle in the lower eyelid.

18. **What are the possible causes of Horner's syndrome?**
    The course of the sympathetic innervation to the eye was discussed in question 3. A lesion anywhere along this course may cause Horner's syndrome. Isolated third-order neuron lesions are generally benign. Second-order neuron lesions are more ominous and may be caused by apical lung tumors or carotid artery dissection. First-order neuron lesions are uncommon in isolation. They are found in demyelinating disease, cerebrovascular accidents, and neoplasms.

19. **How do you test for Horner's syndrome?**
    A cocaine test. Cocaine blocks the reuptake of norepinephrine. A normal pupil dilates in response to a drop of cocaine, whereas in Horner's syndrome the pupil fails to dilate.

20. **What pharmacologic testing helps to localize the lesion in Horner's syndrome?**
    Localization is important because the etiology and possibly the focus of the work-up are quite different, depending on whether the lesion is a first-, second-, or third-order neuron. Hydroxyamphetamine 1% causes release of epinephrine from the third-order neuron junction with the iris. Thus, in third-order neuron lesions there is no pupillary response to hydroxyamphetamine drops. In a first- or second-order neuron lesion, the pupil dilates in response to hydroxyamphetamine drops.

21. **What is the appropriate evaluation for a patient with Horner's syndrome?**
    Patients suspected of having Horner's syndrome should have cocaine testing to confirm the diagnosis. If testing confirms the syndrome, imaging studies should be performed to evaluate the entire course of the sympathetic innervation of the eye, which would include head, neck, and chest. We do not recommend hydroxyamphetamine testing because it is an imperfect localizer; therefore, we would not rely on it to guide further testing.

22. **What is light/near dissociation? What are its possible causes?**
    In light/near dissociation a pupil does not constrict to light but will constrict as part of the near response. Causes include Adie's syndrome, dorsal midbrain syndrome (Parinaud's syndrome), Argyll-Robertson pupils, and blindness from any anterior afferent cause.

23. **What is an Argyll-Robertson pupil?**
    Argyll-Robertson pupils are small, often irregular pupils that do not react to light but have a brisk near response. The cause of Argyll-Robertson pupils is almost always tertiary syphilis.

24. **What is Parinaud's syndrome?**

Found in dorsal midbrain disease, the syndrome is composed of light/near dissociation of the pupils, supranuclear paralysis of upward gaze, convergence refraction nystagmus with attempted upward saccades, and eyelid retraction.

BIBLIOGRAPHY

1. Burde RM, Savino PJ, Trobe JD: Clinical Decisions in Neuro-Ophthalmology, 2nd ed. St. Louis, Mosby, 1992.
2. Miller NR: Walsh and Hoyt's Clinical Neuro-Ophthalmology, 5th ed, vol. 2. Baltimore, Williams & Wilkins, 1998.
3. Newell FW: Ophthalmology: Principles and Concepts, 8th ed. St. Louis, Mosby, 1996.

CHAPTER 30

DIPLOPIA

Julian D. Perry, MD

1. **What is diplopia?**
   Diplopia is a symptom in which the patient perceives two images of a single object. Diplopia may be monocular or binocular. You should check if the double vision resolves with each eye closed. If it does not, the patient has monocular diplopia. If it does, the patient has binocular diplopia.

2. **List the causes of monocular diplopia.**
   Start with glasses and work your way posteriorly through the ocular tissues to obtain the following differential:
   - Refractive error: Astigmatism is the most common cause of monocular diplopia
   - Chalazion or other eyelid tumor that produces irregular astigmatism
   - Keratopathy: Keratoconus, irregular astigmatism (use a retinoscope to see scissoring reflex)
   - Iris atrophy, polycoria, large nonreactive pupil
   - Cataract, subluxated lens, intraocular lens decentration, capsular opacity
   - Retinal disease may produce metamorphopsia or aniseikonia
   Also consider a psychogenic etiology.

3. **What are the causes of binocular diplopia?**
   Causes of binocular diplopia may be grouped into three general categories:
   - **Neuropathic:** The pathology may be supranuclear, nuclear, or infranuclear. Signs and symptoms can often localize the lesion, and specific etiologies often affect certain anatomic areas of the nervous system. Specific neuropathic causes include vaso-occlusive infarction, compression, inflammation, demyelination, and degeneration.
   - **Myopathic:** The pathology may exist within the extraocular muscles. Myopathic causes of diplopia include inflammatory pseudotumor or myositis and thyroid-related eye disease (TED).
   - **Neuromuscular junction disorders:** The major etiology in this category is myasthenia gravis (MG).

4. **What are some causes of intermittent diplopia?**
   The most common causes of intermittent double vision are MG, TED, decompensated phoria, and multiple sclerosis (MS). Other causes include spasm of the near reflex, convergence retraction nystagmus, and ocular neuromyotonia.

5. **What is the most important sign to check for in a third-nerve (oculomotor) palsy?**
   The presence or absence of a dilated, nonreactive pupil. An oculomotor palsy involving the pupil is an emergency. An aneurysm must be ruled out.

6. **What is the work-up of a pupil-involving third-nerve palsy?**
   In adults, perform magnetic resonance imaging/angiography (MRI/A) or spiral computed tomographic (CT) angiography. If the results are consistent with an aneurysm, or even if the results are negative, perform an angiogram. In children, perform MRI/A regardless of the state of the pupil. If the results are negative, children usually do not need an angiogram.

7. **Why do aneurysms involve the pupil in oculomotor nerve palsies, whereas infarctions generally do not?**
   Pupillary parasympathetic fibers travel superficially and dorsomedially in the third nerve as it traverses the subarachnoid space. These fibers are often affected first in a compressive lesion. Ischemic infarction often occurs in the center of the nerve, so the superficial fibers remain unaffected.

8. **What is the work-up of an isolated pupil-sparing but otherwise complete oculomotor nerve palsy in the vasculopathic age group?**
   A lesion that compresses the central third-nerve fibers sufficiently to produce a complete paresis should affect the peripheral pupillary fibers sufficiently to produce at least some degree of pupil involvement. If not, the likelihood of an aneurysm or other compressive etiology is extremely low. The patient may be treated for an assumed vaso-occlusive etiology. Diagnostic work-up includes at least the measurement of systemic blood pressure and a 2-hour postprandial glucose level (or fasting blood sugar). If the patient has symptoms of giant cell arteritis, check erythrocyte sedimentation rate, administer corticosteroids, and perform a temporal artery biopsy; otherwise, the patient may be seen again in 6 weeks. Some physicians reexamine the patient within 5 days to ensure the pupil remains uninvolved.

9. **What are the causes of isolated cranial neuropathies?**
   Many cranial neuropathies are idiopathic, but the causes of isolated cranial neuropathies are summarized in Table 30-1.

TABLE 30-1. CAUSES OF ISOLATED CRANIAL NEUROPATHIES	
Cranial Neuropathy	**Cause**
III (pupil-sparing)	Adults: Infarction, trauma, giant cell arteritis (GCA), tumor; rarely, an aneurysm Children: Congenital, trauma, tumor, aneurysm, migraine
III (pupil-involving)	Usually posterior communicating artery (rarely, basilar artery) aneurysm
IV	Adults: Trauma, infarction, congenital, GCA Children: Congenital, trauma
VI	Adults: Infarction, tumor, trauma, multiple sclerosis, Wernicke's, sarcoid, GCA, herpes zoster, Lyme disease, increased intracranial pressure as in pseudotumor cerebri Children: Trauma, tumor, postviral

10. **How do you test for trochlear nerve palsy in the presence of oculomotor nerve palsy?**
    It is important to specifically test trochlear, abducens, and trigeminal nerve function in a patient with oculomotor nerve palsy in order to localize the lesion. Because the third-nerve palsy may prevent adduction, it may be difficult to test fourth nerve function. When the patient attempts to look down and in with the paretic eye, you will observe intorsion if the trochlear nerve is intact.

11. **Describe the three-step test.**
    This is a test to determine if a hypertropia is a result of superior oblique palsy or other causes (Fig. 30-1).
    - **Step 1:** Which eye is hyperdeviated? A right hyperdeviation could be caused by palsy of any of the muscles circled in step 1. Determine which muscles might cause this.

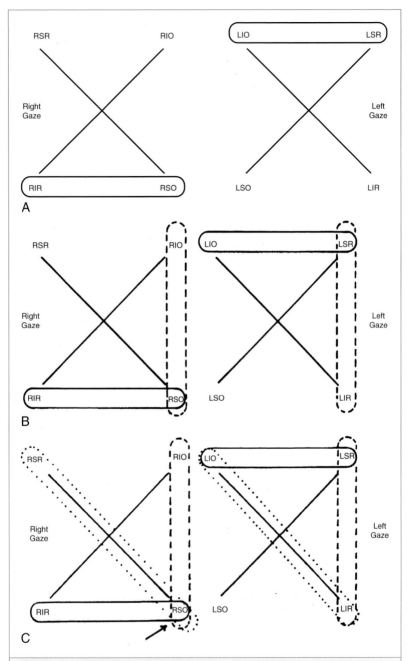

Figure 30-1. The three-step test to determine if hypertropia is a result of superior oblique palsy or other causes. **A,** Step one. **B,** Step two. **C,** Step three. (See question 11 for explanations.) (From American Academy of Ophthalmology: Pediatric Ophthalmology and Strabismus. Section 8. San Francisco, American Academy of Ophthalmology, 1992–1993.)

- **Step 2:** Is the hyperdeviation worse in right gaze or left gaze? Isolate these muscles. A right superior oblique palsy reveals worsening of the right hyperdeviation in the left gaze.
- **Step 3:** Is the hyperdeviation worse on right head tilt or left head tilt? The muscle isolated in all three steps is the palsied muscle. A right superior oblique palsy reveals increased hyperdeviation on head tilt to the right. A double Maddox rod can then be used to determine if the trochlear nerve palsy is bilateral. If excyclotorsion is more than 10 degrees, bilateral superior oblique palsies exist.

12. **What is the best procedure to treat unresolved superior oblique palsy? Do you have to memorize Knapp's rules?**
    Knapp published his treatment scheme several years ago, and many surgeons use similar schemes. You do not need to memorize his particular scheme, but you should understand the principles. Generally, there are three possible surgical approaches:
    - Strengthen (tuck) the palsied superior oblique muscle.
    - Weaken (recess) the antagonist ipsilateral inferior oblique muscle.
    - Weaken the yoke contralateral inferior rectus muscle.

    Typically the surgeon operates on the muscle or muscles that act in the field of gaze where the diplopia is worst. For example, if the left hyperdeviation in a left superior oblique (LSO) palsy is worst in downgaze, one would consider an LSO tuck or a right inferior rectus recession. The latter procedure may be favored because an adjustable suture technique can be used and there is no chance of producing an iatrogenic Brown's syndrome.

13. **Explain the Harada-Ito procedure.**
    The Harada-Ito procedure involves anterior and lateral displacement of the anterior portion of the palsied superior oblique muscle. This procedure is used primarily for correction of excyclotorsion but will correct a small degree of hyperdeviation. The amount of incyclotorsion created is variable, but the procedure is generally successful.

14. **What else should you know about trochlear nerve palsy?**
    - The trochlear nerve is the longest and most commonly injured cranial nerve in trauma.
    - Patients of all ages with trochlear nerve palsy and increased vertical fusional amplitudes do not need further evaluation; they have decompensated "congenital" trochlear nerve palsies.
    - Always consider MG and TED in the evaluation of diplopia, even if the palsy "maps out" to a specific cranial nerve.

15. **List the major causes of abduction deficit other than cranial neuropathy.**
    - Restricted medial rectus muscle
      - □ Trauma (entrapment, damage)
      - □ Inflammatory pseudotumor or myositis
      - □ Thyroid-related eye disease
    - Spasm of the near reflex
    - Myasthenia gravis

16. **How do you treat an unresolved abducens nerve palsy?**
    - Weaken the ipsilateral medial rectus with strengthening of the ipsilateral lateral rectus muscle.
    - Use the vertical transposition procedure.
    - Botulinum toxin (Botox) injections may be used with the above procedures.

17. **What else should you know about abducens nerve palsy?**
    - Abducens palsy may occur as a nonspecific sign of increased intracranial pressure. Abducens palsy may also occur after lumbar puncture.

- In the case of bilateral abducens paresis, you must consider tumor, MS, subarachnoid hemorrhage, or infection. Do not write it off as being due to infarction without doing a work-up.
- In children with bilateral abducens paresis, reconsider strabismus and check for "doll's eyes," which should be incomplete in a paretic disorder.
- Third-order sympathetic fibers briefly join the abducens nerve in the cavernous sinus. Horner's syndrome with abducens nerve palsy localizes to this region.
- Always consider MG and TED in the evaluation of diplopia, even if the palsy maps out to a specific cranial nerve (sound familiar?).

18. **What are the localizing symptom complexes of nerve palsy?**
See Table 30-2.

TABLE 30-2. LOCALIZING SYMPTOM COMPLEXES OF NERVE PALSY

Symptoms/Signs	Syndrome	Anatomic Location
Ipsilateral III-nerve palsy with a contralateral fascicle hemiplegia	Weber's syndrome	Midbrain third nerve and cerebral peduncle
Ipsilateral III-nerve palsy with contralateral choreiform movements	Benedikt's syndrome	Midbrain third nerve fascicle and red nucleus
Ipsilateral VI-nerve palsy with hearing loss and facial pain	Gradenigo's syndrome	Petrous apex
Ipsilateral gaze palsy with facial palsy, Horner's syndrome, and deafness	Foville's, anterior inferior cerebellar artery syndrome	Dorsolateral pons
Ipsilateral VI- and VII-nerve palsies with contralateral hemiparesis	Millard-Gubler syndrome	Anterior paramedical pons
III-, IV-, and VI-nerve (V_1, V_2) palsies with Horner's syndrome and primary aberrant regeneration	Cavernous sinus syndrome	Cavernous sinus
II-, IV-, and VI-nerve (thus, [V_1]) palsies, often with proptosis	Superior orbital fissure syndrome	Superior orbital fissure
V-, VI-, VII-, and VIII-nerve palsies	Cerebellopontine angle syndrome	Cerebellopontine angle tumor

19. **What is internuclear ophthalmoplegia (INO)?**
The medial longitudinal fasciculus carries nerve fibers from the abducens nucleus on each side to the contralateral medial rectus subnucleus to coordinate horizontal gaze. This area of the brain stem may be damaged by demyelination, ischemia, or tumor; ipsilateral decreased adduction and contralateral abduction nystagmus are observed on attempted contralateral gaze. Saccadic velocity may be decreased in the adducting eye and may be the only sign of a subtle INO. Bilateral INO is common, often presenting with esotropia and upward beating nystagmus on attempted convergence, in addition to the aforementioned findings.

KEY POINTS: OCULOMOTOR PALSY

1. A pupil-sparing palsy is probably vasculopathic in adults. In children, obtain an MRI/A to rule out tumor and aneurysm.

2. To test for trochlear nerve palsy in a patient with an oculomotor palsy, have the patient look down and in to check for intorsion.

3. A total of 35% of diabetic patients with oculomotor palsies have anisocoria.

20. **What is ocular myasthenia gravis?**
Intermittent diplopia and ptosis are common symptoms of this condition, and diurnal variability increases suspicion. On examination, ptosis will frequently worsen with prolonged upgaze, and orbicular strength is frequently affected. Myasthenia may mimic any isolated ocular motor nerve palsy or an INO.

21. **What is the work-up for myasthenia gravis?**
Tensilon (edrophonium chloride) is a short-acting anticholinesterase that can cause improvement of symptoms and signs of MG. A positive acetylcholine receptor antibody test supports the diagnosis. Work-up includes MRI of the chest and thyroid studies to rule out associated thymomas and hyperthyroidism. Myasthenia that is purely ocular after 2 years is likely to remain so. Treatment includes the long-acting cholinesterase inhibitors, corticosteroids, and plasmapheresis.

22. **How is the Tensilon test performed?**
Ten mg of Tensilon is drawn into a syringe. A 2-mg IV is given initially to observe for adverse reactions or a positive response. If neither occurs after 2 minutes, the remainder is given either incrementally or as a single bolus. A positive test result shows improved facial expression, eyelid position, or double vision within 3 minutes of injection. A positive test result is quite specific for MG; however, false-negative tests occur. An electromyogram may also show improvement after Tensilon administration. Atropine must be readily available in case adverse reactions occur (abdominal cramps and bradycardia are common).

KEY POINTS: MYASTHENIA GRAVIS

1. Always suspect MG in any patient with diplopia, especially if it is variable and associated with ptosis.

2. Have atropine available for adverse reactions if Tensilon tests are performed.

3. Thymomas and hyperthyroidism are common in patients with MG. Patients need a chest MRI and thyroid function tests.

23. **What is convergence insufficiency?**
Typical convergence insufficiency presents with asthenopia and double vision at near. It is diagnosed by observing an exotropia at 33 cm, an abnormally remote near point of convergence (>3–6 cm for patients younger than age 20; >12 cm for patients older than age 40), and

inadequate amplitudes of fusion. Patients can fully adduct during conjugate gaze movements, and the deviation is comitant for a given distance. The isolated condition is rarely associated with tumor or other serious pathology.

Patients are treated with near point exercises such as focusing on the end of a pencil while moving it from arm's length toward the face.

24. **What is skew deviation?**

Skew deviation is a vertical deviation that cannot be isolated to a single extraocular muscle or muscles. It is almost always associated with other manifestations of posterior fossa disease.

25. **What other supranuclear conditions commonly produce diplopia?**

Progressive supranuclear palsy produces a variety of systemic and ocular motility disturbances, including bradykinesia, axial rigidity, and difficulty with vertical eye movements. If diplopia is present, it is typically caused by convergence difficulty. Similarly, patients with Parkinsonism, Huntington's disease, and Parinaud's dorsal midbrain syndrome may also have diplopia at near because of convergence difficulty.

26. **Explain divergence paresis.**

Patients with divergence paresis present with an exodeviation at distance causing diplopia. Patients are able to fuse at near. The exodeviation is comitant, and horizontal versions are normal. This condition tends to be benign and self-limited; however, it may be associated with infection, demyelinating disease, and tumor. A thorough neurologic evaluation should be performed, and consideration should be given to MR imaging, especially if any neurologic signs or symptoms are present.

27. **Do vaso-occlusive nerve palsies present with aberrant regeneration?**

No. Aberrant regeneration of the third nerve does not occur after a vaso-occlusive (e.g., diabetic) third-nerve palsy. Primary oculomotor aberrant regeneration is highly suggestive of a lesion that is slowly compressing the third nerve, such as an intracavernous meningioma or aneurysm.

28. **To what anatomic region does Horner's syndrome with abducens nerve palsy localize?**

The cavernous sinus. Third order sympathetic fibers briefly join the abducens nerve in the cavernous sinus.

29. **What is the ice test?**

The ice test is a noninvasive test for MG. The palpebral fissure is measured before and immediately after a 2-minute application of ice to the ptotic eyelid. Many patients with MG (approximately 80%) will show an improvement in the ptosis after ice application. The sensitivity of the ice test in patients with complete ptosis decreases considerably.

30. **Can patients who have diabetes with third-nerve palsy have anisocoria?**

Yes. One prospective study found that 38% of diabetic patients with third-nerve palsies had anisocoria up to 2.5 mm.

BIBLIOGRAPHY

1. Bellusci C: Paralytic strabismus. Curr Opin Ophthalmol 12:368–372, 2001.
2. Barton JJ, Fouladuand M: Ocular aspects of myasthenia gravis. Semin Neurol 20:7–20, 2000.
3. Brazis PW, Masdeu JC, Biller J: Localization in Clinical Neurology, 3rd ed. Boston, Little, Brown, 1994.

4. Burde RM, Savino PJ, Trobe JD: Clinical Decisions in Neuro-Ophthalmology, 2nd ed. St. Louis, Mosby-Year Book, 1992.

5. Golnick KC, Pena R, Lee AG, Eggenberger ER: An ice test for the diagnosis of myasthenia gravis. Ophthalmology 106:1282–1286, 1999.

6. Larner AJ, Thomas JD: Can myasthenia gravis be diagnosed with the "ice pack test?" A cautionary note. Postgrad Med J 76:162–163, 2000.

7. Mein J, Trimble R: Diagnosis and Management of Ocular Motility Disorders, 2nd ed. London, Blackwell Scientific Publications, 1991.

8. Miller NR, Newman NJ: Walsh and Hoyts' Clinical Neuro-Ophthalmology, 5th ed. Baltimore, Williams & Wilkins, 1998.

9. von Noorden GK: Binocular Vision and Ocular Motility: Theory and Management of Strabismus, 5th ed. St. Louis, Mosby, 1996.

CHAPTER 31

OPTIC NEURITIS

Barry Schanzer, MD, and Peter J. Savino, MD

1. **What is optic neuritis?**
   Optic neuritis is any inflammation of the optic nerve. It may be idiopathic or associated with systemic disease.

2. **Which systemic diseases are associated with optic neuritis?**
   The most common disease associated with optic neuritis is multiple sclerosis (MS). However, syphilis, sarcoidosis, Lyme disease, and other collagen vascular diseases such as Wegener's granulomatosis and systemic lupus erythematosus are less commonly associated.

3. **Who most commonly gets optic neuritis?**
   Women between the ages of 15 and 45 years are most commonly affected.

4. **What are the typical clinical findings in optic neuritis?**
   Optic neuritis causes acute or subacute visual loss that is preceded or accompanied by pain on eye movement and that may progress over 10–14 days. Visual acuity may range from 20/20 to no light perception. However, even if visual acuity is 20/20, the patient usually has a defect in color vision, contrast sensitivity, and visual field. If the neuritis is unilateral, an afferent pupillary defect is present. The optic disc may be normal or swollen.

5. **Which clinical test is most sensitive for patients with optic neuritis?**
   The most sensitive test—that is, the test most likely to be abnormal in a patient with optic neuritis—is contrast sensitivity.

6. **How common is pain on eye movement in patients with optic neuritis?**
   Pain around the eye or pain exacerbated with eye movement was present in 92% of patients in the Optic Neuritis Treatment Trial (ONTT).

7. **What visual field defects are found in patients with optic neuritis?**
   The classic visual field defect in optic neuritis is central scotoma. However, results of the ONTT showed that any optic nerve visual field defect is compatible with optic neuritis, including altitudinal defects and arcuate defects as well as diffuse visual field defects.

8. **What is the natural history of optic neuritis?**
   The visual loss of optic neuritis may progress over 10–14 days. At that point it should stabilize and shortly thereafter begin to improve.

9. **What is the expected visual outcome for patients with optic neuritis?**
   The ONTT found that at 12 months, 93% of patients were 20/40 or better; 69% were 20/20 or better; and 3% were 20/200 or worse. At 10 years, 91% of patients had acuity of 20/40 or better and 74% were 20/20.

10. **Are there any predictors of poor visual outcome?**
    The ONTT found that the only predictor for poor visual outcome was poor visual acuity at presentation. Nevertheless, all patients with an initial visual acuity of 20/200 or less showed some improvement. However, 5% of the patients were still 20/200 or less at 6 months.

11. **What were the objectives of the ONTT?**
    The ONTT was a multicentered, randomized, prospective clinical trial to determine whether corticosteroid treatment of optic neuritis was beneficial. A secondary objective was to determine the risk of developing MS in patients with optic neuritis. The patients who participated in the ONTT were randomized to three treatment arms. One group of patients received oral placebo; one group received oral prednisone, 1 mg/kg for 14 days; and one group received IV solumedrol, 250 mg every 6 hours for 3 days, followed by oral prednisone, 1 mg/kg for 11 days.

12. **What were the conclusions of the ONTT regarding treatment of optic neuritis?**
    No treatment group had statistically significant better visual acuity at 6 months. However, patients treated with IV solumedrol began to recover vision more quickly. The surprising result was that patients treated with oral prednisone, 1 mg/kg for 14 days, had an increased incidence of recurrence of optic neuritis in the affected or contralateral eye. The researchers concluded that oral prednisone in a dose of 1 mg/kg is contraindicated in the treatment of optic neuritis.

13. **What was the strongest predictor for the development of MS?**
    An abnormal magnetic resonance imaging (MRI) scan (Fig. 31-1) was found to be the strongest predictor for development of clinically definite MS at 2 years. Placebo-treated patients whose MRI scan at study entry showed two or more periventricular white matter lesions >3 mm had a 36% chance of developing MS within 2 years. Patients with one lesion had a 17% chance, and patients with no signal abnormalities had only a 3% chance.

14. **What were the other predictors for developing MS?**
    Previous optic neuritis in the fellow eye, previous nonspecific neurologic symptoms, race (white), and family history of MS were associated with an increased risk of developing MS. Although young age and female gender have been reported to be risk factors for MS, they were not shown to increase the risk within 2 years in the ONTT.

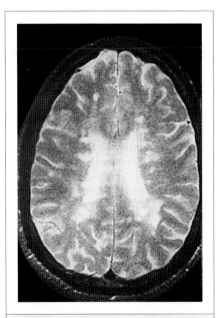

Figure 31-1. Abnormal MRI in a patient with multiple sclerosis. Classic periventricular white matter lesions appear bright on T2-weighted image.

15. **What were the conclusions of the ONTT about the effect of treatment on the risk of developing MS?**
    The results of the ONTT showed that IV solumedrol significantly decreased the risk of developing MS at 2 years. Most of the beneficial effect was seen in patients with abnormal MRI scans, because patients with normal MRI scans had a low incidence of MS, regardless of treatment. Among patients with two or more signal abnormalities on MRI, MS developed in 36% treated with placebo, 32% treated with prednisone, and 16% treated with IV solumedrol. Thus the risk of developing MS at 2 years was cut in half by treatment with IV solumedrol. After 2 years, the beneficial effect seemed to wear off, and at 3 years the three groups had a similar incidence of MS.

16. **What is the 10-year risk of developing MS after optic neuritis?**
A total of 38% of patients enrolled in the ONTT developed MS in a 10-year period. White matter lesions on MRI were the most potent predictor of MS. Patients with one or more lesions had an incidence of MS of 56%. Those with no lesions on MRI had a 22% incidence of MS.

KEY POINTS: OPTIC NEURITIS

1. Optic neuritis causes vision loss that may progress over 10–14 days.

2. Pain is present in more than 90% of patients with optic neuritis.

3. A total of 93% of patients with optic neuritis will recover vision of 20/40 or better.

4. Patients with at least one white matter lesion on MRI scan have a 56% chance of developing MS at 10 years.

17. **What is the 10-year risk of recurrence of optic neuritis?**
A total of 35% of patients in the ONTT who completed the examination at 10 years had a documented recurrence of optic neuritis in the previously affected eye or an attack in the fellow eye. Patients who had a diagnosis of MS had a higher recurrence rate (43%) than those who did not have MS (24%).

18. **Are there any other medications that may influence the risk of developing MS?**
The Controlled High-Risk Subjects Avonex Multiple Sclerosis Prevention Study (CHAMPS) group conducted a randomized double-blind trial to determine whether treatment with interferon beta-1a (Avonex) would affect the risk of developing MS in patients who have a first demyelinating event involving the optic nerve, spinal cord, brain stem, or cerebellum. The patients studied had an acute demyelinating event and an MRI that demonstrated two or more lesions 3 mm or larger in diameter, at least one of which was periventricular or ovoid. All patients were treated with 1 gm intravenous methylprednisolone for 3 days, followed by an oral prednisone taper. They were then randomized to receive weekly intramuscular injections of Avonex or placebo. The results demonstrated that at 3 years the probability of developing clinically definite MS was significantly lower in the patients treated with Avonex (35%) than in patients receiving placebo (50%).

19. **Describe the appropriate workup and treatment for patients with optic neuritis.**
Patients presenting with optic neuritis should have an MRI scan. If the scan is normal, no further workup is warranted and sequential follow up is indicated. If the scan shows two or more typical white matter lesions, the patient should be offered treatment with IV solumedrol and should be referred to a neurologist to discuss treatment with Avonex. The ONTT found no significant benefit in blood tests for antinuclear antibody or fluorescent titer antibody in patients with typical optic neuritis and no other signs of collagen vascular disease.

BIBLIOGRAPHY

1. Beck RW, Cleary PA, Anderson MM Jr, et al: A randomized, controlled trial of corticosteroids in the treatment of acute optic neuritis. N Engl J Med 326:581–588, 1992.

2. Beck RW, Clearly PA, Trobe JD, et al: The effect of corticosteroids for acute optic neuritis on the subsequent development of multiple sclerosis. N Engl J Med 329:1764–1769, 1993.

3. Beck RW, Trobe JD: What we have learned from the Optic Neuritis Treatment Trial. Ophthalmology 102:1504–1508, 1995.

4. Burde RM, Savino PJ, Trobe JD: Clinical Decisions in Neuro-Ophthalmology, 2nd ed. St. Louis, Mosby, 1992.

5. Jacobs LD, Beck RW, Simon JH, et al: Intramuscular interferon beta-1a therapy initiated during a first demyelinating event in multiple sclerosis. N Engl J Med 343:898–904, 2000.

6. Optic Neuritis Study Group: High and low risk profiles for the development of multiple sclerosis within 10 years after optic neuritis. Arch Ophthalmol 121:944–949, 2003.

7. Optic Neuritis Study Group: Visual function more than 10 years after optic neuritis: experience of the optic neuritis treatment trial. Am J Ophthalmol 137:77–83, 2004.

CHAPTER 32

MISCELLANEOUS OPTIC NEUROPATHIES AND NEUROLOGIC DISTURBANCES

Janice A. Gault, MD

1. **A young woman complains of headaches. Her vision is 20/20 in each eye with no evidence of afferent pupillary defect. She has a bitemporal visual field cut. What do you suspect?**
   A chiasmal lesion. Schedule a magnetic resonance imaging (MRI) scan to make an evaluation.

2. **What may simulate a bitemporal field defect?**
   Sector retinitis pigmentosa, coloboma, or a tilted disc.

3. **A patient has 20/20 vision in her right eye and 20/400 in her left eye. Her left eye has an afferent pupillary defect and decreased color plates. What should you evaluate in her right eye?**
   Check visual fields in both eyes. A central scotoma in one eye may be accompanied by a superior temporal field loss in the other. This condition, called a *junctional scotoma,* is also found in chiasmal lesions. See the chapter on visual fields (Chapter 6).

KEY POINTS: DIFFERENTIAL DIAGNOSIS OF CHIASMAL VISUAL DEFECTS

1. Pituitary lesion–tumor or apoplexy

2. Craniopharyngioma

3. Meningioma

4. Glioma

5. Aneurysm

6. Trauma

7. Infection

4. **Is there a difference in the treatment of secreting and nonsecreting symptomatic pituitary tumors?**
   Yes. A prolactinoma secretes prolactin and may be treated successfully with bromocriptine. A nonsecreting tumor probably requires surgery. Of course, an endocrinologist should fully evaluate the patient for other hormonal imbalances.

5. **What visual field is often seen in a toxic or metabolic optic neuropathy?**
   Bilateral central or centrocecal scotomas. Optic nerves show temporal pallor (Fig. 32-1). Alcohol, tobacco, and vitamin B_{12} deficiency, as well as drugs such as chloramphenicol,

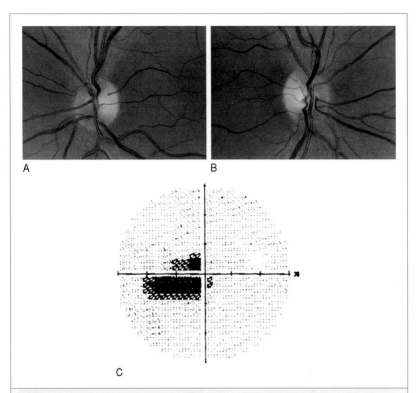

Figure 32-1. Fundus views reveal mild temporal optic disc pallor in right optic disc *(A)* and left optic disc *(B)*. More interesting in *B*, however, is the loss of the nerve fiber layer in the papillomacular bundle. This patient, who had tobacco–alcohol amblyopia (mixed toxic and nutritional deficiency optic neuropathy), also had visual acuities of 20/400 in each eye, which recovered to only 20/100 after changes in habit and diet and vitamin therapy. In this class of optic neuropathies, relatively severely compromised visual acuities and dyschromatopsia often are found with minimal optic disc atrophy. (From Sadun AA, Gurkan S: Hereditary, nutritional, and toxic optic atrophies. In Yanoff M, Duker JS [eds]: Ophthalmology, 2nd ed. St. Louis, Mosby, 2004, 1275–1278.) *C,* Visual field exam reveals centrocecal scotoma. A lesion of the papillomacular bundle (nerve fiber layer or optic nerve) is the usual cause of this defect. (From Burde RM, Savino PJ, Trobe JD: Unexplained visual loss. In Burde RM, Savino PJ, Trobe JD [eds]: Clinical Decisions in Neuro-Ophthalmology, 3rd ed. St. Louis, Mosby, 2002, pp 1–26.)

ethambutol, digitalis, chloroquine, and isoniazid, have been implicated. Check for heavy metals, and order a complete blood count as well as serum levels of vitamins B_{11}, B_{12}, and folate. Consider Leber's hereditary optic neuropathy as a diagnosis.

6. **A 60-year-old man presents with gradual vision loss to 20/400 in his right eye. On examination, the right optic nerve is pale and dot-and-blot retinal hemorrhages are seen. The left eye is normal. What history may be helpful?**
   A history of radiation treatment. The patient reports radiation to his right frontal sinus 3 years earlier. There is no treatment for radiation optic neuropathy or retinopathy except panretinal photocoagulation for neovascular disease, if necessary.

7. **What may cause a constricted visual field?**
   - Retinitis pigmentosa
   - End-stage glaucoma

- Thyroid ophthalmopathy
- Optic nerve drusen
- Vitamin A deficiency
- Occipital strokes
- Panretinal photocoagulation
- Hysteria
- Malingering

8. **How do you differentiate hysteria and malingering from real disease?**
Have the patient do a tangent screen at two different distances. The closer the patient stands, the smaller the field should be. The fields are often of equal size with nonphysiologic visual loss. Patients also may demonstrate spiraling with kinetic visual field testing (see Chapter 6).

9. **A 55-year-old man notices that the vision in his left eye has worsened suddenly. He has 20/50 vision in his right eye and 20/100 in his left eye. The left eye also shows an afferent pupillary defect and decreased color plates. Visual field examination reveals an inferior altitudinal defect on the left with a normal full field on the right. On fundus examination, the left optic nerve appears pale and swollen superiorly. What is your concern?**
An altitudinal defect is a classic finding with ischemic optic neuropathy (ION). The two types are arteritic and nonarteritic (Fig. 32-2). Because they are treated differently, you must differentiate the two. First, it is important to ask about symptoms of giant cell arteritis, such as weight loss, anorexia, fever, jaw claudication, headache, scalp tenderness, and proximal joint and muscle pain. Check for a palpable, tender, nonpulsatile temporal artery. Immediately order an erythrocyte sedimentation rate (ESR) and C-reactive protein (CRP) if you believe that giant cell arteritis is a consideration. The upper limits of normal for an ESR is age divided by 2 for men and age $+10$ divided by 2 for women. The CRP is not affected by age.

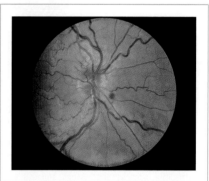

Figure 32-2. Leber's optic neuropathy, acute. Note hyperemic appearance of disc and opacification of the peripapillary nerve fiber layer. (From Burde RM, Savino PJ, Trobe JD: Clinical Decisions in Neuro-Ophthalmology, 3rd ed. St. Louis, Mosby, 2004.)

Both are nonspecific tests; any inflammatory process can elevate them.

The patient denied any of the symptoms, and his ESR was 20. He was diagnosed with nonarteritic ION. Because 50% of these patients have cardiovascular disease, diabetes, and/or hypertension, he was sent to his internist. He was told that his prognosis for significantly improved vision was low. Forty percent of patients may have a mild improvement in vision over 6 months. However, some patients note an initial decrease in visual acuity and field, which is followed by a second decrease in visual acuity or field days to weeks later. Unfortunately, there is no proven treatment. A study recently showed no improvement with optic nerve sheath decompressions. With time, the patient's optic nerve should atrophy in the area of damage. He has a 35% risk of involvement of the other eye.

10. **An 80-year-old man presents with the same history of sudden vision loss and the same visual field as the man in question 9. However, his vision consists of counting fingers at 10 feet, and his optic nerve is pale and swollen with flame-shaped hemorrhages. He admits to pain in his jaw when he chews, weight loss of 10 pounds, and difficulty in getting up from a chair. He has a tender temporal artery without pulses. His ESR is 120. What do you do?**
First, you make a diagnosis of giant cell arteritis and place him on 250 mg of methylprednisolone every 6 hours IV for 12 doses, followed by 80–100 mg/day of prednisone orally for 2–4 weeks after reversal of symptoms and normalization of ESR. Treatment may last for 1 year or more. (Evidence suggests that such high doses can prevent the same process in the other eye, of which there is a 30% risk.) The patient is then scheduled for temporal artery biopsy.

11. **Should the biopsy be done before the steroids are started in order to ensure that the diagnosis can be made?**
Absolutely not. The steroids will not affect the biopsy results for at least 7 days. The therapeutic effect of the steroids is necessary immediately, because the second eye can become involved in as little as 24 hours.

12. **What biopsy finding makes the diagnosis?**
Disruption of the internal elastic lamina. Giant cells are often present but are not necessary for the diagnosis.

13. **What if the temporal artery biopsy is normal?**
Giant cell arteritis is a diagnosis based mainly on symptoms. The ESR may be normal, and your suspicion should be extremely high because of the patient's history. Because skip areas also occur, make sure to get a significant length of artery for biopsy. Sometimes it is necessary to also biopsy the other side. In a patient with less classic symptoms, a negative biopsy warrants discontinuing steroids. Ocular pneumoplethysmography may help if it shows reduced ocular blood flow.

14. **What else may herald giant cell arteritis?**
Amaurosis fugax, cranial nerve palsies, or central retinal artery occlusion.

KEY POINTS: DIFFERENTIAL DIAGNOSIS OF OPTOCILIARY SHUNT VESSELS

1. Meningioma

2. Glaucoma

3. Old central retinal vein occlusion

4. Optic nerve glioma

5. Chronic papilledema

6. Idiopathic disease

15. **A 35-year-old woman says that she has binocular diplopia. On examination, you find weakness of nasal eye movement in her right eye and horizontal jerk nystagmus of the left eye with attempted temporal movement. What does she have?**
    Internuclear ophthalmoplegia (INO). She also may have a skew deviation in which either eye can have a hypertropia that does not map to a specific muscle on the three-step test.

16. **INO can be bilateral or unilateral. What might you find in bilateral disease?**
    Upbeat nystagmus in upgaze and exotropia.

17. **What causes INO?**
    Multiple sclerosis, ischemic vascular disease, or masses of the brain stem. The differential diagnoses that mimic weakness of inward eye movement include the following:
    - **Myasthenia gravis:** Ptosis and orbicularis muscle weakness are common; symptoms worsen with fatigue. Results of a Tensilon test are often positive.
    - **Orbital disease:** Nystagmus is usually not seen. Pain, ptosis, and/or globe displacement may coexist. Orbital computed tomography (CT) reveals the cause.

18. **An obese 30-year-old woman presents with severe headaches and occasional double vision. Her vision is 20/20 in both eyes. How do you evaluate her?**
    Check pupillary responses, color plates, visual fields, and extraocular motility; do a full slit-lamp and dilated examination. You notice that she has bilateral swollen optic nerves.

19. **What do you do after the evaluation?**
    You must emergently evaluate the patient for increased intracranial pressure. First, she needs a CT or MRI of the head and orbit to rule out a mass. Provided the scan is normal, a lumber puncture should follow. If the only abnormality is an increased opening pressure, the diagnosis is pseudotumor cerebri (Fig. 32-3), also known as idiopathic intracranial hypertension.

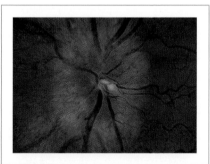

Figure 32-3. Developed papilledema. This is the optic disc of a 30-year-old woman who suffered headaches and blurred vision for 2 months. Disc edema is fully developed. Note the engorged veins and peripapillary hemorrhages. (From Brodsky MC: Congenital optic disc anomalies. In Yanoff M, Duker JS [eds]: Ophthalmology, 2nd ed. St. Louis, Mosby, 2004, pp 1255–1258.)

20. **How should the patient be treated?**
    If she has no optic nerve damage on visual fields, encourage her to lose weight. If the headaches continue or she has evidence of decreased visual acuity or visual field loss, treatment is indicated. Medications include a diuretic, such as acetazolamide, or systemic steroids. Optic nerve sheath decompression is used for worsening visual fields, and lumboperitoneal shunts have been used for headaches. The intraocular pressure should be treated if elevated.

KEY POINTS: CAUSES OF PSEUDOTUMOR CEREBRI ✓

1. Obesity

2. Pregnancy

3. Drug use: Steroids (use or withdrawal), oral contraceptives, nalidixic acid, tetracycline, vitamin A

4. Idiopathic disease

21. **Why did the patient have double vision?**
    Increased intracranial pressure may cause sixth-nerve palsies.

22. **A mother brings in her firstborn for his first exam. He is 6 months old and appears not to see well. Dilated exam reveals optic nerve hypoplasia. What is the differential diagnosis?**
    Optic nerve hypoplasia (Fig. 32-4) seems to occur in the firstborn of young mothers who may have diabetes or who may have used lysergic acid diethylamide (LSD), phenytoin, or alcohol during pregnancy. Patients also may have optic nerve hypoplasia in association with Goldenhar's syndrome or septo-optic dysplasia of de Morsier. The latter patients have seesaw nystagmus and chiasmal anomalies. Because of the risk of growth retardation, diabetes insipidus, and other pituitary abnormalities, patients with optic nerve hypoplasia should have a scan of the optic chiasm and an endocrine evaluation.

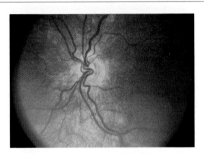

Figure 32-4. Hypoplasia of the left optic nerve. Note the double ring sign. (From Sadun AA: Differentiation of optic nerve from retinal macular disease. In Yanoff M, Duker JS [eds]: Ophthalmology, 2nd ed. St. Louis, Mosby, 2004, pp 1253–1254.)

23. **How do you differentiate between papilledema and pseudopapilledema?**
    Pseudopapilledema is not true disc swelling. The vessels surrounding the disc are not obscured, the disc is not hyperemic, and the peripapillary nerve fiber layer is normal. Spontaneous venous pulsations, if present, strongly suggest pseudopapilledema. Nerve fiber layer hemorrhages are not present in pseudopapilledema. Causes of pseudopapilledema include optic nerve drusen and congenitally anomalous discs.

24. **A patient has a bilateral, right-sided superior field defect. Where do you suspect the lesion is located?**
    A "pie-in-the-sky" defect is located in the temporal lobe. The inferior fibers loop around the temporal lobe (Meyer's loop).

25. **What other symptoms may the patient have?**
    Formed hallucinations, déjà vu experiences, or uncinate fits.

26. **What if the patient has a bilateral, inferior right-sided visual field loss?**
This "pie-on-the-floor" defect is typical for the parietal lobe. Patients have spasticity of conjugate gaze and optokinetic nystagmus abnormalities.

27. **A patient presents with the visual field illustrated in Fig. 32-5. Where is the lesion located?**
The right occipital lobe. The more congruous the defects, the more posterior their location. In addition, the nasal retina is larger and allows a temporal crescent in the visual field in the contralateral eye. Macular sparing or splitting also may occur.

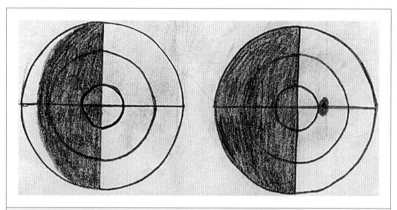

Figure 32-5. Left homonymous hemianopia with temporal crescent in left eye.

28. **What else may the patient experience?**
Patients with occipital lobe lesions often do not experience other neurologic abnormalities. If they do, they may have unformed hallucinations, dyschromatopsia, prosopagnosia, and alexia without agraphia.

29. **What causes pseudo–Foster Kennedy syndrome?**
Pseudo–Foster Kennedy syndrome is optic atrophy with contralateral optic disc edema. A frontal lobe tumor causes true Foster Kennedy syndrome. The pseudosyndrome is usually the result of an acute ischemic optic neuropathy in one eye with contralateral atrophy caused by a past episode of the same process. An olfactory groove meningioma also may cause the pseudosyndrome.

30. **An 18-year-old man presents with sudden vision loss in one eye, followed by the other eye within days. He denies pain. He has 20/20 vision in both eyes with decreased color plates and bilateral mild disc swelling with peripapillary telangiectatic microangiopathy. Affected vessels do not leak on fluorescein angiography. What does he have?**
Leber's hereditary optic neuropathy. The patient's history is typical. The disorder is transmitted by mitochondrial DNA; all female carriers transmit it to their offspring. Ten percent of daughters and 50–70% of sons manifest the disease. All daughters are carriers. None of the sons are carriers. Young men present with symptoms at 15–30 years old. No effective treatment is known, but some mutations are more likely to have spontaneous improvement in the future; thus genetic evaluation of the mitochondria is worthwhile. Because patients have a higher incidence of cardiac conduction defects, referral to a cardiologist is indicated.

BIBLIOGRAPHY

1. Burde RM, Savino PJ, Trobe JD: Clinical Decisions in Neuro-Ophthalmology, 3rd ed. St. Louis, Mosby, 2002.
2. Kunimoto DY, Kanitkar KD, Makar M: The Wills Eye Manual, 4th ed. Philadelphia, Lippincott Williams &Wilkins, 2004.
3. Kline LB, Bajandas FJ: Neuro-Ophthalmology Review Manual, 5th ed. Thorofare, NJ, Slack, 2003.

VII. OCULOPLASTICS

CHAPTER 33

TEARING AND THE LACRIMAL SYSTEM

Nancy G. Swartz, MS, MD, and Marc S. Cohen, MD

1. What are the causes of tearing?

Tearing, also called *epiphora,* can be caused by an increase in the amount of tears produced or by a problem with the tear drainage system. Excess tears are produced as a reflex when there is corneal irritation. Corneal irritation can be mechanical, secondary to a tear film deficiency, or caused by exposure or allergies. Inadequate tear drainage can result from a blockage in the tear drainage system, as in punctal stenosis, canalicular stenosis, and nasolacrimal duct obstructions. Eyelid malpositions (e.g., ectropion or punctal ectropion) and laxity of the lower eyelid with resultant poor tear pump function will also cause inadequate drainage of tears. For many patients, tearing is multifactorial.

KEY POINTS: PRIMARY CAUSES OF TEARING

1. Dry eyes

2. Lower eyelid laxity

3. Blockage of the lacrimal drainage system

---

2. Describe the normal path of tear drainage in the eyelids.

Tears travel across the cornea and conjunctiva to the medial canthus, where they enter small openings in the eyelid called *puncta,* which are located approximately 6–7 mm from the medial canthus. The tears then enter the canaliculi, which are mucosa-lined ducts approximately 10 mm in length that carry the tears to the lacrimal sac. The first portion of the canaliculus is a 2-mm dilated, vertical segment called the *ampulla.* The canaliculus then bends acutely and runs parallel to the eyelid margin toward the medial canthus. In most patients the upper and lower canaliculi join to form the common canaliculus. In some patients, however, the canaliculi enter the lacrimal sac separately.

3. Where do tears go after leaving the eyelids?

Tears enter the lacrimal sac, which lies in a bony fossa of the medial orbital wall formed by the maxillary and lacrimal bones. The sac is generally in a collapsed state. It extends vertically for approximately 10 mm beginning a few millimeters superior to the medial canthal tendon and extending inferiorly to the nasolacrimal duct.

    The nasolacrimal duct travels through a 12-mm bony canal in the maxillary bone and then continues inferiorly for 3–5 mm before opening into the inferior meatus of the nose. The ostium is located 30 mm from the external nares in an adult. In young children, this distance is approximately 20 mm.

4. What is the tear pump?

It is a muscular "pump" that drives the tears through the drainage system by peristalsis. In the resting state the lacrimal sac is collapsed. Initially, tears enter the punctum by capillary action.

During a blink, the orbicularis oculi muscle contracts, causing the puncta to close, the canaliculi to shorten and move medially, and the lacrimal sac to expand. This forces the tears medially through the canaliculi and creates a negative pressure in the sac, drawing the tears into it. When the muscle relaxes, the lacrimal sac again collapses. A valve between the canaliculi and sac, the valve of Rosenmüller, prevents the tears from reentering the canaliculi, so they are forced down the nasolacrimal duct into the nose.

5. **How does lower eyelid laxity affect tear drainage?**
Normal drainage of tears requires normal structure and function of the eyelids. The pretarsal orbicularis muscle surrounds the canaliculi and attaches to the wall of the lacrimal sac. Contraction and relaxation of this muscle help draw the tears into the canaliculus and the sac, and eventually force the tears down the nasolacrimal duct. When lower eyelid laxity is present, contraction of the orbicularis muscle does not force open the lacrimal sac, and the lacrimal pump mechanism cannot function adequately.

6. **How can you tell if a patient has lower eyelid laxity?**
Stretching of the medial and/or lateral canthal tendon causes lower eyelid laxity. In the distraction test, if the lower eyelid can be pulled more than 6 mm from the globe, it is lax.
   Poor orbicularis oculi tone, most obvious in patients with palsy of the seventh cranial nerve, also causes laxity of the lower eyelid. This is best demonstrated with the snap back test, in which the lower eyelid is pulled down inferiorly and allowed to "snap back" into place. If the eyelid returns to its correct position immediately, the muscle tone is good. If the patient must blink to place the eyelid back in its normal position, eyelid tone is poor.

7. **How do you correct lower eyelid laxity?**
If there is laxity of the lateral canthal tendon, a horizontal lid shortening procedure is performed to tighten the eyelid. The best way to do this is with a lateral tarsal strip procedure. In this operation the inferior limb of the lateral canthal tendon is disinserted from the periosteum of the lateral orbital rim, and a new lateral canthal tendon is created from the lateral portion of the tarsus. The newly formed lateral canthal tendon is sutured back to the periosteum of the lateral orbital rim. This effectively shortens the lower eyelid, making the eyelid margin more stable and improving tear pump function.

8. **Why do patients with dry eyes complain of tearing?**
Patients tear when they have dry eyes for the same reason that they tear when cutting an onion. Onion fumes cause corneal irritation, which, in turn, causes reflex tearing.
   Likewise, abnormalities in the tear film coating the cornea cause an irritation of the cornea. Tear film abnormalities can be caused by a decrease in the overall production of tears or to an imbalance in the composition of the tears. Inadequacies in any of the components of the tears cause a tear film deficiency that can result in tearing.

9. **Of what are tears composed?**
Tears are composed of three layers. **Mucin,** made by the conjunctival goblet cells, covers the epithelium, assuring a smooth, uniform tear film. The middle layer of **aqueous,** made by the main and accessory lacrimal glands, provides the oxygen and nutrients to the cornea. The surface **lipid** layer, made in the meibomian glands of the eyelids, prevents rapid evaporation of the tears and provides a smooth surface for the eyelids to move across the cornea.

10. **How can you determine if a patient produces enough tears?**
The volume of tears can be indirectly assessed by visualization of the tear meniscus, the tear layer between the lower eyelid and globe, which should be approximately 1 mm in height. The Schirmer test directly tests production. Gently dry the palpebral conjunctiva with a cotton swab and then place the small, folded end of a 5-mm wide strip of Whatman #41 filter

paper into the inferior conjunctival fornix at the junction of the middle and lateral third of the lower eyelid. In 5 minutes, measure the amount of wetting of the filter paper. If performed on an anesthetized cornea, measure basal tear secretion. A normal result is at least 10 mm. If performed on a nonanesthetized cornea, measure both basal and reflex tearing. Less than 15 mm of wetting is abnormal.

11. **How do you know if the tear composition is inadequate?**
A decrease in the tear break-up time or the presence of protein, mucus, or debris in the tears indicates a tear inadequacy. The tear break-up time is the time between a blink and the development of a dry spot on the cornea. It is measured by touching the palpebral conjunctiva with a moistened fluorescein strip and observing the tear film through the slit lamp with a cobalt-blue filter. It is important not to use other eye drops mixed with fluorescein, because this will change the composition of the tear film you observe. Once the patient blinks, time is measured until the tear film begins to break up on the cornea, causing a dry spot. Less than 10 seconds is considered abnormal.

12. **What are ectropion and entropion? How do they cause tearing?**
Ectropion is an outward rotation of the eyelid margin. Entropion is an inward rotation of the eyelid margin. When an ectropion or entropion is present, patients tear. This occurs because the resultant corneal irritation causes reflex tearing, and tears do not reach the displaced punctum.

KEY POINTS: TESTS FOR PATIENTS WITH TEARING

1. Tear quantity and quality evaluation

2. Evaluation of eyelid position

3. Evaluation of lid laxity

4. Probing and irrigation of lacrimal drainage system

13. **What causes obstructions of the punctum, canaliculus, or lacrimal sac?**
   - **Punctal obstructions** can result from a congenital agenesis, inflammation, infection, or trauma, or they can result from iatrogenic closure in the treatment of dry eyes.
   - **Canalicular stenoses** can occur in one or both canaliculi or in the common canaliculus. These can be congenital or acquired from trauma, infections, inflammation, certain chemotherapeutic agents, or the long-term use of topical medications.
   - **Lacrimal sac obstructions** occur most frequently from scarring as a result of a prior infection. Dacryoliths may develop from infections or chronic use of topical medications. Lacrimal sac tumors are rare.

14. **What causes nasolacrimal duct obstructions?**
Nasolacrimal duct obstructions can be congenital, traumatic, inflammatory, infectious, or neoplastic. Primary acquired nasolacrimal duct obstruction is the most common cause of obstructions in this location. The cause of these is poorly understood. However, it is commonly believed that obstruction of the ostium of the duct most likely is caused by inflammation of the nasal mucosa.

15. **How do I evaluate the lacrimal system for obstructions?**
Obstructions can occur anywhere in the lacrimal system. Punctal obstructions can be visualized on examination. To determine the presence of an obstruction in the canaliculus, lacrimal sac, and nasolacrimal duct, perform a dye disappearance test or a Jones dye test.

Obstruction in the canaliculus can also be determined directly by probing the canaliculus and feeling for stenoses and complete obstructions. Irrigation of the system will uncover obstructions in the lacrimal sac and nasolacrimal duct.

Imaging techniques of the lacrimal system, including ultrasound, computed tomographic scans, contrast dacryocystography, and radionuclide dacryoscintigraphy, are rarely necessary.

16. **What is a dye disappearance test?**
In the dye disappearance test, a drop of fluorescein is placed in the inferior conjunctival fornix. After 5 minutes, the amount present in the tear lake is assessed using a cobalt-blue light. The presence of little or no fluorescein indicates a normal functioning system. If most of the fluorescein remains, the system is not functioning properly.

17. **What is a primary Jones dye test?**
A primary Jones dye test involves placing fluorescein in the inferior conjunctival fornix. A cotton swab is placed under the inferior turbinate at 2 minutes and 5 minutes. If dye is recovered on the swab, the system is patent and functioning well. If no dye is recovered, this indicates a poorly functioning system.

18. **What is a secondary Jones dye test?**
In a secondary Jones dye test the inferior fornix is first irrigated to remove all residual fluorescein from the primary test. Clear saline is then irrigated through the canaliculus with a cannula. If fluorescein-stained fluid is recovered from the nose, the fluorescein must have passed freely through the punctum, canaliculus, and to the lacrimal sac during the primary Jones test, indicating a partial block of the nasolacrimal duct. If clear fluid is recovered, a partial obstruction or functional disorder of the punctum or canaliculus is indicated. If no fluid is recovered from the nose but instead regurgitates from the adjacent punctum, an obstruction at or distal to the common canaliculus is present.

19. **How do you treat obstructions of the eyelid portion of the lacrimal system?**
When the punctum is not patent, this can frequently be opened with a sharp probe or cut-down procedure to find the proximal canaliculus. In most patients, placement of a temporary silicone stent is helpful to prevent the punctum from reclosing. This office-based procedure is performed with local infiltrative anesthesia. If the canaliculus is scarred closed, a canaliculo-dacryocystorhinostomy (CDCR) is performed. In this surgery a fistula is created between the caruncle and the nasal mucosa and a permanent glass tube (Jones tube) is placed in this tract to maintain its patency. A CDCR can be performed on an outpatient basis under general anesthesia or with monitored sedation.

20. **How do you treat obstructions of the nasolacrimal duct?**
The majority of lacrimal system obstructions occur in the nasolacrimal duct, which connects the lacrimal sac to the nose. When the obstruction is in the nasolacrimal duct, a dacryocystorhinostomy (DCR) is performed. In this procedure the lacrimal sac is marsupialized to the nasal passages, so the tears can bypass the blocked nasolacrimal duct and drain directly from the lacrimal sac into the nose.

21. **Describe acute dacryocystitis.**
An acute infection of the lacrimal sac is called *dacryocystitis*. Patients typically present with a painful, erythematous swelling in the medial canthus just inferior to the medial canthal

tendon. A purulent discharge from the punctum may be seen with gentle pressure on the lacrimal sac. Acute dacryocystitis is nearly always the result of a blocked nasolacrimal duct.

22. **What is the appropriate treatment for acute dacryocystitis?**
Dacryocystitis is a serious infection that must be treated as an emergency. If not adequately treated, an orbital cellulitis may develop. There is also the potential for the infection to spread intracranially. Appropriate systemic antibiotics should be given, and warm compresses should be applied to the medial canthus. Patients should be watched carefully to assure improvement. After resolution of the acute infection, a DCR should be performed to avoid future infection.

23. **What are the signs of congenital nasolacrimal duct obstructions?**
Approximately 6% of newborns have a congenital obstruction of the nasolacrimal system. Infants may present with epiphora, conjunctivitis, amniocele formation, or a dacryocystitis. The lacrimal drainage system begins embryologically as a cord in the medial canthus that expands laterally to the punctum and inferiorly to the nasal mucosa of the inferior meatus. The lumen also forms first in the medial canthus, and canalization develops laterally and inferiorly. The distal end of the duct is the last portion to canalize. This may not yet be patent at birth and is the most common site of congenital obstructions.

KEY POINTS: TREATMENT OF CONGENITAL EPIPHORA

1. Treat initially with massage.

2. Then undertake probing of the nasal lacrimal duct under anesthesia, often with balloon dacryoplasty.

3. Then use silicone intubation.

4. Finally, perform a DCR.

24. **How are congenital obstructions first managed?**
Most clinicians recommend massaging the infant's lacrimal sac (in the medial canthus) in an inferior direction to increase the hydrostatic pressure in the nasolacrimal duct and hopefully force open any obstruction. If there is an associated conjunctivitis or discharge, topical antibiotics are also used. Systemic antibiotics are used when a dacryocystitis is present.

25. **What if this doesn't work?**
If a child has a persistent tearing because of blockage of the nasolacrimal duct, a probing of the system should be performed in the first 13 months of life. Katowitz and Welsh have shown that the success rates of probing drop significantly if performed after 13 months of age. In this procedure the child is placed under general anesthesia and a Bowman probe is passed into the punctum, through the lacrimal system, and out through the nasolacrimal duct. Some surgeons elect to perform a balloon dacryoplasty at the time of the initial probing. In this procedure a deflated balloon is passed into the duct and then inflated to dilate the duct and the ostium.

26. **What if the tearing is still present after a probing?**
Approximately 90–95% of infants who undergo a probing enjoy a resolution of their symptoms. When the problem persists after probing or balloon dacryoplasty, intubation with silicone

tubes is indicated. Tubes are generally left in place for approximately 6 months and serve to keep the passageway open. Durso et al. reported an 84% success rate for patients intubated for nasolacrimal duct obstruction. When probing and intubation are unsuccessful, a DCR is performed.

BIBLIOGRAPHY

1. Durso F, Hand SI Jr, Ellis FD, Helveston EM: Silicone intubation in children with nasolacrimal obstruction. J Pediatr Ophthalmol Strabismus 17:389–393, 1980.

2. Kanski JJ: Clinical Ophthalmology. Oxford, England, Butterworth-Heinemann, 1989.

3. Katowitz JA, Welsh MG: Timing of initial probing and irrigation in congenital nasolacrimal duct obstruction. Ophthalmology 94:698–705, 1987.

4. Welham RAN, Hughes SM: Lacrimal surgery in children. Am J Ophthalmol 99:27–34, 1985.

CHAPTER 34

PROPTOSIS

David G. Buerger, MD

1. **What is proptosis?**

   Proptosis is a forward protrusion of one or both eyeballs. Unilateral proptosis is frequently defined as asymmetric protrusion of one eye by at least 2 mm. Normal upper limits for proptosis are approximately 22 mm in Caucasians and 24 mm in African Americans.

2. **How is proptosis diagnosed?**

   Clinically, proptosis can be recognized by observing the globes from above, over the patient's forehead. It is measured with an exophthalmometer, which is usually based at the lateral orbital rim. The amount of proptosis can also be quantified by measuring globe protrusion on a computed tomographic (CT) scan (Fig. 34-1).

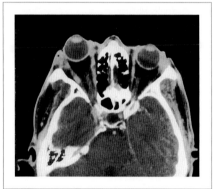

Figure 34-1. Computed tomographic scan demonstrating proptosis of the right globe secondary to thyroid-related enlargement of the rectus muscles.

3. **List common problems associated with proptosis.**

   - **Exposure keratopathy** frequently develops secondary to a poor blink mechanism over the protruding globe. Patients can have mild symptoms of irritation and foreign body sensation, or they may experience more severe symptoms associated with corneal abrasions and ulcers (Fig. 34-2).

   - **Diplopia** (double vision) can result from unilateral or bilateral proptosis from displacement of the globes or poor extraocular muscle function.

   - **Optic nerve compression** can occur with space-occupying lesions of the orbit, which cause proptosis. Indications of nerve compression include decreased visual acuity, relative afferent pupillary defect, color vision deficit, and visual field defect of the affected eye. This is a medical emergency and requires prompt therapeutic intervention, surgically or medically.

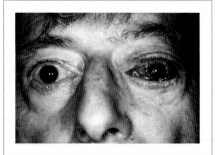

Figure 34-2. Severe conjunctival chemosis with corneal erosion secondary to proptosis caused by an orbital lymphoma.

4. **What is the most common cause of unilateral proptosis?**
   Thyroid eye disease (Graves' ophthalmopathy).

5. **What is the most common cause of bilateral proptosis?**
   Thyroid eye disease.

6. **What are other causes of proptosis?**
   - Orbital inflammatory pseudotumor
   - Orbital infectious cellulitis
   - Orbital tumors (benign or malignant)
   - Lacrimal gland tumors
   - Trauma (retrobulbar hemorrhage)
   - Orbital vasculitis (i.e., polyarteritis nodosa, Wegener's granulomatosis)
   - Mucormycosis
   - Carotid–cavernous fistula
   - Orbital varix

7. **List the causes of pseudoproptosis.**
   - Unilateral high axial myopia can mimic proptosis, owing to the increased length of the myopic eye.
   - Actual enophthalmos of one eye may cause apparent proptosis of the contralateral eye (Fig. 34-3).
   - Upper eyelid retraction produces a more prominent appearing eye. This often coexists in cases of thyroid ophthalmopathy.

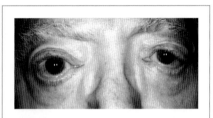

Figure 34-3. Patient with enophthalmos of the left eye secondary to old trauma, which is causing apparent proptosis of the right eye.

8. **Which neuroimaging test is best to evaluate the etiology of proptosis?**
   CT scans are superior in most cases of proptosis, because the relationship of the orbital process to the orbital bones is better visualized. Magnetic resonance imaging (MRI) may be desirable in certain cases when optic nerve dysfunction is present. Plain films are not used for diagnostic accuracy in cases of proptosis.

9. **Which clinical entity is frequently associated with unilateral or bilateral painless proptosis, eyelid retraction, eyelid lag on downward gaze, and motility disturbances?**
   Thyroid ophthalmopathy associated with Graves' disease (Fig. 34-4) is a complex, multisystem, autoimmune disorder. Patients can be hyperthyroid, hypothyroid, or euthyroid when manifesting ophthalmic symptoms. Eye problems develop as a result of inflammation and enlargement of various extraocular muscles (most

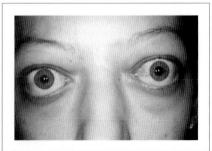

Figure 34-4. Proptosis and eyelid retraction caused by thyroid ophthalmopathy.

frequently the inferior rectus and medial rectus) and peribulbar tissues. CT scan or MRI results often show fusiform enlargement of the involved extraocular muscles with sparing of the tendon that attaches the muscle to the globe. Proptosis and eyelid retraction cause corneal problems, and muscle enlargement in the orbit causes diplopia and possibly optic nerve compression. Treatment is in stages, depending on the severity of the eye disease. Systemic and laboratory evaluation is mandatory.

KEY POINTS: CLINICAL SIGNS OF GRAVES' DISEASE

1. Unilateral or bilateral proptosis

2. Eyelid retraction with lateral flare

3. Lagophthalmos

4. Diplopia

10. **Which clinical entity is frequently associated with unilateral proptosis, pain, conjunctival injection, and motility disturbances in an adult?**
Orbital inflammatory pseudotumor is a nonspecific idiopathic inflammatory disease of the orbit. Inflammation may be localized to a muscle, the lacrimal gland, or sclera, or may be diffuse. Other possible signs include eyelid erythema or edema, palpable mass, decreased vision, uveitis, hyperopic shift, and optic nerve edema. Bilateral disease is more common in children. CT scan results may show thickening of one or more extraocular muscles (including the tendons), lacrimal gland enlargement, or thickening of the posterior sclera. Treatment is primarily with corticosteroids and possibly radiation therapy.

11. **Which clinical entity is characterized by unilateral proptosis, pain, fever, decreased ocular motility, erythema, and edema of the eyelids?**
Infectious orbital cellulitis involves an infection (usually bacterial) that has extended posterior to the orbital septum. Once past the orbital septum barrier, infection can spread rapidly and cause serious complications such as meningitis or cavernous sinus thrombosis. The most common organisms include staphylococci, streptococci, anaerobes, and *Haemophilus influenzae* (in children younger than 5 years of age). The most common source of infectious spread to the orbit is an ethmoid sinusitis. Treatment is with intravenous antibiotics.

12. **What should be done for persistent proptosis or progression of infection despite adequate antibiotic treatment in a case of orbital cellulitis?**
The situation is highly suggestive of an orbital subperiosteal abscess. CT scanning should be performed to confirm this diagnosis and locate the abscess. Definitive treatment consists of surgical drainage and continued intravenous antibiotics.

13. **Which clinical entity is characterized by a child younger than 6 years of age with gradual, painless, progressive, unilateral axial proptosis with visual loss?**
Optic nerve glioma (juvenile pilocytic astrocytoma) is a slow-growing tumor of the optic nerve that causes axial proptosis. Decreased visual acuity is usually associated with a relative afferent pupillary defect. CT scan or MRI results show fusiform enlargement of the optic nerve. Many cases are associated with neurofibromatosis and may be bilateral. Systemic evaluation and genetic counseling for neurofibromatosis are essential.

14. **What clinical entity is characterized by a child with rapidly progressive unilateral proptosis, displacement of the globe inferiorly, and edema of the upper eyelid?**
Rhabdomyosarcoma is the most common primary orbital malignancy of childhood. This malignant growth of striated muscle tissue typically produces a rapidly progressive mass in the superior orbit with proptosis, globe displacement, and eyelid swelling. The average age of presentation is 7 years. Prompt diagnosis with orbitotomy and biopsy is crucial, because **overall mortality is 60%** once the disease has extended to orbital bones. Current treatment strategies with radiation and chemotherapy have lowered mortality rates to 5–10% for orbital rhabdomyosarcoma.

15. **What is the most common benign orbital tumor in adults that causes unilateral proptosis?**
The cavernous hemangioma (Fig. 34-5) is a slow-growing vascular tumor that is usually diagnosed in young adulthood to middle age. CT scanning usually shows a well-defined orbital mass within the ocular muscle cone. Visual acuity is often not affected. Treatment is observation or surgical excision.

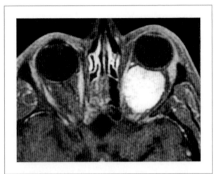

Figure 34-5. Cavernous hemangioma of the left orbit, which is causing proptosis.

16. **What is the most common malignant orbital tumor in adults that causes unilateral proptosis?**
Orbital lymphomas typically develop in the superior orbit with a slow onset and progression. These lesions may be associated with a subconjunctival "salmon-colored" mass in the fornix. CT scanning shows a poorly defined mass conforming to the shape of the orbital bones and globe without bony erosion. Diagnosis is made following orbital biopsy, and definitive treatment is radiation therapy. Orbital lymphoma can be associated with systemic lymphoma; therefore a medical consult and systemic evaluation are necessary for all patients.

17. **Of the various orbital tumors causing proptosis, list those tumors that are encapsulated or appear well circumscribed on neuroimaging.**
   - Cavernous hemangioma
   - Fibrohistiocytoma
   - Hemangiopericytoma
   - Schwannoma
   - Neurofibroma

BIBLIOGRAPHY

1. Dolman PJ, Glazer LC, Harris GJ, et al: Mechanisms of visual loss in severe proptosis. Ophthal Plast Reconstr Surg 7:256–260, 1991.

2. Frueh BR, Garber F, Grill R, Musch DC: Positional effects on exophthalmometric readings in Graves' eye disease. Arch Ophthalmol 103:1355–1356, 1985.

3. Frueh BR, Musch DC, Garber FW: Exophthalmometer readings in patients with Graves' eye disease. Ophthalmic Surg 17:37–40, 1986.

4. Henderson JW: Orbital Tumors. New York, Raven Press, 1994.
5. Hornblass A: Oculoplastic, Orbital and Reconstructive Surgery. Baltimore, Williams & Wilkins, 1988.
6. Rootman J: Diseases of the Orbit. Philadelphia, J.B. Lippincott, 1988.
7. Zimmerman RA, Bilaniuk LT, Yanoff M, et al: Orbital magnetic resonance imaging. Am J Ophthalmol 100:312–317, 1985.

CHAPTER 35

THYROID-RELATED OPHTHALMOPATHY

Robert B. Penne, MD

1. **What is thyroid-related ophthalmopathy?**

   Thyroid-related ophthalmopathy (TRO) is a chronic inflammatory disease of the orbits that often occurs in patients with a systemic thyroid imbalance. Chronic inflammation results in scarring and dysfunction of the orbit. The course and severity are variable.

2. **Who develops TRO?**

   TRO may occur in a wide range of ages. It has been reported from 8 to 88 years of age, with the average age of onset in the forties. Females are affected 3–6 times more often than males. Children are rarely affected.

3. **Is everyone with TRO hyperthyroid?**

   Eighty percent of patients who develop TRO do so while they have been hyperthyroid or after they are diagnosed with hyperthyroidism. Ten percent of patients have some form of hypothyroidism, and up to 10% may not develop a clinically detectable thyroid abnormality. A study found that as many as a third of patients do not develop clinical hyperthyroidism for more than 6 months after onset of symptoms of TRO. This finding suggests that a significant number of patients who present with TRO have not yet developed hyperthyroidism.

   Bartley GB, Fatourechi V, Kadrmas EF: The chronology of Graves' ophthalmopathy in an incidence cohort. Am J Ophthalmol 121:426–434, 1996.

4. **What causes TRO?**

   We do not know. TRO appears to be an immunologically mediated process with the extra ocular muscles as the end organs. Many theories link the orbit and thyroid gland by shared antigens, with some defect in immune surveillance initiating the process. Research continues.

   www.emedicine.com/radio/topic485.htm

5. **Do environmental factors affect TRO?**

   Smoking is the one environmental factor that has been shown definitely to affect TRO. Multiple studies have shown a higher incidence of smoking in patients with TRO than in patients with Graves' disease who do not have TRO. Evidence also suggests that smokers with TRO have more severe disease than nonsmokers. The effects of secondhand smoke can only be speculated.

   Nunery WR, Martin RT, Heintz GW, Gavin TJ: The association of cigarette smoking with subtypes of ophthalmic Graves' disease. Plast Reconstr Surg 9:77–82, 1993.

6. **Does TRO improve when the systemic thyroid imbalance is treated?**

   Treatment of the systemic thyroid dysfunction has little predictable effect on the course of TRO. An equal number of patients improve, worsen, or stay the same. The effects of systemic treatment on TRO are still debated. Also debated is whether radioactive iodine, surgery, and medical treatment have different effects on the course of TRO. A large study suggests that treatment with radioactive iodine has a greater chance of causing progression of TRO. The study also showed that giving systemic steroids during the treatment eliminates this risk.

   Bartalena L, Marcocci C, Bogazzi F, et al: Relation between therapy for hyperthyroidism and the course of Graves' ophthalmopathy. N Engl J Med 1338:73–78, 1998.

7. **Should all patients who receive radioactive iodine be treated with systemic steroids?**
   Unless the patient has specific contraindications or until further studies show otherwise, we recommend that patients undergoing radioactive iodine treatment receive a course of systemic steroids. The dosage and length of treatment are controversial.

8. **What are the early signs of TRO?**
   Many patients initially present with intermittent eyelid swelling along with nonspecific ocular irritation, redness, and swelling (Fig. 35-1). All of these symptoms are so nonspecific that early onset is often missed. The disease is not recognized until the appearance of more obvious clinical signs, such as eyelid retraction, eyelid lag, or early proptosis (Fig. 35-2). Suspecting TRO in patients with the aforementioned nonspecific symptoms is important, especially if they have symptoms or history of a thyroid imbalance.

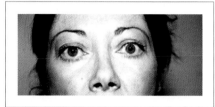

Figure 35-1. Early thyroid-related ophthalmopathy with mild eyelid retraction of the left upper eyelid and the right lower eyelids.

9. **What studies need to be done in the work-up for TRO?**
   The most effective screening tool for systemic thyroid imbalance in patients with TRO is the level of thyroid-stimulating hormone. An internist or endocrinologist can do further evaluation and work-up. A complete ophthalmic exam is needed. Special attention is paid to visual function, including acuity, pupils, color vision, and visual fields, if indicated. Ocular motility with note of any diplopia needs evaluation, along with corneal exposure, proptosis, and eyelid position.

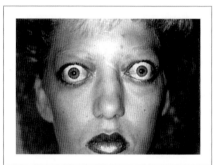

Figure 35-2. Thyroid-related ophthalmopathy with proptosis and eyelid retraction.

10. **Which patients require orbital imaging?**
    Not all patients with TRO require orbital imaging. Indications for imaging include suspicion of optic nerve compression, evaluation for orbital decompression surgery and/or orbital irradiation, unclear diagnosis, and need to rule out other orbital processes. I prefer a computed tomographic scan without contrast in patients with TRO who require imaging.

11. **What findings are present on orbital imaging?**
    Enlargement of the rectus muscle belly with sparing of the tendon is the classic finding (Fig. 35-3). The inferior rectus is the most commonly involved muscle, followed by the medial rectus and the superior rectus. The lateral rectus is least likely to be involved.

12. **Does everyone with proptosis have TRO?**

    No. TRO is the most common cause of both unilateral and bilateral proptosis in adults, but it is not the only cause. Patients with systemic thyroid disease may develop orbital tumors and nonthyroid orbital inflammation. TRO is a bilateral disease, whereas most orbital tumors are unilateral. TRO may present asymmetrically and appear unilateral, especially early in the disease. In rare cases the disease may remain unilateral. If the entire clinical picture is not consistent with TRO, orbital imaging is indicated.

13. **How do the tissues of the orbit change in TRO?**

    The extraocular muscles are the main targets for TRO. Infiltration by inflammatory cells results in fibroblasts that produce mucopolysaccharides in early disease and collagen in later stages. Orbital and eyelid swelling are common early in the disease. Late in the disease the inflammation resolves and the enlarged muscles become fibrotic and scarred.

14. **How long does the disease last?**

    Most patients go through a period of active inflammation and changes in their eyes. This period lasts from 6 months to more than 2 years. In some patients the process may involve slow, mild changes over many months, whereas in others the process is more acute with rapid changes over weeks. Once the disease activity has quieted and the eyes are stable, reactivation is rare. Careful examinations that note changes in motility, eyelid position, proptosis, and general inflammation help to determine disease activity.

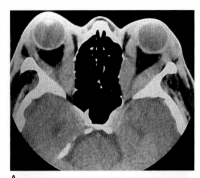
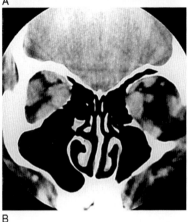

Figure 35-3. Axial *(A)* and coronal *(B)* computed tomographic scans showing enlargement of all four rectus muscles.

15. **Is everyone who develops TRO affected in the same way?**

    No. There is a wide variation from mild irritation and eyelid retraction that resolve totally to severe orbital infiltration with visual loss. Visual loss may result from optic nerve compression or corneal scarring due to corneal exposure. More severe disease involves older patients (average age of 52 versus 36 for milder disease) and has less of a gender difference (female-to-male ratio of 1.5:1 in severe disease versus 8.6:1 in mild disease).

16. **What can be done to treat TRO?**

    Many patients do not require any treatment, but monitoring during the active phase of the disease is important. Ocular lubrication often relieves symptoms. Systemic steroids decrease inflammation. Because of their side effects, systemic steroids are best used as a temporizing measure until more definitive treatment is given. Cessation of steroids generally results in return of orbital inflammation. Orbital irradiation decreases inflammation in the orbit. Surgical treatment is also used.

17. **When are systemic steroids used?**
Systemic steroids are used to decrease orbital inflammation acutely, usually on a temporary basis until other treatment can be started. The most common indication is visual loss from optic nerve compression. Severe proptosis with resultant corneal exposure is a second indication. Both short-term and long-term side effects of steroids limit their usefulness as long-term treatment.

18. **Is orbital irradiation standard treatment for TRO?**
The use of orbital radiation is controversial. A study published in 2001 from the Mayo Clinic concluded that orbital irradiation does not improve TRO. Subsequent smaller studies have shown stabilization of disease progression when compared to controls. Most oculoplastic specialists believe that orbital irradiation has a role in treatment of TRO and that it stops progression of the disease but does not improve preexisting changes. The Mayo Clinic does not use orbital irradiation for treatment of patients with TRO. How it is used varies with the individual physician.

> Gorman CA, Garrity JA, Fatourechi V: A prospective, randomized, double-blind, placebo-controlled study of orbital radiotherapy for Graves' ophthalmopathy. Ophthalmology 108:1523–1534, 2001.

19. **How does orbital irradiation affect TRO?**
The exact mechanism of action of irradiation in the orbit is unclear. Multiple theories of localized immunosuppression in the orbit have been postulated, but all remain unproved. Many patients have a definite decrease in orbital inflammation and edema after orbital irradiation. Irradiation seems to be most effective at stopping disease progression and less effective at reversing changes that have already occurred.

20. **Does orbital irradiation work immediately?**
No. It takes 2–4 weeks to see the initial effects of irradiation, and improvement may continue well beyond that time. If steroids are stopped immediately after completion of irradiation, inflammation may recur rapidly.

21. **Which patients are candidates for orbital irradiation?**
Any patient with *active* TRO is a candidate. Early treatment, if effective, prevents the chronic orbital changes associated with TRO. Later in the disease, irradiation can quiet the active disease and allows earlier and more effective surgical rehabilitation. The use of orbital irradiation has resulted in fewer patients with severe TRO.

22. **Which patients require surgery?**
Surgery may be indicated on an emergent basis because of optic nerve compression or corneal exposure. More often, patients require nonemergent surgery because of severe disfiguring proptosis, double vision from restrictive myopathy, or eyelid retraction.

23. **What kinds of surgery are done in patients with TRO?**
Surgery falls into three basic categories: orbital decompression, eye muscle surgery, and eyelid surgery. Surgery needs to be done in this order because earlier surgeries affect the results of later surgeries. Decompression should be done before eye muscle surgery. Decompression affects ocular motility and may alter muscle surgery. Likewise, muscle surgery should be completed before eyelid surgery is done.

> Shorr N, Seiff SR: The four stages of surgical rehabilitation of the patient with dysthyroid ophthalmopathy. Ophthalmology 93:476–483, 1986.

24. **What is orbital decompression?**

Orbital decompressive surgery involves removal of bone and/or fat to allow the eye to settle back in the orbit. Bone is removed from the inferior and medial walls of the orbit to let the expanded orbital tissue move partially into the sinus space. Lateral wall decompression can also be done. Removal of orbital fat has a decompressive effect to a much lesser degree. The amount of decompression is related to the amount of fat removed.

   Rootman J, Stewart B, Goldberg RA: Orbital Surgery: A Conceptual Approach. Philadelphia, Lippincott-Raven, 1996.

25. **Which patients require orbital decompression?**

Patients with optic nerve compression require decompressive surgery to relieve pressure on the optic nerve. Patients with severe proptosis resulting in corneal exposure or disfigurement are also candidates for orbital decompressive surgery.

26. **What is optic nerve compression?**

Optic nerve compression involves squeezing of the optic nerve at the apex of the orbit. When the extraocular muscles swell in TRO, there is relatively little space at the apex of the orbit; therefore enlargement of muscles exerts pressure on the nerve lying in the center of the muscles. Pressure decreases vision because the function of the optic nerve is affected. This loss of function can manifest as decreased vision, decreased color vision, or visual field loss.

27. **What are the complications of orbital decompression?**

The most common complication is worsening of existing diplopia or new double vision. Patients with preexisting motility problems have a much higher risk of postoperative diplopia. Many patients have infraorbital hypesthesia postoperatively, but it usually improves with time. Risk of visual loss is small. Bleeding and infection, as with any surgery, must be considered.

28. **When do patients require muscle surgery?**

Patients with double vision in their functional field of vision require muscle surgery. Every effort must be made to ensure that the inflammation is quiet and the patient's motility pattern is stable. Repeated stable measurements over months help to ensure that motility is stable.

KEY POINTS: THYROID-RELATED OPHTHALMOPATHY

1. Suspect the diagnosis of TRO in nonspecific ocular irritation even without a systemic thyroid imbalance.

2. Eyelid retraction is often the earliest clinical sign of TRO.

3. Monitor visual function closely in progressive TRO.

4. Get patients who are smokers to stop smoking.

5. TRO patients will take extra time during an office visit.

29. **What are the alternatives to muscle surgery?**

The use of prisms in glasses works for patients with double vision and relatively small deviations. Larger deviations or patterns of diplopia in which the deviation changes with small changes in the direction of gaze are poor candidates for prisms. It is also important that the motility is stable before prisms are prescribed. Temporary Fresnel prisms may be helpful during periods of instability.

30. **What type of muscle surgery is required?**
   Recession of muscles, usually on an adjustable suture. Because the muscles are tight and scarred, resection is not done. The inferior and medical rectus muscles are the most common targets of surgery. Surgery can be done under local or general anesthesia with adjustment of the sutures later in the day or on the following day.

31. **Does eye muscle surgery affect the eyelids?**
   Recession of the tight inferior rectus muscle often improves upper eyelid retraction. The superior rectus muscle has to work against the tight inferior rectus; thus the associated levator muscle is overactive, causing eyelid retraction. When the inferior muscle is recessed, the overactivity ends and often the upper eyelid retraction is less. Large recessions of the inferior rectus muscle may worsen inferior eyelid retraction.

32. **What kind of eyelid surgery is done?**
   Eyelid retraction is the main problem in patients with TRO. In patients undergoing orbital decompression, the eye is lowered, often improving the lower eyelid retraction. For mild eyelid retraction, recession of the eyelid retractors (upper or lower) is adequate. For more severe retraction, spacers are needed, such as hard palate or acellular dermis in the lower eyelids and fascia in the upper eyelids. Patients also may require a blepharoplasty and/or brow lift to deal with the excessive skin that results from stretching caused by chronic swelling. This goal may be met at the time of eyelid repositioning or at a later date.

33. **How many surgeries do patients with TRO require?**
   Most patients with TRO do not require surgery. Patients who do need surgery may need from one to as many as eight to ten operations. Patients with severe disease may require many operations over 2–3 years of reconstruction.

CHAPTER 36

ORBITAL INFLAMMATORY DISEASES

Roberta E. Gausas, MD, and Madhura Tamhankar, MD

1. **What is inflammation?**
   The concept of inflammation is ancient and was used to describe a combination of rubor (redness), dolor (pain), tumor (swelling), calor (heat), and *functio laesa* (loss of function). We now recognize inflammation as a tissue response governed by multiple cellular processes.

2. **How does inflammation affect the orbit?**
   Inflammation is the most common problem that affects the adult orbit, leading to a spectrum of clinical presentations with variable onset and variable orbital tissues affected, causing mass effect, inflammation, and/or infiltration resulting in variable deficits in function or vision.

   Cockerham KP, Hong SH, Browne EE: Orbital inflammation. Curr Neurol Neurosci Rep 3:401–409, 2003.

3. **What does "orbital pseudotumor" mean?**
   It refers to a clinical setting that simulates a tumor but resolves spontaneously or is revealed by biopsy as only inflammation without evidence of malignancy. However, it is an outdated term that fails to include or explain a variety of inflammatory disease processes that can be identified.

   Rootman J: Why "orbital pseudotumour" is no longer a useful concept. Br J Ophthalmol 82:339–340, 1998.

4. **What are the best terms to describe orbital inflammation?**
   For purposes of better understanding and better management, orbital inflammation should be classified based on pathology, anatomic location, and/or associated systemic disease as either specific or nonspecific in nature. **Nonspecific orbital inflammation,** or idiopathic orbital inflammatory syndrome, is a more accurate term that replaces orbital pseudotumor.

5. **What is specific orbital inflammation?**
   The diagnosis of specific orbital inflammation is based on the identification of a specific etiology causing the disorder, such as a specific pathogen (infection, as in orbital cellulitis), specific histopathology (granulomatous disease, as in sarcoidosis), or a specific local and/or systemic constellation of findings that define a distinct entity (vasculitis, as in Wegener's granulomatosis) (Box 36-1).

   Rootman J: Inflammatory diseases of the orbit. Highlights. J Fr Ophthalmol 24:155–161, 2001.

6. **How is nonspecific orbital inflammation (NSOI) different?**
   Orbital inflammation that has no identifiable cause is considered nonspecific. It is a diagnosis of exclusion.

7. **What, then, is the etiology of NSOI?**
   It is generally believed to be an immune-mediated process, although postinfectious and post-traumatic origins have been proposed. Its etiology remains unknown.

   Atabay C, Tyutyunikov A, Scalise D, et al: Serum antibodies reactive with eye muscle membrane antigens are detected in patients with nonspecific orbital inflammation. Ophthalmology 102:145–253, 1995.
   Cockerham KP, Hong SH, Browne EE: Orbital inflammation. Curr Neurol Neurosci Rep 3:401–409, 2003.

BOX 36-1.   DIFFERENTIAL DIAGNOSIS OF ORBITAL INFLAMMATION

SPECIFIC INFLAMMATION
Thyroid-associated orbitopathy
Infection/infestation
Bacterial
   Contiguous spread from sinusitis
   Retained orbital foreign body
Fungal
   Rhino-orbital mucormycosis
   Aspergillosis
Parasitic
   Echinococcosis
   Cysticercosis
Tuberculosis and syphilis
Vasculitis
Wegener's granulomatosis
Polyarteritis nodosa
Hypersensitivity angiitis
   Orbital vasculitis secondary to systemic lupus erythematosus
Giant cell arteritis
Granulomatous inflammation
Sarcoidosis/sarcoidal reactions
Xanthogranulomatous disorders of orbit
Foreign-body granuloma
Erdheim-Chester disease
Sjögren's syndrome

NONSPECIFIC ORBITAL INFLAMMATION
Sclerosing inflammation of the orbit
Idiopathic granulomatous inflammation

NONINFLAMMATORY DISORDERS
Neoplasia
Lymphoid disorder
Vascular disorder
Dural–cavernous sinus arteriovenous fistula

8. **Describe a typical clinical presentation of NSOI.**
Acute onset of painful periorbital swelling and erythema, S-shaped eyelid deformity, and chemosis that may be unilateral or bilateral. However, the symptoms and physical findings will vary based on the degree and anatomic location of the inflammation, which may include diffuse involvement of multiple tissues (e.g., sclerosing) or preferential involvement of specific orbital tissues (e.g., periscleritis, perineuritis).

9. **Is NSOI always acute in onset?**
No. Onset of NSOI may be acute (hours to days), subacute (days to weeks), or chronic (weeks to months).

10. **Is the symptom of pain necessary to make the diagnosis?**
Although pain or discomfort is very typical, atypical cases may occur in which pain is absent.

Mahr MA, Salomao DR, Garrity JA: Inflammatory orbital pseudotumor with extension beyond the orbit. Am J Ophthalmol 138:396–400, 2004.

11. **How is NSOI in children different?**

Bilateral manifestation is much more common, as well as uveitis, elevated erythrocyte sedimentation rate (ESR), and eosinophilia. Uveitis in particular, when present, appears to portend a poor outcome in children.

Bloom JN, Graviss ER, Byrne BJ: Orbital pseudotumor in the differential diagnosis of pediatric uveitis. J Pediatr Ophthalmol Strabismus 29:59–63, 1992.

Mottow-Lippa L, Jakobiec FA, Smith M: Idiopathic inflammatory orbital pseudotumor in childhood. II. Results of diagnostic tests and biopsies. Ophthalmology 88:565–574, 1981.

12. **Name the five most common anatomic patterns of NSOI.**
    1. Extraocular muscle (myositis)
    2. Lacrimal gland (dacryoadenitis)
    3. Anterior
    4. Apical
    5. Diffuse

13. **How is the diagnosis of NSOI made?**

Ultimate diagnosis and treatment relies on complete history and detailed clinical examination followed by judicious use of ancillary diagnostic testing and a comprehensive treatment plan. Diagnostic testing includes neuroimaging, laboratory testing, and biopsy when appropriate.

14. **What is the best imaging technique for NSOI?**

Orbital computed tomography (CT), magnetic resonance image (MRI), or ultrasound can all provide useful information, but orbital MRI with fat saturation is the imaging study with the highest yield. Subtle edema of the retrobulbar fat is often one of the earliest changes seen in NSOI.

Uehara F, Ohba N: Diagnostic imaging in patients with orbital cellulitis and inflammatory pseudotumor. Int Ophthalmol Clin 42:133–142, 2002.

15. **What blood tests can be ordered to evaluate NSOI?**

Complete blood count, electrolytes, ESR, antinuclear antibody, anti–double-stranded DNA, antineutrophil cytoplasmic antibody (ANCA), angiotensin-converting enzyme level, and rapid plasma reagin.

Jacobs DA, Galetta SL: Orbital inflammatory disease. Curr Treat Opt Neurol 4:289–295, 2002.

16. **When should an orbital biopsy be performed?**

The role of orbital biopsy has been an area of controversy, with one school of thought advocating empiric steroid treatment as both a diagnostic and a therapeutic measure, whereas the other school of thought advocates biopsy of all infiltrative lesions to obtain an accurate and definitive diagnosis. Most orbital surgeons advocate biopsy, except for two clinical scenarios—orbital myositis and orbital apex syndrome—in which the risk of biopsy must be weighed against the risk of a missed diagnosis. However, recurrent or nonresponsive orbital myositis and orbital apex syndrome warrant orbital biopsy.

Papalkar D, Sharma S, Francis IC, et al: A rapidly fatal case of T-cell lymphoma presenting as idiopathic orbital inflammation. Orbit 24:131–133, 2005.

17. **What is the histopathology of NSOI?**

In the acute phase, pathology reveals a diffuse polymorphous infiltrate composed of mature lymphocytes, plasma cells, macrophages, eosinophils, and polymorphonuclear leukocytes. In the subacute and chronic phases, an increasing amount of fibrovascular stroma is seen.

18. **Name two subtypes of orbital inflammation.**
    A distinct sclerosing form of orbital inflammation exists, which is characterized by dense fibrous replacement. Another distinct form is one that displays granulomatous inflammation similar to sarcoidosis but is not associated with systemic sarcoidosis.

    Raskin EM, McCormick SA, Maher EA, Della Rocca RC: Granulomatous idiopathic orbital inflammation. Ophthal Plast Reconstr Surg 11:131–135, 1995.
    Weissler MC, Miller E, Fortune MA: Sclerosing orbital pseudotumor: A unique clinicopathologic entity. Ann Otol Rhinol Laryngol 98:496–501, 1989.

19. **How is NSOI treated?**
    High-dose oral corticosteroids are the mainstay of treatment. The recommended starting dose for prednisone is 1 mg/kg/day with a maximum adult dose of 60–80 mg/day, tapering to 10 mg/day every 1–2 weeks. The response is usually quick with resolution of pain and proptosis within 24–48 hours of onset of the treatment.

    Cockerham KP, Hong SH, Browne EE: Orbital inflammation. Curr Neurol Neurosci Rep 3:401–409, 2003.

20. **What if a patient fails to respond to or is intolerant of steroids?**
    Alternative therapies include antimetabolites (azathioprine, methotrexate), T-cell inhibitors (cyclosporine), and alkylating agents (cyclophosphamide). Low-dose external beam radiation has also been shown to be effective.

    Cockerham KP, Hong SH, Browne EE: Orbital inflammation. Curr Neurol Neurosci Rep 3:401–409, 2003.

KEY POINTS: NONSPECIFIC ORBITAL INFLAMMATION

1. Nonspecific orbital inflammation is a diagnosis of exclusion.
2. Onset is usually acute and painful.
3. Inflammation may be unilateral or bilateral.
4. Children often have uveitis and eosinophilia concurrently.
5. Subtle edema of retrobulbar fat is an early finding on imaging.

21. **What is the most common specific orbital inflammation?**
    Thyroid-associated orbitopathy.

22. **How can thyroid-associated orbitopathy be differentiated from orbital myositis?**
    Radiographically, myositis, a nonspecific inflammation of an extraocular muscle, can be distinguished from thyroid-related orbitopathy, a specific orbital inflammation. Both demonstrate thickening of the muscle belly, but only myositis shows thickening of the tendon insertion as well.

23. **What infections can occur in the orbit?**
    Microbial, fungal (e.g., rhino-orbital mucormycosis, aspergillosis), parasitic (e.g., echinococcosis, cysticercosis, trichinosis), tuberculosis, and syphilis.

24. **Name the most common source of orbital cellulites.**
    Contiguous spread of bacterial infection from the sinuses, often the ethmoid sinus.

25. **In adults, what pathogens usually cause orbital cellulitis?**
    Staphylococcus aureus or streptococci.

26. **In a 2-year-old patient, what pathogen might be a likely cause of orbital cellulitis?**
Haemophilus influenzae.

27. **How is orbital cellulitis treated?**
Medical care consists of the proper use of the appropriate antibiotics. Preseptal cellulitis may be treated with oral antibiotics. Orbital cellulitis requires intravenous administration of antibiotics.

28. **When should surgery be undertaken?**
If the response to appropriate antibiotic therapy is poor within 48–72 hours or if the CT scan shows the sinuses to be completely opacified, surgical drainage should be considered. Subperiosteal or intraorbital abscess formations are other indications for surgical drainage if there is a decrease in vision, development of an afferent pupillary defect, or failure of proptosis to resolve despite appropriate antibiotic therapy.

29. **What are the major categories of orbital vasculitis?**
Wegener's granulomatosis, hypersensitivity vasculitis, periarteritis nodosa, Churg-Strauss syndrome.

30. **Are orbital and ocular involvement common in Wegener's granulomatosis?**
Yes, involvement is seen in approximately 50% of cases in both systemic and limited Wegener's granulomatosis.

31. **Describe the features of orbital Wegener's granulomatosis.**
   - **Clinical:** Bilaterality, respiratory tract/sinus/mastoid involvement, scleritis, limbal corneal infiltrates
   - **Imaging:** Three patterns; diffuse orbital involvement (may or may not be bilateral), lacrimal involvement, or midline involvement associated with bone erosion
   - **Laboratory:** Positive c-ANCA (although initially not positive in limited form)
   - **Pathology:** Mixed inflammation "cuffing" vessels, fat necrosis, lipid-laden macrophages, granulomatous microabsesses

   Perry C, Shevland JJE: Limited Wegener's granulomatosis. Austral Radiol 28:106–113, 1984.

CHAPTER 37

PTOSIS

Carolyn S. Repke, MD

1. **How is ptosis classified?**
   Ptosis is classified by either time of onset or etiology. By onset, ptosis is either congenital or acquired. By etiology, ptosis may be neurogenic, aponeurotic, mechanical, myogenic, or traumatic.

2. **What is the most common cause of acquired ptosis?**
   Acquired ptosis is most often the result of disinsertion or attenuation of the levator aponeurosis, which is most commonly related to aging but can be related to chronic ocular inflammation or eyelid edema (Fig. 37-1).

3. **What clinical findings help to differentiate congenital ptosis from acquired aponeurotic ptosis?**
   Patients with aponeurotic ptosis have a ptotic eyelid in all positions of gaze. In downgaze the ptotic eyelid remains ptotic. Patients with congenital ptosis, however, demonstrate eyelid lag in downgaze. The ptotic eyelid frequently appears higher than the normal eyelid as the patient moves toward downgaze. This finding is caused by the maldevelopment of the levator muscle, with poor ability to contract in elevation as well as inability to relax as the eyelid moves to downgaze.

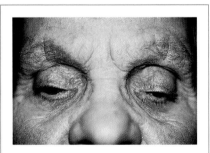

Figure 37-1. Involutional (aponeurotic) ptosis is characteristically mild to moderate with high upper eyelid crease. Deep sulci are seen in severe cases. Levator function is essentially normal. (From Kanski JJ: Clinical Ophthalmology: A Synopsis. New York, Butterworth-Heinemann, 2004.)

KEY POINTS: FEATURES OF APONEUROTIC PTOSIS

1. High eyelid crease

2. Moderate ptosis (3–4 mm)

3. Good levator function (>10 mm)

4. No eyelid lag on downgaze

4. **What are the features of congenital ptosis?**
   Congenital ptosis is dystrophy or maldevelopment in the levator muscle/superior rectus complex (Fig. 37-2). Most patients demonstrate poor levator function on examination and, at surgery, have fatty infiltration of the levator muscle. This myogenic abnormality causes an inability

of the levator to relax on downgaze, resulting in eyelid lag. Patients may or may not demonstrate motility defects because of superior rectus dysfunction. Approximately 75% of cases are unilateral.

Ahmadi AJ, Sires BS: Ptosis in infants and children. Int Ophthalmol Clin 42:15–29, 2002.

5. **What causes pseudoptosis?**
Causes of pseudoptosis (Fig. 37-3) include the following:
- Hypotropia on the ptotic side
- Eyelid retraction on the opposite side
- Enophthalmos/phthisis bulbi
- Anophthalmos/microphthalmos
- Severe dermatochalasis

6. **What is the primary cause of ptosis after intraocular surgery?**
It is thought that levator dehiscence causes ptosis related to previous intraocular surgery. The exact etiology is uncertain; however, it has been linked to superior rectus bridal sutures, eyelid speculums, retrobulbar and peribulbar injections, and other draping maneuvers associated with manipulation of the eyelids. Affected patients probably had a tendency toward levator dehiscence preoperatively.

7. **What is the anatomic cause for the eyelid crease?**
The eyelid crease is formed by the levator aponeurotic attachments that travel through the orbicularis muscle to the skin. With aponeurotic ptosis, these attachments are disinserted, causing the eyelid crease to elevate.

8. **What neurologic conditions are associated with ptosis?**
Neurologic conditions that must be considered in a ptosis evaluation include third-nerve palsy, Horner's syndrome, myasthenia gravis, Marcus Gunn's jaw-winking syndrome, ophthalmoplegic migraine, and multiple sclerosis.

9. **What are the myogenic causes of ptosis?**
Muscular abnormalities associated with ptosis include myasthenia gravis,

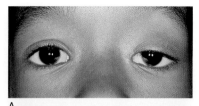

A

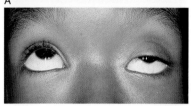

B

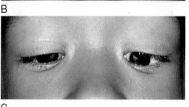

C

Figure 37-2. Simple congenital ptosis. *A,* Decreased levator muscle function occurs along with an indistinct upper eyelid crease. *B,* The ptosis is exaggerated in upgaze because of the poor function of the levator muscle. *C,* In downgaze the ptosis is reduced or absent because the fibrotic levator muscle cannot stretch. (From Custer PL: Blepharoptosis. In Yanoff M, Duker JS [eds]: Ophthalmology, 2nd ed. St. Louis, Mosby, 2004.)

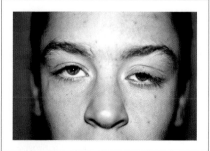

Figure 37-3. Left pseudoptosis caused by ipsilateral hypotropia. (Kanski JJ: Clinical Ophthalmology: A Systematic Approach, 5th ed. New York, Butterworth-Heinemann, 2003.)

muscular dystrophies, chronic progressive external ophthalmoplegia, oculopharyngeal dystrophy, and congenital maldevelopment of the levator.

10. **What are the features of blepharophimosis syndrome?**
Blepharophimosis syndrome (Fig. 37-4) is a congenital autosomal dominant disorder characterized by ptosis, epicanthus, blepharophimosis (narrowing of the palpebral fissure in all dimensions), and telecanthus (widening of the distance between the medial canthi). Some patients also may demonstrate a flat nasal bridge, lower eyelid ectropions, and hypoplastic orbital rims.

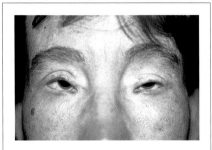

Figure 37-4. Blepharophimosis with bilateral ptosis, eyelid phimosis, telecanthus, and epicanthus inversus. (From Kanski JJ: Clinical Ophthalmology: A Test Yourself Atlas, 2nd ed. New York, Butterworth-Heinemann, 2002.)

11. **What are the signs and symptoms of myasthenia gravis?**
The history of any patient with acquired ptosis should include questions searching for symptoms of myasthenia gravis. Patients may comment on variability in the degree of ptosis from day to day. They also may notice increased ptosis during periods of fatigue or toward the end of the day. They may give a history of diplopia or difficulty with swallowing as well as other muscular weakness.

On examination, patients may demonstrate eyelid fatigue on sustained upgaze, with curtaining of the eyelid on returning to the primary position. They also may demonstrate a Cogan's eyelid twitch after attempted upgaze. On return to primary position, the eyelid may show an upward twitch before it settles to its final resting place. Orbicularis strength may be weak, allowing the examiner to open the patient's eyelids even during attempted forceful closure.

KEY POINTS: FEATURES OF OCULAR MYASTHENIA GRAVIS

1. Ptosis

2. Ocular misalignment

3. Fatigability of eyelids

4. Cogan's lid twitch

5. Orbicularis weakness

12. **What measurements should be taken during the preoperative examination of patients with ptosis?**
   - **Marginal reflex distance:** The distance from the corneal light reflex in primary gaze to the upper eyelid margin; demonstrates the distance of the upper eyelid from the visual axis; evaluated in primary position with the action of the frontalis muscle negated.
   - **Levator function:** Measures the entire excursion of the eyelid in millimeters from extreme downgaze to upgaze; with the action of the frontalis muscle manually negated; determines the

surgical procedure to be performed; function is considered to be normal (>15 mm), good (>8 mm), fair (5–7 mm), or poor (>4 mm).

- **Eyelid crease height:** The crease height is the distance from the eyelid margin to the skin crease.
- **Palpebral fissure width:** This is not an accurate measurement of ptosis because the lower eyelid position can affect this value (e.g., Horner's syndrome with reverse ptosis of the lower eyelid).

Other critical parts of the preoperative evaluation include a careful pupillary examination for anisocoria, a cover test for strabismus, and evaluation of corneal sensation and tear film. Often a Schirmer test is performed to measure basal tear production. The lid position is carefully evaluated in primary position with the action of the frontalis muscle negated. The eyelid position is also evaluated in downgaze, looking for eyelid lag that suggests congenital ptosis or previous thyroid ophthalmopathy. The eyelid is evaluated in upgaze for signs of muscle fatigue and curtaining, which suggest myasthenia gravis. Finally, it is important to document the presence of a good Bell's phenomenon (upshoot of the cornea with eyelid closure).

Kersten RA: Orbit, Eyelids, and Lacrimal System: Basic and Clinical Science Course. San Francisco, American Academy of Ophthalmology, 2006.

13. **How does Hering's law affect ptosis?**
Hering's law of equivalent innervation of yoke muscles applies to the two levator muscles. It needs to be considered during the preoperative evaluation to determine accurately the degree of ptosis on each side. The normal eyelid in a patient with unilateral ptosis may become ptotic when bilateral stimulation is broken. The eye with which the patient prefers to fixate affects the degree to which Hering's law contributes to ptosis. If the ptotic eye is preferred for fixation, the opposite eyelid may develop a retracted position because of increased stimulation during attempts to open the ptotic eyelid. On occluding the ptotic fixating eye, the previously retracted eyelid may resume a more normal position.

Gausas RE, Goldstein SM: Ptosis in the elderly patient. Int Ophthalmol Clin 42:61–74, 2002.

14. **What is the Neosynephrine test?**
The Neosynephrine test is an evaluation of the effect of Müller's muscle contraction on the degree of ptosis. One drop of 2.5% phenylephrine is placed in the eye. After 5 minutes, the degree of ptosis is reevaluated. The phenylephrine causes contraction of the sympathetic Horner's muscle, sometimes causing dramatic improvement in the degree of ptosis. If phenylephrine corrects the ptosis completely, many surgeons elect to perform a Müller's muscle resection as opposed to a levator resection.

Bassin RE, Putterman AM: Ptosis in young adults. Int Ophthalmol Clin 42:31–43, 2002.

15. **What are the surgical and nonsurgical approaches to the correction of ptosis?**
The most common surgical approaches to ptosis correction include levator resection, either from an internal or external approach; Müller's muscle resection; and frontalis suspension. A nonsurgical option is ptosis eyelid crutches, which may be secured to spectacle lenses. Although rarely used, spectacle adaptations are a reasonable option for patients with neurologic ptosis who have a poor Bell's phenomenon and are considered to be at high risk for exposure keratopathy.

McCord CD Jr, Tannebaum M, Nunery WR: Oculoplastic Surgery, 3rd ed. Philadelphia, Lippincott-Raven, 1995.

16. **What are the complications of ptosis surgery?**
The most common complication is overcorrection or undercorrection of the ptosis and/or abnormalities in eyelid contour. Other complications include eyelid lag on downgaze and lagophthalmos on eyelid closure. These complications may result in corneal exposure and superficial keratopathy or even corneal ulceration and scarring. Abnormalities in the eyelid

crease and eyelid fold, loss of eyelashes, conjunctival prolapse, and upper eyelid ectropion also may complicate surgery. In addition, retrobulbar hemorrhage is a risk with all eyelid surgery, and, although rare, infection is a potential complication.

Schaefer AJ, Schaefer DP: Classification and correction of ptosis. In Stewart WB (ed): Surgery of the Eyelid, Orbit, and Lacrimal System, vol. 2. San Francisco, American Academy of Ophthalmology, 1994, pp 128–131.

17. **What is Marcus Gunn's jaw-winking syndrome?**
Marcus Gunn's syndrome is a unilateral congenital ptosis with synkinetic innervation of the levator and ipsilateral pterygoid muscle. Patients demonstrate retraction of the ptotic eyelid on stimulation of the ipsilateral pterygoid muscles by either opening the mouth or moving the jaw to the opposite side.

18. **Describe the anatomy of Whitnall's ligament and its significance in ptosis.**
Whitnall's ligament, also known as the superior transverse ligament, is a condensation of collagen and elastic fibers on the anterior levator sheath as it changes from muscle to aponeurosis. It attaches medially near the trochlea and laterally traverses through the lacrimal gland, attaching to the lateral orbital wall approximately 10 mm above the lateral orbital tubercle. It serves as a suspensory ligament for the upper eyelid and is the point where the vector forces of the levator muscle transfer from an anterior-posterior direction to a superior-inferior direction. It is an important landmark for performing large levator resections.

Kersten RC: Orbit, Eyelids, and Lacrimal System: Basic and Clinical Science Course. San Francisco, American Academy of Ophthalmology, 2006.

19. **What is the concern when Horner's syndrome presents with pain?**
Patients with neck pain, facial pain, or headache and acute Horner's syndrome should be suspected of having a carotid artery dissection. Work-up should be urgent and include magnetic resonance imaging or angiography and carotid Doppler ultrasound of the neck. A carotid dissection usually requires urgent anticoagulation and neurovascular consultation.

Chan C, Paine M, O'Day J: Carotid dissection: A common cause of Horner's syndrome. Clin Exper Ophthalmol 29:411–415, 2001.

KEY POINTS: FEATURES OF HORNER'S SYNDROME

1. Mild ptosis (1–2 mm)
2. Miosis
3. Anhydrosis
4. Reverse ptosis of the lower eyelid
5. Hypopigmentation of iris (congenital cases)

20. **Name some useful tests for diagnosing myasthenia gravis.**
   - Ice test (in office)
   - Acetylcholine receptor antibody blood test: False-negative results in 50% of cases
   - Edrophonium chloride (Tensilon) test
   - Single-fiber electromyography (orbicularis muscle)

Kerrison JB, Newman NJ: Five things oculoplastic surgeons should know about neuro-ophthalmology. Ophthal Plast Reconstr Surg 15:372–377, 2002.

21. **Name some causes of acquired ptosis in young adults.**

Levator aponeurosis dehiscence can certainly occur in a younger age group, but ptosis in younger adults should prompt thought of other causes as well. History and clinical exam should look for obvious neurologic, myogenic, and mechanical causes. Old photographs should be viewed to rule out a longstanding problem. In addition, consideration should be given to the following:

- Contact lens wear (ptosis from manipulation of eyelids or a lost lens under the eyelid)
- Allergies, blepharochalasis, or other source of recurrent eyelid edema
- Eyelid rubbing
- Botox—ptosis is a possible side effect of treatment and is being seen more frequently due to the rise in popularity of cosmesis in younger patients. (Patients should be assured that the ptosis will not be permanent.)

Bassin RE, Putterman AM: Ptosis in young adults. Int Ophthalmol Clin 42:31–43, 2002.

22. **Describe the ice test and its use in the diagnosis of ptosis.**

An ice pack is held over the ptotic eyelid for 10 minutes, and the patient is then reexamined. The cold temperature inhibits acetylcholinesterase at the neuromuscular junction, therefore enhancing neuromuscular transmission and raising the ptotic eyelid in myasthenics (poor man's Tensilon test). A positive result should prompt a further work-up.

Sethi KD, Rivner MH, Swift TR: Ice pack test for myasthenia gravis. Neurology 37:1383–1385, 1987.

CHAPTER 38

EYELID TUMORS

Janice A. Gault, MD

1. **What clues are helpful in determining whether an eyelid lesion is benign or malignant?**

    The size, location, age of onset, rate of growth, presence of bleeding or ulceration, any color change, history of malignancy, or prior radiation therapy are important. A thorough examination is necessary. Malignant or inflammatory lesions may cause loss of eyelashes and distortion of meibomian gland orifices, but only malignant lesions destroy the orifices. If a lesion is near the lacrimal punctum, evaluate for invasion to the lacrimal system. Probing and irrigation may be necessary. Palpate lesions for fixation to deep tissues or bone. Regional lymph nodes also should be examined for enlargement. Restriction of extraocular motility and proptosis are clues to localized invasion. If a sebaceous adenocarcinoma or melanoma is diagnosed, system evaluation should target lung, liver, bones, and neurologic systems. Any lesion to be treated or observed needs photographic documentation.

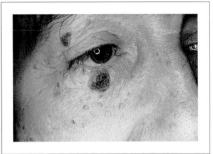

Figure 38-1. Seborrheic keratosis is a greasy, brown, flat lesion with a verrucous surface and a "stuck-on" appearance. (From Kanski JJ: Clinical Ophthalmology: A Synopsis. New York, Butterworth-Heinemann, 2004.)

2. **What is the difference between seborrheic keratosis and actinic keratosis?**

    Both are papillomas, an irregular frondlike projection of skin with a central vascular pedicle. These lesions are more common in elderly patients.

    - **Seborrheic keratosis** is pigmented, oily, and hyperkeratotic. It appears stuck onto the skin (Fig. 38-1). A shaved biopsy is all that is needed to diagnose and treat. It has no increased risk for malignant change.

    - **Actinic keratosis** is found in sun-exposed areas and appears as a flat, scaly, or papillary lesion (Fig. 38-2). This premalignant lesion may evolve into either a basal cell or squamous cell carcinoma.

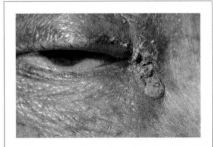

Figure 38-2. Actinic keratosis is a dry, scaly lesion caused by sun exposure and occurring in fair-skinned people. (From Spalton DJ, Hitchings RA, Hunter PA: Atlas of Clinical Ophthalmology, 2nd ed. St. Louis, Mosby, 1994.)

3. **What eyelid lesion is associated with a chronic follicular conjunctivitis?**
   Molluscum contagiosum. A virus causes the multiple waxy nodules with umbilicated centers. They may resolve spontaneously but frequently require surgical excision or cautery to prevent reinfection.

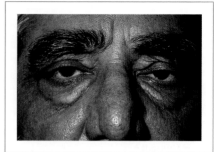

Figure 38-3. Patient with xanthelasma. (From Kanski JJ: Clinical Ophthalmology: A Systematic Approach, 5th ed. New York, Butterworth-Heinemann, 2003.)

4. **What blood tests should you order in young patients with the lesions shown in Fig 38-3?**
   The appropriate tests are cholesterol level, triglyceride level, and fasting blood sugar. Xanthelasma are yellowish plaques found at the medial canthal area of the upper and lower eyelids. They are collections of lipid. In older patients, xanthelasma are common and no cause for concern. In younger patients they may be a sign of hypercholesterolemia, a congenital disorder of cholesterol metabolism, or diabetes mellitus. They may be removed for cosmetic purposes, but they may recur.

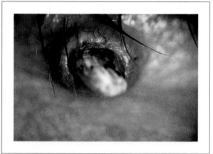

Figure 38-4. Keratoacanthoma is a fast-growing nodule with a keratin-filled crater that spontaneously involutes after several months. (From Kanski JJ: Clinical Ophthalmology: A Synopsis. New York, Butterworth-Heinemann, 2004.)

5. **What is a keratoacanthoma? What malignancy does it simulate?**
   A keratoacanthoma is a rapidly growing lesion that appears over several weeks. It is hyperkeratotic with a central crater that often resolves spontaneously (Fig. 38-4). Clinically, the lesion simulates a "rodent ulcer" basal cell carcinoma. Microscopically, the lesion appears similar to squamous cell carcinoma. It may occur near the edge of areas of chronic inflammation, such as a burn, or on the periphery of a true malignant neoplasm. If you are sure of the diagnosis, it is reasonable to observe. However, because it may cause destruction of the eyelid margin, lesions in this area are often removed surgically. In addition, steroids may be injected into the lesion to hasten resolution.

6. **What is the most common malignant eyelid tumor?**
   Basal cell carcinoma, which is most common in middle-aged or elderly patients.

7. **What are its two clinical presentations?**
   Nodular (Fig. 38-5) and morpheaform (Fig. 38-6) tumors. A nodular tumor is a firm, raised, pearly, discrete mass, often with telangiectasias over the tumor margins. If the center of the lesion is ulcerated, it is called a *rodent ulcer*. Morpheaform tumors are firm, flat lesions with indistinct borders. They tend to be more aggressive and have a worse prognosis than the nodular variety.

8. **In order of frequency, where do basal cell carcinomas present?**
   The most common location is the lower eyelid, followed by the medial canthus, lateral canthus, and upper eyelid.

9. **Do basal cell carcinomas metastasize?**
   Lesions grow only by local extension.

10. **If basal cell carcinomas do not metastasize, why be concerned with them?**
    Ocular adnexal basal cell carcinomas have a 3% mortality rate. The vast majority of patients have canthal area disease, prior radiation therapy, or clinically neglected tumors. Tumors near the medial canthus may invade the orbit via the lacrimal drainage system. Extension to the brain also may occur. Removal of the tumor can be quite disfiguring in some cases.

11. **How do you treat tumors with a suspicious lesion?**
    First, do an incisional biopsy of the lesion to confirm the diagnosis. Permanent sections must be done, not merely frozen sections. If a basal cell lesion is found, there are several possibilities for treatment.
    - **Large surgical resection:** A large surgical resection with frozen sections is performed to confirm the entire tumor has been removed. If the lacrimal system must be removed, do not perform a dacryocystorhinostomy at the same time as the primary surgery. Wait at least 1 year to prevent iatrogenic seeding of the nose.
    - **Mohs' lamellar resection:** The complete tumor is removed, sparing as much healthy tissue as possible. The excised bits of tissue are sent to pathology during the procedure to confirm the presence or absence of tumor and therefore direct the subsequent course of the surgery. This procedure preserves a larger amount of normal tissue, allowing improved function and cosmesis. Sometimes it even saves the globe, whereas conventional surgery may require exenteration. This time-consuming procedure is not available everywhere.
    - **Radiation:** Basal cell carcinoma is radiosensitive, but treatment is not curative, only palliative (see question 10). Radiation should be reserved for elderly patients who are unable to undergo surgery.
    - **Cryotherapy:** This treatment is not curative and should be used only palliatively.

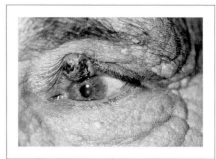

Figure 38-5. Nodular basal cell carcinoma of the eyelid. A firm, pink-colored basal cell carcinoma of the left upper eyelid with raised border, superficial telangiectatic vessels, and characteristic central ulceration These lesions are more commonly seen on the lower eyelid. (From Vaughan GJ, Dortzbach RK, Gayre GS: Eyelid malignancies. In Yanoff M, Duker JS [eds]: Ophthalmology, 2nd ed. St. Louis, Mosby, 2004, pp 711–719. Courtesy of Dr. Morton Smith.)

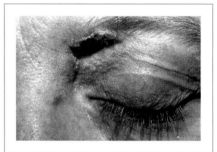

Figure 38-6. Unlike nodular basal cell tumors, morpheaform basal call carcinomas have less clearly defined surgical margins. (From Spalton DJ, Hitchings RA, Hunter PA: Atlas of Clinical Ophthalmology, 2nd ed. St. Louis, Mosby, 1994.)

12. **How do you treat a recurrent tumor that has limited the extraocular motility from invasion of the orbit?**
   Exenteration.

13. **Describe basal cell nevus syndrome.**
   This autosomal dominant disease is characterized by development of multiple basal cell carcinomas at an early age. Patients also have skeletal, endocrine, and neurologic abnormalities.

14. **What are the complications of radiation to the area around the eye?**
   Keratitis sicca, cataracts, radiation retinopathy (if more than 3000 rads are used), optic neuropathy, entropion, lacrimal stenosis, and dermatitis. In young children the bones of the orbit may not grow normally, causing a significant cosmetic deformity.

KEY POINTS: COMPLICATIONS OF RADIATION TREATMENT AROUND THE OCULAR AREA

1. Keratitis sicca

2. Cataracts

3. Radiation retinopathy

4. Optic neuropathy

5. Entropion

6. Lacrimal stenosis

7. Dermatitis

8. Cosmetic deformity in children (orbital bones may not develop normally)

15. **Where do squamous cell carcinomas usually present around the eye?**
   The upper eyelid (Fig. 38-7). However, basal cell carcinomas are 40 times more common.

16. **How are patients with squamous cell carcinomas treated?**
   Similarly to patients with basal cell carcinomas. However, squamous cell carcinomas are more aggressive locally and metastasize via the blood or lymph system. Neuronal spread is described and can be fatal. Exenteration is suggested for recurrences.

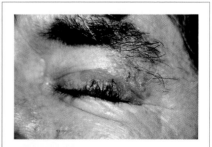

Figure 38-7. Squamous cell carcinoma of the upper eyelid. (From Kanski JJ: Clinical Ophthalmology: A Synopsis. New York, Butterworth-Heinemann, 2004.)

17. **A 60-year-old man has had a chalazion removed from his left upper eyelid three times. It has recurred yet again. How do you treat it?**

A sebaceous gland carcinoma must be suspected. Lesions arise from the meibomian glands in the tarsal plate, Zeis' glands near the lashes, and sebaceous glands in the caruncle and brow. Any recurrent chalazia must be biopsied for pathologic evaluation. The lesion can mimic benign ocular diseases such as chronic blepharoconjunctivitis, corneal pannus, and superior limbic keratitis. Patients who do not respond to treatment should be biopsied, especially those with loss of lashes and destruction of meibomian gland orifices.

18. **How is the biopsy performed? How is the specimen sent to the lab? What stains should be requested?**

Sebaceous cell carcinoma is multicentric and undergoes pagetoid spread. Multiple sites must be biopsied, including bulbar and palpebral conjunctiva, even if they appear uninvolved. A full-thickness eyelid biopsy may be necessary to make the diagnosis because the lesion originates deep in the tissues. The tissue should not be placed in alcohol, which will dissolve the fat from the specimen and make the diagnosis more difficult. Oil red O stain will stain the fat red.

19. **How are patients with sebaceous cell carcinoma treated?**

Because sebaceous cell carcinoma is an aggressive and potentially fatal disease, wide surgical excision is mandatory. Some physicians prefer exenteration as a primary treatment. Mohs' microsurgery should be used with caution because the disease is multicentric with skip areas and some lesions may be missed. The tumor may spread hematogenously, lymphatically, or by direct extension.

20. **What is the most common type of malignant melanoma of the eyelid?**

Superficial spreading melanoma accounts for 80% of cases; lentigo maligna and nodular melanoma each occur in 10% of cases. However, all are rare and represent less than 1% of eyelid tumors. Superficial spreading melanoma occurs both in sun-exposed and in nonexposed areas. Lentigo maligna, also known as melanotic freckle of Hutchinson, is sun induced. Both have a long horizontal growth phase before invading the deeper tissues. Nodular melanoma is more aggressive with earlier vertical invasion. Treatment is wide surgical excision and lymph node dissection if microscopic evidence of lymphatic or vascular involvement is noted.

21. **How do you follow a patient who has had an eyelid malignancy?**

Once the patient has healed from the initial treatment, reevaluate every 6–12 months. Patients are at risk for additional malignancies. A thorough examination by a dermatologist may reveal cutaneous malignancies elsewhere.

BIBLIOGRAPHY

1. Albert DM, Jakobiec FA: Principles and Practice of Ophthalmology, vol. 3. Philadelphia, W.B. Saunders, 1999.
2. American Academy of Ophthalmology: Basic and Clinical Science Course on Orbit, Eyelids, and Lacrimal System. San Francisco, 1999.
3. Kunimoto DY, Kanitkar KD, Makar M: The Wills Eye Manual, 4th ed. Philadelphia, Lippincott, Williams & Wilkins, 2004.

UVEITIS

Tamara R. Vrabec, MD, Caroline R. Baumal, MD, Vincent F. Baldassano, Jr., MD, Vinay N. Desai, MD, and Jay S. Duker, MD

CHAPTER 39

UVEITIS IN THE IMMUNOCOMPETENT PATIENT

1. **What is uveitis?**
   Uveitis is inflammation of the pigmented middle layer of the eye, the uvea. Clinically, it may be classified as follows:
   - Anterior uveitis (iritis)
   - Panuveitis, or inflammation of both the anterior and posterior segments
   - Intermediate uveitis, an inflammation of the anterior segment with associated vitreous cells but no retinal or choroidal involvement
   - Posterior uveitis, in which inflammation of the retina, choroids, or sclera is predominant
   The incidence of uveitis may differ in different patient populations. This chapter focuses on uveitis in the developed Western world.

2. **Name and describe the typical clinical signs of anterior uveitis.**
   Cells and flare in the anterior chamber's aqueous fluid and keratic precipitates (KP). Flare is leakage of protein into the aqueous secondary to increased permeability of iris vessels. Keratic precipitates are accumulations of white blood cells on the endothelial surface of the cornea. They may vary in size and location. Depending on the duration and severity of uveitis, adhesions can develop between the iris and lens surface (posterior synechiae [PS]) and between the iris and peripheral cornea (peripheral anterior synechiae [PAS]).

3. **How is granulomatous uveitis distinguished from nongranulomatous uveitis?**
   Uveitis may be classified as granulomatous or nongranulomatous based on pathologic features. Histopathologically, granulomatous uveitis is characterized by nodular collections of epithelioid cells and giant cells surrounded by lymphocytes, whereas nongranulomatous uveitis is characterized by diffuse infiltration of lymphocytes and plasma cells are present. Both of these entities have relatively distinct clinical appearances.

4. **What are the *distinctive* clinical features of granulomatous anterior uveitis?**
   Granulomatous uveitis is often chronic (greater than 4 months' duration). Anterior segment examination may reveal "mutton-fat" (large, "greasy") KP, nodules on the iris surface (Busacca nodules), and PAS. Anterior chamber cells and flare are also present (Table 39-1).

5. **What are the clinical features of nongranulomatous anterior uveitis (NGAU)?**
   NGAU is often acute with an abrupt onset of symptoms that in most cases are self-limited, lasting less than 4 months. Clinical signs include fine KP most often located on the inferior cornea, anterior chamber cells, and flare. PS may or may not be present, depending on the duration and severity of the inflammation. Certain forms of NGAU may present with hypopyon (Table 39-1).

6. **Can iris nodules occur in nongranulomatous anterior uveitis?**
   Koeppe nodules, which are grayish-white nodules that appear on the pupillary margin, may be present in either granulomatous or nongranulomatous anterior uveitis.

TABLE 39-1. FEATURES OF GRANULOMATOUS AND NONGRANULOMATOUS ANTERIOR UVEITIS

Features	Granulomatous	Nongranulomatous
Onset	Often insidious	Acute (usually)
Course	Chronic	Acute or chronic
Injection	+	+++ (usually)
Pain	+/−	+++ (usually)
Iris nodules	+++ (Busacca and Koeppe)	− (Koeppe on occasion)
Keratic precipitates	Large, mutton-fat	Small, fine
Other	Dense posterior synechiae	+/− posterior synechiae, hypopyon

+ = present, − = absent.

7. **Is the distribution of KP helpful in narrowing a differential diagnosis?**
   Yes. In Fuchs' heterochromic iridocyclitis, the fine "stellate" KP are found scattered diffusely on the entire posterior surface of the cornea, unlike most KP, which are located in the inferior cornea.

8. **Is dilated fundus examination indicated in all patients with anterior uveitis?**
   Yes. All patients who appear to have anterior uveitis require dilated examination to identify potentially blinding posterior segment disease that may otherwise be missed.

9. **What is the most common cause of NGAU?**
   Human leukocyte antigen (HLA)-B27–associated conditions account for approximately 45% of acute NGAU. These conditions include ankylosing spondylitis (AS), Reiter's disease, psoriatic arthritis, and inflammatory bowel disease. Review of systems is useful in differentiation (Table 39-2).

   Brewerton DA, Hart FD, Nicholls A, et al: Ankylosing spondylitis and HL-A 27. Lancet. 1:904–907, 1973.
   Tay-Kearney ML, Schwam BL, Lowder C, et al: Clinical features and associated systemic diseases of HLA-B27 uveitis. Am J Ophthalmol 121:47–56, 1996.

10. **Describe the typical NGAU seen in HLA-B27 disease.**
    Typically, the anterior uveitis is unilateral and self-limited. It may present in alternate eyes over time. A fibrinous response in the anterior chamber and, in some cases hypopyon, may occur.

11. **What is the incidence of HLA-B27 in the general population?**
    The incidence of HLA-B27 in the general population is 8%. In contrast, it is present in 90% of patients with AS and 80% of those with Reiter's disease.

12. **What other conditions are in the differential diagnosis of acute NGAU?**
    More than 50% of cases are idiopathic. Other uveitides that may present with clinical findings consistent with NGAU are listed in Tables 39-3 and 39-4. Note that some forms of granulomatous uveitis (e.g., sarcoidosis, syphilis, Lyme disease, and toxoplasmosis) may present with nongranulomatous features. Nongranulomatous conditions do not present in a granulomatous fashion.

13. **Discuss the most common cause of uveitis in children.**
    Juvenile idiopathic arthritis (JIA) is the most common identifiable cause of uveitis in children. The uveitis is anterior and chronic and can lead to serious visual loss. The eye is white and

TABLE 39-2. DIFFERENTIATION OF HLA-B27–ASSOCIATED CONDITIONS

HLA-B27–associated Disease	Symptoms	Systemic Clinical Findings
Ankylosing spondylitis	Stiffness and low back pain worsen with inactivity	Spinal fusion, sacroiliac joint disease No skin findings 25% develop NGAU
Reiter's disease	Same plus painless mouth ulcers, heel pain, painful urination	Keratoderma blennorrhagica, circinate balanitis, urethritis, polyarthritis Conjunctivitis is typically bilateral and papillary
Psoriatic arthritis	Skin rash, arthritis	Psoriasis
Inflammatory bowel disease	Gastrointestinal symptoms	Erythema nodosum

HLA = human leukocyte antigen, NGAU = nongranulomatous anterior uveitis.

quiet externally, and children often do not complain of symptoms, which causes a delay in diagnosis. Young girls (age 4 years) with pauciarticular JIA, who are rheumatoid factor-negative and antinuclear antibody (ANA)-positive, are at highest risk. These children should be screened every few months for uveitis. Boys may develop more acute recurrent inflammation at a later age (9 years). A majority of children with JIA are HLA-B27–positive and may develop ankylosing spondylitis (AS) later in life.

14. **Which condition may produce spontaneous hyphema in a child?**
    Juvenile xanthogranuloma is a systemic condition that consists of one or more nonmalignant inflammatory tumors. Ocular lesions include iris xanthogranuloma masses, recurrent anterior chamber cellular reaction, and spontaneous hyphema (Fig. 39-1). Diagnosis is made with iris biopsy or by finding similar lesions on the skin.

    Clements DB: Juvenile xanthogranuloma treated with local steroids. Br J Ophthalmol 50:663–665, 1966.
    Zimmerman LE: Ocular lesions of juvenile xanthogranuloma. Nevoxanthoendothelioma. Trans Am Acad Ophthalmol Otolaryngol 69:412–439, 1965.

15. **What is the most common cause of granulomatous anterior uveitis?**
    Sarcoidosis is the most common cause of granulomatous anterior uveitis in adults. Differential diagnosis includes syphilis, Lyme disease, *Propionibacterium acnes* (pseudophakic patients), tuberculosis, and herpes virus infection. Other more common causes are also listed in Tables 39-3 and 39-4.

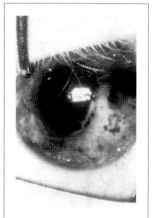

Figure 39-1. Large, solitary juvenile xanthogranuloma that had given rise to a spontaneous hyphema in a 7-month-old patient. (From Shields JA, Shields CL: Intraocular Tumors: A Text and Atlas. Philadelphia, W.B. Saunders, 1992.)

TABLE 39-3. MORE COMMON INFECTIOUS CAUSES OF UVEITIS

Disease	Granulomatous Versus Nongranulomatous	Clinical Presentation	Infectious Agent
Syphilis	Granulomatous*	Anterior, pan, or posterior	*Treponema pallidum*
Acute retinal necrosis	Granulomatous	Panuveitis	Herpes simplex or zoster viruses
Chronic postoperative endophthalmitis	Granulomatous	Anterior or intermediate	*Propionibacterium acnes*
Lyme disease	Granulomatous*	Predominantly intermediate	*Borrelia burgdorferi* via *Ixodes* tick bite
Tuberculosis	Granulomatous	Panuveitis	*Mycobacterium tuberculosis*
Toxoplasmosis	Granulomatous*	Pan or posterior	*Toxoplasma gondii*
Cat-scratch disease	Granulomatous	Panuveitis	*Bartonella henselae*
Toxocariasis	Granulomatous	Panuveitis	*Toxocara canis*
Onchocerciasis	Nongranulomatous	Panuveitis	*Onchocerca volvulus*
Ocular histoplasmosis	No anterior chamber or vitreous cells	Posterior	*Histoplasma capsulatum*
Fungal choroiditis	Granulomatous	Predominantly posterior	*Cryptococcus, Aspergillus, Candida* species
Diffuse unilateral subacute neuroretinitis (DUSN)	Nongranulomatous	Posterior	*Baylisascaris procyonis*

*May also have nongranulomatous anterior uveitis.

TABLE 39-4. MORE COMMON NONINFECTIOUS CAUSES OF UVEITIS

Disease	Granulomatous Versus Nongranulomatous	Clinical Presentation	Secrets
JIA	Nongranulomatous	Anterior	See text
HLA-B27–associated uveitis	Nongranulomatous	Anterior	See text
Fuchs' iridocyclitis	Nongranulomatous	Anterior	Iris heterochromia
			No PAS/PS
Kawasaki syndrome	Nongranulomatous	Anterior	Rash, lymphadenopathy, fever, cardiac disease in children
TINU syndrome	Nongranulomatous	Anterior	Cellular casts in urine
Sarcoidosis	Chronic granulomatous	Anterior, posterior, or panuveitis	Clinical findings depend on age
	Acute nongranulomatous		
Pars planitis	Nongranulomatous	Intermediate	16% may develop MS
	If granulomatous, suspect MS		
Juvenile xanthogranuloma	Nongranulomatous	Anterior or intermediate	See text
Phacoanaphylactic uveitis	Granulomatous	Intermediate uveitis	Autoimmunity to lens proteins post trauma or cataract surgery
Multifocal choroiditis	Nongranulomatous	Panuveitis	Myopia
			30% develop CNVM

Continued

TABLE 39-4. MORE COMMON NONINFECTIOUS CAUSES OF UVEITIS—CONT'D

Disease	Granulomatous Versus Nongranulomatous	Clinical Presentation	Secrets
Birdshot chorioretinitis	Nongranulomatous	Posterior or panuveitis	HLA-A29 in more than 90%
APMPPE	Nongranulomatous	Posterior or panuveitis	Young patients, viral prodrome, bilateral
			Recurrence and CNVM rare
MEWDS	Nongranulomatous	Posterior	IVFA wreath
			Hyperfluorescence
Serpiginous choroiditis	Nongranulomatous	Posterior	Older patients, lesions contiguous to disc, unilateral
			Recurrence common, CNVM 30%
Behçet's disease	Nongranulomatous	Anterior	Hypopyon iritis
		Posterior	
		Panuveitis	
Vogt-Koyanagi-Harada syndrome	Granulomatous	Panuveitis	Starry sky
Sympathetic ophthalmia	Granulomatous	Panuveitis	See text

APMPPE = acute posterior multifocal placoid pigment epitheliopathy, CNVM = choroidal neovascular membrane, IVFA = fluorescein angiography, JIA = juvenile idiopathic arthritis, MEWDS = multiple evanescent white dot syndrome, MS = multiple sclerosis, PAS = peripheral anterior synechiae, PS = posterior synechiae, TINU = tubulo-interstitial nephritis–uveitis.

16. **What is the leading cause of blindness in the world?**
Onchocerciasis (river blindness), caused by *Onchocerca volvulus,* which is transmitted by the bite of a Simulium black fly, is the most common cause of world blindness. Sclerosing keratitis and extensive chorioretinal and optic atrophy cause severe visual impairment. The disease predominantly affects people in western and central Africa and Central America. Treatment of at-risk populations with antifilarial agents, including ivermectin, can dramatically reduce disease.

Cupp EW, Duke BO, Mackenzie CD, et al: The effects of long–term community level treatment with ivermectin (Mectizan) on adult *Onchocerca volvulus* in Latin America. Am J Trop Med Hyg 71:602–607, 2004.

17. **When is a systemic work-up indicated in uveitis?**
A systemic evaluation should be performed in patients with granulomatous uveitis, a second episode of nongranulomatous uveitis, positive review of systems, or severe disease.

18. **What studies should be ordered?**
A chest x-ray for sarcoidosis, fluorescent treponemal antibody absorption (FTA–ABS), urinalysis, and a complete blood count should be ordered in all patients. HLA-B27 titers should be ordered in patients with NGAU. Additional diagnostic tests may be appropriate based on clinical history and ocular and physical examination and positive review of systems.

19. **When are ocular tests helpful?**
Ocular tests including intravenous fluorescein angiography, B-scan ultrasound, and ocular coherence tomography (OCT) may help to characterize uveitis with posterior segment findings, or to detect complicating reasons for visual loss, such as cystoid macular edema.

20. **What may confound interpretation of serology for infectious agents?**
Because of its localized nature, an active intraocular infection is not always accompanied by a significant rise in systemic antibody titers. As well, serology may be unreliable in immunocompromised patients. Specimens from aqueous, vitreous, iris, retina, or choroid may be needed in cases of progressive sight-threatening uveitis in one or both eyes that is unresponsive to therapy. Antibody titers and polymerase chain reaction (PCR) of ocular fluids are useful when unusual infections are suspected and systemic antibody titers are nondiagnostic.

21. **What is the most common cause of intermediate uveitis?**
Pars planitis, an inflammation of unknown etiology, is the most common cause of intermediate uveitis. It is recognized by the typical inflammatory "snow bank" in the inferior pars plana. The clinical course is variable. Approximately 16% of patients may develop multiple sclerosis (MS). HLA-DR15 may play a role in both diseases. Granulomatous anterior uveitis may be present in MS-associated uveitis.

Raja SC, Jabs DA, Dunn JP, et al: Pars planitis: Clinical features and class II HLA associations. Ophthalmology 106:594–599, 1999.
Zein G, Berta A, Foster CS: Multiple sclerosis-associated uveitis. Ocul Immunol Inflamm 12:137–142, 2004.

22. **What are the causes of visual loss in pars planitis?**
Cystoid macular edema is the most common cause of visual loss. Other causes include cataract, glaucoma, vitreous hemorrhage, epiretinal membrane (ERM), and tractional retinal detachment.

23. **What are the indications for treatment in pars planitis?**
Patients who have cystoid macular edema (CME) with visual loss less than or equal to 20/40 should be treated.

24. **Describe the most common causes of posterior uveitis.**
Ocular toxoplasmosis is characterized by necrotizing retinochoroiditis, which appears as a white infiltrate; most commonly adjacent to a pigmented retinal scar is typical. A diffuse vitritis may

make the retinitis appear as a "headlight in the fog." In immunocompromised patients, including the elderly, the retinitis may be multifocal, bilateral, and may not be associated with a scar.

Smith JR, Cunningham ET Jr: Atypical presentations of ocular toxoplasmosis. Curr Opin Ophthalmol 13:387–392, 2002.

25. **How is the diagnosis of ocular toxoplasmosis made?**
In most cases, diagnosis is based on clinical history and fundus examination. Positive IgG or IgM titers, even in very low concentrations (undiluted serum), are supportive of the diagnosis. Interpretation may be confounded by a high prevalence of positive titers in the population. A negative titer excludes the diagnosis except in immunosuppressed patients.

Weiss MJ, Velazquez N, Hofeldt AJ: Serologic tests in the diagnosis of presumed toxoplasmic retinochoroiditis. Am J Ophthalmol 109:407–411, 1990.

26. **How is ocular toxoplasmosis managed?**
Treatment is recommended for active lesions that threaten the macula or optic nerve and for severe vitritis. Although sulfonamides, clindamycin, pyrimethamine, folinic acid, and corticosteroids have been used in various combinations, there is no universally accepted treatment regimen, and the effectiveness of toxoplasmosis therapy has been questioned. Observation is recommended for small peripheral lesions.

Engstrom RE Jr, Holland GN, Nussenblatt RB, Jabs DA: Current practices in the management of ocular toxoplasmosis. Am J Ophthalmol 111:601–610, 1991.

Stanford MR, See SE, Jones LV, Gilbert RE. Antibiotics for toxoplasmic retinochoroiditis: An evidence-based systematic review. Ophthalmology 110:926–931, 2003.

27. **What serious side effects may occur with oral antibiotic therapy for toxoplasmosis?**
   - Pseudomembranous colitis (clindamycin)
   - Hematologic toxicity (pyrimethamine)
   - Erythema multiforme and Stevens-Johnson's reactions (sulfonamides)

28. **What are the features of ocular sarcoidosis?**
The eye is involved in approximately 20% of individuals. Uveitis is the most common ocular manifestation. Anterior segment inflammation is classically bilateral, chronic, and granulomatous, although acute and asymmetric anterior uveitis may occur. Posterior segment inflammation including choroidal or optic nerve granulomas, vitritis, retinal vasculitis or vascular occlusions, and neovascularization are less common, but do threaten sight. Conjunctival and eyelid nodules and enlarged lacrimal glands may be noted and are useful tissues for confirmatory biopsy.

Jabs DA, Johns CJ: Ocular involvement in chronic sarcoidosis. Am J Ophthalmol 102:297–301, 1986.

29. **How does the presentation of sarcoidosis differ with age?**
In children younger than 5 years, uveitis, arthritis, and skin rash are typical and the presentation may resemble JIA. In patients 20–40 years old, bilateral chronic granulomatous iritis or panuveitis and hilar adenopathy are most common, whereas in elderly patients, lesions resembling multifocal choroiditis or birdshot chorioretinitis and interstitial lung disease may be seen.

Vrabec TR, Augsburger JJ, Fischer DH, et al: Taches de bougie. Ophthalmology 102:1712–1721, 1995.

30. **What testing may be helpful in making the diagnosis of sarcoidosis?**
   - Chest x-ray is positive in 90% of patients with sarcoidosis.
   - Angiotensin-converting enzyme and lysozyme are sensitive but not very specific indicators of sarcoidosis.
   - In cases with high suspicion and a negative chest x-ray, gallium scan and computed tomographic (CT) scan of chest can be considered.

- Biopsy of normal-appearing conjunctiva in patients with presumed sarcoidosis is positive in 12% of cases. Lacrimal biopsy in presumed sarcoidosis is positive in 22% of cases.

    Weineb RN: Diagnosing sarcoidosis by transconjunctival biopsy of the lacrimal gland. Am J Ophthlamol 97:573–576, 1984.

KEY POINTS: MOST COMMON FORMS OF UVEITIS

1. Children—JIA

2. NGAU—HLA-B27

3. Granulomatous anterior uveitis—sarcoidosis

4. Intermediate uveitis—pars planitis

5. Posterior uveitis—toxoplasm

31. **What are the features of ocular syphilis?**
    Salt-and-pepper chorioretinitis, vitritis, uveitis, and interstitial keratitis typify congenital syphilis. The clinical findings of acquired syphilis are protean. Anterior uveitis, vitritis, choroiditis, retinitis, retinal vasculitis, optic neuropathy, and Argyll Robertson pupils are most common. Others have been reported.

    Margo CE, Hamed LH: Ocular syphilis. Surv Ophthalmol 37:203–220, 1992.

32. **Which diagnostic tests are used to assess for syphilitic uveitis?**
    Nontreponemal tests, including serial venereal disease research laboratory (VDRL) titers, are useful in monitoring response to therapy, but they may be negative in late-stage syphilis. For this reason, syphilitic uveitis must be evaluated with specific treponemal tests, that is, FTA-ABS test or the microhemagglutination test (MHA-TP). Examination of cerebrospinal fluid for elevated protein, lymphocytic pleocytosis, or VDRL may reveal neurosyphilis. Human immunodeficiency virus (HIV) testing should be performed in all patients with syphilis.

    Tramont EC: Syphilis in HIV-infected persons. AIDS Clin Rev 61–72, 1993–1994.

33. **How is syphilitic uveitis treated?**
    Ocular syphilis is treated as neurosyphilis with 12–24 million units/day of intravenous penicillin G for 14 days followed by intramuscular benzathine penicillin G, 2.4 million units/week for 3 weeks. Doxycycline, tetracycline, and erythromycin have been used in penicillin-allergic patients.

34. **What are the most common features of ocular histoplasmosis?**
    Peripapillary atrophy or pigmentation, peripheral chorioretinal lesions, and macular choroidal neovascular membrane (CNVM).

35. **What is Vogt-Koyanagi-Harada (VKH) syndrome?**
    This is an idiopathic multisystem disorder that primarily affects heavily pigmented individuals. Clinical manifestations are present in the skin (alopecia, vitiligo, poliosis), eye (granulomatous uveitis, exudative retinal detachment), and central nervous system (CNS) (encephalopathy, cerebrospinal fluid lymphocytosis). Symptoms may include dysacousis, headache, and stiff neck. Fluorescein angiography (IVFA) is notable for a characteristic "starry sky" pattern of early hyperfluorescence. Treatment usually requires systemic immune suppression.

36. **Name five other conditions that have uveitis and CNS manifestations.**
    Sarcoidosis, syphilis, Behçet's disease, acute posterior multifocal placoid pigment epitheliopathy, and MS.

37. **What is sympathetic ophthalmia?**
This is a bilateral, diffuse granulomatous T-cell–mediated uveitis that develops from 5 days to many years after perforating ocular injury (0.2%) or ocular surgery (0.01%). Eighty percent of cases occur within 2 weeks to 3 months after the inciting event. Clinical findings include panuveitis, papillitis, and in some cases exudative retinal detachment. Dalen-Fuchs' nodules or collections of sub–retinal pigment epithelium (RPE) lymphocytes may be recognized clinically as grayish-white lesions scattered throughout the posterior fundus. Treatment usually requires systemic immune suppression. Enucleation of the traumatized eye after the onset of the uveitis is not typically recommended.

38. **Describe acute retinal necrosis (ARN) syndrome.**
Acute retinal necrosis (ARN) is a clinical syndrome caused by herpes virus infections (varicella-zoster, herpes simplex types 1 and 2). The typical triad includes peripheral retinitis, arteritis, and vitritis. Long-term complications include retinal detachment, glaucoma, cataract, and optic atrophy. Intravenous acyclovir for 14 days, followed by 3 months of oral therapy, is recommended to limit retinal necrosis, as well as the occurrence of ARN in the fellow eye. Prophylactic laser coagulation may decrease risk of secondary retinal detachment. Acute retinal necrosis may occur in the fellow eye in approximately 30% of patients at an average interval of 4 weeks.

Duker JS, Blumenkranz MS: Diagnosis and management of the acute retinal necrosis (ARN) syndrome. Surv Ophthalmol 35:327–343, 1991.

39. **What other types of retinitis may have a similar clinical presentation?**
Toxoplasmosis, syphilis, Behçet's disease, aspergillus, and lymphoma.

Balansard B, Bodaghi B, Cassoux N, et al: Necrotising retinopathies simulating acute retinal necrosis syndrome. Br J Ophthalmol 89:96–101, 2005.

40. **What are the major diagnostic characteristics of Behçet's disease?**
Recurrent anterior and posterior uveitis, skin lesions (erythema nodosum, thrombophlebitis), genital ulcers, and painful oral ulcers.

41. **What is unusual about the clinical course of Behçet's disease?**
Behçet's disease is characterized by periodic relapse and spontaneous remission. Remissions may be misunderstood as a response to intermittent steroid therapy. Unlike most other causes of retinal vasculitis, including sarcoidosis, which may have similar clinical findings, Behçet's disease requires chronic systemic immunosuppression to prevent relapses and blindness.

42. **Describe the ocular features of Lyme disease.**
Ocular Lyme disease is usually bilateral. In stage one, conjunctivitis may occur. A migratory rash (erythema migrans) or arthritis may also be described. In later stages an atypical intermediate uveitis with granulomatous KP and PS may be present. Inflammation may affect almost any ocular tissue. Diagnosis requires a history of outdoor activity in an endemic area in the late spring or summer and positive indirect immunofluorescent antibody (IFA) and/or the enzyme-linked immunosorbent assay (ELISA). Western blot, which is very specific, may be confirmatory. False-negative results occur in the early stages or following incomplete antibiotic treatment. The spirochete may be identified in skin rash biopsy or cerebrospinal fluid.

Aaberg TM: The expanding ophthalmologic spectrum of Lyme disease. Am J Ophthalmol 107:77–80, 1989.
Zaidman GW: The ocular manifestations of Lyme disease. Int Ophthalmol Clin 33:9–22, 1993.

43. **Describe the most common features of ocular tuberculosis.**
The most common feature of ocular tuberculosis is choroiditis. Inflammation is typically unilateral. Associated anterior uveitis is chronic and granulomatous. Ocular involvement may occur without signs of active pulmonary involvement.

Helm CJ, Holland GN: Ocular tuberculosis. Surv Ophthalmol 38:229-256, 1993.

44. **What form of uveitis may present with enlarged lymph glands?**
Primary inoculation with *Bartonella henselae* produces regional lymphadenopathy and conjunctivitis (Parinaud's oculoglandular syndrome). Additional findings may include Leber's neuroretinitis and a retinal white dot syndrome. Patients with sarcoidosis may also present with lymphadenopathy.

> Ormerod LD, Dailey JP: Ocular manifestations of cat-scratch disease. Curr Opin Ophthalmol 10:209–216, 1999.

45. **Why do patients with uveitis develop glaucoma?**
The most common mechanism of acute glaucoma is direct inflammation of the trabecular meshwork or trabeculitis. Chronic glaucoma may result from closure of the trabecular meshwork by peripheral anterior synechia or angle closure glaucoma from iris bombé (360 degrees of PS). In addition, topical, intraocular, and periocular corticosteroids can cause glaucoma.

> Moorthy RS, Mermoud A, Baerveldt G, et al: Glaucoma associated with uveitis. Surv Ophthalmol 41:361–394, 1997.

46. **Name the uveitis entities that are associated with an acute elevation in intraocular pressure (IOP).**
   - Herpes simplex and zoster
   - Toxoplasmosis
   - Sarcoidosis
   - Syphilis

47. **What is the approach to the treatment for uveitis?**
   1. Identify and treat the underlying causes. This is especially important in immunocompromised individuals, in whom most uveitis cases are infectious.
   2. Prevent vision-threatening complications. Anti-inflammatory agents are the mainstay of treatment to prevent or reverse vision-threatening complications, including retinal ischemia, retinal scarring, cataract, and macular edema, among others.
   3. Relieve ocular discomfort and improve vision. Cycloplegic agents relax the ciliary body and reduce pain. In addition, they stabilize the blood aqueous barrier and help to break or prevent PS.

48. **What should be the general approach to the use of steroids to treat uveitis?**
Corticosteroids should be used intensely initially until inflammation is suppressed and then tapered. A common mistake is too-infrequent dosing initially, which results in a smoldering, extended course. Topical corticosteroids are best suited for anterior uveitis, but they do not reach the posterior segment. Prednisolone acetate achieves the highest anterior chamber (AC) concentrations. Posterior segment disease must be treated with periocular (posterior subtenon or preseptal) or intravitreal injection, and/or systemic corticosteroids. Systemic steroids are typically reserved for severe or bilateral disease. In patients unresponsive to steroids, one must suspect an infectious or neoplastic masquerade syndrome.

49. **When are alternate immunosuppressives indicated to treat autoimmune uveitis?**
   - When the systemic steroids required to suppress ocular inflammation are higher than can be safely administered over extended periods. In these cases a steroid-sparing agent is indicated.
   - When the systemic or local steroids are causing intolerable side effects.
   - When steroids do not significantly alter the nature of the uveitis or underlying condition.

50. **In which conditions with uveitis or scleritis are immunosuppressive agents indicated?**
Behçet's disease, Wegener's granulomatosis, and rheumatoid arthritis-associated vasculitis. They are often required in cases of sympathetic ophthalmia, VKH syndrome, serpiginous choroiditis, and multifocal choroiditis.

51. **Name major categories of alternate immunosuppressives.**
    - Antimetabolites (e.g., methotrexate): Often used for their steroid-sparing effect
    - T-cell inhibitors (e.g., cyclosporine)
    - Alkylating agents (e.g., cyclophosphamide): Typically reserved for severe, sight-threatening uveitis not adequately responsive to aforementioned agents
    - Biologicals (e.g., infliximab): Tumor necrosis factor (TNF) inhibitors are one example of this expanding arsenal of immunosuppressant and anti-inflammatory agents

    Jabs DA, Rosenbaum JT, Foster CS, et al. Guidelines for the use of immunosuppressive drugs in patients with ocular inflammatory disorders: recommendations of an expert panel. Am J Ophthalmol 130:492–513, 2000.

MASQUERADE SYNDROMES

52. **Define masquerade syndrome.**
    The term *masquerade syndrome* refers to ophthalmic disorders that are not primarily inflammatory in nature but may present clinically as either anterior or posterior uveitis (Table 39-5). These entities may be mistaken for, or masquerade as, primary uveitis. Extensive evaluation is often initiated because patients manifest with atypical features, recurrent episodes of uveitis, or uveitis that is unresponsive to standard therapy.

KEY POINTS: COMMON MASQUERADE SYNDROMES

1. Retinoblastoma in children

2. Leukemia in children

3. Primary intraocular lymphoma in the elderly

4. Ocular ischemic syndrome in the elderly

5. Peripheral retinal detachment in any age group

53. **In what age groups should one have the highest suspicion for masquerade syndromes?**
    In the very young and in the elderly.

54. **Describe the clinical features of retinoblastoma.**
    Retinoblastoma is the most common primary intraocular malignancy in children, usually presenting before age 2. The most common signs are leukocoria (white pupillary reflex) and strabismus. Occasionally, tumor necrosis may produce significant inflammation. Tumor cells layered in the anterior chamber may produce a pseudohypopyon (Fig. 39-2). Retinoblastoma cells may enter the vitreous, as vitreous seeds, and simulate vitritis. Calcification on ultrasonography and CT scan may help

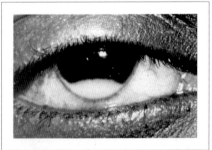

Figure 39-2. Pseudohypopyon caused by seeding of retinoblastoma cells in the anterior chamber. (From Shields JA, Shields CL: Intraocular Tumors: A Text and Atlas. Philadelphia, W.B. Saunders, 1992.)

TABLE 39–5. MOST COMMON MASQUERADE SYNDROMES THAT MAY MIMIC UVEITIS				
Disease	Location	Age (yr)	Signs of Inflammation	Diagnostic Tests
Retinoblastoma	Anterior	<15	Flare, cells, pseudohypopyon	Aqueous tap for LDH levels and cytology
Leukemia	Anterior	<15	Flare, cells, heterochromia	Bone marrow, peripheral blood smear, aqueous cytology
Intraocular foreign body	Anterior	Any age	Flare, cells	X-ray, ultrasound, CT scan
Malignant melanoma	Anterior	Any age	Flare, cells	Angiography (fluorescein, ICG), ultrasound, MRI
Ocular ischemic syndrome	Anterior	50+	Cell, flare, redness	IVFA, carotid Doppler
Peripheral retinal detachment	Anterior	Any age	Flare, cells	Ophthalmoscopy, ultrasound
Retinitis pigmentosa	Posterior	Any age	Cells in vitreous	ERG, EOG, visual fields
Primary intraocular lymphoma	Posterior	15+	Vitreous cells, retinal hemorrhage or exudates, RPE infiltrates	Cytology of aqueous/vitreous fluid
Lymphoma	Posterior	15+	Retinal hemorrhage, exudates, vitreous cells	Biopsy of lymph node/bone marrow, physical examination
Retinoblastoma	Posterior	<15	Vitreous cells, retinal exudate	Ultrasound, aqueous tap
Malignant melanoma	Posterior	15+	Vitreous cells	Fluorescein ultrasound

CT = computed tomography, ERG = electroretinogram, EOG = electro-oculogram, ICG = indocyanine green, IVFA = fluorescein angiography, LDH = lactate dehydrogenase, MRI = magnetic resonance imaging, RPE = retinal pigment epithelium.
Adapted from American Academy of Ophthalmology: Ophthalmology Basic and Clinical Science Course, Section 6. San Francisco, American Academy of Ophthalmology, 1997.

to differentiate retinoblastoma from various forms of childhood uveitis, including toxoplasmosis, toxocariasis, cysticercosis, and pars planitis.

Shields JA, Augsburger JJ: Current approaches to the diagnosis and management of retinoblastoma. Surv Ophthalmol 25:347–372, 1981.

55. **What may present with chronic steroid-resistant panuveitis in a patient older than age 50?**
Primary intraocular lymphoma, formerly known as reticulum cell sarcoma (Fig. 39-3). Elderly individuals may present with bilateral vitreous cells, anterior chamber reaction, and retinal and choroidal infiltrates. The retinal infiltrates may be patchy and associated with hemorrhage and exudate. Dense vitritis may be the only presenting sign. Most patients eventually develop some form of CNS involvement. CT or magnetic resonance imaging (MRI) may demonstrate CNS tumors. Vitreous aspirate or lumbar puncture may establish the diagnosis. Therapy may include ocular and CNS irradiation combined with intrathecal chemotherapy.

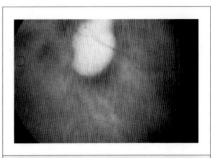

Figure 39-3. Yellow-white chorioretinal infiltrates in intraocular lymphoma. (From Shields JA, Shields CL: Intraocular Tumors: A Text and Atlas. Philadelphia, W.B. Saunders, 1992.)

Char DH, Ljung BM, Miller T, Phillips T: Primary intraocular lymphoma (ocular reticulum cell sarcoma): Diagnosis and management. Ophthalmology 95:625–630, 1988.

56. **Describe the ocular findings associated with leukemia.**
Clinically, the retina is the most commonly affected (Fig. 39-4). Retinal vascular dilation and tortuosity, hemorrhages, cotton-wool spots, and peripheral neovascularization occur. Roth spots are hemorrhages with white centers composed of leukemic cells or platelet-fibrin aggregates. Histopathologically, the choroid is the most commonly involved and may cause exudative retinal detachment. IVFA demonstrates multiple areas of hyperfluorescence similar to that found in VKH syndrome. Anterior segment findings include conjunctival mass, iris heterochromia, anterior chamber cell and flare, pseudohypopyon, spontaneous hyphema, and elevated intraocular pressure. Optic nerve infiltration and orbital involvement are common.

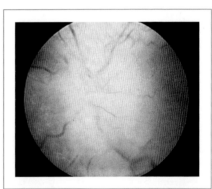

Figure 39-4. Leukemic infiltration of the optic nerve head, retina, and choroid in an 8-year-old child. (From Shields JA, Shields CL: Intraocular Tumors: A Text and Atlas. Philadelphia, W.B. Saunders, 1992.)

Kincaid MC, Green WR: Ocular and orbital involvement in leukemia. Surv Ophthalmol 27:211–232, 1983.

57. **How can a malignant melanoma produce inflammatory signs?**
Necrotic tumors may elicit an intense inflammatory response associated with seeding of tumor cells into the vitreous cavity and anterior segment. Occasionally, melanophages or tumor cells that contain melanin produce a brown pseudohypopyon. Blockage of the

trabecular meshwork by tumor cells may result in elevated intraocular pressure (melanomalytic glaucoma). Necrosis of the tumor may result in spontaneous vitreous hemorrhage. Other clinical findings include iris heterochromia and exudative retinal detachment with shifting subretinal fluid. Ultrasound examination and IVFA help to establish the diagnosis.

Fraser DJ Jr, Font RL: Ocular inflammation and hemorrhage as initial manifestations of uveal malignant melanoma: Incidence and prognosis. Arch Ophthalmol 97:1311–1314, 1979.

58. **Describe other entities that may simulate anterior and/or posterior uveitis.**
   - **Long-standing peripheral rhegmatogenous retinal detachment** may produce a cellular reaction in the anterior or posterior chamber as well as PS.
   - **Retained intraocular foreign body** associated with trauma may cause persistent anterior and/ or posterior segment inflammation. CT or ultrasonography results should demonstrate the abnormality.
   - **Retinitis pigmentosa** may present with vitreous cells and posterior subcapsular cataract. The "bone spicule" pigment deposition in the retina, attenuated retinal vessels, mottling and atrophy of the RPE, and waxy pallor of the optic nerve help to distinguish this disease from other disorders. The diagnosis can be confirmed with an extinguished electroretinogram and ring scotoma on visual field testing.

Heckenlively JR (ed): Retinitis Pigmentosa. Philadelphia, J.B. Lippincott, 1988.

OCULAR MANIFESTATIONS OF ACQUIRED IMMUNE DEFICIENCY SYNDROME (AIDS)

59. **Who is at greatest risk for developing AIDS-related eye disease?**
   Patients with severely reduced $CD4^+$ T-lymphocyte counts and associated immunosuppression are most likely to develop AIDS-related eye disease. For this reason, screening for opportunistic infections with dilated fundus examination is recommended every 3 months in patients with $CD4^+$ counts less than 100 cells/μL.

Baldassano V, Dunn JP, Feinberg J, Dabs BA: Cytomegalovirus retinitis and low $CD4^+$ T-lymphocyte counts. N Engl J Med 333:670, 1995.

60. **What is the most common ocular manifestation of AIDS?**
   Retinal microvasculopathy that manifests clinically as cotton-wool spots (CWS) (Fig. 39-5). Retinal microaneurysms and hemorrhages may be present. Most patients are asymptomatic. CWS become more common as the $CD4^+$ T-lymphocyte count declines, reaching a prevalence of 45% in patients with counts <50 cells/μL.

Freeman WR, Chen A, Henderly DE, et al: Prevalence and significance of acquired immunodeficiency-related retinal microvasculopathy. Am J Ophthalmol 107:229–235, 1989.

61. **What is the most common ocular opportunistic infection in patients with AIDS?**
   Cytomegalovirus (CMV) is by far the most common cause of opportunistic ocular infection and most frequently results in necrotizing retinitis (Fig. 39-6). Other less common ocular

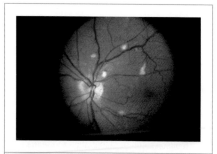

Figure 39-5. Cotton-wool spots are infarcts of the nerve fiber layer. Unlike early infiltrates of cytomegalovirus retinitis, they do not enlarge, do not have associated hemorrhage, and may resolve in several weeks.

opportunistic infectious agents in patients with AIDS include herpes zoster, toxoplasmosis, and *Mycobacterium avium*. Syphilis may be observed in patients with less severe immunosuppression (CD4$^+$ counts >100 cells/μL). Because it occurs at higher CD4$^+$ counts, syphilitic retinitis is not considered strictly an opportunistic infection.

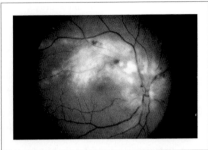

Figure 39-6. Cytomegalovirus retinitis is characterized by areas of retinal infiltrate with associated hemorrhage. Note the optic nerve involvement.

62. **What is the incidence of CMV retinitis?**
    Among patients whose CD4$^+$ count is less than 50 cells/μL, 20% per year develop CMV retinitis.

63. **Describe the early symptoms of CMV retinitis.**
    Floaters that appear as numerous tiny black specks are often present early in the course of CMV retinitis. Pain and redness are not associated. Scotomas (blind spots) or visual loss may develop with more advanced stages of the disease.

64. **How does CMV retinitis present clinically?**
    Classic ophthalmologic findings of fulminant CMV retinitis include white areas of retinal necrosis with associated hemorrhage and minimal vitreous inflammation (see Fig. 39-6). The indolent or granular form, which is often less symptomatic, is characterized by peripheral retinal whitening with minimal associated hemorrhage.

    Jabs DA, Enger C, Bartlett JG: Cytomegalovirus retinitis and acquired immunodeficiency syndrome. Arch Ophthalmol 107:75–80, 1989.

65. **What are the more common entities in the differential diagnosis of CMV retinitis?**
    - Progressive outer retinal necrosis (PORN)
    - Toxoplasmosis
    - Syphilis
    - HIV retinitis
    - CWS

66. **How is the diagnosis of CMV retinitis made?**
    The diagnosis of CMV retinitis is made clinically when characteristic findings of fulminant or indolent retinitis are found in an immunosuppressed patient with CD4$^+$ count <100 cells/μL. In the unusual case when the diagnosis is in question, a vitreous biopsy with or without retinal biopsy for PCR analysis may be performed.

67. **What is the initial treatment strategy for CMV retinitis?**
    Treatment of CMV retinitis is given in two stages. The first stage is 2–6 weeks of induction therapy with ganciclovir (Fig. 39-7), valganciclovir, foscarnet, or cidofovir, which are antiviral agents that inhibit viral DNA polymerase. Induction is discontinued after a healing response (consolidation or stabilization of the margins) begins. The second stage, maintenance therapy, consists of a lower dose of the medication that is continued until relapse occurs.

68. **What is the strategy in the event of a relapse?**
    Despite maintenance therapy, CMV retinitis relapses in most patients who remain immunosuppressed. The mean interval to relapse varies from 2 to 8 months and depends on the

medication used and the route of administration. When relapse occurs in patients taking oral or IV medication, reinduction with the same medication (2–6 weeks of high-dose IV or multiple intraocular injections) is indicated. When relapse develops in patients with ganciclovir implants, the implant is replaced.

69. Does resistance to antiviral medication develop?

Drug resistance is an emerging problem of great concern because of the limited number of available agents that are effective against CMV. Ganciclovir-resistant CMV has been reported in 27.5% of urine samples at 9 months. CMV UL97 mutations (a CMV DNA polymerase mutation that confers

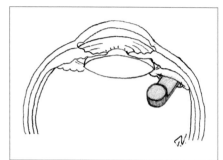

Figure 39-7. The intraocular ganciclovir implant is sutured to the sclera and extends into the vitreous cavity. The drug delivery system slowly releases ganciclovir over 8 months. It may be replaced when the drug supply is exhausted. Although it is not associated with the systemic toxicity seen with oral or intravenous therapy, the implant provides no prophylaxis against systemic cytomegalovirus (CMV) or CMV retinitis in the fellow eye.

ganciclovir resistance) were detected in 30.8% of patients treated with ganciclovir over 3 months and in none treated less than 3 months. Cidofovir-resistant CMV was observed after treatment with either cidofovir or ganciclovir. Foscarnet resistance also has been reported.

Gilbert C, Handfield J, Toma E, et al: Emergence and prevalence of cytomegalovirus UL97 mutations associated with ganciclovir resistance in AIDS patients. AIDS 12:125–129, 1998.

Jabs DA, Enger C, Dunn JP, Forman M: Cytomegalovirus retinitis and viral resistance: Ganciclovir resistance. CMV Retinitis and Viral Resistance Study Group. J Infect Dis 177:770–773, 1998.

70. What is clinical resistance? How is it managed?

Clinical resistance is recognized when there is no clinical response to 6 weeks of reinduction therapy. A change in medication or combination therapy is indicated.

71. How long should treatment be continued in patients with CMV retinitis?

Length of therapy depends on the immune status of the patient. For patients who remain severely immunosuppressed (CD4$^+$ count <100 cells/μL), treatment must be continued indefinitely. In patients whose immune status is improved by highly active antiretroviral therapy (HAART) (see question 73), maintenance therapy may be discontinued if the retinitis is completely quiescent and CD4$^+$ counts are >100 cells/μL.

72. Name the main toxicities of the antiviral therapies.

The main toxicity of ganciclovir is bone marrow toxicity with neutropenia and/or thrombocytopenia. Neutropenia may be limited by concurrent use of granulocyte colony-stimulating factor (G-CSF). The main toxicity of foscarnet is renal toxicity. The principal toxicity associated with cidofovir is nephrotoxicity, which may be ameliorated by concurrent probenecid. In addition, severe hypotony may develop after either intravenous or intravitreal administration of cidofovir.

73. How has HAART affected the natural history and treatment of CMV retinitis?

HAART uses a combination of protease inhibitors plus other antiretroviral agents. HAART has resulted in significant and sustained increases in CD4$^+$ counts and remission of CMV retinitis. Discontinuation of maintenance therapy has been recommended for patients with completely quiescent retinitis, $CD4^+$ count greater than 100 cells/μL. Other criteria include $CD4^+$ elevation for at least 3 months, prolonged relapse-free intervals, HAART therapy longer than 18 months, and reduced HIV and CMV viremia.

Vrabec TR, Baldassano VF, Whitcup SM: Discontinuation of maintenance therapy in patients with quiescent CMV retinitis and elevated CD4+ counts. Ophthalmology 105:1259–1264, 1998.

74. **What is progressive outer retinal necrosis?**
PORN is an extremely aggressive form of retinitis in the AIDS population (Fig. 39-8). Caused by herpes zoster virus, it is temporally associated with herpes zoster skin lesions, which may or may not be in the periocular region. Blindness develops in >80% of patients because of either relentless progression of infection despite therapy or secondary retinal detachment.

Engstrom RE Jr, Holland GN, Margolis TP, et al: Progressive outer retinal necrosis syndrome. Ophthalmology 101:1488–1452, 1994.

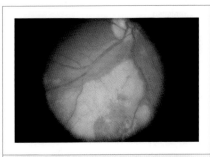

Figure 39-8. Progressive outer retinal necrosis typically affects the outer retina with sparing of the retinal vessels. Note the areas of perivascular clearing and absence of associated hemorrhage.

75. **Why do retinal detachments develop in cases of infectious retinitis? Who is at risk?**
Retinal infections may cause multiple necrotic retinal holes that over time lead to retinal detachment. Retinal detachments occur in 34% of patients with CMV. However, patients with PORN are at highest risk; retinal detachments occur in 60–70% of these cases.

76. **How are most AIDS-related retinal detachments repaired?**
Lasers may be used to demarcate or wall off macula-sparing retinal detachments, especially in patients who are not well enough to tolerate surgery. Vitrectomy with silicone oil injection is often required in cases when the macula is detached or retinitis is active. The silicone oil replaces the vitreous and tamponades the multiple necrotic holes to prevent redetachment.

Lim JI, Enger C, Haller JA, et al: Improved visual results after surgical repair of cytomegalovirus-related retinal detachments. Ophthalmology 101:264–269, 1994.
Vrabec TR: Laser demarcation of macula-sparing cytomegalovirus-related retinal detachment. Ophthalmology 104:2062–2067, 1997.

77. **Describe the unique characteristics of ocular syphilis in patients with AIDS.**
Syphilis is not an opportunistic infection by definition, because most patients who develop it have $CD4^+$ T-cell counts >250 cell/μL. Ocular findings may range from iritis to necrotizing retinitis. CNS syphilis is present in 85% of HIV-positive patients with ocular syphilis. Hence, evaluation of cerebrospinal fluid is mandated for all HIV-positive patients with ocular syphilis. Syphilis may be seronegative (negative rapid plasmin reagin test despite active infection) in the AIDS population. Regardless of clinical findings, syphilis in patients with AIDS should be treated as tertiary disease with a 10-day course of intravenous antibiotics.

Passo MS, Rosenbaum JT: Ocular syphilis in patients with human immunodeficiency virus infection. Am J Ophthalmol 106:1–6, 1988.

KEY POINTS: OCULAR MANIFESTATIONS OF AIDS

1. Microvasculopathy is the most common ocular manifestation.

2. CMV is the most common ocular opportunistic infection.

3. PORN is the most potentially blinding ocular complication.

4. Kaposi's sarcoma is the most common periocular malignancy.

5. Cryptococcus is the most common cause of neuro-ophthalmologic abnormalities in ambulatory patients.

78. **What is the most common cause of neuro-ophthalmologic abnormalities in the ambulatory population, and what are the clinical findings?**
Cryptococcal meningitis causes papilledema and cranial nerve palsies (Fig. 39-9). Papilledema is defined as disc swelling that is secondary to increased intracranial pressure. The central disc tissue remains pink. Early optic nerve dysfunction is minimal, and vision is usually preserved in contrast to papillitis (see question 80). Other more common causes of papilledema include CNS infection by toxoplasmosis or malignancy (lymphoma).

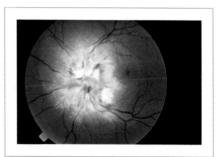

Figure 39-9. Papilledema caused by cryptococcal meningitis is characterized by optic disc swelling and blurring of the disc margins

79. **How should retrobulbar optic neuritis be diagnosed and managed in AIDS patients?**
The etiology of retrobulbar optic neuritis in an AIDS patient is almost always infectious. Idiopathic optic neuritis is a diagnosis of exclusion. Prompt evaluation and aggressive treatment is paramount in this potentially blinding condition. Evaluation must include serology for Cryptococcus, syphilis, and herpes zoster virus. A history of syphilis or previous herpes zoster infection should be recorded. A lumbar puncture is also indicated. Work-up for optic neuropathy should include a review of medications. Ethambutol and didanosine may cause toxic optic neuropathy. Treatment with corticosteroids is contraindicated.

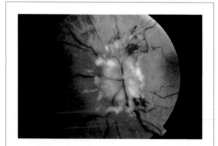

80. **What is papillitis?**
Papillitis is direct infection of the visible intraocular portion of the optic nerve. The optic nerve appears white and necrotic (Fig. 39-10), and vision is severely compromised. CMV may

Figure 39-10. Note white, necrotic appearance and associated hemorrhage of entire optic disc in this example of papillitis secondary to cytomegalovirus.

cause papillitis, often in association with adjacent retinitis. Vision may improve after treatment with antiviral medications.

81. **What is the most common malignancy in the periocular region in AIDS patients?**
Kaposi's sarcoma is the most common periocular malignancy (Fig. 39-11). This aggressive tumor affects 35% of bisexual HIV-positive males and is viscerally disseminated in 70% of cases. Ocular findings are observed in 20% of patients with visceral disease. Skin lesions are more common than conjunctival lesions. Orbital tumors are rare. Treatment is indicated in patients with cosmetic or functional problems. Local ocular treatment is reserved for lesions that persist following systemic therapy. Conjunctival lesions may be excised, and skin lesions may be treated with cryotherapy (flat lesions) or external beam radiation (nodular lesions).

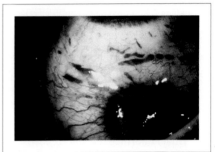

Figure 39-11. Kaposi's sarcoma of the conjunctiva most often occurs in the inferior cul-de-sac. Flat lesions may be easily mistaken for subconjunctival hemorrhage. (Courtesy Drs. Carol and Jerry Shields.)

Dugel PU, Gill PS, Frangieh GT, Rao NA: Ocular adnexal Kaposi's sarcoma in AIDS. Am J Ophthalmol 110:500–503, 1990.

Dugel PU, Gill PS, Frangieh GT, Rao NA: Treatment of ocular adnexal Kaposi's sarcoma in AIDS. Ophthalmology 99:1127–1132, 1992.

82. **What other periocular malignancies may develop?**
Squamous cell carcinoma of the conjunctiva has been reported with increasing frequency in patients with AIDS. The lesions may mimic papillomas or be more characteristic masses with associated leukoplakia. Young patients with conjunctival squamous cell carcinoma should be tested for HIV.

Karp CL, Scott IU, Chang TS, Pflugfelder SC: Conjunctival intraepithelial neoplasia: A possible marker for HIV infection? Arch Ophthalmol 114:257–261, 1996.

83. **Which medications may be associated with ocular toxicity?**
Rifabutin, when used in combination with clarithromycin and fluconazole, has been reported to cause severe hypopyon iritis and, in rare instances, sterile endophthalmitis. Ethambutol may cause optic neuropathy. Side effects of cidofovir include uveitis, hypotony, and nephrotoxicity.

Saran BR, Maguire AM, Nichols C, et al: Hypopyon uveitis in patients with AIDS treated for systemic *Mycobacterium avium* complex infection with rifabutin. Arch Ophthalmol 112:1159–1165, 1994.

TOXIC RETINOPATHIES

Sobha Sivaprasad and Philip G. Hykin

CHAPTER 40

1. **Describe the clinical features of chloroquine retinopathy.**
   Patients notice paracentral scotomas, nyctalopias, color vision defects, and blurred vision. In the early stages of toxicity, mild mottling of the perifoveal retinal pigment epithelium is seen in conjunction with a reduced foveal reflex. Peripheral pigmentary changes often occur at this stage but may be overlooked. Macular pigmentary changes progress to a classic bull's eye maculopathy (Fig. 40-1). In the later stages, generalized retinal pigmentary changes occur with vascular attenuation and optic disc pallor.

2. **What doses of chloroquine and hydroxychloroquine cause retinopathy?**
   Retinopathy is extremely unlikely with a total dose <100 gm of chloroquine or <300 gm of hydroxychloroquine and rare with a total dose <300 gm or 700 gm, respectively. Perhaps more important, retinopathy is unlikely with a daily dose of <4 mg/kg/day of chloroquine or <6.5 mg/kg/day of hydroxychloroquine. A daily dose of >8 mg/kg/day of hydroxychloroquine produces retinopathy in 40% of cases.

3. **How should patients taking chloroquine and hydroxychloroquine be monitored?**
   Before commencing hydroxychloroquine therapy, a baseline assessment should include a detailed clinical examination with special attention to pigmentary changes in the macular area. Threshold static perimetry with a red light in scotopic conditions may elicit parafoveal scotomata

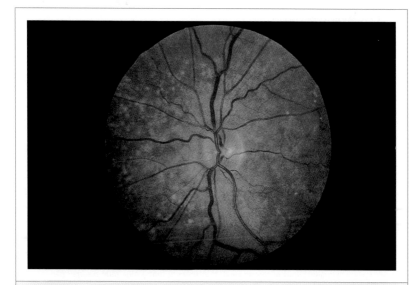

Figure 40-1. Bull's eye lesion (chloroquine retinopathy).

before clinical or fluorescein angiographic evidence of retinal damage. Abnormalities may be found in electroretinography (ERG), electro-oculography (EOG), and dark adaptation tests, but they generally indicate more widespread retinal damage. Annual review by an ophthalmologist is adequate in most cases. However, a review every 6–12 months is recommended in those taking >6.5 mg/kg/day hydroxychloroquine and/or those with renal impairments, or in the elderly population or when duration of treatment exceeds 10 years.

4. **What management is advised for chloroquine retinopathy?**
   If retinal toxicity is present, hydroxychloroquine or chloroquine should be stopped immediately. Clinical improvement may be noted, but progression typically continues because of slow excretion of the drugs. Studies in laboratory animals suggest that NH_4Cl and dimercaprol increase renal excretion of chloroquine, but they have not been proven effective in the clinical setting.

5. **Is the pathogenesis of chloroquine and hydroxychloroquine retinopathy understood?**
   The earliest histopathologic changes of chloroquine retinopathy include membranous cytoplasmic bodies in ganglion cells and degenerative changes in the outer segments of the photoreceptors. However, chloroquine has a selective affinity for melanin, and it has been suggested that this affinity reduces the ability of melanin to combine with free radicals and protect visual cells from light and radiation toxicity. Other authors believe that direct damage to photoreceptors occurs.

KEY POINTS: CHLOROQUINE/HYDROXYCHLOROQUINE TOXICITY ✔

1. Screening should include threshold static perimetry with a red light (i.e., Humphrey field 24-2).

2. Early stages of toxicity cause mild mottling of the perifoveal retinal pigment epithelium.

3. The classic bull's eye maculopathy is a later finding.

4. Annual screening should be increased to every 6 months if high doses are used, the patient has renal impairment, or usage exceeds 10 years.

6. **How may thioridazine affect the retina?**
   Thioridazine (Mellaril) may cause complaints of nyctalopia, dyschromatopsia, and blurred vision. The earliest retinal changes are a fine mottling or granularity to the retinal pigment epithelium posterior to the equator, which may progress to marked pigmentary atrophy and hypertrophic pigment plaques (Fig. 40-2). Vascular attenuation and optic atrophy may follow. Toxicity is said to be uncommon with daily doses <800 mg/day but may develop rapidly with doses over 1200 mg/day.

7. **What other phenothiazines cause retinopathy?**
   Retinal toxicity has been reported with other phenothiazines, including chlorpromazine. However, these compounds are less likely to cause retinopathy, probably because they lack the piperidinylethyl side group of thioridazine. It is thought that 1200–2400 gm/day of chlorpromazine for at least 12 months is required before toxicity occurs.

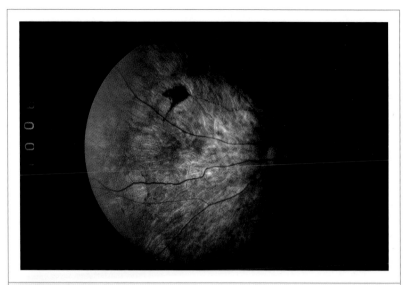

Figure 40-2. Thioridazine retinopathy.

8. **How may quinine sulphate cause retinopathy?**
   Quinine sulphate is used for nocturnal cramps and malarial prophylaxis. It may cause retinal toxicity after a single large ingestion (4 gm). The therapeutic window is narrow with some patients taking a daily dose of 2 gm. Patients develop blurred vision, nyctalopia, nausea, tinnitus, dysacusis, and even coma within 2–4 hours of ingestion. The acute findings include dilated pupils, loss of retinal transparency caused by ganglion cell toxicity (Fig. 40-3), and dilated retinal vessels. As the acute phase resolves, vessel attenuation and optic disc pallor result. Visual acuity may improve after the acute phase.

9. **What are the similarities and differences in electrophysiologic tests between chloroquine and phenothiazine retinopathy?**
   The ERG in chloroquine toxicity may show an enlarged A wave and depressed B wave, whereas it is generally depressed in phenothiazine toxicity. The EOG is decreased in both, but only progressive disease is significant in chloroquine retinopathy because some decrease is common shortly after starting chloroquine therapy. Dark adaptation may remain normal in chloroquine toxicity even in late cases, whereas adaptation is delayed in phenothiazine toxicity.

10. **What are the retinal toxic effects of sildenafil (Viagra)?**
    Sildenafil is an effective drug for erectile dysfunction, acting to inhibit phosphodiesterase type 5 (PDE-5) isoenzyme. It can also inhibit PDE-6 isoenzyme, an important enzyme in the retinal phototransduction cascade, and can cause reversible reduced amplitude of the A and B waves in ERG.

11. **How does cocaine abuse affect the retina?**
    Cocaine has both dopaminergic and adrenomimetic effects. Dopamine is found in high concentrations in the retina and plays an important role in color vision. Cocaine-withdrawn patients have significantly reduced blue cone B-wave amplitude responses on the electroretinogram and blue-yellow color vision defects. The adrenomimetic response and sudden increase in blood pressure associated with the intranasal use of cocaine may also cause retinal arterial occlusions.

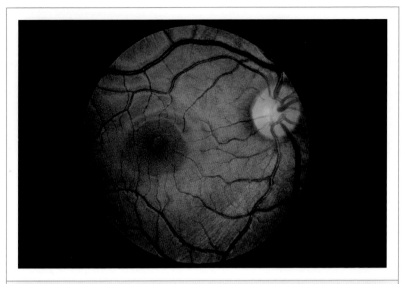

Figure 40-3. Mild loss of retinal transparency caused by quinine sulphate toxicity.

12. **What is vigabatrin retinotoxcity?**
    Vigabatrin (VGB) is an irreversible inhibitor of gamma-aminobutyric acid (GABA) transaminase and is a highly effective antiepileptic drug for treating partial-onset seizures and infantile spasms. It causes a characteristic form of peripheral retinal atrophy and nasal or "inverse" optic disc atrophy in approximately 10% of children being treated with VGB resulting in severely constricted visual fields. Discontinuation of VGB should be strongly considered in these children.

13. **How does fetal alcohol syndrome affect the retina?**
    Alcohol-induced malformations include hypoplastic optic discs and tortuous retinal vessels.

14. **What is unusual about cystoid macular edema caused by nicotinic acid?**
    Nicotinic acid is used in conjunction with dietary restriction of fats for the treatment of hyperlipidemia in doses of 1–3 gm/day. Although typical cystoid macular edema is seen clinically, fluorescein angiography shows no leakage, suggesting that the edema is caused by intracellular edema in Müller cells.

15. **Name the substances that may cause crystalline retinopathy.**
    - Tamoxifen
    - Canthaxanthin
    - Talc (often used with intravenous drug abuse) (Fig. 40-4)
    - Drugs that cause secondary oxalosis
      - Methoxyflurane anesthesia
      - Ethylene glycol
      - Salicylate ingestion in the presence of renal failure

16. **What is the mechanism of the retinopathy caused by talc?**
    Talc is used as filler in methylphenidate hydrochloride (Ritalin) pills that drug addicts may crush and inject intravenously. Initially, the talc particles embolize the lungs, but after prolonged abuse (=12,000 pills), pulmonary arteriovenous shunts allow talc into the systemic circulation.

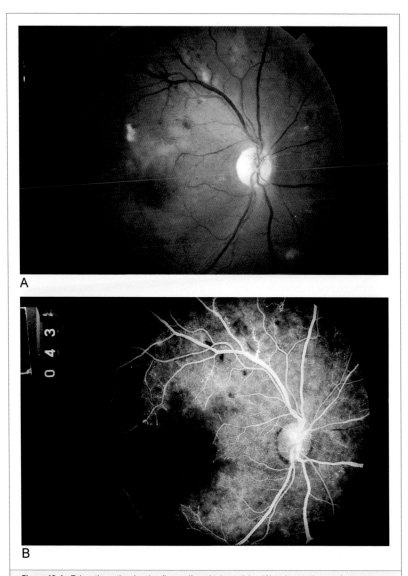

Figure 40-4. Talc retinopathy showing fine perifoveal talc particles *(A)* and extensive resultant posterior pole retinal vascular closure on fluorescein angiography *(B)*.

Emboli to the retinal arterioles may lead to marked peripheral and posterior closure, resulting in retinal neovascularization, vitreous hemorrhage, and ischemic maculopathy.

17. **How should talc retinopathy be managed?**
    Immediate cessation of Ritalin abuse is essential. If retinal neovascularization and vitreous hemorrhage are present, peripheral panretinal photocoagulation should be considered. There is no effective treatment for ischemic maculopathy.

18. **What is xanthopsia? Which drug may cause it?**
   Xanthopsia is the unusual symptom of yellow vision. Along with hemeralopia (reduced visual acuity in the presence of increased background illumination), blurred vision, poor color vision, and paracentral scotomas, it is caused by digitalis toxicity.

19. **What are the clinical features of tamoxifen retinopathy? How much drug is necessary to cause symptoms?**
   Patients are typically asymptomatic, although significantly reduced visual acuity has been reported. Small crystals are seen deposited in the inner retina in the macular area. Punctate retinal pigment epithelial changes and cystoid macular edema may occur. Toxicity has been reported in patients taking between 20 and 320 mg/day.

20. **Can intraocular injection of antibiotics cause retinopathy?**
   Inadvertent intraocular injection of gentamicin may result in rapid onset of retinal whitening in the macular area. Optic atrophy and retinal pigment epithelial changes develop later. The visual prognosis is poor and neovascular glaucoma may develop. Macular infarction has been reported after intravitreal injection of 400 μg, although 200 μg is probably safe. Similar problems may occur with tobramycin and amikacin.

21. **What is interferon retinopathy?**
   Interferon may cause retinal changes that include cotton-wool spots, retinal hemorrhages, macular edema, capillary nonperfusion, and vascular occlusions. The mechanism may be immune complex deposition in the retinal vasculature, followed by leukocyte infiltration and vascular closure. Interferon alpha may aggravate autoimmune thyroiditis and polyarthropathy in 10% of cases by stimulating antibody production.

22. **What effects may iron overload have on the retina?**
   A retained iron intraocular foreign body may lead to darkening of the iris, orange deposits in the anterior subcapsular region of the lens, anterior and posterior vitritis, pigmentary retinopathy, and progressive loss of field. The intraocular foreign body should be removed as soon as possible.

23. **What drugs can cause retinal thromboembolic events?**
   Oral contraceptives have been associated with central, branch, and cilioretinal artery occlusions and central retinal vein occlusion. Considerable controversy surrounds the role of oral contraceptives in causing these events, but stopping the oral contraceptive seems advisable. Talc retinal emboli are discussed in question 16 and periorbital steroid injection with inadvertent arterial penetration may result in extensive embolization of the retinal circulation.

24. **What chelating agents may cause maculopathy?**
   Desferrioxamine, a chelating agent used to treat iron overload, particularly in thalassemia major, may cause blurred vision, nyctalopia, and ring scotoma. The fundus may show bilateral widespread retinal pigment derangement.

BIBLIOGRAPHY

1. Browning DJ: Hydroxychloroquine and chloroquine retinopathy: Screening for drug toxicity. Am J Ophthalmol 133:649–656, 2002.
2. Campochiaro PA, Lim JI: Aminoglycoside toxicity in the treatment of endophthalmitis. The Aminoglycoside Toxicity Study Group. Arch Ophthalmol 112:48–53, 1994.
3. Gass JDM: Toxic diseases affecting the pigment epithelium and retina. In Gass JDM (ed): Stereoscopic Atlas of Macular Diseases, 4th ed. St. Louis, Mosby, 1997, pp 775–808.

4. Haimovici R, D'Amico DJ, Gragoudas ES, Sokol S: Deferoxamine Retinopathy Study Group. The expanded clinical spectrum of deferoxamine retinopathy. Ophthalmology 109:164–171, 2002.

5. Laties A, Zrenner E: Viagra (sildenafil citrate) and ophthalmology. Prog Retin Eye Res 21:485–506, 2002.

6. Roy M, Roy A, Williams J, et al: Reduced blue cone electroretinogram in cocaine-withdrawn patients. Arch Gen Psych 54:153–156, 1997.

7. Swartz M: Other diseases: Drug toxicity, metabolic and nutritional conditions. In Ryan SJ (ed): Retina, 2nd ed. St. Louis, Mosby, 1994.

8. Urey JC: Some ocular manifestations of systemic drug abuse. J Am Optom Assoc 62:834–842, 1991.

9. van der Torren K, Graniewski-Wijnands HS, Polak BC: Visual field and electrophysiological abnormalities due to vigabatrin. Doc Ophthalmol 104:181–188, 2002.

10. Weiner A, Sanberg MA, Raudie AR, et al: Hydroxychloroquine retinopathy. Am J Ophthalmol 106:286–292, 1988.

CHAPTER 41

COATS DISEASE

William Tasman, MD

1. **What is Coats disease?**
   Exudation and retinal telangiectasia are hallmarks of the disorder, which is named for the British ophthalmologist who first described this condition in 1908. It comes on painlessly and may be slow and insidious in its development. In many instances, Coats disease is not discovered until it is in a well-advanced stage.

2. **List the clinical characteristics of Coats disease.**
   - It occurs most frequently in young males.
   - It is usually unilateral.
   - It is not familial and not known to be associated with any systemic disease.
   - Characteristic retinal vascular lesions are telangiectatic-like "light bulb" aneurysms that are associated with capillary dropout and sometimes vascular sheathing, usually in the fundus periphery (Fig. 41-1, B and F).
   - Exudation, a prominent feature, has a predilection to accumulate in the posterior pole of the fundus (Fig. 41-1, A); it contains cholesterol.
   - It may lead to retinal detachment, cataract, glaucoma, and phthisis bulbi.

3. **What is the incidence in women?**
   Between 8% and 10% in women.

4. **What is the most common age at which Coats disease becomes apparent?**
   Between 8 and 10 years of age. However, it can be noted in infancy and later in life. It is often much more severe when noted early in life.

5. **What percentage of cases are unilateral versus bilateral?**
   Approximately 80–90% of the cases are unilateral. When bilateral cases do develop, there is usually asymmetry, with one eye being much more involved than the other.

6. **Are the retinal vascular changes easy to detect?**
   Usually if the patient is cooperative, it is not hard to diagnose the peripheral retinal telangiectasia. In younger patients, however, these changes can be subtle. With the patient under anesthesia, it is possible to perform fluorescein angiography, which usually helps to confirm the diagnosis.

7. **How does this condition differ from Leber's miliary aneurysms?**
   Leber described retinal miliary aneurysms within a couple of years of Coats disease. He suggested that the conditions were one and the same, and that is the generally accepted thinking at the present time.

8. **Do we know the etiology of Coats disease?**
   The precise etiology for Coats disease has not been determined. Some studies suggest that the retinal changes are not predominantly inflammatory in nature. We have few additional insights into the underlying cause, and at this point one would have to say that the etiology remains obscure.

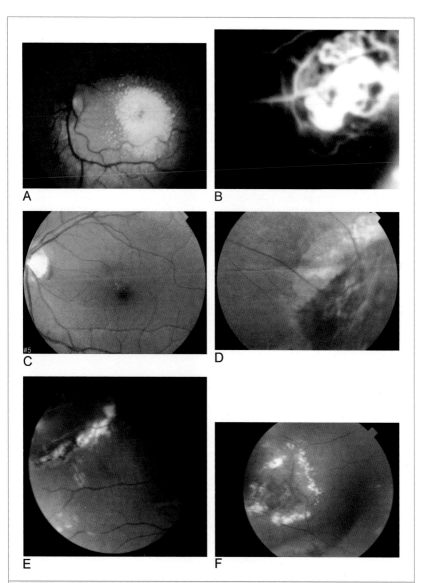

Figure 41-1. *A*, Exudate in the posterior pole of a 9-month-old girl before treatment. *B*, Peripheral retinal telangiectasia seen on fluorescein angiography in the temporal periphery of patient shown in *A*. *C*, The exudate has not recurred 12 years after treatment. *D*, Area of peripheral cryotherapy 12 years later. *E*, Recurrent Coats disease 13 years after original treatment. *F*, Recurrent Coats disease 27 years after original treatment.

9. **Are there any conditions with which Coats disease can be confused?**
   When there is exudation in the macula and peripheral retinal telangiectasia, but no retinal detachment, the disease can frequently be competently diagnosed. In advanced stages there are a number of conditions that Coats disease may simulate, most notably retinoblastoma, the

malignant intraocular tumor that occurs in infancy and childhood. It has been estimated that approximately 3.9% of eyes originally diagnosed as harboring retinoblastoma were subsequently discovered to have Coats disease.

10. **Can conditions other than retinoblastoma simulate Coats disease?**
    Angiomatosis retinae (von Hippel-Lindau syndrome), one of the phakomatoses, can cause exudation in the macula. This condition is inherited in an autosomal dominant fashion and has visceral and central nervous system hemangioblastomas as part of the syndrome. In addition, visceral cysts and tumors, including renal cell carcinoma, may occur. Early in its onset, the fundus picture is different from Coats disease in that angiomatosis retinae demonstrates a dilated and tortuous afferent arteriole and an efferent draining venule that enters and leaves a reddish balloon-like mass, usually in the fundus periphery. If the capillary angioma is on the disc, it may be associated with macular exudation, making the differential diagnosis from Coats disease more difficult. Other conditions to be considered in the diagnosis are familial exudative vitreoretinopathy, which is a dominantly inherited condition that may have a Coats disease–like response, hyperplastic primary vitreous, which is usually unilateral and occurs in a microphthalmic eye, and retinopathy of prematurity, which may present with retinal detachment but usually in patients with a history of significant prematurity.

KEY POINTS: DIFFERENTIAL DIAGNOSIS OF COATS DISEASE

1. Angiomatosis retinae

2. Retinoblastoma

3. Familial exudative vitreoretinopathy

4. Hyperplastic primary vitreous

5. Retinopathy of prematurity

11. **Other than fluorescein angiography, what may be helpful in confirming the diagnosis?**
    Ultrasonography may help to differentiate between Coats disease and retinoblastoma by detecting the presence or absence of subretinal calcifications. Calcification is found in retinoblastoma, but it is extremely rare in Coats disease.

12. **Is it advisable to obtain a computed tomographic (CT) scan?**
    CT scanning is perhaps the single most valuable test in diagnosing Coats disease, because of its ability to delineate intraocular morphology, to qualify retinal densities, and to detect associated orbital or intracranial abnormalities. However, this does expose a young patient to low levels of radiation if studies are repeated periodically.

13. **Can aspiration of subretinal exudates aid in diagnosis?**
    The key diagnostic findings in the analysis of subretinal aspirates are the presence of cholesterol crystals and pigment-laden macrophages and the absence of tumor cells. Reserve this technique for patients in whom retinoblastoma has been ruled out by all other noninvasive means, because tumor seeding can occur.

14. **How is Coats disease managed?**
    It is desirable to treat the condition before exudate accumulates in the macular area. Treatment is directed at the peripheral telangiectatic vascular abnormalities. Photocoagulation can be used to eliminate these abnormal vessels. In patients with exudation under the peripheral vascular telangiectasia, cryotherapy may be preferable (Fig. 41-1, D). Elimination of the defective vessels prevents further leakage and is followed by resorption of the exudate.

15. **How long does it take for the exudate to disappear?**
    Resorption of the exudate may take up to a year or more before it is completely gone.

16. **Is more than one treatment necessary?**
    If more than two quadrants have retinal telangiectasia, two to three treatments may be required.

17. **Once the abnormal vessels are gone, is the patient considered cured?**
    Recurrence, which is usually heralded by the reappearance of exudate and is almost always associated with new vascular abnormalities, can occur even many years later. It is recommended that patients be scheduled for follow-up appointments at 6-month intervals.

18. **Can this condition be managed once the retina has detached?**
    The drainage of subretinal exudative fluid and the placement of a scleral buckle may, in some cases, help to reattach the retina. Less commonly, vitrectomy may be performed, and internal drainage of fluid and cholesterol may be accomplished through a retinotomy. At the same time, it is necessary to treat the abnormal vessels by photocoagulation or cryotherapy. The vision in these eyes, however, is usually quite limited, and sometimes, despite reattachment of the retina, there is no light perception.

19. **If left untreated, what is the outcome?**
    Untreated Coats disease does not invariably lead to intractable glaucoma. However, retinal detachment and neovascular glaucoma are the ultimate complications that may lead to loss of the globe.

20. **When should an eye with Coats disease be enucleated?**
    When retinoblastoma cannot be ruled out or when neovascular glaucoma is present in blind, painful eyes.

21. **Can Coats disease occur with any other retinal conditions?**
    Coats disease may occur in conjunction with retinitis pigmentosa. Autoimmunity toward retinal antigens may play a role in specific types of retinitis pigmentosa.

BIBLIOGRAPHY

1. Char DH: Coats' syndrome: Long-term follow up. Br J Ophthalmol 84:37–39, 2000.
2. Coats G: Forms of retinal disease with massive exudation. R Lond Ophthalmol Hosp Rep 17:440–525, 1908.
3. Coats G: Über retinitis exsudativa (retinitis haemorrhagica externa). Albrecht von Graefes Arch Klin Exp Ophthalmol 18:275–327, 1912.
4. Egerer I, Tasman W, Tomer TL: Coats disease. Arch Ophthalmol 92:109–112, 1974.
5. Haik BG, Saint Louis L, Smith ME, et al: Computed tomography of the nonrhegmatogenous retinal detachment in the pediatric patient. Ophthalmology 92:1133–1142, 1985.
6. Howard GM, Ellsworth RM: Differential diagnosis of retinoblastoma: A statistical survey of 500 children: I. Relative frequency of the lesions which simulate retinoblastoma. Am J Ophthalmol 60:610–617, 1965.
7. Leber T: Über eine durch Vorkommen multipler Miliaraneurysmen charakterisierte Form von Retinaldegeneration. Arch Ophthalmol 81:1–14, 1912.

8. Matsuura S, Shiragami C, Takasu I, et al: Retinal attachment achieved by vitrectomy in two cases of bullous exudative retinal detachment. Folia Ophthalmol Jpn 50:786–790, 1999.

9. Ridley ME, Shields JA, Brown GC, et al: Coats disease: Evaluation of management. Ophthalmology 898:1381–1387, 1982.

10. Shields JA, Shields CL, Honavar SG, Demirci H: Clinical variations and complications of Coats disease in 150 cases: The 2000 Sanford Gifford memorial lecture. Am J Ophthalmol 131:561–571, 2001.

11. Solomon A, Banin E, Anteby I, Benezra D: Retinitis pigmentosa, Coats disease and uveitis. Eur J Ophthalmol 9:202–205, 1999.

12. Tarkkanen A, Laatikainen L: Coats disease: Clinical, angiographic, histopathological findings and clinical management. Br J Ophthalmol 67:766–776, 1983.

CHAPTER 42

FUNDUS TRAUMA

Jeffrey P. Blice, MD

1. **What are the mechanisms of injury to the fundus in blunt trauma?**
   Blunt trauma to the sclera can produce a direct effect on the underlying choroid and retina. In addition, a concussive effect from force transmitted through the vitreous may be seen away from the initial point of impact. The sudden deformation of the globe may cause stretching of the retina and retinal pigment epithelium (RPE) and traction on the vitreous base. The shearing forces generated by this traction may tear the retina in the area of the vitreous base or result in avulsion of the vitreous base. Forces can be severe enough to avulse the optic nerve (Fig. 42-1).

   Delori F, Pomerantzeff O, Cox MS: Deformation of the globe under high-speed impact: Its relation to contusion injuries. Invest Ophthalmol 8:290–301, 1969.

2. **What clinical entity is caused by the contrecoup mechanism?**
   Indirect damage from the concussive effect of an injury tends to occur at the interfaces of tissue with the greatest differences in density, most commonly the lens–vitreous interface and posterior vitreoretinal interface. The transmitted force may cause fragmentation of photoreceptor outer segments and damage to the receptor cell bodies. Clinically, these areas appear as opacified retina and are termed *commotio retinae*. Although the retinal whitening is only temporary, resolving over 3–4 weeks, permanent damage may occur. Loss of vision depends on the amount and location of early photoreceptor loss. The RPE underlying an area of commotio may develop a granular hyperpigmentation

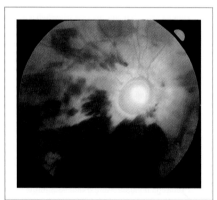

Figure 42-1. Optic nerve avulsion after severe blunt trauma.

   or atrophic appearance and lead to decreased vision. The eponym associated with this entity is Berlin's edema; however, there is no true intracellular or extracellular edema, and no fluorescein leakage is seen.

3. **Name the five types of retinal breaks seen in fundus trauma.**
   - Retinal dialyses
   - Horseshoe tears
   - Operculated holes
   - Macular holes
   - Retinal dissolution (necrosis)

   Cox MS, Schepens CL, Freeman HM: Retinal detachment due to ocular contusion. Arch Ophthalmol 76:678–685, 1966.

4. **Where are retinal dialyses most commonly seen?**
Retinal dialyses are usually located in the superonasal or inferotemporal quadrants (Fig. 42-2). Trauma is more clearly related to the superonasal than inferotemporal dialyses. Dialyses may be associated with avulsion of the vitreous base. Because they can lead to retinal detachment, a careful depressed exam of all patients with a history of blunt trauma is essential. Prophylactic treatment of all dialyses with cryopexy or laser photocoagulation is recommended in the hope of decreasing the likelihood of future retinal detachments.

Hollander DA, Irvine AR, Poothullil AM, Bhisitkul RB: Distinguishing features of nontraumatic and traumatic retinal dialyses. Retina 24:669–675, 2004.

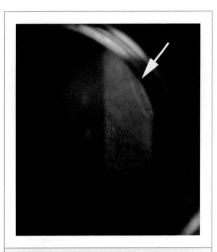

Figure 42-2. Retinal dialysis *(arrow)* with associated chronic retinal detachment through contact lens.

5. **When do retinal detachments occur with dialyses?**
Retinal detachments present at variable intervals after injury; however, the dialysis is usually detectable early or immediately at the time of injury. Approximately 10% of dialysis-related detachments present immediately, 30% within 1 month, 50% within 8 months, and 80% within 2 years. Most trauma victims are young with a formed vitreous that tamponades a break or dialysis, but as the vitreous eventually liquefies, fluid passes through retinal breaks causing detachments. The nature of the vitreous in such cases may explain the delay in presentation of the detachments.

Tasman W: Peripheral retinal changes following blunt trauma. Trans Am Ophthalmol Soc 70:190–198, 1972.

6. **Besides retinal dialyses, do other trauma-related breaks need to be treated prophylactically?**
Horseshoe tears and operculated holes in the setting of acute trauma are usually treated by cryopexy or laser photocoagulation. Macular holes require pars plana vitrectomy with gas exchange if closure of the hole is attempted; however, macular holes usually do not progress to retinal detachments. Surgery is not performed for the purposes of prophylactic closure. Direct injury with necrosis of the retina is usually associated with underlying choroidal injury so that a chorioretinal adhesion may be formed spontaneously. However, any accumulation of subretinal fluid or persistent traction on damaged retina makes prophylactic treatment reasonable.

7. **What is the prognosis for repair of a retinal detachment associated with a dialysis?**
Dialysis-related detachments are usually smooth, thin, and transparent. Intraretinal cysts are common, and half have demarcation lines. In addition, proliferative vitreoretinopathy is rare. The characteristics of the detachment are suggestive of its chronic nature and insidious onset; however, the prognosis for repair with conventional scleral buckling techniques is good.

8. **Describe the clinical features of a choroidal rupture.**
The retina is relatively elastic, and the sclera is mechanically strong. Bruch's membrane, the structure between the retinal pigment epithelium and choriocapillaris, is neither elastic nor

strong. Consequently, it is susceptible to the stretching forces exerted on the globe in blunt trauma. Bruch's membrane usually tears along with the choriocapillaris and RPE. Choroidal ruptures may be found at the point of contact with the globe or in the posterior pole as a result of indirect forces. Clinically, choroidal rupture appears as a single area or multiple areas of subretinal hemorrhage, usually concentric and temporal to the optic nerve (Fig. 42-3). The hemorrhage may dissect into the vitreous. As the blood resolves, a crescent-shaped or linear white area is seen where the rupture occurred. With time, surrounding RPE hyperplasia or atrophy may be seen.

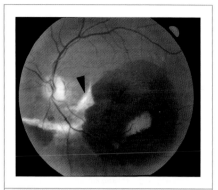

Figure 42-3. Choroidal ruptures *(large arrows)* located concentric to the optic nerve. The *small arrow* demonstrates the center of associated subretinal hemorrhage.

Kelley JS, Dhaliwal RS: Traumatic choroidopathies. In Ryan SJ (ed): Retina, vol. 2. St. Louis, Mosby, 1994, pp 1783–1796.

9. **Are there any long-term complications of choroidal ruptures?**
   The visual consequences of a choroidal rupture depend on its location with respect to the fovea. A patient with a choroidal rupture near the fovea may have good vision; however, the break in Bruch's membrane predisposes him or her to the development of a choroidal neovascular membrane, which may threaten vision long after the initial injury. Therefore, patients at risk should be followed regularly and advised of the potential complication.

10. **Can orbital adnexal trauma result in fundus abnormalities?**
    High-velocity missile injuries may cause an indirect concussive injury to the globe, resulting in retinal breaks and ruptures in Bruch's membrane that resemble a claw. A fibroglial scar with pigment proliferation forms, but retinal detachment is rare, possibly because a firm adhesion develops, acting as a retinopexy. Chorioretinitis sclopetaria is the name given to this clinical entity.

KEY POINTS: RETINAL BREAKS IN BLUNT TRAUMA

1. The five types of breaks are horseshoe tears, operculated tears, dialyses, retinal dissolution, and macular holes.

2. Retinal dialyses usually occur superonasally in trauma.

3. A total of 50% of dialysis-related detachments present within 8 months.

4. A dialysis-related detachment has a very high success rate with treatment by scleral buckling.

11. **What are the signs of a scleral rupture?**
    When a laceration or obvious deformation of the globe is not visible, other findings raise the index of suspicion that an injury may be more serious than initially thought. The presence of an

afferent pupillary defect (APD), poor motility, marked chemosis, and vitreous hemorrhage raise the suspicion of an open globe. Other findings that may be helpful include a deeper than normal anterior chamber and a low intraocular pressure; however, in an eye with a posterior rupture and incarcerated uvea the intraocular pressure may be normal.

12. **Why is the initial exam of a severely traumatized eye important?**
A poor outcome is associated with initially poor visual acuity, presence of an APD, large wounds (>10 mm) or wounds extending posterior to the rectus muscles, and vitreous hemorrhage. The first person to evaluate the traumatized eye may have the only opportunity to assess the best visual acuity. The delay often associated with referral to other institutions or dealing with life-threatening complications may result in diffusion of vitreous hemorrhage and corneal or other anterior segment abnormalities that preclude an adequate view of the posterior segment. The first look may be the only look at a traumatized eye.

Pieramici DJ, MacCumber MW, Humayun MU, et al: Open-globe injury. Update on types of injuries and visual results. Ophthalmology 103:1798–1803, 1996.

13. **Where is the most likely place for a globe to rupture?**
The globe may rupture anywhere, depending on the nature of the injury. However, the globe most often ruptures at the limbus, beneath the recti muscles, or at a surgical scar. The sclera is thinnest and therefore weakest behind the insertions of the recti muscles. The site of a previous cataract extraction or glaucoma procedure is weaker than normal sclera.

14. **Outline the goals of managing a ruptured globe.**
   1. Identify the extent of the injury. Perform a 360-degree peritomy, inspecting all quadrants. If necessary, disinsert a muscle to determine the extent of a laceration.
   2. Rule out a retained foreign body. In any case of projectile injury, sharp lacerations, uncertain history, or questionable mechanism of injury, consider a computed tomographic (CT) scan to detect a foreign body.
   3. Close the wound, and limit reconstruction as much as possible. Close the sclera with a relatively large suture (e.g., 8-0 or 9-0 nylon), and reposit any protruding uvea. If vitreous is protruding, cut it flush with the choroidal tissues, using fine scissors and a cellulose sponge or automated vitreous cutter.
   4. Guard against infection. Start prophylactic systemic antibiotic treatment using an IV aminoglycoside or third-generation cephalosporin in combination with vancomycin (e.g., ceftriaxone, 1–2 mg every 12 hours and vancomycin, 1 mg every 12 hours). Clindamycin can be added if coverage for *Bacillus* sp. is desired.
   5. Protect the remaining eye. Place a shield over the fellow eye during the repair procedure to prevent accidental injury. Counsel the patient at the earliest opportunity about the need for protective eyewear to prevent future injury.

KEY POINTS: GLOBE RUPTURES

1. Vitreous hemorrhage, poor vision, APD, and massive chemosis/subconjunctival hemorrhage are the hallmarks of a ruptured globe.

2. The globe is most likely to rupture at the limbus, underneath a rectus muscle, or at a previous surgical site.

3. Large ruptures (>10 mm) are associated with a poor prognosis.

4. Sympathetic ophthalmia is an exceedingly rare complication.

5. Remember to protect the remaining eye during repair and afterward.

15. **Discuss the role of CT and magnetic resonance imaging (MRI) in the detection of intraocular foreign bodies.**

The best method of detecting intraocular foreign bodies is indirect ophthalmoscopy (Fig. 42-4). If a view of the posterior segment is impossible, CT is the next best alternative. A CT scan is excellent for the detection of metallic foreign bodies but also detects glass or even plastic foreign bodies in some instances (Fig. 42-5). When an organic foreign body is suspected, MRI offers the advantage of better soft tissue discrimination and is an excellent supplement to CT. However, any suspicion of a metallic foreign body prevents the use of MRI. Ultrasonography also supplements the information provided by a CT, possibly detecting a radiolucent foreign body as well as providing information about the status of the retina and vitreous. Plain films of the orbit are still useful for the detection of a foreign body if a CT scanner is not available; however, the ability to localize and detect nonmetallic foreign bodies is more limited.

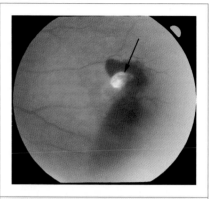

Figure 42-4. Fundus photograph of intraocular foreign body *(arrow)* resting on surface of retina.

16. **What ultrasound artifacts are important to recognize in evaluation of the traumatized globe?**

The appearances of intraocular foreign bodies on ultrasonography are related to the nature, shape, and size of the foreign body, in addition to the angle of incidence of the sound waves.

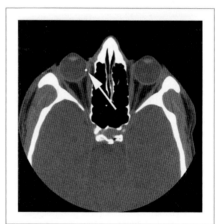

Figure 42-5. Computed tomographic scan demonstrating the presence of a small intraocular foreign body *(arrow)* located nasally.

Reverberations and shadowing are characteristic ultrasound artifacts seen with intraocular foreign bodies. Reverberations are the multiple echoes that appear behind the initial reflection from a foreign body. Shadowing is the absence of echoes seen behind the initial reflection from a foreign body. Both of these artifacts may be demonstrable on the same patient by altering the angle of incidence of the ultrasound.

17. **Do all intraocular foreign bodies need to be removed immediately? Which ones require early vitrectomy for removal?**

All foreign bodies do not require immediate removal. The decision to remove a foreign body at the time of initial repair is complex and depends somewhat on the preferences of the surgeon and the specific situation. However, in a patient with acute traumatic endophthalmitis or a known toxic or reactive foreign body, vitrectomy with removal of any intraocular foreign bodies at the time of initial repair, or soon after, is a reasonable option.

Wani VB, Al-Ajmi M, Thalib L, et al: Vitrectomy for posterior segment intraocular foreign bodies: Visual results and prognostic factors. Retina 23:654–660, 2003.

18. **Which metals are toxic to the eye?**
    The toxicity of a metal is related to the reduction-oxidation potential (redox potential).
    Metals such as copper and iron have a low redox potential and tend to dissociate into their
    respective ionic forms, which makes them more toxic. Pure forms are more reactive than alloys.
    The ocular toxicity from an iron foreign body is called *siderosis*. When copper is the offending
    agent, the condition is named *chalcosis*. Other metals such as gold, platinum, silver, and
    aluminum are relatively inert. Nonmetallic substances such as glass, plastic, porcelain, and
    rubber are also relatively inert and pose no threat of toxicity on the basis of their chemical
    composition.

19. **List the clinical findings in siderosis bulbi.**
    Iron tends to be deposited in epithelial tissues. Hyperchromic heterochromia of the involved
    iris and a mid-dilated, minimally reactive pupil are seen. Brownish dots are visible in the lens
    from iron deposition in the lens epithelium, along with generalized yellowing of the lens from
    involvement of the cortex. The retinal effects of iron toxicity can be detected and followed by
    electroretinography (ERG). Pure iron particles may cause a flat ERG in 100 days. Clinically, a
    pigmentary degeneration with sclerosis of vessels, retinal thinning, and, later, atrophy develops
    in the periphery and progresses posteriorly. If not removed initially, the potential toxic effects
    of a foreign body can be monitored by clinical exam and serial ERG. However, siderosis
    generally causes progressive gradual permanent visual loss unless the foreign body is removed.

20. **Do all copper foreign bodies cause chalcosis?**
    Foreign bodies composed of less than 85% pure copper cause chalcosis; greater than 85% pure
    copper foreign bodies cause sterile endophthalmitis. Copper ions are deposited in basement
    membranes. In the cornea, Descemet's membrane may be affected, causing a Kaiser Fleischer
    ring, a brownish discoloration of the peripheral cornea. The iris may be sluggishly reactive to
    light and have a greenish color. Deposition of copper in the anterior capsule results in a
    "sunflower" cataract, and the vitreous may become opacified. ERG findings are similar but may
    improve if the foreign body is removed.

KEY POINTS: INTRAOCULAR FOREIGN BODIES

1. The best method of detection is indirect ophthalmoscopy whenever possible.

2. An intraocular foreign body does not usually require immediate removal.

3. Topical and systemic antibiotics are required as prophylaxis against endophthalmitis.

4. MRI is contraindicated in any patient with a suspected metallic intraocular foreign body.

5. Iron can cause siderosis and copper can cause chalcosis or sterile endophthalmitis.

21. **Which organisms most commonly cause posttraumatic endophthalmitis?**
    The most common organism associated with endophthalmitis in the setting of acute
    trauma is *Staphylococcus aureus*. Skin flora are the most likely source of contamination of a
    traumatic ocular wound. Infections caused by *Bacillus cereus*, although much less common
    (estimates range from 8% to 25%), are important because of the severity and damage caused
    by the infection. In any ocular injury contaminated by soil, the possibility of infection with
    B. cereus needs to be considered and the regimen of prophylactic antibiotics adjusted
    accordingly.

22. **Outline the role of prophylactic antibiotics.**
    Posttraumatic endophthalmitis is a relatively rare complication of penetrating ocular trauma, occurring in only 7% of cases; however, the potential for devastation to the eye warrants prophylactic treatment. In cases of obvious endophthalmitis, a grossly contaminated wound, or contaminated foreign body, initial intravitreal antibiotic injection may be considered. Although no definitive evidence exists for a clinical benefit, postoperatively, all ruptured or lacerated globes are usually treated with prophylactic topical and systemic antibiotics for 3–5 days. Although the Endophthalmitis Vitrectomy Study (EVS) showed no benefit to systemic antibiotic treatment in postoperative endophthalmitis, the issue of prophylaxis in trauma was not specifically addressed.

    Meredith TA: Posttraumatic endophthalmitis. Arch Ophthalmol 117:520–521, 1999.

23. **What regimen of antibiotics is used to treat posttraumatic endophthalmitis?**
    The choice of intravitreal injections is directed at covering a broad spectrum of organisms. Although a number of combinations are possible, a regimen with coverage for typical pathogens is vancomycin, 1 mg/0.1 mL, or clindamycin, 1 mg/0.1 mL, in combination with amikacin, 0.2–0.4 mg/0.1 mL, or gentamicin, 0.1 mg/0.1 mL. Frequently applied topical treatment with a fluoroquinolone should be initiated postoperatively in addition to systemic antibiotics for 7–10 days.

24. **Does injury to one eye place the other eye at risk for visual loss?**
    Granulomatous inflammation may affect both the noninjured and injured eye weeks to years after a penetrating injury. Sympathetic ophthalmia (SO) is a bilateral granulomatous uveitis manifested by anterior segment inflammation and multiple yellow-white lesions in the peripheral fundus. Complications include cataract, glaucoma, optic atrophy, exudative retinal detachments, and subretinal fibrosis. Exposure of the immune system to a previously immunologically isolated antigen in the uvea probably triggers the response. Eighty percent of cases develop within 3 months of injury, and 90% develop within 1 year. Rare cases of SO have occurred after ocular surgery. Therapy is directed at immunosuppression with steroids, cyclosporin, and/or cytotoxic agents. Most patients retain 20/60 vision or better at 10-year follow-up, but complications limit vision in many patients.

25. **How can the uninjured eye be protected from the long-term sequelae of penetrating ocular injury?**
    The incidence of SO is extremely rare (<0.5% of penetrating trauma). The only known way to prevent the disease absolutely is enucleation of the injured eye 10–14 days after the injury. With modern repair techniques, the potential for vision in severely injured eyes has improved; therefore, enucleation as prophylactic treatment for SO should be reserved only **for eyes confirmed to have no visual potential**. Removal of the inciting eye after inflammation has developed may improve the final acuity of the noninjured eye, but the inciting eye may eventually retain the best visual acuity. Enucleation as a treatment is reserved for inciting eyes with **no visual potential**.

    Chu DS, Foster CS: Sympathetic ophthalmia. Int Ophthalmol Clin 42:179–185, 2002.

26. **Can trauma elsewhere in the body cause fundus abnormalities?**
    Cotton-wool spots, usually in the peripapillary distribution, retinal hemorrhages, and optic disc edema have been described after severe head injury or compressive chest trauma. Purtscher's retinopathy, the name given to this entity, is a result of microvascular occlusion presumed to be embolic in nature and related to complement activation; however, the true pathogenesis is unknown. A similar appearance in other conditions, such as acute pancreatitis, collagen vascular disease, renal dialysis, and eclampsia, suggests a systemic process with secondary retinal capillary occlusion. The fundus manifestations in severe trauma may be related to the generally

poor condition of patients who sustained such trauma rather than the trauma itself. Vitreous, preretinal, and retinal hemorrhages may be seen in birth trauma; however, if seen in the absence of such trauma or other causes (leukemia or bleeding diathesis), nonaccidental trauma should be suspected. Ocular manifestations are present in 40% of abused children, and the ophthalmologist is first to recognize the abuse in 6% of cases. Suspicious injuries need to be reported to protect children from further abuse.

CHAPTER 43

AGE-RELATED MACULAR DEGENERATION

Joseph I. Maguire, MD

1. **What is age-related macular degeneration?**
   Age-related macular degeneration (ARMD) is the leading cause of significant, irreversible central visual loss in the Western world. It is characterized by age-dependent alterations of the sensory retina, retinal pigment epithelium, and choriocapillaris complex in the central retina (macula). The macula is defined clinically by the area roughly within the major temporal vascular arcades and serves our sharp, discriminating vision (Fig. 43-1). Incidence of disease is age dependent, and prevalence steadily increases past age 55. A common international classification exists, but most clinicians still divide ARMD into exudative (wet) and nonexudative (dry) forms.

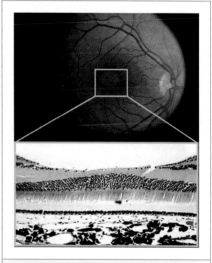

Figure 43-1. The clinical macula describes that area of the retina encompassed by the temporal arcade vessels.

2. **Who develops ARMD?**
   Anyone can. The greatest statistical association with macular degeneration development is increasing age. All long-term epidemiologic studies indicate an increasing prevalence of exudative and nonexudative macular changes, as well as visual loss, with increasing age. Most reports point to a greater incidence of disease in women over men. In addition, skin pigmentation plays an important role in exudative disease; African Americans have a significantly smaller incidence of choroidal neovascularization compared with Caucasians.

   Framingham Study: VI. Macular degeneration. Surv Ophthalmol 24:428–435, 1980.

3. **Why will ARMD become such an enormous challenge in the next 25 years?**
   The number of Americans in the 65 and over age group will double in the next 25 years. The visual morbidity and mortality associated with ARMD will affect a huge number of elderly Americans socially, emotionally, and economically. The loss of reading and driving vision, the increased need for social and familial support, the cost of treatment, and the resultant emotional consequences will have a multifaceted impact on our resources.

4. **Describe etiologic factors involved in the development of ARMD.**
   The exact cause of ARMD is unknown and appears to be multifactorial. In addition to increasing age, smoking is a consistent risk predictor. The discovery of a genetic link in the complement factor H gene has exposed a single nuclear polymorphism responsible for nearly 50% of ARMD risk.

This supports the hypothesis of ARMD being an inflammatory disease. Female gender, white race, smoking, nutrition, scleral rigidity, photic exposure, previous cataract surgery, and hypertension have been implicated as well.

Age-Related Eye Disease Study Research Group: Risk factors for the incidence of advanced age-related macular degeneration in the age-related eye disease study (AREDS). AREDS report no. 19. Ophthalmology 112:533–539, 2005.

Edwards AO, Ritter R, Abel KJ, et al: Complement factor H polymorphism and age-related macular degeneration. Science 308:421–424, 2005.

Young R: Pathophysiology of age-related macular degeneration. Surv Ophthalmol 31:291–306, 1987.

5. **Name common visual symptoms in ARMD patients.**
   - Visual blurring
   - Central scotomas
   - Metamorphopsia

   Metamorphopsia is visual distortion. Images may appear smaller (micropsia) or larger (macropsia) than they really are. Patients frequently comment that straight lines such as door jams, tile patterns, telephone poles, or other straight-edged surfaces appear curved. Special graphs called *Amsler grids*—which test the central 20 degrees of vision—are effective home-testing devices for eyes at higher risk for development of exudative ARMD.

6. **What is dry or nonexudative ARMD?**
   Nonexudative ARMD is characterized by drusen, pigmentary changes, and atrophy. Drusen are the most common and earliest dry ARMD changes (Fig. 43-2). Drusen represent metabolic by-products of retinal pigment epithelial cell metabolism. They vary in shape, size, and color. Hard drusen are small, discrete, yellow-to-white nodules, whereas soft drusen tend to be larger and more amorphous. Soft drusen may coalesce with neighboring drusen and are frequently associated with overlying pigmentary changes either from photoreceptor dysfunction or retinal pigment epithelial demise. Progressive retinal pigment epithelial disruption eventually causes loss of overlying sensory retina and underlying choriocapillaris. Such developments result in localized atrophic regions that extend and coalesce around the fovea and eventually involve the fovea itself.

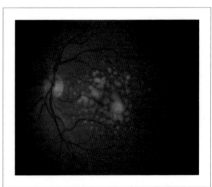

Figure 43-2. Drusen are the by-product of retinal metabolism and manifest as focal yellow-white deposits deep to the retinal pigment epithelium. They serve as markers of nonexudative age-related macular degeneration.

7. **What is wet or exudative ARMD?**
   Exudative ARMD is characterized by the development of vascular changes and fluid under the sensory retina and retinal pigment epithelium (RPE). Choroidal neovascular membranes and pigment epithelial detachments progressing to end-stage disciform macular scarring are the classic presentations of wet ARMD. Clinically, choroidal neovascular membranes are slate green–hued subretinal lesions associated with hard exudate, hemorrhage, or fluid. These vessels originate from the normal choriocapillaris and enter the subretinal space through defects in Bruch's membrane, a collagenous layer separating the choroidal circulation from the retina (Fig. 43-3). Pigment epithelial detachments are dome-shaped clear, turbid, or blood-filled

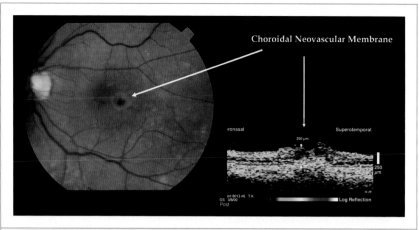

Choroidal Neovascular Membrane

Figure 43-3. Choroidal neovascular membranes gain access to the subretinal space via defects in Bruch's membrane *(arrow)*. Once there, these vessels may cause bleeding and disciform scar formation, resulting in overlying retinal dysfunction.

KEY POINTS: CLINICAL FINDINGS ASSOCIATED WITH ARMD

1. Nonexudative changes
   a. Drusen
   b. Pigmentary alterations
   c. Atrophy: Incipient, geographic

2. Exudative changes
   a. Hemorrhage
   b. Hard exudate
   c. Subretinal, sub-RPE, and intraretinal fluid

elevations of the retinal pigment epithelium; they may or may not be associated with choroidal neovascular ingrowth.

Gass JDM: Drusen and disciform macular detachment and degeneration. Arch Ophthalmol 90:206–217, 1973.

8. **Describe the difference between occult and classic choroidal neovascularization.**
   Classic choroidal neovascularization is clinically well defined. Fluorescein angiography demonstrates discrete hyperfluorescent lesion with a cartwheel configuration that increases in intensity over the course of the study (Fig. 43-4). Occult neovascularization usually demonstrates a poorly defined, stippled, pigmented appearance with associated retinal thickening. It is not well localized with fluorescein angiography, exhibiting diffuse punctate hyperfluorescence (Fig. 43-5).

9. **How does ARMD cause visual loss?**
ARMD ultimately leads to visual loss via permanent alterations in the sensory retina, retinal pigment epithelium, and choroid within the macula. These changes may arise from the development of disciform scarring secondary to choroidal neovascularization or atrophy in which areas of retina cease to exist.

10. **What is fluorescein angiography?**
Fluorescein angiography is a photographic test used in the diagnosis and treatment of ARMD. Fluorescein dye is injected via an antecubital vein while simultaneous photographs of the macula are taken with a fundus camera. Fluorescein dye demonstrates fluorescence when stimulated with visible light in the blue frequency range. This property, along with anatomic constraints in the retinal and choroidal circulations, allows the identification and localization of abnormal vascular processes, such as choroidal neovascularization, that are found frequently in ARMD.

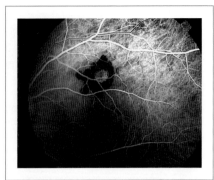

Figure 43-4. Angiographically, classic neovascular membranes appear as focal hyperfluorescent lesions deep to the retina. This example shows a corona of hyperfluorescence, which is associated hemorrhage.

11. **What is indocyanine green video-angiography?**
Indocyanine green (ICG) videoangiography is a photographic technique stylistically similar to fluorescein angiography. The major difference is the use of ICG dye, which has a peak absorption and emission in the infrared range, whereas the spectral qualities of fluorescein dye are in the visible range. ICG angiography's advantage is allowing visualization through pigment and thin blood, which facilitates viewing of the choroid.

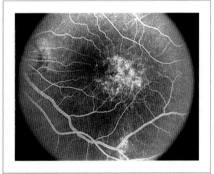

Figure 43-5. Unfortunately, the majority of choroidal neovascularization is nondiscrete or occult in character. This presentation is often not fully localized with fluorescein angiography. It has a punctuate hyperfluorescent pattern with nondiscrete borders.

Yannuzzi LA, Slakter JS, Sorenson JA, et al: Digital indocyanine green videoangiography and choroidal neovascularization. Retina 12:191–223, 1992.

12. **What is optical coherence tomography (OCT)?**
OCT uses the property of optical coherence to give a cross-sectional representation of the macula. Its high resolution allows localization of choroidal neovascular processes and secondary effects such as retinal edema, sensory retinal detachment, and atrophy. Its articulation of retinal edema may make it an able or even superior diagnostic test in eliciting and following choroidal neovascular membrane activity.

Voo I, Mavrofrides EC, Puliafito CA. Clinical applications of optical coherence tomography for the diagnosis and management of macular disease. Ophthalmol Clin North Am 17:21–31, 2004.

13. **Name proven therapies for exudative ARMD.**
    Current proven therapies for ARMD involve thermal laser photocoagulation, photodynamic therapy (PDT), and intravitreal injection of vascular endothelial growth factor (VEGF) inhibitors (e.g., pegaptanib [Macugen], ranibizumab [Lucentis], and bevacizumab [Avastin]).

    Macular Photocoagulation Study Group: Argon laser photocoagulation for neovascular maculopathy: Three year results from randomized clinical trials. Arch Ophthalmol 104:694–701, 1986.

14. **What is the Macular Photocoagulation Study (MPS)?**
    The MPS is a multicenter study sponsored by the National Institutes of Health to evaluate the utility of laser in the treatment of extrafoveal exudative ARMD, ocular histoplasmosis, and idiopathic choroidal neovascular membranes. Over time it has also established the benefits of laser treatment in juxtafoveal and subfoveal neovascularization, as established in its guidelines.

15. **How does conventional laser treatment affect exudative ARMD?**
    Conventional laser treatment works by creating a thermal burn and coagulating abnormal vasculature. However, local environmental effects, such as retinal pigment epithelial stimulation and increased oxygenation, also may play crucial roles.

16. **What percentage of patients with exudative ARMD can be effectively treated with laser photocoagulation?**
    Using MPS guidelines, no more than 25% of current patients with ARMD are candidates for laser photocoagulation. Because more than a third of eyes that are treatable have subfoveal lesions and more than 50% of successfully treated lesions recur within 3 years, the capacity of laser in the treatment and preservation of vision becomes even more limited.

17. **Describe the role of vitamins in the treatment and prophylaxis of ARMD.**
    The Age-related Eye Disease Study (AREDS) is sponsored jointly by the National Institutes of Health and the National Eye Institute, and has proved the benefit of high-dose vitamins in the prophylaxis of ARMD. Individuals with intermediate or high risk of developing ARMD had a 25% reduction in developing visual loss from either exudative or nonexudative forms of ARMD. Theoretically, the intake of certain vitamins and trace elements act directly, or indirectly through association with certain enzymes in free radical scavenging, thereby modulating the aging process.

    AREDS vitamins include high concentrations of vitamins C and E, betacarotene, zinc, and copper. Smoking and a previous history of lung cancer are contraindications for vitamin therapy; betacarotene increases lung carcinoma risk. However, a formula that substitutes lutein for betacarotene is available.

    AREDS summary: www.nei.nih.gov/amd/summary.asp

18. **What is the role of additional nutritional supplements in ARMD therapy?**
    The AREDS did not investigate other nutritional compounds such as macular pigments lutein and zeaxanthin and omega fatty acids. The AREDS II will prospectively investigate these supplements and their utility in ARMD prevention. Photic-protective macular pigments lutein and zeaxanthin are readily found in vegetables with green, yellow, or red pigmentation such as spinach, sweet potatoes, and carrots.

19. **What is photodynamic therapy? How does it differ from laser photocoagulation?**
    PDT is a Food and Drug Administration (FDA)-approved intervention for predominantly discrete subfoveal choroidal neovascular membranes secondary to ARMD. It involves the intravenous

administration of a porphyrin-based medication that is absorbed by abnormal subretinal vessels. The drug is then activated by wavelength-specific, low-energy, nonthermal infrared laser exposure. Activation of the photosensitizing compounds produces localized vascular damage via generation of free radicals. Its action, however, is local, thereby sparing the overlying sensory retina while destroying abnormal neovascularization. Because so many exudative features of ARMD are foveal, PDT has the ability to eliminate subfoveal choroidal neovascular changes while preserving fixation.

Treatment of Age-related Macular Degeneration with Photodynamic Therapy (TAP) Study Group. Photodynamic therapy of subfoveal choroidal neovascularization in age-related macular degeneration with verteporfin: Two-year results of two randomized clinical trials-TAP report 2. Arch Ophthalmol 119:198–207, 2001.

20. **What is the role of surgery in ARMD?**
The Submacular Surgery Trial (SST) was a prospective randomized trial that evaluated the benefits of invasive surgical techniques in the treatment of ARMD. For ARMD, removal of choroidal neovascular membranes was not found beneficial. Removal or displacement of submacular hemorrhage was found to be helpful in selected cases where visual acuity was less than 20/200.

21. **What is macular translocation?**
Macular translocation surgery is performed for exudative foveal ARMD. It has not been evaluated in prospective clinical trials. It involves physically "picking up" and moving macular retina away from the underlying choroidal neovascularization. This allows placement of the fovea in areas of healthy retinal pigment epithelium and choroid. Currently, there are two methods of translocation—limited translocation and 360-degree macular translocation.

22. **What is the role of pharmacologic management in ARMD?**
Currently, medical management involves the inhibition of angiogenic growth factors and associated modulators. Inhibition of VEGF has assumed primary importance. These agents can cause successful regression or inhibition of neovascular membranes in selected vascular neoplasms and animal models of neovascularization. Several vascular inhibitors and their delivery systems are currently available or under development and investigation.

Ferris FL: A new treatment for ocular neovascularization. N Engl J Med 351:2863–2865, 2004.

23. **Describe VEGF and its role in ocular neovascularization.**
Vascular endothelial growth factor is a homodimeric glycoprotein with multiple isomers, split products, and receptor sites. It is essential in the development and proper maintenance of normal body vasculature. It is influenced by multiple growth factors, cofactors, and environmental influences such as ischemia. Loss of normal VEGF homeostasis can result in its up-regulation with resultant neovascularization.

D'Amato RJ, Adamis AP: Angiogenesis inhibition in age-related macular degeneration. Ophthalmology 102:1261–1262, 1995.

24. **What is combination therapy?**
Combination therapy involves the use of more than one treatment regimen or treatment modality. Similar to the evolution of oncologic therapeutics, treatment of ARMD may come to involve laser, photodynamic therapy, and/or combinations of vascular growth inhibitors (Box 43-1). A current example involves the use of PDT with intravitreal injection of triamcinolone steroid.

25. **Name the three processes necessary for choroidal neovascular membrane development.**
- Increased vascular permeability
- Extracellular matrix breakdown
- Endothelial budding and vascular proliferation

> **BOX 43-1. ADDITIONAL ARMD TREATMENT STRATEGIES PREVIOUSLY OR CURRENTLY UNDER INVESTIGATION**
>
> 1. Radiation therapy
>   a. External beam
>   b. Radioactive plaque therapy
>   c. External probe application
> 2. Submacular surgery
>   a. Removal of choroidal neovascular membranes
>   b. Removal of submacular hemorrhage
> 3. Laser treatment
>   a. Prophylactic laser for drusen in nonexudative disease
>   b. Transpupillary thermotherapy for treatment of occult choroidal neovascularization
>   c. High-speed ICG-guided laser therapy for feeder vessels in occult and classic choroidal neovascularization
> 4. Pharmacologic management with inhibitors of angiogenesis
>   a. Anti-VEGF agents
>   b. Steroids
>   c. Angiostatic steroids
> 5. Combination therapies
>
> ICG = indocyanine green, VEGF = vascular endothelial growth factor.

26. **What are low vision AIDS?**

    Low vision support involves the use of devices that maximize a visually deficient eye's visual function through magnification, lighting, and training. It allows patients to take advantage of near peripheral vision. Such aids take many forms, including special spectacles, magnifiers, closed-circuit television devices, digitally enhanced cameras, and overhead viewers. People often can read print and carry out important functions not possible without such support. In patients with untreatable bilateral visual loss, evaluation for low vision support is critical.

CHAPTER 44

RETINOPATHY OF PREMATURITY

J. Arch McNamara, MD

1. **What is retinopathy of prematurity?**
   Retinopathy of prematurity (ROP) is a vasoproliferative retinal disease that affects infants born prematurely. It has two phases. In the acute phase, normal vascular development goes awry with the development of abnormal vessels that proliferate, occasionally with associated fibrous proliferation. In the chronic or late proliferation phase, retinal detachment, macular ectopia, and severe visual loss may occur. More than 90% of cases of acute ROP go on to spontaneous regression.

2. **Who gets retinopathy of prematurity?**
   Infants weighing less than 1500 grams at birth and those born at a gestational age of 32 weeks or less are at risk for developing ROP. The disease is more likely to affect the smallest and most premature of infants. The incidence of acute ROP in infants weighing less than 1 kg at birth is 3 times greater than that of infants weighing between 1 and 1.5 kg. Infants born at 23–27 weeks of gestation have a particularly high chance of developing ROP.

3. **Who should be screened for ROP?**
   Guidelines published by the American Academy of Pediatrics, Section on Ophthalmology; the American Association of Pediatric Ophthalmology and Strabismus; and the American Academy of Ophthalmology recommend that all infants weighing less than 1500 grams at birth or those with a gestational age of 28 weeks or less should be examined. Selected infants with a birth weight between 1500 and 2000 grams with an unstable clinical course should also be examined. Infants at particularly high risk are those who weigh less than 1000 grams at birth and those born at less than 27 weeks' gestation. The first exam should take place 4–6 weeks after birth or between 31 and 33 weeks of postconceptional or postmenstrual age. The frequency of follow-up examinations is based on the retinal status at the time of the first exam. Exams should be done every 1–2 weeks, either until there is complete retinal vascularization or until two successive 2-week examinations show stage 2 ROP in zone III (more on staging is discussed later in this chapter). Infants should then be examined every 4–6 weeks until the retina is fully vascularized. If there is prethreshold disease (see further discussion), examinations should be done every week until threshold disease occurs (at which point treatment should be offered) or until the disease regresses.

KEY POINTS: INDICATIONS FOR SCREENING INFANTS FOR ROP

1. All infants weighing less than 1500 grams at birth

2. All infants with a gestational age of 28 weeks

3. Infants with a birth weight between 1500 and 2000 grams with an unstable clinical course

4. Any infant that the neonatologist considers at risk because of an unstable clinical course

4. **How is ROP classified?**

The International Classification of Retinopathy of Prematurity (ICROP) is the system used for describing the findings in ROP. ICROP defines the location of disease in the retina and the extent of involvement of the developing vasculature. It also specifies the stage of involvement with levels of severity ranging from 1 (least affected) to 5 (severe disease).

For the purpose of defining location, the retina is divided into three zones, with the optic nerve as the center because vascularization starts from the optic nerve and progresses peripherally (Fig. 44-1). Zone I consists of a circle, the radius of which subtends an angle of 30 degrees and extends from the disc to twice the distance from the disc to the center of the macula (twice the disc-to-fovea distance in all directions from the optic disc). Zone II extends from the edge of zone I peripherally to a point tangential to the nasal ora serrata and around to an area near the temporal anatomic equator. Zone III is the residual temporal crescent of retina anterior to zone II.

Staging pertains to the degree of abnormal vascular response observed. Staging for the eye as a whole receives the stage of the most severe manifestation present. Stage 1 (demarcation line) is defined as a thin but definite structure that separates avascular retina anteriorly from the vascularized retina posteriorly. Abnormal branching of vessels can be seen leading up to the line. It is flat and white and is in the plane of the retina. Stage 2 (ridge) is present when the line of stage 1 has height and width and occupies a volume extending out of the plane of the retina. The ridge may be pink or white. Vessels may leave the plane of the retina to enter it. Small tufts of new vessels may be seen on the surface of the retina posterior to the ridge. These vessels do not constitute fibrovascular growth. Stage 3 (ridge with extraretinal fibrovascular proliferation) is present when fibrovascular proliferation is added to the ridge of stage 2 (Fig. 44-2). Stage 4 ROP exists when there is subtotal retinal detachment. Retinal detachments in ROP are concave, tractional retinal detachments. Stage 4A ROP is a subtotal retinal detachment that does not involve the central macula. Typically, it is present in the temporal region of zones II and III. Stage 4B ROP is a subtotal retinal detachment that involves the central macula. Lastly, stage 5 ROP is a total retinal detachment. These retinal detachments are funnel-shaped but may have an open or closed configuration in their anterior and posterior areas. The old term for ROP, "retrolental fibroplasia," was coined because of the most severe form of retinal detachment in which the retina is totally detached and drawn up into a fibrous mass behind the lens.

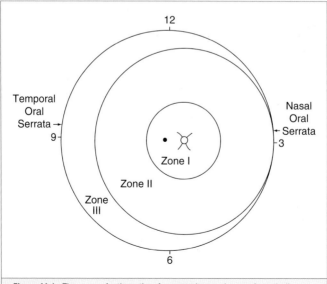

Figure 44-1. The zones of retinopathy of prematurity are shown schematically.

Improved imaging techniques have allowed for more detailed clinical examination of premature infants' eyes. This has resulted in a refinement of the ICROP. The committee added the concept of a more virulent retinopathy usually observed in the lowest-birth–weight infants, which they called aggressive posterior ROP (AP-ROP). This form of ROP is posteriorly located and has prominent plus disease with ill-defined retinopathy. The plus disease is out of proportion to the peripheral retinopathy and usually progresses rapidly to stage 5 disease. AP-ROP typically extends circumferentially and is associated with a circumferential vessel.

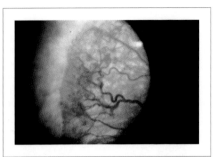

Figure 44-2. Stage 3 retinopathy of prematurity.

5. **What is plus disease?**
Plus disease is indicative of progressive vascular incompetence and is a strong risk factor for development of more severe ROP. Anteriorly, plus disease manifests itself as iris vascular engorgement and pupillary rigidity. Posteriorly, plus disease appears as retinal venous dilation and arterial tortuosity in the posterior pole. It is

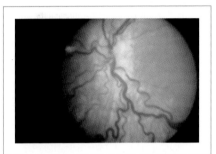

Figure 44-3. Moderately severe plus disease.

graded as mild, moderate, or severe (Fig. 44-3). When plus disease is present in the posterior pole, a plus sign (i.e., +) is added to the number stage of the disease, for example, stage 3+. Before the appearance of plus disease, increasing dilation and tortuosity of the posterior vessels manifests increasing activity of ROP. Pre–plus disease is present when there are vascular abnormalities of the posterior pole that are insufficient for the diagnosis of plus disease, but that demonstrate more venous dilation and arterial tortuosity than normal.

6. **When should acute ROP be treated?**
Because ROP can lead to blindness from retinal detachment, treatment to prevent progression to retinal detachment is indicated. However, 90% of infants who develop acute ROP undergo spontaneous regression. Treatment should therefore only be performed for those infants who have a high risk of developing retinal detachment. The Cryotherapy for Retinopathy of Prematurity (Cryo-ROP) study set out to determine whether or not treatment for ROP would prevent poor outcomes. For the purposes of that study, a level of disease (called *threshold disease*) was chosen at which 50% of infants were predicted to go blind without treatment. This prediction was appropriate for the Cryo-ROP study and remains the level of clinical disease at which treatment is recommended.

Threshold disease is defined as the presence of at least five contiguous or eight cumulative 30-degree sectors (clock hours) of stage 3 ROP in zone I or II, in the presence of plus disease (Fig. 44-4). Thus, prethreshold ROP is defined as zone I, any stage; zone II, stage 2 with plus disease; or zone II with extraretinal fibrovascular proliferation less than threshold. When ROP reaches prethreshold, examinations should be performed weekly.

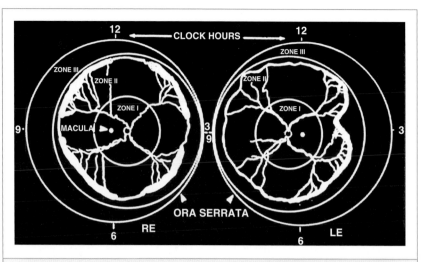

Figure 44-4. The Cryo-ROP definition of threshold disease is shown schematically.

Analysis of natural history data from the Cryo-ROP study indicated that certain infants are at high risk for an unfavorable outcome. Infants with zone I ROP are included as infants at high risk for an unfavorable outcome. The Early Treatment for Retinopathy of Prematurity (ETROP) study used a risk model (RM-ROP2) based on the natural history data from the Cryo-ROP study to identify infants at high risk for an unfavorable outcome. The model used demographic characteristics of the infants and clinical features of ROP to classify eyes with prethreshold ROP at high or low risk. High-risk prethreshold eyes that received conventional management had a much higher likelihood of unfavorable structural outcome (10% versus 1% at 6 months).

Using the RM-ROP2 computer model and an analysis of the visual fields from those treated within the ETROP study, a clinical algorithm for which eyes should be treated was developed. High-risk eyes (termed *type 1 ROP*) were those with the following findings: zone I, any stage ROP with plus disease; zone I, stage 3 ROP with or without plus disease; and zone II, stage 2 or 3 ROP with plus disease. Plus disease requires that there be at least two quadrants of dilation and tortuosity of the posterior pole vessels. With these criteria to apply laser treatment to the anterior avascular zone of affected high-risk prethreshold eyes, there was a reduction from 19.5% to 14.5% in an unfavorable grating visual acuity measurement and from 15.6% to 9.1% in an unfavorable structural outcome at 9 months compared to the control group that was not treated until threshold was reached. Less severely advanced, low-risk prethreshold eyes (termed *type 2 ROP*) included the following: zone I, stage 1 or 2 ROP without plus disease; and zone II, stage 3 ROP without plus disease. It was recommended that infants with type 2 ROP should be monitored closely and treated if they progress to type 1 ROP or to threshold disease. The recommendation to treat type 1 eyes and adopt a "wait-and-watch" approach for type 2 eyes (treat if the eyes progress to type 1 or threshold) was supported by the final results of the ETROP study.

7. **How do you treat acute ROP?**
   Cryotherapy was the standard of care for treating acute ROP. More recently, multiple studies have reported on the efficacy of treating ROP with laser photocoagulation delivered by the indirect ophthalmoscope. Indirect laser has become the most common form of treatment for acute ROP.

Indirect laser can be delivered in the intensive care nursery without having to take the infant to an operating room. An "isolation room" in the nursery is a desirable location because it allows for others to be shielded from the laser energy. Intravenous sedation is administered at the discretion of the neonatologist, who should be immediately available to manage any possible systemic complications. The pupils are dilated and an eyelid speculum is inserted. Diode or argon laser is then applied to the entire peripheral avascular zone, with the use of a laser indirect ophthalmoscope. The peripheral retina is brought into view with the aid of a pediatric scleral depressor. The laser spot desired is a dull white or gray spot, and the spots are placed approximately 1–1.25 lesion-widths apart (Fig. 44-5). With the IRIS Medical (Mountain View, CA) diode laser, it is advisable to start with a power of 200 milliwatts and duration of 200 milliseconds. Critical focus on the retina is essential. If the desired lesion is not obtained, increase the power in 50-milliwatt increments until you get the desired result.

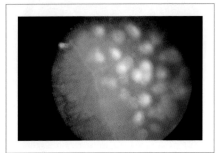

Figure 44-5. Appearance of the peripheral fundus immediately after laser treatment.

8. **How is cryotherapy applied?**
Cryotherapy is still preferred by some ophthalmologists for managing acute ROP. As for laser treatment, intravenous sedation can be administered at the discretion of the neonatologist. Some ophthalmologists prefer general anesthesia because of the greater stress on the infant and the greater risk of cardiopulmonary complications with cryotherapy than with laser photocoagulation. The pupils are dilated and an eyelid speculum is inserted. Cryotherapy is applied to the entire peripheral avascular zone using a hand-held cryo-pencil. The peripheral retina is brought into view using the cryo-pencil as a scleral depressor. A white freeze spot seen for 1–2 seconds is the desired endpoint. The lesions are placed contiguously.

9. **Does posterior ROP respond to treatment?**
Zone I and posterior zone II disease have a worse prognosis than more anterior ROP. In the Cryo-ROP study the beneficial effect of treatment for zone I threshold ROP was limited to a reduction in unfavorable anatomic outcome rate from 92% to 75% at 3 months' follow-up. Studies have shown that 100% of eyes with any amount of extraretinal fibrovascular proliferation in zone I and approximately 70% of eyes with vascularization limited to zone I or posterior zone II and stage 1 or stage 2 ROP will progress to threshold disease. Investigations have shown that laser photocoagulation for posterior disease can limit the likelihood of an unfavorable anatomic outcome to approximately 20%. Applying the criteria of the ETROP noted previously will result in a better prognosis for zone I disease.

10. **What is the expected result after laser treatment for ROP?**
Various reports have quoted a regression rate of approximately 90% after laser photocoagulation for threshold ROP. If regression is to occur, plus disease is usually less on the first week's follow-up visit. There may not be much change in the extraretinal fibrovascular proliferation (ERFP). By 2 weeks, one should start to see a reduction in the ERFP.

11. **When should you consider re-treatment for ROP?**
Laser photocoagulation for threshold ROP is successful at inducing regression of the acute disease in approximately 90% of cases. Occasionally (approximately 10% of the time),

supplemental treatment after the initial session is necessary to induce regression. Re-treatment should be considered if there is worse disease (worse plus disease and increased extraretinal fibrovascular proliferation) at the 1-week visit or persistently active disease (ERFP with plus disease) and the presence of "skip lesions" (areas of apparently missed treatment) or widely spaced laser lesions at the 2-week follow-up visit. Additional treatment should be applied to previously untreated areas rather than treating over old laser spots. In a similar fashion, supplemental cryotherapy can be applied to "skip areas" if there has not been an adequate response to initial cryotherapy treatment.

KEY POINTS: INDICATIONS FOR LASER TREATMENT OF ROP

1. Eyes with type 1 ROP

2. Zone I, any stage ROP with plus disease

3. Zone II, stage 2 or 3 ROP with plus disease

4. Eyes with threshold ROP: At least five contiguous or eight cumulative 30-degree sectors (clock hours) of stage 3 ROP in zone I or II, in the presence of plus disease

12. **What can be done for more advanced stages of ROP?**
Stage 4B and progressive stage 4A retinal detachments may be managed with lens-sparing vitrectomy. There is a 70–85% rate of retinal reattachment. Vitrectomy surgery may be tried for more advanced stage 5 ROP. However, the anatomic and visual success rates are extremely poor.

13. **What are some of the late complications of ROP?**
The late complications of ROP include myopia, retinal pigmentation, dragging of the retina (Fig. 44-6), lattice-like vitreoretinal degeneration, retinal holes, retinal detachment, and angle-closure glaucoma. Obviously, these children need long-term follow-up by both a retina specialist and a pediatric ophthalmologist. Amblyopia and strabismus are also common.

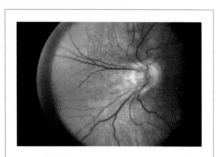

Figure 44-6. Moderate temporal dragging of the macula caused by regressed retinopathy of prematurity.

14. **What is the differential diagnosis for ROP?**
The differential diagnosis differs depending on the extent of the disease (Table 44-1). In less severe ROP, conditions that lead to peripheral retinal vascular changes and retinal dragging should be considered. In more severe disease the differential diagnosis of a white pupillary reflex must be considered.

TABLE 44-1. DIFFERENTIAL DIAGNOSIS OF RETINOPATHY OF PREMATURITY

Less Severe Disease	More Severe Disease
Familial exudative vitreoretinopathy	Congenital cataract
Incontinentia pigmenti (Bloch-Sulzberger syndrome)	Persistent hyperplastic primary vitreous/persistent fetal vasculature (PHPV/PFV)
X-linked retinoschisis	Retinoblastoma
	Ocular toxocariasis
	Intermediate uveitis
	Coats disease
	Advanced x-linked retinoschisis
	Vitreous hemorrhage

BIBLIOGRAPHY

1. American Academy of Pediatrics: Screening examination of premature infants for retinopathy of prematurity. Pediatrics 108:809–811, 2001.

2. An International Committee for the Classification of Retinopathy of Prematurity: The International Classification of Retinopathy of Prematurity Revisited. Arch Ophthalmol 123:991–999, 2005.

3. Capone AJ, Diaz-Rohena R, Sternberg PJ, et al: Diode laser photocoagulation for zone I threshold retinopathy of prematurity. Am J Ophthalmol 116:444–450, 1993.

4. Committee for the Classification of Retinopathy of Prematurity: An international classification of retinopathy of prematurity. Arch Ophthalmol 102:1130–1134, 1984.

5. Cryotherapy for Retinopathy of Prematurity Cooperative Group: Multicenter trial of cryotherapy for retinopathy of prematurity: Preliminary results. Arch Ophthalmol 106:471–479, 1988.

6. Cryotherapy for Retinopathy of Prematurity Cooperative Group: Multicenter trial of cryotherapy for retinopathy of prematurity: Three-month outcome. Arch Ophthalmol 108:195–204, 1990.

7. Cryotherapy for Retinopathy of Prematurity Cooperative Group: Multicenter trial of cryotherapy for retinopathy of prematurity: One-year outcome—structure and function. Arch Ophthalmol 108:1408–1416, 1990.

8. Cryotherapy for Retinopathy of Prematurity Cooperative Group: Multicenter trial of cryotherapy for retinopathy of prematurity: 3½ year outcome—structure and function. Arch Ophthalmol 111:339–344, 1993.

9. Cryotherapy for Retinopathy of Prematurity Cooperative Group: The natural ocular outcome of premature birth and retinopathy: Status at one year. Arch Ophthalmol 112:903–912, 1994.

10. Cryotherapy for Retinopathy of Prematurity Cooperative Group: Multicenter trial of cryotherapy for retinopathy of prematurity: Snellen visual acuity and structural outcome at 5½ years after randomization. Arch Ophthalmol 114:417–424, 1996.

11. Early Treatment For Retinopathy of Prematurity Cooperative Group: Revised indications for the treatment of retinopathy of prematurity: Results of the early treatment of retinopathy of prematurity randomized trial. Arch Ophthalmol 121:1684–1694, 2003.

12. Fleming T, Runge P, Charles S: Diode laser photocoagulation for prethreshold, posterior retinopathy of prematurity. Am J Ophthalmol 114:589–592, 1992.

13. Flynn J, Tasman W: Retinopathy of Prematurity: A Clinician's Guide. New York, Springer-Verlag, 1992.

14. Goggin M, O'Keefe M: Diode laser for retinopathy of prematurity: Early outcome. Br J Ophthalmol 77:559–562, 1993.

15. Hartnett ME, Maguluri S, Thompson HW, McColm JR: Comparison of retinal outcomes after scleral buckling or lens-sparing vitrectomy for stage 4 retinopathy of prematurity. Retina 24:753–757, 2004.

16. International Committee for the Classification of the Late Stages of Retinopathy of Prematurity: An international classification of retinopathy of prematurity. II: The classification of retinal detachment. Arch Ophthalmol 105:906–912, 1987.

17. Iverson D, Trese M, Orgel I, Williams G: Laser photocoagulation for threshold retinopathy of prematurity. Arch Ophthalmol 108:1342–1343, 1991.

18. Lakhanpal RR, Sun RL, Albini TA, Holz ER: Anatomic success rate after 3-port lens-sparing vitrectomy in stage 4A or 4B retinopathy of prematurity. Ophthalmology 112:1569–1573, 2005.

19. Landers M, Toth C, Semple H, Morse L: Treatment of retinopathy of prematurity with argon laser photocoagulation. Arch Ophthalmol 110:44–47, 1992.

20. McNamara J: Laser treatment for retinopathy of prematurity. Curr Opin Ophthalmol 4:76–80, 1993.

21. McNamara J, Tasman W: Retinopathy of prematurity. Ophthalmol Clin North Am 3:413–427, 1990.

22. McNamara J, Tasman W, Brown G, Federman J: Laser photocoagulation for stage 3+ retinopathy of prematurity. Ophthalmology 98:576–580, 1991.

23. McNamara J, Tasman W, Vander J, Brown G: Diode laser photocoagulation for retinopathy of prematurity: Preliminary results. Arch Ophthalmol 110:1714–1716, 1992.

24. Quinn G, Dobson V, Barr C, et al: Visual acuity in infants after vitrectomy for severe retinopathy of prematurity. Ophthalmology 98:5–13, 1991.

25. Quinn G, Dobson V, Barr C, et al: Visual acuity of eyes after vitrectomy for ROP: Follow-up at 5½ years. Ophthalmology 103:595–600, 1996.

26. Schaffer D, Palmer E, Plotsky D, et al: Prognostic factors in the natural course of retinopathy of prematurity. Ophthalmology 100:230–236, 1993.

27. Seiberth V, Linderkamp O, Vardarli I, et al: Diode laser photocoagulation for stage 3+ retinopathy of prematurity. Graefes Arch Clin Exp Ophthalmol 233:489–493, 1995.

28. Vander J, Handa J, McNamara J, et al: Early laser photocoagulation for posterior retinopathy of prematurity: A randomized controlled clinical trial. Ophthalmology 104:1731–1734, 1997.

CHAPTER 45

DIABETIC RETINOPATHY

James F. Vander, MD

1. **How is diabetic retinopathy classified? What fundus features are characteristic of each category?**
   - **Nonproliferative diabetic retinopathy (NPDR):** This form is arbitrarily divided into three categories based on severity: mild, moderate, and severe. Features of mild and moderate nonproliferative retinopathy result predominantly from loss of capillary integrity (i.e., microaneurysms, dot-and-blot hemorrhages, hard yellow exudates, and macular edema) (Fig. 45-1). Cotton-wool spots are also seen. Features of more severe NPDR are related to early signs of ischemia. In addition to the features found in mild nonproliferative disease, the fundus shows venous beading and intraretinal microvascular abnormalities (IRMA). Intraretinal hemorrhages are more extensive as well (Fig. 45-2).
   - **Proliferative diabetic retinopathy (PDR):** Typical features are related to the consequences of extensive retinal capillary nonperfusion. Fundus findings include those of NPDR as well as the development of neovascularization of the disc (NVD; Fig. 45-3), neovascularization elsewhere in the retina (NVE), preretinal and/or vitreous hemorrhage, and vitreoretinal traction with tractional retinal detachment.

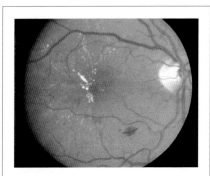

Figure 45-1. Nonproliferative diabetic retinopathy with exudates, hemorrhages, and edema.

2. **What is the most common cause of vision loss in diabetic retinopathy?**
   Macular edema.

3. **Who is at risk for the development of diabetic retinopathy?**
   All patients with diabetes mellitus are at risk for diabetic retinopathy. Relative risk factors include the following:
   - **Duration of diabetes:** The longer diabetes has been present, the greater the risk of some manifestation of diabetic retinopathy. After 10–15 years, more than 75% of patients show some signs of retinopathy.

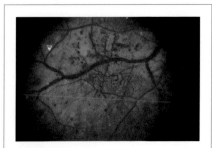

Figure 45-2. Severe nonproliferative retinopathy with venous beading and intraretinal microvascular abnormalities.

- **Age:** Diabetic retinopathy is uncommon before puberty even in patients who were diagnosed shortly after birth. NPDR appears sooner in patients diagnosed with diabetes after the age of 40. This may be related to duration of disease before diagnosis.
- **Diabetic control:** The Diabetic Control and Complications Trial (DCCT) clearly demonstrated a correlation between poor long-term glucose control and subsequent development of diabetic retinopathy as well as other complications of diabetes.

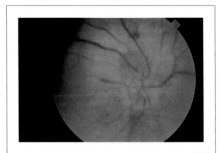

Figure 45-3. Neovascularization of the disc in proliferative retinopathy.

- **Renal disease:** Proteinuria is a particularly good marker for the development of diabetic retinopathy. This association may not be causal, but a patient with renal dysfunction should be followed more closely.
- **Systemic hypertension:** Again, the causal nature of the relationship is not certain.
- **Pregnancy:** Diabetic retinopathy may progress rapidly in patients who are pregnant. Patients with preexisting retinopathy are at particular risk.

KEY POINTS: MECHANISMS OF VISION LOSS IN DIABETES

1. Macular edema

2. Macular ischemia

3. Vitreous hemorrhage

4. Macular traction detachment

5. Combined rhegmatogenous/tractional retinal detachment

4. **What is the significance of the hemoglobin A_1C? What is its correlation with the development of diabetic retinopathy?**
   Hemoglobin A_1C measures serum glycosylated hemoglobin, which is an indicator for the average level of serum glucose for the preceding 3 months. Thus it provides a report card of the adequacy of glucose control for the preceding 3 months without identifying peaks, valleys, or timing of glucose fluctuation. The hemoglobin A_1C has been found to correlate most closely with the development of diabetic retinopathy. Nondiabetic patients typically have a level of 6 or less. The DCCT demonstrated that hemoglobin A_1C less than 8 was associated with a significantly reduced risk of retinopathy when compared with a value greater than 8.

5. **What is the recommendation for screening patients with diabetes?**
   Patients with juvenile insulin-dependent diabetes should have a dilated ophthalmologic examination 5 years after diagnosis. Patients with type II adult-onset diabetes should be examined at diagnosis. All diabetic patients should have an annual dilated funduscopic examination; more frequent examinations depend on the findings.

6. **What are the fluorescein angiographic features of nonproliferative and proliferative diabetic retinopathy?**

- In **mild-to-moderate nonproliferative retinopathy** the large vessels fill normally. Pinpoint areas of early hyperfluorescence correspond to microaneurysms, whereas dot-and-blot hemorrhages show hypofluorescence. Microaneurysms leak in the later frames with blurring of margins and diffusion of fluorescein dye, whereas hemorrhages remain hypofluorescent throughout the study. Telangiectasis also shows early hyperfluorescence with late leakage. Hard yellow exudate generally does not appear on a fluorescein angiogram unless it is extremely thick, in which case it reveals hypofluorescence. Macular edema usually is apparent as fluorescein leaks into the retina as the angiogram progresses (Figs. 45-4 and 45-5).

- In **more severe nonproliferative retinopathy** the features outlined previously are usually noted. In addition, patients show evidence of retinal capillary loss. Cotton-wool spots are usually hypofluorescent, sometimes with late hyper-fluorescence along the margins. Areas of capillary dropout appear as smooth, hypofluorescent "ground-glass" patches, often with staining at the margins in the later frames of the angiogram. IRMA fills in the arterial phase of the angiogram and does not leak significantly in the later frames (Fig. 45-6).

- **Proliferative retinopathy.** Extensive retinal capillary loss is seen early in the angiogram with diffuse leakage at the edges of the ischemic areas in the later frames. NVD and NVE show intense early hyperfluorescence with marked leakage developing rapidly (Fig. 45-7).

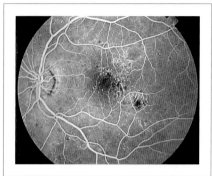

Figure 45-4. Early-phase fluorescein angiogram shows pinpoint hyperfluorescence corresponding to microaneurysms.

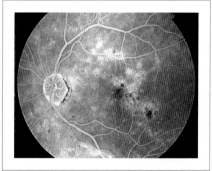

Figure 45-5. Later phase fluorescein angiogram shows leakage with diffusion of dye and blurring of the microaneurysms.

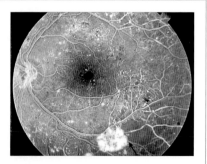

Figure 45-6. Neovascularization *(arrow)* is markedly hyperfluorescent early and develops at the border of perfused and nonperfused retina.

7. **What is the definition of clinically significant macular edema (CSME)?**

CSME, as defined in the Early Treatment Diabetic Retinopathy Study (ETDRS), is present in patients with any one of the following:

- Retinal thickening within 500 microns of the center of the fovea
- Hard yellow exudate within 500 microns of the center of the fovea with adjacent retinal thickening (Fig. 45-8)
- At least one disc area of retinal thickening, any part of which is within 1 disc diameter of the center of the fovea

CSME describes the fundus features as seen on stereoscopic high-magnification viewing of the macula. Visual acuity is not relevant; a patient with 20/20 vision may still have CSME. The fluorescein angiographic appearance is not relevant for the definition of CSME. Monocular viewing of the macula with a direct ophthalmoscope or a solitary color photograph is not adequate for diagnosing CSME, nor is the low-magnification view provided by the indirect ophthalmoscope.

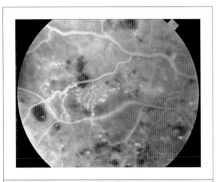

Figure 45-7. Intraretinal microvascular abnormalities do not leak on fluorescein angiography.

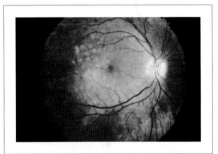

Figure 45-8. Clinically significant macular edema with thickening and exudate within 500 microns of the center of the fovea.

KEY POINTS: CLINICAL FEATURES OF CLINICALLY SIGNIFICANT MACULAR EDEMA

1. Macular thickening = 500 microns center of fovea **or**

2. Hard exudates = 500 microns center of fovea with adjacent thickening **or**

3. Macular thickening = one disc area any part of which within one disc diameter of center of fovea

8. **What are the results of the ETDRS concerning treatment of diabetic macular edema?**

The ETDRS showed that macular laser treatment for patients with CSME reduced the risk of doubling of the visual angle (for example, 20/40 worsening to 20/80) from 24% to 12% over a 3-year period. This benefit was detected over all levels of visual acuity. Significant visual improvement is uncommon after macular laser treatment. The goal is to prevent worsened vision in the future. Treatment is directed at areas of diffuse leakage by using a grid pattern and at areas of focal leakage by treatment of the leaking abnormality (Fig. 45-9). Resolution of macular edema may take several months and re-treatment is occasionally necessary.

9. **What other findings did the ETDRS report?**
The ETDRS also was designed to determine whether aspirin use was helpful or harmful in patients with diabetic retinopathy; the study concluded that it was neither. The study also assessed the role of early panretinal laser treatment for proliferative disease (see further discussion).

10. **What is the definition of high-risk characteristics (HRC)?**
HRC was used by the Diabetic Retinopathy Study (DRS) to describe patients at a high risk of severe vision loss from PDR. The study found that patients with (1) NVE and vitreous hemorrhage, (2) mild NVD and vitreous hemorrhage, and (3) moderate or severe NVD with or without vitreous hemorrhage are at high risk for severe vision loss over the ensuing 3 years. Initiation of full-scatter panretinal photocoagulation (PRP) greatly reduced the risk of severe vision loss in patients with HRC (Fig. 45-10). Subsequently, the EDTRS found that for patients with severe nonproliferative retinopathy and/or early proliferative retinopathy without HRC, there was no clear-cut benefit to initiation of full-scatter PRP. So long as careful follow-up can be assured, PRP may be safely withheld in such cases.

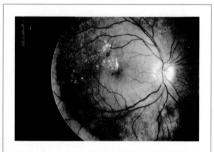

Figure 45-9. Four months after focal laser, the edema and exudate are gone.

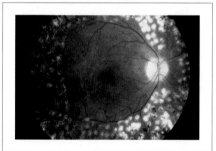

Figure 45-10. Panretinal photocoagulation several months after treatment.

KEY POINTS: DRS HIGH-RISK CHARACTERISTICS

1. Neovascularization of the disc (NVD) = ¼ to ⅓ of disc area

2. NVD <¼ disc area with any vitreous hemorrhage

3. Neovascularization elsewhere in the retina with any vitreous hemorrhage

11. **What are the side effects of PRP?**
PRP does not improve vision but is performed to prevent the blinding complication of proliferative retinopathy. Loss of peripheral vision and night vision are the major concerns. Loss of central vision also may result from exacerbation of macular edema. Thus, if possible, macular focal laser should be performed before PRP when both are indicated. Other complications include impaired accommodation, papillary dilation, and inadvertent macular burns.

12. **Do all patients treated with PRP show resolution of HRC?**
No. As many as one-third of patients do not show resolution of NVD or NVE, and in some cases there will be no apparent regression.

13. **What is the role of supplemental PRP?**
The DRS evaluated the placement of 2000 spots of PRP. For patients who do not show regression of high-risk characteristics or who have persistent vitreous hemorrhage, it is not clear whether additional PRP improves the long-term visual prognosis. Patients have been reported with 7000 or more spots of PRP, and in some cases recurrent vitreous hemorrhage persists.

14. **What are the indications for fluorescein angiography in diabetic retinopathy?**
Fluorescein angiography is not part of the definition of either clinically significant macular edema for patients with nonproliferative retinopathy or HRC for patients with proliferative disease. The indications for treatment are based on clinical rather than angiographic features. Nevertheless, fluorescein angiography is important, particularly for patients with diabetic maculopathy. Most patients considered for treatment of macular edema should have a fluorescein angiogram to determine the focal and diffuse areas of leakage and thus to guide the treating physician during placement of the laser. Areas of capillary nonperfusion also are treated with a grid pattern, which can be determined angiographically. The proximity of focal areas of leakage to the foveal avascular zone (FAZ) also can be demonstrated on fluorescein angiography. Treatment too close to the FAZ carries a higher risk of vision loss and therefore should be done with caution. In patients with unexplained vision loss the cause may be macular ischemia, which is nicely demonstrated on fluorescein angiography. Finally, patients with a vitreous hemorrhage of uncertain etiology may benefit from a fluorescein angiogram. In patients with significant media opacity a fluorescein angiogram may demonstrate retinal neovascularization that was not apparent clinically.

15. **What are the possible uses of optical coherence tomography (OCT) in the management of diabetic retinopathy?**
OCT provides a noninvasive, photographic method for obtaining a cross-sectional view of the macula. Macular thickness and volume may be quantified, providing an objective measurement that can be especially useful when serial studies are available and progression or response to treatment is being evaluated. The presence of significant vitreomacular traction can be demonstrated, lending insight into a possible mechanism for the presence of macular edema and pointing toward vitrectomy as a therapeutic option. OCT may also show significant macular thinning as can sometimes occur after treatment of macular edema. This may explain a poor visual result in an eye after resolution of intraretinal fluid.

16. **What is the differential diagnosis of diabetic retinopathy?**
The differential diagnosis includes branch or central retinal vein obstruction, ocular ischemic syndrome, radiation retinopathy, hypertensive retinopathy, and miscellaneous proliferative retinopathies such as sarcoidosis, sickle cell hemoglobinopathy, and other less common causes. In patients with typical macular features of nonproliferative retinopathy such as microaneurysms and macular edema, but no evidence of diabetes mellitus, the disease usually is categorized as idiopathic juxtafoveal telangiectasia.

17. **What is the significance of neovascularization of iris (NVI) in diabetes?**
Neovascularization of iris is an ominous sign of severe PDR and generally requires urgent treatment. NVI may progress to occlude the trabecular meshwork in a relatively short period, leading to severe neovascular glaucoma. This dreaded complication of proliferative disease usually can be avoided if heavy PRP can be placed before the angle has become occluded.

18. **What are the indications for vitrectomy in diabetic retinopathy?**
    - **Vitreous hemorrhage:** Vitreous hemorrhage obscuring the visual axis causes severe vision loss. Although it generally clears spontaneously, for patients with more extensive hemorrhage, vitrectomy may be indicated. The Diabetic Retinopathy Vitrectomy Study (DRVS) concentrated on eyes with vitreous hemorrhage reducing vision to 5/200 or worse. The study demonstrated a strong benefit for patients with type I diabetes, perhaps related to extensive fibrovascular proliferation. Guidelines are variable, but most surgeons wait at least 3 months for patients to clear spontaneously unless occupational or personal needs demand early intervention or extensive untreated fibrovascular proliferation is known to be present. The development of NVI also may prompt earlier vitrectomy.
    - **Tractional retinal detachment:** Most surgeons agree that tractional retinal detachment involving the macula is an indication for diabetic vitrectomy. If the vitreoretinal traction can be relieved within weeks or a few months of onset, visual results are excellent. Long-standing tractional retinal detachments generally do not respond favorably in terms of visual recovery. Progressive extramacular tractional retinal detachment moving toward the fovea is occasionally an indication for surgery, although this indication is controversial.
    - **Combined tractional-rhegmatogenous retinal detachment:** The development of combined retinal detachment with an open retinal break is an indication for vitrectomy. Such detachments are notoriously difficult to fix and usually are taken to surgery shortly after diagnosis.
    - **Refractory macular edema:** Patients with a taut posterior hyaloid face producing chronic macular edema that is not responsive to focal laser therapy can undergo surgery, sometimes with significant visual improvement. It is believed that the chronic traction of the vitreous face on the macula produces persistent leakage and that the edema can resolve only after traction is released.

19. **What are the complications of vitrectomy for diabetes?**
    - **Progression of cataract:** Progressive nuclear sclerotic or posterior subcapsular cataracts occur frequently after vitrectomy. The risk of secondary neovascular glaucoma may be higher in patients in whom the lens is removed intraoperatively.
    - **Nonhealing corneal epithelial defects:** The cornea may swell, and the surface may break down during vitrectomy. Diabetic patients are prone to poor healing of corneal epithelial defects.
    - **Retinal detachment:** Retinal detachment may be related to a peripheral tear near one of the sclerotomy sites or posteriorly as a result of persistent or recurrent vitreoretinal traction.
    - **Vitreous hemorrhage:** Some degree of vitreous hemorrhage is frequently present postoperatively. It generally clears quickly.

20. **Are there any other options for the treatment of diabetic macular edema beyond laser and, occasionally, vitrectomy?**
    Within the past few years there have been numerous reports regarding the use of intraocular steroid injections to manage macular edema from this and other causes (Fig. 45-11). Many cases will show prompt resolution of

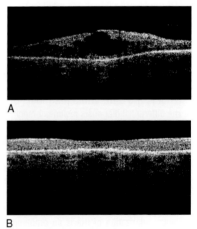

Figure 45-11. *A*, Optical coherence tomography (OCT) shows marked macular edema with cystic spaces. *B*, Repeat OCT taken 3 weeks after injection of intravitreal steroids shows resolution of edema.

macular thickening, even if long-standing edema has been present. Complications such as cataract, elevated intraocular pressure, infection, and retinal detachment may occur. Although severe complications are infrequent, they can be devastating. Furthermore, the benefits of the injection often fade over several months; consideration may be given to repeat injections. Alternative pharmacologic agents such as inhibitors of angiogenesis factors are currently under investigation.

BIBLIOGRAPHY

1. Benson WE, Brown GC, Tasman W: Diabetes and Its Ocular Complications. Philadelphia, W.B. Saunders, 1988.
2. Diabetic Control and Complications Trial Research Group: The effect of intensive diabetes treatment on the progression of diabetic retinopathy in insulin-dependent diabetes mellitus. Arch Ophthalmol 113:36–51, 1995.
3. Diabetic Retinopathy Study Research Group: Photocoagulation treatment of proliferative diabetic retinopathy. Clinical application of Diabetic Retinopathy Study (DRS) findings, DRS report number 8. Ophthalmology 88:583–600, 1981.
4. Diabetic Retinopathy Vitrectomy Study Research Group: Early vitrectomy for severe vitreous hemorrhage in diabetic retinopathy: Two-year results of a randomized trial. Diabetic Retinopathy Vitrectomy Study report 2. Arch Ophthalmol 103:1644–1652, 1985.
5. Early Treatment for Diabetic Retinopathy Study Research Group: Photocoagulation for diabetic macular edema: Early Treatment for Diabetic Retinopathy Study report number 1. Arch Ophthalmol 103:1796–1806, 1985.
6. Martidis A, Duker JS, Greenberg PB, et al: Intravitreal triamcinolone for refractory diabetic macular edema. Ophthalmology 109:920–927, 2002.
7. Pendergast SD, Hassan TS, Williams GA: Vitrectomy for diffuse diabetic macular edema associated with a taut premacular posterior hyaloid. Am J Ophthalmol 130:178–186, 2000.

CHAPTER 46

RETINAL ARTERIAL OBSTRUCTION

Jay S. Duker, MD

1. **What types of retinal arterial obstructions can occur?**

   Retinal arterial obstructions are generally divided into branch retinal arterial obstructions and central retinal arterial obstructions, depending on the precise site of obstruction:

   - A **branch retinal arterial obstruction** (BRAO) occurs when the site of blockage is distal to the lamina cribrosa of the optic nerve; in other words, within the visible vasculature of the retina. A BRAO can involve as large an area as three-quarters of the retina or as small an area as just a few microns.
   - A **central retinal arterial obstruction** (CRAO) occurs when the blockage is within the optic nerve substance itself. The site of obstruction is therefore not generally visible on ophthalmoscopy in a CRAO. In a CRAO most, if not all, of the retina is affected.

   Obstructions more proximal to the central retinal artery, in the ophthalmic artery, or even in the internal carotid artery can cause visual loss as well. Ophthalmic arterial obstructions can be difficult to differentiate from CRAO on a clinical basis.

2. **What causes a retinal artery to become blocked?**

   The typical causes differ for CRAO and BRAO. Because the site of obstruction is not visible on clinical examination and, in general, the central retinal artery is too small to image with most techniques, the precise cause of most CRAOs cannot be definitely determined. It is currently believed that most CRAOs are caused by thrombus formation. Localized intimal damage in the form of atherosclerosis probably incites the thrombus in most cases. In approximately 20% of cases an embolus is visible in the central retinal artery or one of its branches, suggesting an embolic cause (Fig. 46-1). Extrinsic mechanical compression caused by orbital or optic nerve tumor, hemorrhage, or inflammation is a rare cause. Inflammation in the form of vasculitis, optic

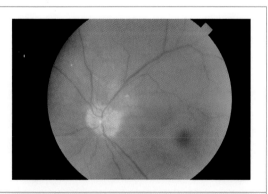

Figure 46-1. A central retinal arterial obstruction caused emboli in this patient. Note the refractile particles in the central retinal artery in the center of the optic disc, as well as in two branch retinal arteries superior to the optic disc.

neuritis, or even orbital disease (e.g., mucormycosis) can cause a CRAO as well. Trauma with direct damage to the optic nerve or blood vessels can lead to CRAO. In addition, system coagulopathies can also be associated with both CRAO and BRAO.

Emboli are the cause of more than 90% of BRAOs. Cholesterol, calcium, fibrin, and platelets have all been implicated individually or together. Emboli are usually visible in the retinal arterial tree. In an older individual the most common source of emboli is the ipsilateral carotid artery. In a younger person it is more likely to be cardiac in origin. Rarely, intraocular inflammations such as toxoplasmosis or herpes retinitis (the acute retinal necrosis syndrome) can lead to BRAO.

3. **Describe the typical symptoms of a retinal arterial obstruction.**
The hallmark symptom of an acute retinal arterial obstruction is abrupt, painless loss of sight in the visual field that corresponds to the territory of the obstructed artery. In a CRAO this would be most, if not all, of the visual field. In some patients an artery derived from the choroidal circulation, called a *cilioretinal artery,* may perfuse a small amount of the central retina. The cilioretinal artery, which is present in up to 20% of individuals, remains patent when the site of obstruction is the central retinal artery. Some of the visual field corresponding to the territory of the patent cilioretinal vessel can be spared in select individuals. Cilioretinal artery sparing can rarely leave a patient with 20/20 (normal) central vision, albeit with a very constricted visual field (Fig. 46-2).

Occasionally, patients report stuttering visual loss or episodes of amaurosis fugax before arterial obstruction. Pain is not generally a part of retinal arterial obstruction unless some other underlying disease is present (e.g., giant cell arteritis, ocular ischemia).

In a BRAO the visual field loss can vary from up to three-quarters of the visual field to as little as a few degrees, depending on the territory of the obstructed vessel. Often, the central vision will be 20/20, therefore sparing the macular area.

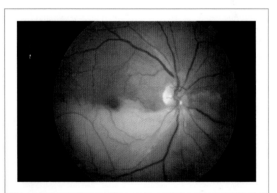

Figure 46-2. Typical inferior hemispheric branch retinal arterial obstruction. The visual acuity was 20/20, but there was a marked superior visual field defect.

4. **What do you see on examination when a retinal arterial obstruction has occurred?**
The decreased blood flow results in ischemic whitening of the retina in the territory of the obstructed artery. Because the retinal vasculature only supplies circulation to the inner retina (the outer retina gets its circulation from the choroid), the ischemia is limited to the inner retina. The retinal whitening is most pronounced in the posterior pole where the nerve fiber layer of the inner retina is thickest.

In an arterial obstruction the retinal arteries distal to the blockage appear thin and attenuated. The blood column may be interrupted in both the distal arteries and the corresponding draining veins. This phenomenon has been labeled "boxcarring." Splinter retinal hemorrhages on the disc are common. Embolic material may be visible in the central retinal artery, where it exits the disc or in one of the branches of the central retinal artery. In most instances a cherry-red spot will be visible in the macular area.

The most common sites of obstruction in a BRAO are the retinal arterial bifurcations. Because there are more bifurcations and more retinal vessels in the temporal retina, temporal BRAOs are more common than nasal BRAOs.

In a CRAO the visual acuity is usually quite poor. The patient typically can only discern motion or, perhaps, count fingers from a distance of several feet. Many episodes of BRAO result in only peripheral visual loss with intact central acuity.

5. **What is a cherry-red spot?**
A cherry-red spot represents a pathologic appearance of the macula, the center of the retina. There are two main causes: ischemia and abnormal depositions. A cherry-red spot occurs in CRAO because of the retinal whitening of the surrounding nerve fiber layer. The fovea itself has no nerve fibers, so its appearance does not change from normal. The retinal whitening surrounding the normal reddish tint of the macular area produces the cherry-red spot.

6. **What other conditions result in a cherry-red spot of the retina? How can you differentiate these from an arterial obstruction?**
Besides CRAO, a cherry-red spot can occur in conditions of abnormal deposition into the cells of the retinal nerve fiber layer. The classic example is Tay-Sachs disease, which is a sphingolipidosis. A cherry-red spot has been reported in other sphingolipidoses as well, such as Farber syndrome, Sandhoff's disease, Niemann-Pick disease, Goldberg's syndrome, Gaucher's disease, and gangliosidase GM1, type 2. A cherry-red spot has also been reported in Hurler's syndrome (MPS I-H), B-galactosidase deficiency (MPS-VII), Hallervorden-Spatz disease, and Batten-Mayou (Vogt-Spielmeyer) disease.

An ischemic cherry-red spot can be differentiated from these other entities by the history of visual loss, concurrent systemic disease, age of the patient, and the appearance of the surrounding retinal blood vessels and retina.

7. **Is there any ancillary testing that can be done to confirm the diagnosis?**
In most cases an experienced observer can accurately diagnose CRAO and BRAO. In cases in which the diagnosis is in doubt, an intravenous fluorescein angiogram can be performed. This will show a significant diminution in dye flow through the obstructed vessels. A color Doppler ultrasound evaluation of the orbital circulation can also be used to determine the degree of obstruction and to differentiate an ophthalmic artery obstruction from CRAO.

8. **Which systemic diseases are associated with retinal arterial obstruction?**
Although many systemic diseases are associated with retinal arterial obstruction, more than 50% of all affected patients will manifest no apparent cause for their retinal disease. The most common association is ipsilateral carotid artery disease, which is present in approximately one-third of affected patients. Approximately 10% of arterial obstructions are associated with giant cell arteritis. This is a critical association to be aware of because visual loss can occur rapidly in the fellow eye in these patients, and prompt administration of intravenous corticosteroids may prevent the contralateral visual loss.

In both CRAO and BRAO, all patients should be evaluated for embolic sources from the carotid artery system and the heart with the use carotid noninvasive testing and echocardiogram. In some instances, esophageal echocardiography is necessary to detect embolic sources. Holter monitoring to detect a cardiac arrhythmia may be appropriate in select patients.

9. **Do you always have to test for giant cell arteritis?**
It is of paramount importance that giant cell arteritis be ruled out in all patients older than age 50 with a CRAO. A stat erythrocyte sedimentation rate should be performed and, if the result is high, or if there is clinical suspicion of giant cell arteritis, then a biopsy should be considered. BRAO associated with giant cell arteritis is exceedingly uncommon.

10. **Which patients are at risk to get a retinal arterial obstruction?**
Patients who have suffered an arterial obstruction in one eye are at more risk for developing an obstruction in the contralateral eye. The risk of bilaterality is approximately 10%. Patients with known carotid artery disease, diseased heart valves, or cardiac arrhythmias are also at increased risk. In addition, conditions that result in abnormal rheologic parameters such as pancreatitis, lupus, pregnancy, and amniotic fluid emboli can result in artery obstructions.

11. **Can any prophylactic treatment be given?**
With the exception of corticosteroid treatment for giant cell arteritis, prophylaxis against arterial obstructions is not generally given. The utility of anticoagulation to prevent retinal arterial obstructions in the setting of known carotid disease is not definitively proven. Extrapolation from studies showing a benefit of the risk of subsequent stroke in this situation suggests that anticoagulation is useful to lower the risk of arterial obstruction as well. The same conclusion may be extrapolated from the studies, proving a benefit for carotid endarterectomy for appropriate patients with carotid arterial disease.

12. **What is the incidence of bilateral retinal arterial obstructions?**
Ten percent.

13. **Is there any proven treatment for retinal arterial obstruction?**
There is no proven treatment for either CRAO or BRAO. Some investigators feel that none of the currently recommended treatments have any value. Because the inner retina is highly sensitive to loss of perfusion, intervention is rarely, if ever, attempted in anyone with an obstruction more than 72 hours old. Proposed therapies for retinal arterial obstructions are as follows:

- Dislodging emboli to a more distal location
- Dissolving thrombi
- Increasing oxygenation to the retina
- Protecting surviving retinal cells from ischemic damage

The traditional approach to CRAO includes paracentesis, ocular massage, and medications to lower the intraocular pressure. All three of these interventions are an attempt to dislodge any embolus that may be present. A paracentesis is the removal of a small amount of aqueous humor via a small needle (30 gauge or 27 gauge). This can be done in an office setting. Although generally simple and safe, it has rarely been reported to cause endophthalmitis.

Increasing oxygenation to the retina is attempted by having patients inhale a mixture of 95% oxygen and 5% carbon dioxide (carbogen) for 10 minutes out of every 2 hours for 24–48 hours after the blockage. The purpose of the carbon dioxide is to counteract the normal retinal arterial vasoconstriction that occurs when pure oxygen is inhaled. This theoretically increases the oxygenation to the ischemic inner retina; however, there is no clinical evidence that any beneficial effect is achieved. Carbogen should not be used to treat any patient suffering from chronic obstructive pulmonary disease.

More recently, both systemic (via intravenous infusion) and local (directly into the ophthalmic artery via an arterial catheter) infusions of clot-dissolving medications (streptokinase, tissue plasminogen activator, urokinase, heparin) have been given for retinal arterial obstruction. Although the initial reports are encouraging, these therapies are not without risk and should be reserved for obstructions less than 48 hours old. These medications should be given only by experienced personnel under close supervision. Because branch retinal arterial obstructions do not usually affect central vision, such invasive procedures probably should not be attempted in these cases.

At present, there are no means to "rescue" ischemic retinal tissue. This is an area of active research and may be possible in the future.

KEY POINTS: RETINAL ARTERIAL OBSTRUCTION

1. Systemic disease must be ruled out in any retinal artery obstruction.

2. Giant cell arteritis should be considered and ruled out in any patient older than age 60 with a central retinal artery obstruction.

3. No proven treatment exists for retinal artery obstruction.

14. **Why is the retina so sensitive to arterial inflow problems?**
    The retina is a highly metabolic organ and is therefore sensitive to ischemia. The central retinal artery is an end artery with no true normal anastomosis. As part of the central nervous system, the retina is unable to regenerate if damaged.

15. **How do you tell a retinal arterial obstruction from a retinal venous obstruction?**
    Simple-white versus red. The hallmark of retinal arterial obstructions is ischemic retinal whitening. The hallmark of retinal venous obstruction is retinal hemorrhage in the territory of the obstructed vessel. In addition, the retinal veins will appear dilated and tortuous as opposed to thin and attenuated.

    Warning: Rarely, a patient may present with a combined obstruction. Obstructions of a branch retinal artery or the central retinal artery in conjunction with a central retinal venous obstruction have been reported. This produces a combined fundus picture (i.e., whitening from ischemia with red from retinal hemorrhage).

16. **Is acute obstruction of a retinal artery an emergency?**
    CRAO is considered a true ophthalmic emergency, even though there is no proven treatment. Because the retina is highly sensitive to ischemia, treatment should be initiated as quickly as possible if contemplated. Although animal studies indicate that more than 90 minutes of ischemia produce irreversible retinal cell death, clinical experience suggests that some eyes can tolerate ischemia for up to 72 hours and still recover. If a potentially risky intervention such as anticoagulation is contemplated, the visual loss should be no more than 48 hours old to maximize the possibility of recovery and the overall risk-to-benefit ratio. Optimal timing for anticoagulation is within 6–8 hours of visual loss.

17. **What does the retina look like months or years after an arterial obstruction?**
    The retinal vessels look attenuated and the optic disc is often pale, owing to the loss of the retinal nerve fiber layer. Because the retina itself is transparent and the underlying retinal pigment epithelium and choroid are unaffected by a pure CRAO or BRAO, the retina itself looks normal.

18. **Are there any other late complications after retinal arterial obstructions?**
    In approximately 15% of patients after being diagnosed with CRAO, neovascularization of the iris occurs. It is usually seen within 3 months of the CRAO and can result in a severe type of glaucoma (elevated intraocular pressure) called *neovascular glaucoma*. If NVI is detected, a laser treatment to the ischemic retina, panretinal photocoagulation, is usually performed. Neovascularization is extremely rare after BRAO.

BIBLIOGRAPHY

1. Arruga J, Sanders MD: Ophthalmologic findings in 70 patients with evidence of retinal embolism. Ophthalmology 89:1336–1347, 1982.

2. Atebara NH, Brown GC, Cater J: Efficacy of anterior chamber paracentesis and carbogen in treating acute nonarteritic central retinal artery obstruction. Ophthalmology 102:2029–2035, 1995.

3. Brown GC, Magargal LE: Central retinal artery obstruction and visual acuity. Ophthalmology 89:14–19, 1982.

4. Brown GC, Magargal LE, Sergott R: Acute obstruction of the retinal and choroidal circulations. Ophthalmology 93:1373–1382, 1986.

5. Duker JS: Retinal arterial obstruction. In Yanoff M, Duker JS (eds): Ophthalmology. St. Louis, Mosby, 1999, pp 856–863.

6. Duker JS, Brown GC: Recovery following acute obstruction of the retinal and choroidal circulations. Retina 8:257–260, 1988.

7. Duker JS, Sivalingham A, Brown GC, Reber R: A prospective study of acute central retinal artery obstruction. Arch Ophthalmol 109:339–342, 1991.

8. Greven CM, Slusher MM, Weaver RG: Retinal arterial occlusions in young adults. Am J Ophthalmol 120:776–783, 1995.

9. Hayreh SS, Podhajsky P: Ocular neovascularization with retinal vascular occlusion. II. Occurrence in central and branch retinal artery obstruction. Arch Ophthalmol 100:1585–1596, 1982.

10. Schmidt D, Schumaker M, Wakhloo AK: Microcatheter urokinase infusion in central retinal artery occlusion. Am J Ophthalmol 113:429–434, 1992.

CHAPTER 47

RETINAL VENOUS OCCLUSIVE DISEASE

Vernon K. W. Wong, MD

BRANCH RETINAL VEIN OCCLUSION

1. **What are the symptoms of a branch retinal vein occlusion (BRVO)?**
    Patients may notice an acute, painless loss of vision if there is macular edema, ischemic maculopathy, or intraretinal hemorrhage involving the fovea. A BRVO in a nasal quadrant may be asymptomatic. A long-standing BRVO can present with floaters or an abrupt decrease in vision from vitreous hemorrhage.

2. **What are the clinical signs of a BRVO?**
    In a recent BRVO, ophthalmoscopy results may reveal a segmental pattern of intraretinal hemorrhages, cotton-wool spots, and macular edema (Fig. 47-1). In a chronic BRVO, collateral vessels on the disc or bridging the horizontal raphe, macular retinal pigment epithelium changes, or neovascularization of the retina or disc can develop.

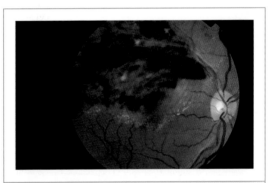

Figure 47-1. Superotemporal branch retinal vein occlusion with intraretinal hemorrhages, cotton-wool spots, hard exudates, and macular edema.

3. **Are there systemic associations in patients with a BRVO?**
    Hypertension, cardiovascular disease, increased body mass index, and glaucoma are risk factors for a BRVO. Approximately 10% of patients with a BRVO will develop a retinal vein occlusion in the fellow eye.

4. **Where does a BRVO most commonly occur?**
    In the superotemporal quadrant.

KEY POINTS: COMMON CHARACTERISTICS OF A BRANCH RETINAL VEIN OCCLUSION

1. Occurs at arteriovenous crossing

2. Segmental pattern of intraretinal hemorrhages

3. Macular edema

4. Majority occur in the superotemporal quadrant

5. **How is a BRVO categorized?**
   A BRVO is categorized as ischemic or nonischemic. A nonischemic BRVO is defined as having less than five disc areas of retinal capillary nonperfusion, as documented by fluorescein angiography. An ischemic BRVO is defined as having more than five disc areas of retinal capillary nonperfusion.

6. **What are the complications of a BRVO?**
   Patients with a nonischemic BRVO may lose vision secondary to macular edema. Patients with an ischemic BRVO most commonly lose vision from macular edema, ischemic maculopathy, or vitreous hemorrhage (VH). If ischemia occurs in the macula, patients complain of central vision loss, and ophthalmoscopy may not reveal macular edema. A fluorescein angiogram will demonstrate an enlarged and irregular foveal avascular zone. Approximately 40% of patients with an ischemic BRVO develop neovascularization of the retina (NVE) or disc. In approximately 60% of the patients who develop neovascularization, traction from the vitreous causes the NVE to bleed, which leads to VH and decreased vision.

7. **What is the treatment for an uncomplicated BRVO?**
   Patients with a nonischemic BRVO without macular edema are followed clinically for the development of macular edema and for progression into an ischemic BRVO and its complications, which include ischemic maculopathy, NVE, and VH.

8. **What were the results of the Branch Vein Occlusion Study in the treatment of macular edema?**
   The Branch Vein Occlusion Study was a multicentered, randomized, controlled clinical trial designed to answer whether argon laser photocoagulation is useful in improving visual acuity in eyes with a BRVO and macular edema that reduced vision to 20/40 or worse. The study found 65% of eyes treated with argon laser photocoagulation compared to 37% of control eyes gained two or more lines of vision. The study investigators recommend argon laser photocoagulation for patients with a BRVO of at least 3 months in duration and vision 20/40 or worse secondary to macular edema.

   Branch Vein Occlusion Study Group: Argon laser photocoagulation for macular edema in branch vein occlusion. Am J Ophthalmol 98:271–282, 1984.

9. **What is the treatment for a patient with an ischemic BRVO before the development of neovascularization?**
   The Branch Vein Occlusion Study was designed to answer whether peripheral scatter argon laser photocoagulation can prevent the development of retinal neovascularization. Significantly less neovascularization developed in patients treated with laser than in control patients. Although the

Branch Vein Occlusion Study was not designed to determine whether peripheral scatter laser treatment should be applied before rather than after the development of neovascularization, data accumulated in the study suggested there was minimal risk for severe vision loss if laser treatment was performed after the development of neovascularization.

Branch Vein Occlusion Study Group: Argon laser scatter photocoagulation for prevention of neovascularization and vitreous hemorrhage in branch vein occlusion. Arch Ophthalmol 104:34–41, 1996.

10. **What is the treatment for a patient with an ischemic BRVO after the development of neovascularization?**
   The Branch Vein Occlusion Study was designed to answer whether peripheral scatter argon laser photocoagulation can prevent vitreous hemorrhage in patients who have already developed neovascularization. Treated patients developed vitreous hemorrhage significantly less than the control patients.

   Branch Vein Occlusion Study Group: Argon laser scatter photocoagulation for prevention of neovascularization and vitreous hemorrhage in branch vein occlusion. Arch Ophthalmol 104:34–41, 1996.

KEY POINTS: MEDICAL EVALUATION OF PATIENTS WITH BRVO

1. Blood pressure

2. Fasting blood glucose

3. Complete blood count with differential

4. Prothrombin time/partial thromboplastin time

5. Erythrocyte sedimentation rate

6. Complete medical exam

11. **What are emerging therapies for a branch retinal vein occlusion?**
   Vitrectomy and vitrectomy with arteriovenous sheathotomy have been reported in small, uncontrolled studies. Intravitreal triamcinolone is currently being studied as a treatment for macular edema in a prospective, randomized, controlled clinical trial (**S**tandard **C**are versus **Co**rticosteroid for **Re**tinal Vein Occlusion Study [SCORE]).

   Yamamoto S, Saito W, Yagi F, et al: Vitrectomy with or without arteriovenous adventitial sheathotomy for macular edema associated with branch retinal vein occlusion. Am J Ophthalmol 138:907–914, 2004.
   http://spitfire.emmes.com/study/score

CENTRAL RETINAL VEIN OCCLUSION

12. **What are the symptoms of a central retinal vein occlusion (CRVO)?**
   Patients may complain of sudden, painless loss of vision. Occasionally, patients complain of a painful red eye because they have developed neovascular glaucoma secondary to an ischemic CRVO.

13. **What are the clinical signs of a CRVO?**
   In an acute CRVO, ophthalmoscopy reveals intraretinal hemorrhages in all four quadrants and dilated, tortuous retinal veins (Fig. 47-2). Other signs include a swollen disc,

cotton-wool spots, and cystoid macular edema. Patients with an ischemic CRVO can develop anterior segment or posterior segment neovascularization, which manifests as new vessels on the iris, angle, disc, or retina. In a long-standing CRVO, patients may develop disc or retinal venous collaterals, cystoid macular edema, and macular retinal pigment epithelium changes.

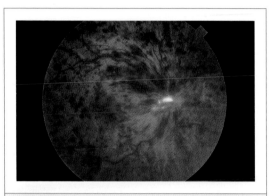

Figure 47-2. Nonischemic central retinal vein occlusion with dilated tortuous veins, disc edema, intraretinal hemorrhages in four quadrants, and macular edema.

KEY POINTS: COMMON CHARACTERISTICS OF A CENTRAL RETINAL VEIN OCCLUSION

1. Intraretinal hemorrhages in all four quadrants

2. Dilated tortuous retinal veins

3. Disc edema

4. Macular edema

14. **What are the risk factors for a CRVO?**
    Hypertension, diabetes mellitus, and glaucoma are risk factors for a CRVO.

15. **How is a CRVO categorized?**
    A CRVO is ischemic or nonischemic. A nonischemic CRVO is defined as having less than 10 disc areas of capillary nonperfusion on fluorescein angiography, whereas an ischemic CRVO is defined as having greater than 10 disc areas of capillary nonperfusion. Clinically, patients with an ischemic CRVO have poor vision, an afferent pupillary defect, and extensive intraretinal hemorrhages.

    Central Vein Occlusion Study Group: Baseline and early natural history report: The central vein occlusion study. Arch Ophthalmol 111:1087–1095, 1993.

16. **What are the complications of a CRVO?**
    Patients with a nonischemic CRVO can lose vision secondary to macular edema. Patients with an ischemic CRVO can lose vision from macular edema, ischemic maculopathy, neovascular

glaucoma (NVG), and vitreous hemorrhage. If ischemia occurs in the macula, a patient complains of central vision loss, and a fluorescein angiogram will demonstrate an enlarged and irregular foveal avascular zone. The most feared complication of an ischemic CRVO is anterior segment neovascularization, which can lead to NVG. Approximately 15% of patients with an ischemic CRVO develop neovascularization of the retina or disc. Traction from the vitreous may cause these new vessels to bleed, leading to VH and decreased vision.

Central Vein Occlusion Study Group: A randomized clinical trial of early panretinal photocoagulation for ischemic central vein occlusion: The Central Vein Occlusion Study Group N report. Ophthalmology 102:1434–1444, 1995.

17. **What is the treatment for an uncomplicated CRVO?**
Patients with a nonischemic CRVO without macular edema are followed clinically for the development of macular edema and for progression into an ischemic CRVO and its complications, including ischemic maculopathy, NVG, and VH.

18. **What is the standard treatment for a patient with a CRVO and macular edema?**
The Central Vein Occlusion Study was a multicentered, randomized, controlled clinical trial designed to answer whether argon laser photocoagulation was useful in improving visual acuity in eyes with a CRVO and macular edema that reduced vision to 20/50 or worse. Patients were randomized to macular grid photocoagulation or no treatment. There was no difference between the visual acuity in treated and untreated eyes. The study investigators do not recommend macular grid photocoagulation for patients who met the study entry criteria.

Central Vein Occlusion Study Group: Evaluation of grid pattern photocoagulation for macular edema in central vein occlusion: The central vein occlusion study group M report. Ophthalmology 102:1425–1433, 1995.

KEY POINTS: MEDICAL EVALUATION OF PATIENTS WITH CRVO

1. See branch retinal vein occlusion evaluation

2. Lipid profile

3. Homocysteine

4. Antinuclear antibody

5. Fluorescent treponemal antibody absorption test

6. Consider hemoglobin electrophoresis, cryoglobulins, antiphospholipid antibodies, lupus anticoagulants, and serum protein electrophoresis if clinically indicated

19. **Are there emerging therapies for macular edema from a central retinal vein occlusion?**
Radial optic neurotomy for central vein occlusion has been reported in an uncontrolled series. Intravitreal triamcinolone is currently being studied as a treatment for macular edema in a prospective, randomized, controlled clinical trial (SCORE).

Opremcak EM, Bruce RA, Lemeo MD, et al: Radial optic neurotomy for central retinal vein occlusion: A retrospective pilot study of 11 consecutive cases. Retina 21:408–415, 2001.
http://spitfire.emmes.com/study/score

20. **What is the recommended treatment for a patient with an ischemic CRVO?**
    The Central Vein Occlusion Study was also designed to answer whether panretinal argon laser photocoagulation could prevent the development of anterior segment neovascularization and NVG. Although prophylactic laser decreased the incidence of anterior segment neovascularization, laser at the time of development of anterior segment neovascularization was effective in preventing NVG. The study investigators recommend careful follow-up of patients with an ischemic CRVO and panretinal photocoagulation at the time a patient develops 2 clock hours of iris neovascularization or any angle neovascularization.

    Central Vein Occlusion Study Group: A randomized clinical trial of early panretinal photocoagulation for ischemic central vein occlusion: The Central Vein Occlusion Study Group N report. Ophthalmology 102:1434–1444, 1995.

    Clarkson JG, Coscas G, Finkelstein D, et al: The CVOS group M and N reports [letter]. Ophthalmology 103:350–354, 1996.

CHAPTER 48

RETINAL DETACHMENT

Michael J. Borne, MD, and James F. Vander, MD

1. **What is retinal detachment?**

   Retinal detachment (RD) is separation of the neurosensory retina from the underlying retinal pigment epithelium with accumulation of fluid in the potential space between the two layers. The types of retinal detachment include rhegmatogenous, traction, and exudative.

   - In **rhegmatogenous retinal detachments (RRDs)**, a break in the retina allows fluid from the vitreous cavity access to the potential space between the retina and retinal pigment epithelium.

   - **Tractional retinal detachment** occurs when epiretinal tissue forms and contracts, pulling the retina away from the pigment epithelial layer. Occasionally the severe traction caused by epiretinal membranes may cause a tear in the retina, creating a combination rhegmatogenous-tractional detachment.

   - **Exudative retinal detachments** are produced by retinal and choroidal conditions that damage the blood–retina barrier and allow fluid to accumulate in the subretinal space (the potential space between the retina and retinal pigment epithelium).

2. **What are the major characteristics of each type of retinal detachment?**

   - **RRDs** typically have a corrugated appearance caused by intraretinal edema (Fig. 48-1). Obviously, they are associated with a retinal break, although in a small percentage of cases the break is not easily identifiable. Decreased intraocular pressure, pigmented cells in the vitreous cavity, and vitreous hemorrhage are also associated with RRDs. Fixed folds and other signs of proliferative vitreoretinopathy (PVR) strongly suggest an RRD. Extension of fluid through the macula is a poor prognostic sign. The intraocular pressure is usually low.

   - **Tractional retinal detachments** are characterized by a smooth and stiff-appearing retinal surface. In most cases the epiretinal membranes that cause the traction may be ophthalmoscopically observed. The detachment is usually concave toward the front of the

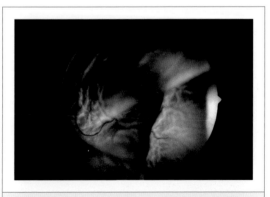

Figure 48-1. Bullous rhegmatogenous retinal detachment with mobile, corrugated appearance.

eye. The most common location of the tractional membranes is in the postequatorial region; the traction detachment rarely extends to the ora serrata.

- **Exudative retinal detachments** are characterized by shifting subretinal fluid. The subretinal fluid accumulates according to gravitational forces and detaches the retina in the area where it accumulates. Thus the fluid is noted to shift when the patient is viewed in an upright compared with a supine position. The surface of the retina is usually smooth in exudative detachments, compared with the corrugated appearance of an RRD. Occasionally the retina may be seen directly behind the lens in exudative detachments. This rarely occurs in RRDs, unless severe vitreoretinal traction is present.

3. **What are the major causes of exudative retinal detachments?**
The major causes of exudative RDs are intraocular tumors, intraocular inflammatory diseases, and congenital abnormalities. Intraocular neoplasms, such as choroidal melanomas, choroidal hemangiomas, and metastatic choroidal tumors, are most likely to produce serous RDs. Intraocular inflammation, such as posterior scleritis, Harada's disease, severe posterior uveitis, and central serous chorioretinopathy, occasionally produce shifting subretinal fluid. The most common congenital abnormalities known to produce exudative RD are optic pits, nanophthalmos, and the morning glory disc syndrome.

4. **How does the retina remain attached?**
The retinal photoreceptors and retinal pigment epithelial (RPE) cells are oriented with the apices of each cell in apposition. An interphotoreceptor matrix between the cells forms a "glue" that helps to maintain cellular apposition. It also has been postulated that the RPE functions as a cellular pump to remove ions and water from the interphotoreceptor matrix, providing a "suction force" that helps to keep the retina attached.

5. **What are the major predisposing factors for RRDs?**
The main predisposing factors for RRDs are previous cataract surgery, lattice degeneration, and myopia. The incidence of RRD after cataract surgery is approximately 2 in 1000. The incidence becomes much higher after complicated cataract surgery, including posterior capsule rupture, vitreous loss, and retained lens fragments. Some studies have shown an incidence of RRDs after complicated cataract surgery as high as 15%. Currently, approximately half of all primary RRDs occur in patients with a history of cataract surgery.

    Lattice degeneration (Fig. 48-2) is a peripheral retinal degeneration characterized by thinning of the retina with liquefaction of the overlying vitreous, which results in a high risk for retinal

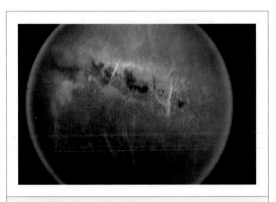

Figure 48-2. Lattice degeneration.

tears and breaks. Lattice degeneration is found in 6–7% of the population and is often bilateral. Lattice degeneration is the direct cause of primary RRD in approximately 25% of eyes.

High myopes have a high risk of RD for several reasons. First, the incidence of lattice degeneration is higher in myopes. Second, myopes tend to have a higher rate of posterior vitreous detachment. Of greater importance, myopic eyes have a higher rate of retinal breaks because of the thin peripheral retina. The rate of retinal breaks tends to be higher with increasing myopia.

6. **What are the signs and symptoms of a retinal break?**
Flashes and floaters are the classic symptoms. Pigmented cells or blood in the vitreous strongly suggests the possibility of a retinal break.

7. **What are the types of retinal breaks?**
   - **Horseshoe tear:** A flap of retina created by vitreous traction gives the appearance of a horseshoe. The open end of the horseshoe is anterior. A retinal vessel may bridge the gap of the tear (Figs. 48-3 and 48-4). The risk of subsequent RD is high, especially with acute tears.
   - **Operculated tear:** When a piece of retina is completely torn away by vitreous traction, the fragment is seen floating over the retinal defect. The risk of RD is lower than with a horseshoe tear.

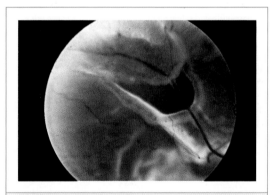

Figure 48-3. Horseshoe retinal tear with a bridging vessel.

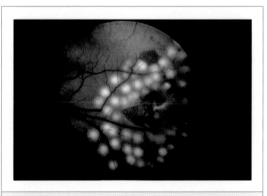

Figure 48-4. Horseshoe retinal tear after laser photocoagulation.

- **Atrophic hole:** A round hole without evidence of retinal traction is often associated with lattice degeneration. The risk of RD is low.
- **Dialysis** (Fig. 48-5): A disinsertion of the retina at the ora serrata, this is most common in the inferotemporal quadrant. The second most common site is superonasal. A frequent cause is trauma.

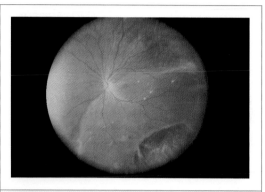

Figure 48-5. Retinal detachment resulting from inferotemporal dialysis.

KEY POINTS: SYMPTOMS AND SIGNS OF RHEGMATOGENOUS RETINAL DETACHMENT

1. Flashes

2. Floaters

3. Pigment in the vitreous

4. Posterior vitreous detachment (usually)

5. Elevated mobile retina

6. Corrugations

7. Loss of retinal transparency

8. Presence of a retinal break

9. Retinal pigment epithelial alterations under detachment

10. Fixed folds

11. Peripheral visual field loss

12. Loss of central vision (with macular involvement)

8. **What are the signs of a chronic RRD?**
   The retina is more transparent than in an acute RD, and the corrugations are minimal or absent. Pigmentary alterations are more prominent including hyperpigmented demarcation lines

(indicative of progression if multiple), RPE atrophy in the bed of the detachment, and abundant pigment in the vitreous. Retinal cysts, sometimes very large, may develop. The causative retinal break may be difficult to identify. PVR may also be present. The intraocular pressure may be low, normal, or high.

9. **What is degenerative retinoschisis?**
   Sometimes called senile retinoschisis, this is a dome-shaped elevation of the inner retina caused by a splitting within the outer plexiform layer. In contrast to an RRD, this rarely progresses and is usually observed. Occasionally, outer wall holes will form and create a progressive retinoschisis-related RRD. The inferotemporal quadrant is most commonly affected, and 80% are bilateral.

KEY POINTS: SIGNS OF CHRONIC RETINAL DETACHMENT VERSUS RETINOSCHISIS

1. Presence of retinal break most reliable method to distinguish the two but is often difficult to find

2. Pigment in the vitreous

3. Pigment alterations in the retinal pigment epithelium

4. Retinal folds

5. Absence of schisis in the fellow eye

10. **What are the options for repair of retinal detachment?**
    First, consideration of the type of RD is important before identifying the modality of treatment. Exudative RDs are approached differently from rhegmatogenous or traction detachments. Exudative detachments are repaired by treating the primary cause of the fluid extravasation into the subretinal space. For example, an RD associated with choroidal melanoma is addressed by treatment of the tumor with radiation, thermotherapy, or resection. Exudative RDs related to intraocular inflammatory conditions are generally treated by aggressive anti-inflammatory regimens. Rarely does an exudative detachment require primary surgical repair.
    On the other hand, treatment of rhegmatogenous and tractional RD is primarily surgical. Tractional RDs caused by diabetes or proliferative vitreoretinopathy require relief of all traction membranes before the retina will remain reattached.
    Small, localized RRDs are usually treated by cryotherapy or barrier laser photocoagulation. Rarely, an asymptomatic localized detachment may be treated with close observation only. If significant vitreous traction is present on the retinal tear, especially if the tear is superior in location, or if a large amount of subretinal fluid is found, more definitive treatment is usually indicated. Options include pneumatic retinopexy, Lincoff balloon, scleral buckling, and pars plana vitrectomy. Scleral buckling surgery is the time-honored approach and has been applied routinely since the 1950s. Pars plana vitrectomy was first performed in the late 1960s and has become the operation of choice for some surgeons. Pneumatic retinopexy has gained popularity since the early 1980s.

11. **Which patients are the best candidates for pneumatic retinopexy?**
    Pneumatic retinopexy involves injection of an inert gas or sterile air into the vitreous cavity; strict positioning is required to place the gas bubble in contact with the retinal break. If the break is

closed by the surface tension from the gas bubble, the retinal pigment epithelium can pump the subretinal fluid back into the choroid and allow retinal reattachment. The break is sealed either with cryotherapy at the time of gas injection or with laser photocoagulation after the retina is flattened. The ideal candidates are patients with a detachment caused by a single retinal break in the superior 8 clock hours or multiple breaks if all of the tears are within 1–2 clock hours of each other. Obviously the patient must not have a systemic disease or mechanical problem that precludes the positioning requirements. Phakic patients tend to fare slightly better than patients with a history of cataract surgery.

12. **Which patients are poor candidates for pneumatic retinopexy?**
Patients with RDs caused by multiple tears in several locations are poor candidates, as well as patients with a detachment resulting from a single tear but with tears in other areas of attached retina. Proliferative vitreoretinopathy, especially if fixed folds are present, lessens the chances for reattachment with pneumatic retinopexy. And, as previously stated, patients with rheumatoid arthritis or other systemic conditions who are unable to obey the strict postoperative positioning requirements are poor candidates.

KEY POINTS: FACTORS THAT INFLUENCE THE DECISION TO TREAT RETINAL BREAKS PROPHYLACTICALLY

1. Type of break.

2. Presence of symptoms of vitreoretinal traction.

3. Horseshoe tears are usually treated. All symptomatic horseshoe tears should be treated.

4. Operculated tears are generally not treated unless symptomatic.

5. History of retinal detachment in the fellow eye.

6. Family history of retinal detachment.

7. Anticipated prolonged inaccessibility to care.

13. **What are the advantages of scleral buckling and pars plana vitrectomy?**
Scleral buckling and pars plana vitrectomy reduce vitreous traction mechanically. Scleral buckling involves the surgical placement of a silicone band or sponge, either sewn to the sclera as an exoplant or implanted in the sclera after a partial-thickness scleral bed is surgically created (Fig. 48-6). Scleral buckles provide smooth, broad relief of vitreous traction. Subretinal fluid may be drained at the time of placement of the scleral buckle via an external sclerostomy, and intraocular gas may be injected into the vitreous cavity as an adjunct to aid in retinal reattachment. Scleral buckles are especially effective in anterior retinal breaks. This is the most common site for postcataract retinal breaks. Another advantage of scleral buckling is the opportunity to repair the RD from a purely external approach with no intraocular invasion.

With vitrectomy, it is possible to relieve vitreous traction directly with the vitrectomy cutter. This technique is especially useful in cases with very posterior breaks. Vitrectomy is advantageous in cases of RD with vitreous hemorrhage or vitreous opacities that obscure a view of the retinal breaks. Vitrectomy also allows the surgeon to remove epiretinal membranes when proliferative vitreoretinopathy is present. When vitrectomy is performed, the vitreous cavity must be filled with gas to reattach the retina. The presence of intravitreal gas hastens the development of cataract in phakic patients.

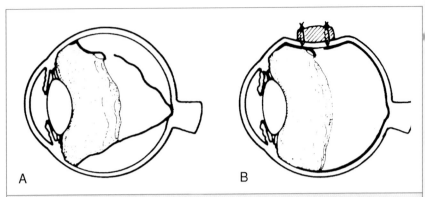

Figure 48-6. Placement of a scleral buckle. **A,** Rhegmatogenous retinal detachment. **B,** The retina is unattached after placement of a scleral buckle supenaly.

14. **What are the major risks and complications with scleral buckling and pars plana vitrectomy?**

Risks of infection and hemorrhage are found with any invasive ocular procedure. The risk of an infection with a scleral buckle is less than 3%. Other risks and complications from scleral buckles include angle-closure glaucoma, acute glaucoma from intraocular gas injection, intraocular hemorrhage from perforation during drainage of subretinal fluid, and anterior segment ischemia and necrosis. The surgically placed buckles may cause extrusion or intrusion over time, and, if the buckle is placed under an extraocular muscle, strabismus may result.

Vitrectomy involves the risks of endophthalmitis, iatrogenic retinal breaks, retinal or vitreous incarceration in the sclerostomy sites, and glaucoma from the use of intraocular gases.

15. **What intraoperative findings should be confirmed at the time of scleral buckle placement?**

The most important intraoperative decisions at the time of scleral buckling procedures are to find and treat all retinal tears and place the scleral buckle in a position to support all retinal breaks. After the buckle has been temporarily placed, the surgeon should confirm that the tears are flat on the buckle. If the tears are not flat, the placement of the buckle should be checked with scleral depression. If the buckle is in the appropriate position but fluid still exists between the retina and the buckle, the decision to drain subretinal fluid or to inject an intravitreal gas bubble should be made. If the detachment is primarily inferior in location, most surgeons prefer to have the retina completely attached before leaving the operating room. Superior detachments may flatten with gas injection and postoperative positioning; the decision to drain subretinal fluid adds potential complications.

16. **What three factors should be confirmed with indirect ophthalmoscopy at the conclusion of scleral buckling surgery?**

Apposition of the scleral buckle to the retinal breaks, absence of complications at the drainage site, and absence of central retinal artery pulsations should be confirmed before final closure. If pulsations are present, the intraocular pressure is high enough to cause a central retinal artery obstruction. The pressure should be lowered by loosening the buckle, removing intraocular fluid or gas until pulsations are no longer seen.

17. **How should cases of RRD be approached if pars plana vitrectomy is the chosen treatment?**

The placement of the infusion cannula must be carefully confirmed to avoid flushing fluid or air into the subretinal space. Vitreous traction on all retinal breaks should be relieved if possible. Care must be taken to avoid damaging retinal blood vessels if they are coursing across the retinal tears. The infusion pressure should be kept low, and instruments should be passed through the sclerostomy sites infrequently to avoid retinal incarceration. A complete posterior vitreous detachment should be created, if possible. Sclerostomy sites should be checked carefully at the end of the case to evaluate for iatrogenic retinal breaks. All retinal tears should be treated completely with laser or cryotherapy. Finally, the intraocular pressure must be measured if intraocular gas is used.

18. **Which gases may be used inside the eye? In what concentrations?**
The inert gases sulfur hexafluoride (SF_6) and perfluoropropane (C_3F_8), along with sterile air, are the most commonly used intraocular gases. Nonexpansile mixtures are composed of approximately 20% sulfur hexafluoride and 14% perfluoropropane. These are the most commonly used mixtures when the vitreous cavity is filled with gas, as in vitrectomy. Pure 100% gas injection allows a larger bubble to form with a smaller volume of injection. This technique is advantageous in patients with pneumatic retinopexy and scleral buckles. Typically, sulfur hexafluoride expands to 2–3 times its initial volume, and perfluoropropane expands to approximately 4 times its initial volume. Thus, injection of 0.4 mL of each gas produces a 20–40% intravitreal gas bubble when they are injected as a pure concentration.

19. **What are the primary causes of failure of initial RD repair?**
Except for cases of severe PVR, in which epiretinal membranes cause traction retinal detachments (Fig. 48-7), failures of RD repair are caused by an open retinal break. With pneumatic retinopexy, the most common reasons for failure include poor patient compliance with positioning requirements, inadequate identification of all retinal breaks, and development of new retinal tears from vitreous traction related to intravitreal gas. After scleral buckling surgery, failure to flatten the retina or to keep it attached results most often from undetected retinal breaks; continued vitreous traction with new, extended, or reopened retinal breaks; or a misplaced scleral buckle. Inadequate photocoagulation or cryotherapy, continued vitreous traction, and new or missed breaks are the most common reasons for failure after pars plana vitrectomy. Ten percent of retinal reattachments have evidence of PVR. However, only 10–25% of these progress to require treatment for detachment.

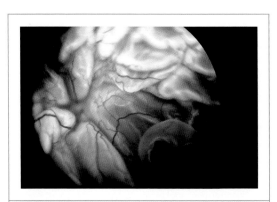

Figure 48-7. Severe proliferative vitreoretinopathy with total retinal detachment.

20. **What are the major objectives in repair of tractional retinal detachment?**
When tractional retinal detachments are caused by proliferative diabetic retinopathy (Fig. 48-8), one of the major aims is to relieve all anteroposterior traction. A complete posterior vitreous separation must be created to remove or segment all retinal traction. Segmentation of diabetic tractional membranes is effective if no anterior traction remains (Fig. 48-9). Delamination of

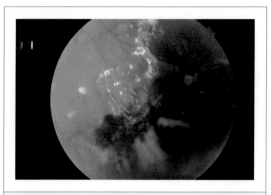

Figure 48-8. Proliferative diabetic retinopathy causing localized tractional retinal detachment.

traction membranes is accomplished by carefully identifying the plane between epiretinal tissue and the retina and by lysing all adhesions. In advanced PVR, retinal traction may be so severe that the retina must be cut to relieve all retinal traction. In cases with such severe traction, especially when a retinotomy must be created, silicone oil is often useful as a long-acting tamponade. The silicone oil is usually removed after 3–6 months but may be left in place longer if the retina appears unstable.

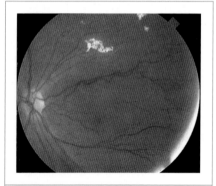

Figure 48-9. Detachment of retina after membrane peeling.

21. **Describe the classification system for PVR.**

The Retina Society published a classification system for PVR in 1983, which was updated in 1991. The three grades—A, B, and C—describe increasing severity of the disease. Posterior or anterior location of the proliferations has been emphasized, along with the number of clock hours involved. Five contraction types also have been described. Focal, diffuse, subretinal, circumferential, and anterior displacement are descriptive terms to quantify the type of contraction.

BIBLIOGRAPHY

1. Benson WE: Retinal Detachment: Diagnosis and Management, 2nd ed. Philadelphia, J.B. Lippincott, 1988.
2. Davis MD: Natural history of retinal breaks without detachment. Arch Ophthalmol 92:183–194, 1974.
3. Hilton GF, McLean EB, Chuang EL: Retinal Detachment: Ophthalmology Monograph Series. San Francisco, American Academy of Ophthalmology, 1989.
4. Kramer SG, Benson WE: Prophylactic therapy of retinal breaks. Surv Ophthalmol 22:41–47, 1977.
5. Machemer R, Aaberg TM, Freeman HM, et al: An updated classification of retinal detachment with proliferative vitreoretinopathy. Am J Ophthalmol 112:159–165, 1991.

CHAPTER 49

RETINOBLASTOMA

Carol L. Shields, MD

1. **What is retinoblastoma?**
   Retinoblastoma is the most common eye cancer in children and is believed to arise from primitive retinoblasts.

2. **How common is retinoblastoma?**
   Retinoblastoma occurs with a frequency of approximately 1 in 14,000 live births. Approximately 250–300 children in the United States each year are diagnosed with retinoblastoma.

3. **What causes retinoblastoma?**
   There are no determined causes for the cancer. Advanced paternal age and excess instances of cancer in relatives have been found to be associated with retinoblastoma. One study found human papilloma virus in some eyes with retinoblastoma.

4. **On what chromosome is the genetic mutation associated with retinoblastoma?**
   The genetic mutation associated with retinoblastoma is found on chromosome 13 in the region 13q14. It is believed that this single locus exists for all forms of retinoblastoma. Theesterase D gene is closely linked to this site.

5. **What syndrome is associated with retinoblastoma?**
   The 13q deletion syndrome is associated with retinoblastoma. The characteristic findings include the following:
   - Microcephaly
   - Broad prominent nasal bridge
   - Hypertelorism
   - Microphthalmos
   - Epicanthus
   - Ptosis
   - Protruding upper incisors
   - Micrognathia
   - Short neck with lateral folds
   - Large, low-set ears
   - Facial asymmetry
   - Imperforate anus
   - Genital malformations
   - Perineal fistula
   - Hypoplastic or absent thumbs
   - Toe abnormalities
   - Psychomotor delay
   - Mental delay

6. **What is the laterality of retinoblastoma?**
   Retinoblastoma is unilateral in approximately 67% of cases and bilateral in 33% of cases.

7. **What is germline mutation retinoblastoma?**
    Germline mutation retinoblastoma is the occurrence of the retinoblastoma (Rb) mutation on all cells in the body, including the retina and systemic sites. These patients typically develop bilateral retinoblastoma and are at risk for pinealoblastoma and second cancers.

8. **Who manifests germline mutation retinoblastoma?**
    All bilateral and familial retinoblastoma by definition have germline mutation. Between 10% and 15% of unilateral sporadic retinoblastoma have germline mutation.

9. **What is somatic mutation retinoblastoma?**
    Somatic mutation retinoblastoma is the occurrence of the Rb mutation only in the retina in one clone of cells. Hence these patients typically develop unilateral sporadic retinoblastoma. These patients are generally not at increased risk for pinealoblastoma or second cancers.

10. **Who manifests somatic mutation retinoblastoma?**
    Only unilateral sporadic retinoblastoma are somatic mutation.

11. **What are the most common presenting findings of retinoblastoma?**
    In the United States, leukocoria is the presenting feature in nearly 50% of cases and strabismus in 20%. Other less common presenting features include poor vision, red eye, glaucoma, and orbital cellulitis.

12. **What are the most common lesions simulating retinoblastoma?**
    Of all patients referred to an ocular oncology center with the diagnosis of possible retinoblastoma, approximately 50% prove to have retinoblastoma and 50% are found to have pseudoretinoblastoma. The most common pseudoretinoblastomas include persistent hyperplastic primary vitreous in 28% of patients, Coats disease in 16%, and ocular toxocariasis in 16%.

13. **At what age does retinoblastoma typically present?**
    Retinoblastoma is diagnosed at an average age of 18 months. Bilateral cases are recognized at an average of 12 months and unilateral cases at 23 months. In 8% of cases the tumor is first diagnosed after age 5 years.

14. **What is trilateral retinoblastoma?**
    Trilateral retinoblastoma is the association of bilateral retinoblastoma with midline brain tumors, especially pinealoblastoma. Trilateral disease represents 3% of all retinoblastoma cases and typically occurs before the age 5.

15. **When is pinealoblastoma diagnosed?**
    Pinealoblastoma is generally diagnosed within 1 year of retinoblastoma diagnosis. In fact, most cases are found before age 5. Keep in mind that benign pineal cyst can resemble malignant pinealoblastoma and magnetic resonance imaging is necessary to differentiate these two conditions.

16. **What second cancers are associated with retinoblastoma?**
    The most common second cancers associated with retinoblastoma include osteosarcoma (especially of the femur), cutaneous melanoma, and other sarcomas. The peak incidence for second cancers is age 13, but these tumors can occur anytime during the patient's life. It is believed that second cancers are related to germline mutation of chromosome 13.

17. **How often do eyes with retinoblastoma present with glaucoma?**
    From a clinical standpoint, 17% of eyes with retinoblastoma have glaucoma, most often neovascular or angle-closure glaucoma. From a pathology standpoint, glaucoma is present in 40% of eyes that come to enucleation.

KEY POINTS: EVALUATION AND DIAGNOSIS OF RETINOBLASTOMA

1. Retinoblastoma is an ocular cancer of childhood, usually detected before age 3 years. However, approximately 5% of newly diagnosed cases are in children older than age 5.

2. The diagnosis of retinoblastoma must be excluded in any child, even a teenager or young adult, who manifests atypical uveitis, vitreous hemorrhage, or nonrhegmatogenous retinal detachment.

3. Do not perform a vitrectomy or intraocular needle aspiration biopsy on an eye with retinoblastoma.

4. Any child with spontaneous hyphema or vitreous hemorrhage should be evaluated for trauma, retinoblastoma, and other intraocular tumors and inflammations.

5. The best way to diagnose retinoblastoma is with indirect ophthalmoscopy by an experienced observer. If uncertain, ultrasonography, fluorescein angiography, and computed tomography can be useful tests.

6. Magnetic resonance imaging is most useful for evaluating tumor invasion into the optic nerve or orbit as well as assessment of the brain for related intracranial neuroblastic malignancy (trilateral retinoblastoma; pinealoblastoma).

18. **How often does retinoblastoma invade the optic nerve?**
    Optic nerve invasion by retinoblastoma occurs in 29% of eyes that come to enucleation. Usually it occurs in the prelaminar area. Risks for optic nerve invasion by retinoblastoma include a large exophytic tumor measuring greater than 15 mm and secondary glaucoma.

19. **What is the survival rate with retinoblastoma?**
    In the twenty-first century in the United States, more than 95% of children with retinoblastoma survive this cancer. Risks for metastatic disease include substantial optic nerve, choroidal, or orbital invasion by the tumor.

20. **What are the growth patterns of retinoblastoma?**
    The growth patterns are endophytic and exophytic. Endophytic retinoblastoma arises from the inner retina and seeds the vitreous. Exophytic retinoblastoma arises from outer retinal layers and causes a solid retinal detachment. A variant of endophytic retinoblastoma is the diffuse infiltrating retinoblastoma. These patterns impart no difference to the patient's life prognosis.

21. **What is the differential diagnosis of endophytic retinoblastoma?**
    The differential diagnosis of endophytic retinoblastoma includes various inflammatory or infectious processes of the eye in children, such as toxocariasis, endophthalmitis, or advanced uveitis.

22. **What is the differential diagnosis of exophytic retinoblastoma?**
    The differential diagnosis of exophytic retinoblastoma includes Coats disease, retinal capillary hemangioma, familial exudative vitreoretinopathy, and other causes of rhegmatogenous or nonrhegmatogenous retinal detachment in children.

23. **Can retinoblastoma spontaneously regress?**
    Yes, approximately 3% of all cases of retinoblastoma are classified as spontaneously regressed. They are also termed *retinoma* and *retinocytoma*. These tumors nevertheless carry the risk for recurrence and the same genetic implications as other retinoblastoma.

24. **What are the pathologic features of a well-differentiated retinoblastoma?**
Flexner-Wintersteiner rosettes and fleurettes represent well-differentiated retinoblastoma (Fig. 49-1).

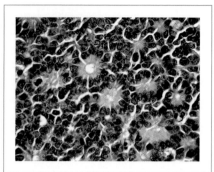

Figure 49-1. Flexner Wintersteiner rosettes in a retinoblastoma.

25. **List the options for management of an eye with intraocular retinoblastoma.**
   - Enucleation
   - Chemoreduction
   - Thermotherapy
   - Cryotherapy
   - Laser photocoagulation
   - Plaque radiotherapy
   - External-beam radiotherapy

26. **What are the conservative options for management of a small retinoblastoma posterior to the equator of the eye?**
Chemoreduction combined with thermotherapy or plaque radiotherapy is the most appropriate therapy for this tumor. Cryotherapy is generally limited to small tumors anterior to the equator of the eye (Fig. 49-2).

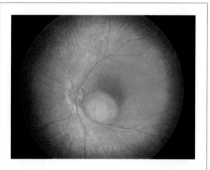

Figure 49-2. Small retinoblastoma adjacent to the optic nerve suitable for conservative treatment with chemoreduction plus thermotherapy or plaque radiotherapy.

27. **What are the conservative options for managing a small (<3 mm) retinoblastoma anterior to the equator of the eye?**
Chemoreduction combined with thermotherapy, laser photocoagulation, cryotherapy, or plaque radiotherapy is the most conservative option. Using the indirect ophthalmoscope delivery system, thermotherapy and laser photocoagulation can be adequately delivered to peripheral tumors.

28. **What are the risks of external-beam radiotherapy to the patient?**
External-beam radiotherapy can cause short-term and long-term effects. The short-term effects include the following:
   - Dry eye
   - Cilia loss
   - Cutaneous erythema
The long-term effects include the following:
   - Persistent dry eye
   - Cataract
   - Retinopathy
   - Papillopathy
   - Orbital fat atrophy
   - Maldevelopment of the orbital bones
   - Second cancers

29. **What are the chances that future offspring of a child with bilateral retinoblastoma will develop retinoblastoma?**
The quoted risk is 40%. See Table 49-1.

TABLE 49-1. CHANCES OF HAVING A BABY WITH RETINOBLASTOMA			
	Parents*	Affected Child	Normal Sibling
No family history			
Bilateral retinoblastoma	6%	40%	1%
Unilateral retinoblastoma	1%	8%	1%
Positive family history			
Bilateral retinoblastoma	40%	40%	7%
Unilateral retinoblastoma	40%	40%	7%

*Chance of having another baby with retinoblastoma.

30. **What is the most used classification scheme for retinoblastoma?**
The Reese Ellsworth classification scheme (Box 49-1) was devised in the 1950s to predict survival of the eye with retinoblastoma, not survival of the patient. At that time, external-beam radiotherapy was the only widely available conservative modality to save the eye.

> **BOX 49-1.   REESE ELLSWORTH CLASSIFICATION SYSTEM**
>
> **Group 1: Very Favorable**
> A. Solitary tumor less than 4 disc diameters (DD), at or behind the equator
> B. Multiple tumors, none over 4 DD, all at or behind the equator
>
> **Group 2: Favorable**
> A. Solitary tumor, 4–10 DD, at or behind the equator
> B. Multiple tumors, 4–10 DD, behind the equator
>
> **Group 3: Doubtful**
> A. Any tumor anterior to the equator
> B. Solitary tumor, larger than 10 DD, behind the equator
>
> **Group 4: Unfavorable**
> A. Multiple tumors, some larger than 10 DD
> B. Any lesion extending anteriorly to the ora serrata
>
> **Group 5: Very Unfavorable**
> A. Massive tumors involving more than half the retina
> B. Vitreous seeding

31. **What is the International Classification of Retinoblastoma?**
This new classification, designed by world experts on retinoblastoma, is a simple and practical classification that is more pertinent for current therapies. It will be used in the upcoming national collaborative studies on retinoblastoma (Table 49-2).

TABLE 49-2. INTERNATIONAL CLASSIFICATION OF RETINOBLASTOMA	
Group A	Small Rb (≤3 mm diameter)
Group B	Bigger Rb (≤3 mm diameter) or
	■ Any Rb in macula
	■ Any Rb with subretinal fluid
Group C	Localized subretinal or vitreous seeds (<3 mm from Rb)
Group D	Diffuse subretinal or vitreous seeds (>3 mm from Rb)
Group E	Extensive Rb involving more than 50% of the fundus
	■ Opaque media
	■ Neovascularization of iris
	■ Suspicion of invasion of optic nerve, choroid, or orbit

Rb = Retinoblastoma.

32. **How does retinoblastoma appear on ultrasound?**
    On ultrasound, retinoblastoma appears as a mass originating from the retina with acoustic solidity and high internal reflectivity. Foci of calcium can be seen as dense echoes.

33. **How does retinoblastoma appear on computed tomography?**
    On computed tomography, retinoblastoma appears as a solid mass within the globe with foci of bone density, representing calcium (Fig. 49-3). Retinal detachment often can be detected.

34. **How does retinoblastoma appear on magnetic resonance imaging?**
    On magnetic resonance imaging, retinoblastoma shows a hyperintense signal to the vitreous on T1-weighted images and a hypointense signal on T2. Contrast enhancement can be seen. The foci of calcium remain hypointense on both T1 and T2 without enhancement. Areas of necrosis appear similar to calcium except that they show enhancement.

35. **Should pars plana vitrectomy be performed to obtain tissue for confirming the diagnosis of retinoblastoma?**
    No. Pars plana vitrectomy should not be performed in any eye with untreated retinoblastoma because it potentially seeds the tumor into the orbit and may lead to retinoblastoma metastasis.

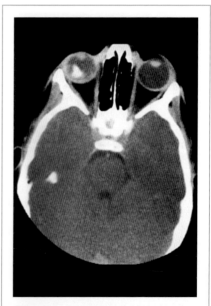

Figure 49-3. Computed tomography of eye with retinoblastoma shows the calcified mass within the right globe.

KEY POINTS: MANAGEMENT OF RETINOBLASTOMA

1. The goal in managing retinoblastoma is first, and most importantly, to save the patient's life, then globe salvage and vision preservation is considered.

2. The most common method for management of unilateral advanced retinoblastoma (Reese Ellsworth group V) is enucleation with a long section of optic nerve.

3. Most bilateral retinoblastoma can be treated with chemoreduction initially. However, enucleation of one eye is often necessary.

4. Fresh retinoblastoma tissue should be harvested for DNA analysis and family genetic counseling.

BIBLIOGRAPHY

1. Shields CL, Honavar SG, Meadows AT, et al: Chemoreduction plus focal therapy for retinoblastoma: Factors predictive of need for treatment with external beam radiotherapy or enucleation. Am J Ophthalmol 133:657–664, 2002.

2. Shields CL, Mashayekhi A, Cater J, et al: Chemoreduction for retinoblastoma. Analysis of tumor control and risks for recurrence in 457 tumors. Am J Ophthalmol 138:329–337, 2004.

3. Shields CL, Mashayekhi A, Demirci H, et al: Practical approach to management of retinoblastoma. Arch Ophthalmol 122:729–735, 2004.

4. Shields CL, Santos C, Diniz W, et al: Thermotherapy for retinoblastoma. Arch Ophthalmol 117:885–893, 1999.

5. Shields CL, Shields JA: Diagnosis and management of retinoblastoma. Cancer Control 11:317–327, 2004.

6. Shields CL, Shields JA: Recent developments in the management of retinoblastoma. J Pediatr Ophthalmol Strabism 36:8–18, 1999.

7. Shields CL, Shields JA, Kiratli H, De Potter P: Treatment of retinoblastoma with indirect ophthalmoscope laser photocoagulation. J Pediatr Ophthalmol Strabism 32:317–322, 1995.

8. Shields JA, Parsons H, Shields CL, Giblin ME: The role of cryotherapy in the management of retinoblastoma. Am J Ophthalmol 108:260–264, 1989.

9. Shields JA, Shields CL: Atlas of Intraocular Tumors. Philadelphia, Lippincott, Williams & Wilkins, 1999, pp 207–242.

10. Shields JA, Shields CL: Intraocular Tumors: A Text and Atlas. Philadelphia, W.B. Saunders, 1992.

CHAPTER 50

PIGMENTED LESIONS OF THE OCULAR FUNDUS

Jerry A. Shields, MD

1. **What is the main differential diagnosis of a relatively flat pigmented fundus lesion?**
   - Choroidal nevus (Fig. 50-1)
   - Congenital hypertrophy of the retinal pigment epithelium (CHRPE) (Fig. 50-2)

2. **What ophthalmoscope features help to differentiate choroidal nevus and CHRPE?**
   Choroidal nevus is generally a slate-gray lesion with a slightly ill-defined border. Drusen may be present on the surface of the lesion. CHRPE is usually black, has a sharply demarcated border, and may have depigmented lacunae through which the underlying choroid can be visualized.

3. **What is the difference in the natural course of a choroidal nevus and CHRPE?**
   Although both lesions are benign and usually stationary, CHRPE has no metastatic potential. However, some cases give rise to elevated, nodular tumors that can be locally invasive. In contrast, choroidal nevus occasionally evolves into malignant melanoma.

4. **What is the main differential diagnosis of an elevated pigmented fundus lesion?**
   - Choroidal melanoma
   - Subretinal hemorrhage
   - Tumor of the retinal pigment epithelium

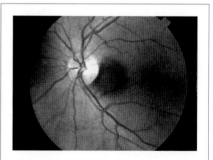

Figure 50-1. Typical choroidal nevus adjacent to the optic disc.

5. **What ophthalmoscopic features help to differentiate a choroidal melanoma from a subretinal hemorrhage?**
   In general a choroidal melanoma is a rather homogeneous brown-to-black lesion with a smooth surface. Subretinal hemorrhage in the macular area (age-related macular degeneration) or in the peripheral fundus (peripheral disciform degeneration) initially has a reddish-blue color; as it undergoes resolution, it has a more heterogeneous color with areas of fresh red blood and older yellow blood.

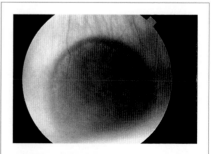

Figure 50-2. Congenital hypertrophy of the retinal pigment epithelium.

6. **What is the most practical ancillary test for differentiating melanoma from subretinal blood?**
Fluorescein angiography. Most melanomas show hyperfluorescence, and most hemorrhages are hypofluorescent.

7. **What is the significance of a mushroom-shaped fundus lesion?**
A mushroom-shaped fundus lesion is strongly suggestive of choroidal melanoma (Fig. 50-3). Even when the mushroom-shaped lesion is nonpigmented, melanoma is still the most likely diagnosis. It is extremely unusual for any other fundus lesion to assume a mushroom shape.

8. **What is the most reliable way to diagnose choroidal melanoma?**
The use of binocular indirect ophthalmoscopy by an experienced ophthalmologist who is familiar with the characteristic features of choroidal melanoma and other lesions that simulate choroidal melanoma. Most melanomas can be readily diagnosed by indirect ophthalmoscopy alone.

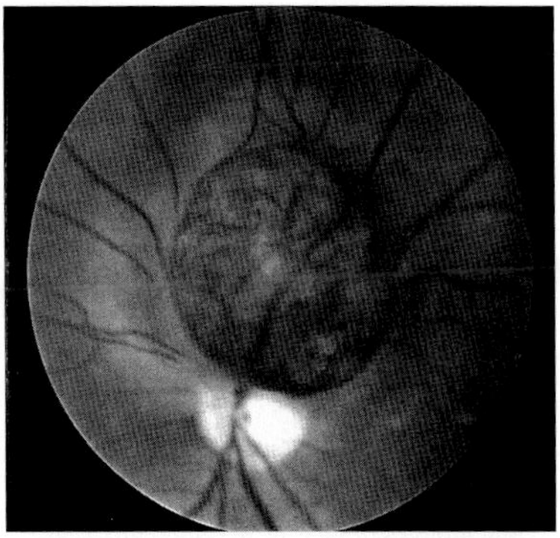

9. **In atypical cases in which the diagnosis is less evident, what are the four most helpful ancillary tests in the diagnosis of uveal melanoma?**
- Transillumination
- Fluorescein angiography
- Ultrasonography
- Fine-needle aspiration biopsy

Figure 50-3. Mushroom-shaped choroidal melanoma.

Most melanomas cast a shadow with transillumination, are hyperfluorescent with angiography, and show low internal reflectivity with ultrasonography. Most simulating lesions show different patterns with these modalities. Fine-needle aspiration biopsy is perhaps the most reliable method, but it is an invasive procedure that requires a skilled and experienced physician.

10. **What clinical signs suggest that a benign choroidal nevus is likely to grow and eventually evolve into a malignant choroidal melanoma?**
Elevation of the lesion, orange pigment on the surface of the lesion, secondary retinal detachment, proximity of the lesion to the optic disc, and presence of visual symptoms.

KEY POINTS: RISK FACTORS FOR CHOROID NEVUS BECOMING MALIGNANT

1. Elevation

2. Orange pigment

3. Associated retinal detachment

4. Proximity to optic disc

5. Visual symptoms

11. **What clinical signs suggest that a small, suspicious pigmented fundus lesion may eventually metastasize?**
   - Elevation of the lesion >2 mm
   - Proximity to the optic disc
   - Visual symptoms
   - Documentation of growth

12. **What congenital ocular conditions are clearly associated with a higher incidence of uveal melanoma?**
   Congenital ocular melanocytosis and oculodermal melanocytosis (nevus of Ota)—perhaps because of the excessive melanocytes in their uveal tract—have a greater chance of developing uveal melanoma.

13. **Does uveal melanoma have a predilection for gender, age, or race?**
   Uveal melanoma has no significant predilection for gender. It generally occurs in patients between 40 and 70 years of age and is relatively uncommon in patients younger than age 20. It has a definite predilection for Caucasians; only 1–2% of cases occur in African Americans and Asians.

14. **What external ocular sign strongly suggests the presence of an underlying ciliary body or peripheral choroidal melanoma?**
   One or more dilated, tortuous episcleral blood vessels in the ciliary body region (sentinel vessels; Fig. 50-4).

15. **What is the main route of distant spread of uveal melanoma?**
   Melanoma spreads to extraocular locations primarily by hematogenous metastasis to liver. Metastatic uveal melanoma to skin, lung, and other organs is considerably less common. Because there are no lymphatic channels in the eye, lymphogenous metastasis does not occur.

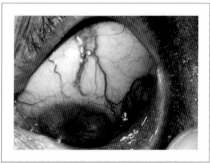

Figure 50-4. Sentinel vessel over a ciliary body melanoma.

16. **What is a melanocytoma?**
   A melanocytoma is a variant of benign nevus that has distinct clinical and histopathologic features. Clinically, it is usually detected on and next to the optic disc as a deeply pigmented lesion that may have a feathery border because of involvement of the nerve fiber layer of the retina (Fig. 50-5). It also may occur as a deeply pigmented nevus in the choroid, not near the optic disc. Histopathologically, it is composed of round-to-oval cells that have densely packed cytoplasmic melanosomes, small uniform nuclei, and few prominent nucleoli. Like other uveal nevi, it rarely gives rise to uveal melanoma.

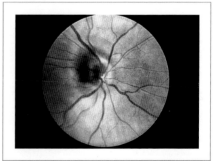

Figure 50-5. Melanocytoma of the optic nerve.

17. **What is the most acceptable method of treating a choroidal melanoma that occupies more than half of the globe and has produced severe visual loss?**
Enucleation.

18. **What is the most often used alternative to enucleation for a medium-sized melanoma located posterior to the equator?**
Brachytherapy with a radioactive plaque.

19. **What is the most common treatment for a melanoma that occupies 2 clock hours of the ciliary body?**
Resection of the tumor by iridocyclectomy or application of radioactive plaque depending on several clinical circumstances.

20. **What is the most acceptable method of management for an asymptomatic pigmented lesion that measures 3 mm in diameter and 1 mm in thickness and has fine drusen on its surface?**
Baseline fundus photographs and examination every 6–12 months. Most such lesions are benign nevi that remain stationary.

BIBLIOGRAPHY

1. Shields CL, Demirci H, Materin MA, et al: Clinical factors in the identification of small choroidal melanoma: The 2004 Torrence A. Makley, Jr., Lecture. Can J Ophthalmol 39:351–357, 2004.
2. Shields CL, Mashayekhi A, Ho T, et al: Solitary congenital hypertrophy of the retinal pigment epithelium: Clinical features and frequency of enlargement in 330 patients. Ophthalmology 110:1968–1976, 2003.
3. Shields CL, Shields JA, Kiratli H, et al: Risk factors for metastasis of small choroidal melanocytic lesions. Ophthalmology 102:1351–1361, 1995.
4. Shields CL, Shields JA: Recent developments in the management of choroidal melanoma. Curr Opin Ophthalmol 15:244–251, 2004.
5. Shields JA, Demirci H, Mashayekhi A, Shields CL: Melanocytoma of the optic disc in 115 cases: The 2004 Samuel Johnson Memorial Lecture. Ophthalmology 111:1739–1746, 2004.
6. Shields JA, Shields CL: Atlas of Intraocular Tumors. Philadelphia, Lippincott, William & Wilkins, 1999.
7. Shields JA, Shields CL, DePotter P, et al: Plaque radiotherapy for uveal melanoma. Ophthalmol Clin 33:129–135, 1993.
8. Shields JA, Shields CL: Diagnostic approaches to posterior uveal melanoma. In Shields JA, Shields CL (eds): Intraocular Tumors: A Text and Atlas. Philadelphia, W.B. Saunders, 1992, pp 155–169.
9. Shields JA, Shields CL: Differential diagnosis of posterior uveal melanoma. In Shields JA, Shields CL (eds): Intraocular Tumors: A Text and Atlas. Philadelphia, W.B. Saunders, 1992, pp 137–153.
10. Shields JA, Shields CL, Ehya H, et al: Fine needle aspiration biopsy of suspected intraocular tumors. The 1992 Urwick Lecture. Ophthalmology 100:1677–1684, 1993.
11. Shields JA, Shields CL: Introduction to melanocytic tumors of the uvea. In Shields JA, Shields CL (eds): Intraocular Tumors: A Text and Atlas. Philadelphia, W.B. Saunders, 1992, pp 45–49.
12. Shields JA, Shields CL: Management of posterior uveal melanoma. In Shields JA, Shields CL (eds): Intraocular Tumors: A Text and Atlas. Philadelphia, W.B. Saunders, 1992, pp 171–205.
13. Shields JA, Shields CL: Melanocytoma. In Shields JA, Shields CL (eds): Intraocular Tumors: A Text and Atlas. Philadelphia, W.B. Saunders, 1992, pp 101–115.
14. Shields JA, Shields CL: Posterior uveal melanoma. Clinical and pathologic features. In Shields JA, Shields CL (eds): Intraocular Tumors: A Text and Atlas. Philadelphia, W.B. Saunders, 1992, pp 117–136.
15. Shields JA, Shields CL, Shah P, Sivalingam V: Partial lamellar sclerouvectomy for ciliary body and choroidal tumors. Ophthalmology 98:971–983, 1991.
16. Shields JA, Shields CL, Singh AD: Acquired tumors arising from congenital hypertrophy of the retinal pigment epithelium. Arch Ophthalmol 118:637–641, 2000.
17. Territo C, Shields CL, Shields JA, Schroeder RP: Natural course of melanocytic tumors of the iris. Ophthalmology 95:1251–1255, 1988.

X. NEOPLASMS

CHAPTER 51

OCULAR TUMORS

Ralph C. Eagle, Jr., MD

1. **What is the most common malignant intraocular neoplasm?**
    Uveal metastasis, usually from a distant primary carcinoma, is thought to be the most common malignant intraocular neoplasm. An estimated 66,000 patients develop uveal metastases each year. However, most of these tumors occur in terminal patients, few of whom are evaluated ophthalmologically or pathologically. In contrast, only 1800 cases of uveal malignant melanoma and 300 cases of retinoblastoma occur in the United States yearly.

    Many textbooks state that uveal malignant melanoma is the most common primary intraocular tumor, but this statement actually applies only to the United States and Europe, because uveal melanoma has a propensity for fair-skinned, blue-eyed persons. Throughout Africa, Asia, and South America, where melanoma is relatively rare, retinoblastoma is the most common primary intraocular tumor.

    Nelson CC, Hertzberg BS, Klintworth GK: A histopathologic study of 716 unselected eyes in patients with cancer at the time of death. Am J Ophthalmol 95:788–793, 1983.

2. **What is the characteristic shape of choroidal malignant melanoma?**
    Approximately 60% of choroidal malignant melanomas have a mushroom or collar-button configuration (Fig. 51-1). Melanomas have a discoid or almond shape when they initially arise in the choroid. The mushroom or collar-button configuration develops after the tumor ruptures or erodes through Bruch's membrane and invades the subretinal space, where it forms a round or ovoid nodule.

3. **Is a mushroom configuration pathognomonic for choroidal melanoma?**
    A mushroom or collar-button configuration almost always signifies that a choroidal tumor is a malignant melanoma. Few things in medicine are pathognomonic, however. Exceedingly rare mushroom-shaped choroidal metastases and hemangiomas have been reported.

    Shields JA, Shields CL, Brown GC, Eagle RC Jr: Mushroom-shaped choroidal metastasis simulating a choroidal melanoma. Retina 22:810–813, 2002.
    Spraul CW, Kim D, Fineberg E, Grossniklaus HE: Mushroom-shaped choroidal hemangioma. Am J Ophthalmol 122:434–436, 1996.

4. **What important prognostic features of uveal melanoma can be assessed during routine histopathologic examination?**
    Tumor size and cell type are two of the most important prognostic factors that can be assessed during routine histopathological evaluation of uveal

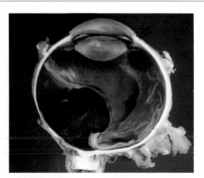

Figure 51-1. Mushroom-shaped choroidal melanoma.

melanoma. Larger tumors and tumors that contain epithelioid cells have a poorer prognosis. Tumor size generally is expressed in millimeters as the largest tumor diameter. Other prognostic features include mitotic activity (expressed as the number of mitoses in 40 high power fields), the presence of extrascleral extension, extracellular matrix patterns called vascular loops and networks, and lymphocytic infiltration.

De la Cruz PO Jr, Specht CS, McLean IW: Lymphocytic infiltration in uveal malignant melanoma. Cancer 65:112–115, 1990.

Folberg R, Mehaffey M, Gardner LM, et al: The microcirculation of choroidal and ciliary body melanomas. Eye 11:227–238, 1997.

McLean IW, Foster WD, Zimmerman LE: Uveal melanoma: Location, size, cell type, and enucleation as risk factors in metastasis. Hum Pathol 13:123–132, 1982.

KEY POINTS: PROGNOSTIC FACTORS IN UVEAL MELANOMA

1. Size

2. Cell type

3. Extraocular extension

4. Mitotic activity

5. Lymphocytic infiltration

6. Vascular patterns

5. **What is the Callender classification?**
   In 1931, Major George Russell Callender reported that there was an association between survival and the histologic characteristics of uveal melanomas called *cell type*. Callender showed that uveal melanomas could contain two types of spindle cells (spindle A and spindle B cells), and less-differentiated epithelioid cells. Dr. Ian McLean modified Callender's classification in 1978. Spindle A and spindle B melanomas were lumped together as spindle melanomas in the modified classification, and necrotic and fascicular variants were deleted.

   Callender G: Malignant melanotic tumors of the eye: A study of histologic types in 111 cases. Trans Am Acad Ophthalmol Otolaryngol 36:131–142, 1931.

   McLean IW, Foster WD, Zimmerman LE, Gamel JW: Modifications of Callender's classification of uveal melanoma at the Armed Forces Institute of Pathology. Am J Ophthalmol 96:502–509, 1983.

6. **What is the most common cell type?**
   Most melanomas that are enucleated and examined histopathologically are mixed-cell tumors that contain a mixture of spindle and epithelioid cells. A total of 89% of the melanomas that were enucleated in the Collaborative Ocular Melanoma Study (COMS) were mixed-cell tumors.

7. **How are melanoma cell types distinguished histopathologically?**
   Melanoma cells are readily differentiated by the characteristics of their nuclei. Spindle A cells have long, tapering cigar-like nuclei, an absent or indistinct nucleolus, and a characteristic longitudinal stripe caused by a fold in the nuclear membrane. Spindle B nuclei are oval and plumper and have less finely dispersed chromatin and a distinct nucleolus (Fig. 51- 2). Epithelioid cell nuclei are typically round and vesicular and have a prominent reddish-purple nucleolus (Fig. 51-3). The chromatin is coarse and often clumps along the inside of the nuclear membrane (peripheral margination of chromatin).

Spindle melanoma cells grow as a syncytium, making it difficult to discern the cytoplasmic margins of the bipolar fusiform cells. Epithelioid cells are poorly cohesive and their cytoplasmic margins are readily discernible.

McLean IW: Uveal nevi and malignant melanomas. In Spencer WH (ed): Ophthalmic Pathology: An Atlas and Textbook, vol. 3. Philadelphia, W.B. Saunders, 1996, pp 2121–2217.

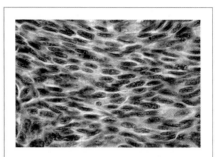

Figure 51-2. Spindle melanoma cells.

8. **Which cell type has the worst prognosis?**
   The presence or absence of epithelioid cells in a uveal melanoma has an important effect on prognosis. If no epithelioid cells are present, the expected survival at 15 years is 72%. If epithelioid cells are present (mixed, epithelioid, or necrotic cell type), the survival at 15 years drops to 37%.
   A tumor composed entirely of spindle A cells is now considered to be a benign nevus incapable of metastasis. Tumors composed entirely of epithelioid cells have the worst prognosis. Overall, approximately 50% of patients with uveal melanoma will die from their tumors.

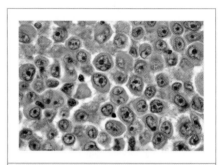

Figure 51-3. Epithelioid melanoma cells.

McLean IW, Foster WD, Zimmerman LE: Uveal melanoma: Location, size, cell type, and enucleation as risk factors in metastasis. Hum Pathol 13:123–132, 1982.

9. **What is the most common site of metastatic uveal melanoma?**
   The liver. Liver metastases occur in 93% of patients who develop metastatic uveal melanoma. Other sites include the lungs (24%) and bone (16%).

   COMS: Assessment of metastatic disease status at death in 435 patients with large choroidal melanoma in the Collaborative Ocular Melanoma Study (COMS). COMS Report No. 15. Arch Ophthalmol 119:670–676, 2001.

10. **Does enucleation of uveal melanoma increase tumor deaths by disseminating tumor cells?**
    Probably not. In 1978, Zimmerman, McLean, and Foster hypothesized that enucleation of uveal melanoma increased tumor deaths by disseminating tumor cells. This became known as the Zimmerman hypothesis. It currently is believed that melanomas have already micrometastasized years before they produce symptoms and are treated. This conclusion is based on studies of tumor doubling times and the observation that increased mortality also occurs after plaque brachyradiotherapy and charged particle therapy.

    Eskelin S, Pyrhonen S, Summanen P, et al: Tumor doubling times in metastatic malignant melanoma of the uvea: Tumor progression before and after treatment. Ophthalmology 107:1443–1449, 2000.
    Singh AD, Rennie IG, Kivela T, et al: The Zimmerman-McLean-Foster hypothesis: 25 years later. Br J Ophthalmol 88:962–967, 2004.
    Zimmerman LE, McLean IW, Foster WD: Does enucleation of the eye containing a malignant melanoma prevent or accelerate the dissemination of tumour cells? Br J Ophthalmol 62:420–425, 1978.

11. **What was the main consequence of the Zimmerman hypothesis?**
The Zimmerman hypothesis stimulated interest in alternate therapies for uveal melanoma, including plaque brachytherapy. It also was a major factor that led to the COMS.

12. **What is the Collaborative Ocular Melanoma Study?**
The COMS is a large prospective, randomized, multicentered study funded by the National Eye Institute that investigated the treatment of choroidal malignant melanoma. The arm of the study that focuses on medium-sized tumor compared survival after enucleation and radioactive iodine 125 (I[125]) plaque therapy. The large tumor study compared survival after standard enucleation and enucleation preceded by external beam radiotherapy.

   COMS: Design and methods of a clinical trial for a rare condition: The Collaborative Ocular Melanoma Study. COMS Report No. 3. Control Clin Trials 14:362–391, 1993.

13. **What did the COMS results reveal?**
The medium-sized tumor arm of the study showed that survival is similar after both enucleation and plaque brachytherapy. The large tumor arm showed that "sterilization" of large melanomas with pre-enucleation external-beam radiotherapy does not improve survival.

   Diener-West M, Earl JD, Fine SL, et al: The COMS randomized trial of iodine 125 brachytherapy for choroidal melanoma. III: Initial mortality findings. COMS Report No. 18. Arch Ophthalmol 119:969–982, 2001.
   Hawkins BS: The Collaborative Ocular Melanoma Study (COMS) randomized trial of pre-enucleation radiation of large choroidal melanoma. IV: Ten-year mortality findings and prognostic factors. COMS Report No. 24. Am J Ophthalmol 138:936–951, 2004.

14. **How are most uveal melanomas treated?**
Today, most posterior uveal melanomas are treated with radioactive plaques. Plaque-treatment failures and eyes with larger tumors and/or tumor-related complications, such as secondary glaucoma or extrascleral extension, are still enucleated. Some smaller tumors are locally resected or treated with transpupillary thermotherapy.

   Shields CL, Shields JA: Recent developments in the management of choroidal melanoma. Curr Opin Ophthalmol 15:244–251, 2004.

15. **How effective is treatment of posterior uveal melanoma?**
Treatment is relatively ineffective from the standpoint of survival. All forms of treatment seem to have little effect on decreasing subsequent death from metastases. Unfortunately, most tumors have already metastasized before they are treated. Treatment for metastatic melanoma is also ineffective.

   Singh AD, Rennie IG, Kivela T, et al: The Zimmerman-McLean-Foster hypothesis: 25 years later. Br J Ophthalmol 88:962–967, 2004.

16. **What clinical features suggest that a small pigmented choroidal tumor is a melanoma?**
The mnemonic **TFSOM** (**T**o **F**ind **S**mall **O**cular **M**elanoma) lists the clinical factors that suggest a small pigmented tumor is a melanoma that is likely to grow, therefore, putting the patient at greater risk for metastasis.
T = **T**hickness greater than 2 mm
F = Subretinal **F**luid
S = **S**ymptoms
O = **O**range pigment
M = **M**argin touching optic disc
   Choroidal melanocytic tumors that display none of these factors have a 3% risk of growth into melanoma at 5 years and most likely represent choroidal nevi. Tumors with two or more factors show growth in more than 50% of cases. Most tumors with two or more risk

factors probably represent small choroidal melanomas, and early treatment is generally indicated.

Shields CL, Demici H, Materin MA, et al: Clinical factors in the identification of small choroidal melanoma. Can J Ophthalmol 39:351–357, 2004.

KEY POINTS: OVERVIEW OF UVEAL MELANOMA

1. Caucasian patients at risk
2. Mushroom shape
3. Spindle and epithelioid cells
4. Liver metastases
5. A 50% mortality rate

17. Do melanomas of the iris behave differently?
The prognosis of iris melanoma generally is excellent (4–10% mortality). Most pigmented tumors of the iris are benign spindle cell nevi. Overall, only 6.5% will enlarge during a 5-year period of observation. Although tumors containing epithelioid cells occasionally are encountered, most iris melanomas are low-grade spindle cell tumors.

Clinical features that suggest a pigmented iris tumor is a melanoma include documented tumor growth, elevated intraocular pressure, hyphema, large tumor size, and tumor vascularity. Although they can occur anywhere, melanomas arise most frequently in the inferior sun-exposed part of the iris.

Harbour JW, Augsburger JJ, Eagle RC Jr: Initial management and follow-up of melanocytic iris tumors. Ophthalmology 102:1987–1993, 1995.
Jakobiec FA, Silbert G: Are most iris "melanomas" really nevi? A clinicopathologic study of 189 lesions. Arch Ophthalmol 99:2117–2132, 1981.

18. What clinical features suggest that a uveal tumor is a metastasis?
Uveal metastases usually are creamy yellow amelanotic tumors that have a placoid or nummular configuration. Pigment mottling may occur on the tumor apex. Metastases are often multiple but can be solitary. Metastases usually cause a nonrhegmatogenous serous detachment of the retina with shifting subretinal fluid.

Shields CL, Shields JA, Gross NE, et al: Survey of 520 eyes with uveal metastases. Ophthalmology 104:1265–1276, 1997.

19. What is the most common site of uveal metastasis?
Uveal metastases involve the choroid 81% of the time. They typically are found in the region of the macula where the choroidal blood supply is richest.

Shields CL, Shields JA, Gross NE, et al: Survey of 520 eyes with uveal metastases. Ophthalmology 104:1265–1276, 1997.

20. What primary tumors are responsible for most uveal metastases?
Breast carcinoma in women and lung carcinoma in men. Breast carcinoma is responsible for more than half of all ocular metastases. Nearly one-fourth are caused by lung cancer. Most women with uveal metastases from breast tumors have a history of breast carcinoma. In contrast, uveal metastasis may herald the presence of an occult lung tumor.

Shields CL, Shields JA, Gross NE, et al: Survey of 520 eyes with uveal metastases. Ophthalmology 104:1265–1276, 1997.

21. **What type of hemangiomas occur in the choroid?**
Choroidal hemangiomas are classified as capillary, cavernous, or mixed. They are composed of thin-walled vessels and have little stroma (Fig. 51-4). Sporadic hemangiomas tend to be discrete, localized, elevated reddish-orange tumors. The choroidal hemangiomas that occur in patients with Sturge-Weber syndrome are typically diffuse, with indistinct tapering margins. These obscure the underlying choroidal architecture and impart a "tomato ketchup" appearance to the fundus.

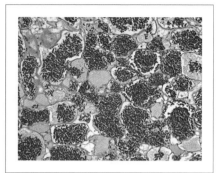

Figure 51-4. Choroidal hemangioma.

Witschel H, Font RL: Hemangioma of the choroid. A clinicopathologic study of 71 cases and a review of the literature. Surv Ophthalmol 20:415–431, 1976.

22. **If choroidal hemangiomas are benign, why are they treated?**
Choroidal hemangiomas are treated to save vision or the eye itself. Although they are benign from a systemic standpoint, choroidal hemangiomas cause retinal detachment and secondary glaucoma via iris neovascularization and/or a papillary block mechanism. The latter can lead to eye loss. Hemangiomas are treated with laser photocoagulation or photodynamic therapy (PDT).

Gunduz K: Transpupillary thermotherapy in the management of circumscribed choroidal hemangioma. Surv Ophthalmol 49:316–327, 2004.

Madreperla SA: Choroidal hemangioma treated with photodynamic therapy using verteporfin. Arch Ophthalmol 119:1606–1610, 2001.

23. **What is the typical clinical presentation of retinoblastoma in the United States?**
Retinoblastoma typically presents with leukocoria (a white pupillary reflex) in the United States and Europe. Smaller tumors that involve the macula initially may present with strabismus. All children with strabismus should have a careful fundus examination to exclude retinoblastoma or other significant macular pathology. In developing countries, children may present in an advanced stage of the disease with a large orbital tumor secondary to extraocular extension.

McLean IW: Retinoblastomas, retinocytomas and pseudoretinoblastomas. In Spencer WH (ed): Ophthalmic Pathology: An Atlas and Textbook, vol. 3. Philadelphia, W.B. Saunders, 1996, pp 1332–1438.

24. **How old are patients when diagnosed with retinoblastoma?**
The mean age at diagnosis is 18 months. Patients who have the familial form of the disease (i.e., who have germline mutations) are diagnosed earlier (mean age of 12 months), probably because only a solitary "hit" or gene inactivation is required. Sporadic somatic cases occur in slightly older patients; they are diagnosed at a mean age of 24 months.

McLean IW: Retinoblastomas, retinocytomas and pseudoretinoblastomas. In Spencer WH (ed): Ophthalmic Pathology: An Atlas and Text book, vol. 3. Philadelphia, W.B. Saunders, 1996, pp 1332–1438.

25. **What does retinoblastoma look like grossly?**
Grossly, retinoblastoma has a distinctly encephaloid or brainlike appearance. This is not surprising because the tumor arises from the retina, which is a peripheral colony of brain cells. Foci of dystrophic calcification occur in many retinoblastomas. These foci of calcification are evident grossly as lighter flecks.

26. **What is an exophytic retinoblastoma?**
Retinoblastoma shows several growth patterns. Exophytic retinoblastoma arises from the outer retina and grows in the subretinal space, causing retinal detachment (Fig. 51-5). Endophytic

retinoblastoma arises from the inner layers of the retina, which remains attached (Fig. 51-6). Endophytic tumors invade the vitreous and may seed the anterior chamber, forming a pseudohypopyon of tumor cells. Most large retinoblastomas exhibit a combined endophytic/exophytic growth pattern. The diffuse infiltrative growth pattern is relatively rare and occurs in older children. The retina is diffusely thickened without a distinct tumefaction.

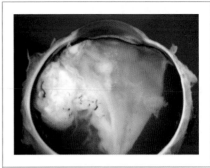

Figure 51-5. Exophytic retinoblastoma with total retinal detachment.

McLean IW: Retinoblastomas, retinocytomas and pseudoretinoblastomas. In Spencer WH (ed): Ophthalmic Pathology: An Atlas and Textbook, vol. 3. Philadelphia, W.B. Saunders, 1996, pp 1332–1438.

27. **Why do retinoblastomas appear blue, pink, and purple under low-magnification light microscopy?**
The blue, pink, and purple areas evident on low-magnification light microscopy of retinoblastoma represent zones of viable, necrotic, and calcified tumor, respectively. Areas of viable tumor are basophilic. Retinoblastoma is composed of poorly differentiated neuroblastic cells that have intensely basophilic nuclei and scanty cytoplasm. Retinoblastoma cells tend to outgrow their blood supply rapidly and undergo spontaneous necrosis. The necrotic

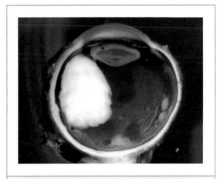

Figure 51-6. Endophytic retinoblastoma.

parts of the tumor are eosinophilic because the dead cells lose their basophilic nuclear DNA. Dystrophic calcification often occurs in necrotic parts of the tumor. The calcium has a purple hue in sections stained with hematoxylin and eosin.

Burnier MN, McLean IW, Zimmerman LE, Rosenberg SH: Retinoblastoma. The relationship of proliferating cells to blood vessels. Invest Ophthalmol Vis Sci 31:2037–2040, 1990.

McLean IW: Retinoblastomas, retinocytomas and pseudoretinoblastomas. In Spencer WH (ed): Ophthalmic Pathology: An Atlas and Textbook, vol. 3. Philadelphia, W.B. Saunders, 1996, pp 1332–1438.

28. **What do rosettes signify in retinoblastoma?**
Rosettes are histologic markers for tumor differentiation in retinoblastoma. Homer Wright rosettes reflect low-grade neuroblastic differentiation. They are nonspecific and occur in other tumors such as neuroblastoma. Flexner-Wintersteiner rosettes represent early retinal differentiation and are highly characteristic for retinoblastoma, but they are not pathognomonic. They are also found in some medulloepitheliomas.

Ts'o MO, Fine BS, Zimmerman LE: The Flexner-Wintersteiner rosettes in retinoblastoma. Arch Pathol 88:664–671, 1969.

29. **How are Homer Wright and Flexner-Wintersteiner rosettes distinguished histopathologically?**
The nuclei of Homer Wright rosettes encircle a central tangle of neural filaments (Fig. 51-7). No lumen is present. Flexner-Wintersteiner rosettes have a central lumen that corresponds to

the subretinal space (Fig. 51-8). The cells that enclose the lumen are joined by a girdle of apical intercellular connections analogous to the retinal external limiting membrane. Cilia, the precursors of photoreceptors, project into the lumen of the rosette.

Shields JA, Eagle RC Jr, Shields CL, Potter PD: Congenital neoplasms of the nonpigmented ciliary epithelium (medulloepithelioma). Ophthalmology 103:1998–2006, 1996.

Ts'o MO, Fine BS, Zimmerman LE: The Flexner-Wintersteiner rosettes in retinoblastoma. Arch Pathol 88:664–671, 1969.

30. **What are fleurettes?**
Fleurettes are aggregates of neoplastic photoreceptors (Fig. 51-9). Photoreceptor differentiation is the highest degree of differentiation found in retinoblastomas. Fleurettes are composed of groups of bulbous eosinophilic cellular processes that correspond to photoreceptor inner segments. They are often aligned along a segment of neoplastic external limiting membrane in a bouquet-like arrangement. A benign retinal tumor composed entirely of fleurettes is called a *retinocytoma* or *retinoma*.

McLean IW: Retinoblastomas, retinocytomas and pseudoretinoblastomas. In Spencer WH (ed): Ophthalmic Pathology: An Atlas and Textbook, vol. 3. Philadelphia, W.B. Saunders, 1996, pp 1332–1438.

Ts'o MO, Fine BS, Zimmerman LE: The nature of retinoblastoma. II. Photoreceptor differentiation: An electron microscopic study. Am J Ophthalmol 69:350–359, 1970.

Ts'o MO, Zimmerman LE, Fine BS: The nature of retinoblastoma. I. Photoreceptor differentiation: A clinical and histopathologic study. Am J Ophthalmol 69:339–349, 1970.

31. **What are the most important prognostic features of retinoblastoma?**
Important prognostic features of retinoblastoma that can be assessed histopathologically include the presence and degree of optic nerve invasion, extrascleral extension, and possibly uveal invasion. Unlike uveal melanoma, the size of the tumor does not appear to be important. Mortality rises as the depth of tumor invasion into the optic nerve increases. Postlaminar optic nerve invasion is equivalent to extraocular extension and is an indication for chemotherapy in many centers.

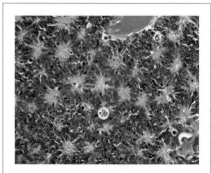
Figure 51-7. Homer Wright rosettes, retinoblastoma.

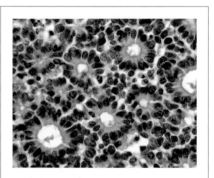
Figure 51-8. Flexner-Wintersteiner rosettes, retinoblastoma.

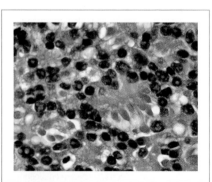
Figure 51-9. Fleurettes, retinoblastoma.

Kopelman JE, McLean IW, Rosenberg SH: Multivariate analysis of risk factors for metastasis in retinoblastoma treated by enucleation. Ophthalmology 94:371–377, 1987.
Singh AD, Shields CL, Shields JA: Prognostic factors in retinoblastoma. J Pediatr Ophthalmol Strabismus 37:134–141; quiz, 168–169, 2000.

32. **How does retinoblastoma become fatal?**
Many children who die from retinoblastoma have some degree of intracranial involvement. This is caused by direct extension of tumor cells along the optic nerve, subarachnoid space, or orbital foramina. Distant hematogenous metastases to bone and viscera can develop after the tumor invades the richly vascularized uvea. Anterior extrascleral extension provides access to conjunctival lymphatics and may be associated with regional lymph node metastases.

McLean IW: Retinoblastomas, retinocytomas and pseudoretinoblastomas. Philadelphia, W.B. Saunders, 1996.

33. **The retinoblastoma gene is located on what chromosome?**
Chromosome 13, found in the segment of the long, or "q," arm, which is designated the 1-4 band (13q1-4).

Murphree AL: Molecular genetics of retinoblastoma. Ophthalmol Clin North Am 8:155–166, 1995.

34. **How is the retinoblastoma gene classified?**
The retinoblastoma (Rb) gene is the paradigmatic example of a recessive oncogene. The Rb gene is called a recessive oncogene because both copies of the gene must be lost or inactivated before a tumor can develop. Normal individuals have two functional copies of the Rb gene, although only one is needed for normal functioning. The gene's protein product, called Rb protein, is found in the nucleus, where it interacts with other transcription factors to control the cell cycle. Absence of Rb protein allows continual cell division and lack of terminal differentiation.

Murphree AL: Molecular genetics of retinoblastoma. Ophthalmol Clin North Am 8:155–166, 1995.

35. **If the RB gene is recessive, why do cases of familial retinoblastoma appear to be inherited in an autosomal-dominant fashion?**
Patients with hereditary retinoblastoma are heterozygous for the Rb gene. The genotype of carriers includes a single functional wild-type gene. The second copy of the Rb gene has been lost, inactivated, or produces a defective gene product. A retinoblastoma will develop when a retinal cell loses its single functional copy of the Rb gene. A mating between a normal individual (RbRb) and a heterozygous carrier (Rbrb) gives rise to 50% normal offspring and 50% heterozygous carriers—a 50/50 ratio that perfectly mimics autosomal dominant transmission.

36. **What does bilateral retinoblastoma signify clinically?**
The presence of bilateral retinoblastoma indicates that the affected patient carries a germline mutation in the Rb gene and is capable of transmitting the tumor to offspring.

37. **Can a child with a unilateral retinoblastoma have hereditary disease?**
Yes. Unfortunately, the presence of a unilateral tumor does not exclude a germline mutation and transmissible disease. Only approximately 60% of patients with familial retinoblastoma actually develop bilateral tumors.

38. **Are most retinoblastomas familial?**
No, most retinoblastomas occur sporadically in infants who have no family history of the disease. Nearly ¾ of sporadic retinoblastomas are caused by somatic mutations in retinal cells, which cannot be passed on to offspring. Such somatic sporadic tumors are invariably unilateral and unifocal. The remaining fourth of sporadic retinoblastomas are caused by germline mutations (i.e., they are new familial cases). The latter can be bilateral and can be passed on to

offspring in what appears to be autosomal dominant transmission. Only 5–10% of retinoblastomas occur in patients with a family history of the tumor.

39. **Why are sporadic retinoblastomas caused by somatic mutations always unilateral and unifocal?**
A sporadic somatic retinoblastoma is caused by the inactivation of both Rb genes in a single retinal cell. The spontaneous mutation rate of the Rb gene is very low. Hence the chance of this occurring in more than a single retinal cell is infinitesimally small. Therefore, sporadic somatic retinoblastomas always are unilateral and unifocal. In contrast, it is highly probable that one or more gene inactivations will occur in both retinas of a heterozygous carrier, because the mutation rate is substantially smaller than the number of mitoses involved in the development of the retina and genes usually are lost during cellular division. That is why familial cases typically are bilateral and may be multifocal.

40. **Are patients with hereditary retinoblastomas at risk for other nonocular tumors?**
Yes. Between 20% and 50% of patients who have germline mutations in the retinoblastoma gene will develop a second malignant neoplasm within 20 years. One of the most interesting and characteristic secondary tumors is a pineoblastoma, a retinoblastoma-like tumor of the pineal gland. The association of pineoblastoma and hereditary retinoblastoma has been termed *trilateral retinoblastoma*. There also is a 500-fold increase in the incidence of osteogenic sarcoma in retinoblastoma gene carriers. Patients also are at risk to develop radiation-induced orbital sarcomas (e.g., osteogenic sarcomas) after external-beam radiotherapy for retinoblastoma, which is why oncologists currently try to avoid this therapy.

KEY POINTS: RETINOBLASTOMA

1. Tumor suppressor gene on chromosome 13 (13q-14)
2. Most cases are sporadic (75% somatic, 25% germline)
3. Bilaterality indicates transmissible germline mutation
4. Heritable cases pass disease to 50% of offspring (autosomal dominant pattern)
5. Heritable cases at risk for second tumors

41. **Name the three diseases that are most often confused with retinoblastoma clinically.**
   - Persistent hyperplastic primary vitreous (also called persistent fetal vasculature)
   - Coats disease
   - Ocular toxocariasis

   Shields JA, Parsons HM, Shields CL, Shah P: Lesions simulating retinoblastoma. J Pediatr Ophthalmol Strabismus 28:338–340, 1991.
   Shields JA, Shields CL: Intraocular Tumors: A Text and Atlas. Philadelphia, W.B. Saunders, 1992.
   Shields JA, Shields CL: Atlas of Intraocular Tumors. Philadelphia, Lippincott, Williams & Wilkins, 1999.
   Shields JA, Shields CL, Parsons HM: Differential diagnosis of retinoblastoma. Retina 11:232–243, 1991.

42. **How does Coats disease differ from retinoblastoma?**
Coats disease is characterized by an exudative retinal detachment caused by leaky congenital vascular anomalies in the retina (Fig. 51-10). The subretinal fluid is rich in lipid-laden

macrophages and cholesterol crystals, which appear as empty clefts in microscopic sections. Histopathologically, the retina contains abnormal telangiectactic vessels, and its outer layers are massively thickened by hard exudates. A bullous retinal detachment may abut the lens, displacing it anteriorly and causing pupillary block glaucoma. Coats disease usually occurs unilaterally in boys between ages 4 and 10. It usually is confused clinically with exophytic retinoblastoma.

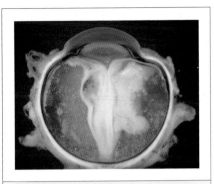

Figure 51-10. Coats disease.

Shields JA, Shields CL, Honavar SG, Demirci H: Clinical variations and complications of Coats' disease in 150 cases: The 2000 Sanford Gifford Memorial Lecture. Am J Ophthalmol 131:561–571, 2001.

Shields JA, Shields CL, Honavar SG, et al: Classification and management of Coats' disease: The 2000 Proctor Lecture. Am J Ophthalmol 131:572–583, 2001.

43. **What are the characteristic features of persistent hyperplastic primary vitreous (persistent fetal vasculature)?**
Persistent hyperplastic primary vitreous (PHPV) is a congenital disorder that is present at birth. It is almost always unilateral, and classically is found in a microphthalmic eye. Leukocoria is caused by a plaque of fibrovascular tissue that adheres to the posterior surface of the lens. The ciliary processes typically are disclosed by dilating the pupil because their tips are attached to the edge of the retrolental plaque and drawn centrally. Persistent fetal vasculature may be a more appropriate term for this disorder. Congenital retroblastomas have been reported but are exceedingly rare. On average, retinoblastomas are diagnosed at age 18 months.

Goldberg MF: Persistent fetal vasculature (PFV): An integrated interpretation of signs and symptoms associated with persistent hyperplastic primary vitreous (PHPV). LIV Edward Jackson Memorial Lecture. Am J Ophthalmol 124:587–626, 1997.

Shields JA, Shields CL: Intraocular Tumors: A Text and Atlas. Philadelphia, W.B. Saunders, 1992.

Shields JA, Shields CL: Atlas of Intraocular Tumors. Philadelphia, Lippincott, Williams & Wilkins, 1999.

44. **What is the second most common primary intraocular tumor of childhood?**
Embryonal medulloepithelioma is the second most common primary intraocular tumor of childhood. Medulloepitheliomas probably are derived from anlagen of the embryonic medullary epithelium, which lines the forebrain and optic vesicle. Most of these rare tumors become symptomatic around age 4 years and are diagnosed at 5 years of age.

Broughton WL, Zimmerman LE: A clinicopathologic study of 56 cases of intraocular medulloepithelioma. Am J Ophthalmol 85:407–418, 1978.

Folberg R, Mehaffey M, Gardner LM, et al: The microcirculation of choroidal and ciliary body melanomas. Eye 11:227–238, 1997.

Shields JA, Eagle RC Jr, Shields CL, Potter PD: Congenital neoplasms of the nonpigmented ciliary epithelium (medulloepithelioma). Ophthalmology 103:1998–2006, 1996.

45. **Where are most medulloepitheliomas located?**
Most medulloepitheliomas are ciliary body tumors that arise from the neuroepithelial layers on their inner surface. Rare medulloepitheliomas of the optic nerve do occur, however.

Green WR, Iliff WJ, Trotter RR: Malignant teratoid medulloepithelioma of the optic nerve. Arch Ophthalmol 91:451–454, 1974.

O'Keefe M, Fulcher T, Kelly P, et al: Medulloepithelioma of the optic nerve head. Arch Ophthalmol 115:1325–1327, 1997.

46. **What is a teratoid medulloepithelioma?**

In addition to bands, cords, and rosettes of neoplastic neuroepithelium and pools of hyaluronic acid, teratoid medulloepitheliomas contain foci of heteroplastic tissue including hyaline cartilage, rhabdomyoblasts, striated muscle, and/or brain. More than a third of medulloepitheliomas are teratoid. Nonteratoid medulloepitheliomas lack heteroplastic elements. Both benign and malignant variants of teratoid and nonteratoid tumors occur.

CHAPTER 52

ORBITAL TUMORS

Jurij R. Bilyk, MD

1. **Should all orbital capillary hemangiomas be excised?**
   No. Orbital capillary hemangioma (hemangioma of infancy) should be treated only if there is evidence of:
   - Amblyopia caused by refractive error (induced myopia or astigmatism) or
   - Ptosis causing visual obstruction or head tilt.
   Treatment options include:
   - Corticosteroid injections or systemic therapy.
   - Excision, usually reserved for cases unresponsive to more conservative therapy.
   - Interferon alpha-2 therapy, especially in large localized or systemic cases. There is a risk of spastic diplegia with this therapy.

   Bilyk JR, Adamis AP, Mulliken JB: Treatment options for periorbital hemangioma of infancy. Int Ophthalmol Clin 32:95–109, 1992.
   Ezekowitz RAB, Mulliken JB, Folkman J: Interferon alfa-2a therapy for life-threatening hemangiomas of infancy. N Engl J Med 326:1456–1463, 1992.
   Loughnan MS, Elder J, Kemp A: Treatment of massive orbital-capillary hemangioma with interferon alfa-2b: Short-term results. Arch Ophthalmol 110:1366–1367, 1992.

2. **What orbital tumors can mimic orbital cellulitis?**
   In **both adults and children,** consider noninfectious inflammation (idiopathic orbital pseudotumor, sarcoidosis, Graves' orbitopathy, Wegener's granulomatosis).
   In **children,** consider:
   - Ruptured dermoid cyst, which causes a fulminant soft tissue inflammation
   - Rhabdomyosarcoma
   - Lymphangioma, especially with rapid expansion from a blood-filled "chocolate cyst"
   - Neuroblastoma, which can present with a rapid onset of proptosis and ecchymosis
   In **adults,** consider:
   - Ruptured dermoid cyst
   - Lymphangioma
   - Extrascleral spread and necrosis of an intraocular melanoma
   - Metastatic disease to the orbit

3. **What are the most common causes of childhood proptosis?**
   - Orbital cellulitis
   - Capillary hemangioma
   - Inflammatory orbital pseudotumor
   - Dermoid cyst
   - Rhabdomyosarcoma
   - Lymphangioma

4. **When and how does cavernous hemangioma usually present?**
   - Cavernous hemangioma is the most common vascular orbital tumor in adults and the most common benign orbital tumor.
   - It typically presents in the fourth and fifth decades of life.
   - It is well circumscribed on imaging (see question 16).

- It is *not* the adult equivalent of capillary hemangioma. Not only are the lesions distinct histopathologically, but also cavernous hemangioma is a slowly proliferating entity.
- Because of its slow growth, it is usually a well-tolerated lesion that causes few symptoms. Visual loss, if any, is slow and limited to lesions of the orbital apex.
- The excision is curative.

Harris GJ, Jakobiec FA: Cavernous hemangioma of the orbit: An analysis of 66 cases. J Neurosurg 51:219–228, 1979.

McNab AA, Wright JE: Cavernous hemangioma of the orbit. Austr N Z J Ophthalmol 17:337–345, 1989.

Mulliken JB, Glowacki J: Hemangiomas and vascular malformations in infants and children: A classification based on endothelial characteristics. Plast Reconstr Surg 69:412–420, 1982.

5. **List some basic facts about fibrous histiocytoma and hemangiopericytoma.**
Because both are spindle cell tumors, histopathologic diagnosis may be difficult.
Fibrous histiocytoma
- Fibrous histiocytoma is the most common mesenchymal tumor that afflicts adults.
- The excision is curative.
- Malignant transformation is rare.
Hemangiopericytoma
- Hemangiopericytoma has reclassified as solitary fibrous tumor with cellularity.
- Histopathologic appearance has little correlation with clinical behavior. In other words, a histologically benign lesion may behave aggressively and recur after excision, whereas a tumor with aggressive features on microscopic examination may never recur.
- Patients need to be followed clinically, even after excision, for possible recurrence or aggressive behavior.

Croxatto JO, Font RL: Hemangiopericytoma of the orbit: A clinicopathologic study of 30 cases. Hum Pathol 13:210–218, 1982.

Font RL, Hidayat AA: Fibrous histiocytoma of the orbit: A clinicopathologic study of 150 cases. Hum Pathol 13:199–209, 1982.

Jacomb-Hood J, Moseley IF: Orbital fibrous histiocytoma: Computed tomography in 10 cases and a review of radiological findings. Clin Radiol 43:117–120, 1991.

Jakobiec FA, Howard G, Jones IS, Tannenbaum M: Fibrous histiocytoma of the orbit. Am J Ophthalmol 77:333–345, 1974.

Jakobiec FA, Howard G, Jones IS, Wolff M: Hemangiopericytoma of the orbit. Am J Ophthalmol 78:816–834, 1974.

6. **What about orbital schwannoma?**
- Orbital schwannoma is a tumor of the Schwann cells that form the lining of peripheral nerves.
- Schwannomas do *not* arise from the optic nerve sheath.
- Within the orbit, most schwannomas arise from sensory nerve sheaths, which may explain their predilection for the superior orbit.
- Antoni A and B patterns are the classic histologic findings in schwannoma. The A pattern is characterized by abundant, tightly packed spindle cells, whereas the B pattern exhibits fewer cells within a myxoid matrix.

Rootman J, Goldberg C, Robertson W: Primary orbital schwannomas. Br J Ophthalmol 66:194–204, 1982.

Schmitt E, Spoerri O: Schwannomas of the orbit. Acta Neurochir 53:79–85, 1980.

7. **How does one order orbital computed tomography?**
- Order axial and coronal cuts in all cases.
- If direct coronals cannot be obtained, coronal reconstructions usually suffice.
- Print and review both soft tissue and bone windows.
- Never order cuts greater than 3 mm.
- Intravenous contrast is helpful in cases of infection or inflammation. It is not necessary for trauma or Graves' orbitopathy.

Wirtschafter JD, Berman EL, McDonald CS: Magnetic Resonance Imaging and Computed Tomography. San Francisco, American Academy of Ophthalmology, 1992.

8. **How does one order orbital magnetic resonance imaging (MRI)?**
   Very carefully, referring to the following rules:
   - *Never* order MRI as the first imaging modality in trauma, unresponsive patients, or in poor historians. Occult metal within the magnetic field can move and cause severe soft tissue damage.
   - Always order axial, coronal, and parasagittal views.
   - Always include the cavernous sinus and paranasal sinuses.
   - Always order gadolinium and fat suppression (Fig. 52-1).
   - In T1, orbital fat is bright and vitreous is dark.
   - In T2, vitreous is brighter than fat.
   - The majority of orbital masses are dark in T1 *before* gadolinium administration. Exceptions to this rule: Lesions containing melanin (e.g., melanoma); lesions containing fat (e.g., lipoma, liposarcoma); lesions containing mucus (mucocele, dermoid cyst); and subacute blood (2–7 days old).

   Newton TH, Bilaniuk LT: Radiology of the Eye and Orbit. New York, Raven Press, 1990.

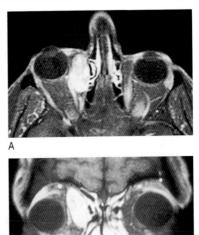

Figure 52-1. *A and B,* T1-weighted magnetic resonance images of the orbit with fat suppression.

9. **Discuss the histologic classification of orbital rhabdomyosarcoma.**
   Orbital rhabdomyosarcoma (RMS) is histologically divided into the following three groups:
   - Embryonal
   - Alveolar
   - Anaplastic (formerly pleomorphic)

   The average age of onset is 9 years, but the span is broad. RMS is thought to arise from pluripotential mesenchymal tissue within the orbit and *not* from extraocular muscle. There are many useful facts to remember about each group.

   Embryonal
   - This group is further subdivided into classic, botryoid, and spindle cell.
   - The most common histology is found in children.
   - The botryoid subtype is defined as an embryonal RMS abutting a mucosal surface (e.g., conjunctiva).

   Alveolar
   - Alveolar RMS appears to affect the inferior orbit most frequently and carries the worst prognosis.
   - Fortunately, findings by the Intergroup Rhabdomyosarcoma Study (IRS) indicate that with more aggressive therapy, the prognosis for alveolar RMS approaches the prognosis for the embryonal form.

   Anaplastic
   - This group of RMS occurs in older adults.

10. **How is orbital RMS best treated? What is the prognosis?**
    Much of what is known about the treatment of orbital rhabdomyosarcoma comes from the four Intergroup Rhabdomyosarcoma Studies.
    - Treatment of orbital RMS consists of a combination of chemotherapy and radiation therapy.
    - Radiation therapy in doses of 4000–6000 cGy definitely carries significant morbidity for the globe, but the third IRS concluded that it is still necessary for adequate treatment. Lower doses of radiation are currently under study.
    - Orbital and genitourinary RMS carry the best prognosis for unclear reasons.
    - Local spread from the orbit into the paranasal sinuses or cranial vault decreases survival rates.

    Crist W, Gehan EA, Ragab AH, et al: The Third Intergroup Rhabdomyosarcoma Study. J Clin Oncol 13:610–630, 1995.

    Regine WF, Fontanese J, Kumar P, et al: Local tumor control in rhabdomyosarcoma following low-dose irradiation: Comparison of group II and select group III patients. Int J Rad Oncol Biol Phys 31:485–491, 1995.

KEY POINTS: IMAGING IN ORBITAL PROCESSES

1. Unilateral or bilateral proptosis usually requires imaging, especially if it is progressive.

2. Computed tomography (CT) of the orbit is generally easier to obtain and interpret than magnetic resonance imaging (MRI).

3. CT is the recommended imaging modality for trauma, infection, and Graves' orbitopathy.

4. MRI is recommended for soft tissue processes, for imaging of the orbital apex/cavernous sinus, and for suspected intracranial processes.

5. Well-tolerated, well-circumscribed lesions of the orbit can be followed conservatively with serial imaging alone in selected cases.

11. **With regard to lacrimal gland lesions, what is "the rule of 50's?"**
    The "rule of 50's" summarizes the incidence of lacrimal gland tumors in an orbital referral practice.
    - A total of 50% of lacrimal gland lesions are nonepithelioid, consisting mostly of inflammatory and lymphoproliferative lesions, and 50% are of epithelial origin.
    - A total of 50% of the epithelial tumors are benign pleomorphic adenomas (benign mixed tumor), and 50% are various malignant types.
    - A total of 50% of the malignant tumors are adenoid cystic carcinomas.
    - A total of 50% of the adenoid cystic carcinomas are of the basaloid variant.

    The final rule is important clinically, because a basaloid histopathology for adenoid cystic carcinoma carries the worst prognosis.

    In a general ophthalmology practice the rule of 50's does not apply. The incidence of infectious and noninfectious inflammatory dacryoadenitis is several times higher than in an orbital referral practice.

    Font RL, Gamel JW: Epithelial tumors of the lacrimal gland: An analysis of 265 cases. In Jakobiec FA (ed): Ocular and Adnexal Tumors. Birmingham, AL, Aesculapius Publishing, 1978, pp 787–805.

    Font RL, Gamel JW: Adenoid cystic carcinoma of the lacrimal gland: A clinicopathologic study of 79 cases. In Nicholson DH (ed): Ocular Pathology Update. New York, Masson Publishing, 1980, pp 277–283.

12. **What factors help to distinguish benign and malignant epithelial lacrimal gland tumors?**
    See Table 52-1.

TABLE 52-1. CLINICAL CHARACTERISTICS OF LACRIMAL GLAND LESIONS

	Pleomorphic Adenoma	Adenoid Cystic Carcinoma
Duration	>1 year	<1 year
Pain	Rare	Common
Diplopia	Uncommon	Common
Computed tomographic findings	No bony destruction ± Fossa formation	Bony destruction common
Surgery	**Ex**cisional biopsy	**In**cisional biopsy
When in doubt, perform total excision of the mass.		
Postsurgical therapy	Clinical follow-up only	Controversial: Radiation, chemotherapy, radical excision

Data from Henderson JW: Adenoid cystic carcinoma of the lacrimal gland, is there a cure? Trans Am Ophthal Soc 85:312–319, 1987; Rose GE, Wright JE: Pleomorphic adenoma of the lacrimal gland. Br J Ophthalmol 76:395–400, 1992; and Wright JE: Factors affecting the survival of patients with lacrimal gland tumours. Can J Ophthalmol 17:3–9, 1982.

13. **What is the most common metastatic tumor to the orbital soft tissue in men and women?**
    - **Men:** Lung
    - **Women:** Breast carcinoma (but the incidence of lung carcinoma is increasing)
    Note that the question asks specifically about orbital soft tissue. Otherwise, prostate carcinoma would be an acceptable alternative in men, depending on the clinical series. Metastatic prostate carcinoma has a propensity for orbital bone.
    Note: Metastatic lesions are approximately 10 times more common to the uvea than the orbit on autopsy studies. This may be caused by the high blood flow through the choroid, which may allow more facile metastatic seeding of uveal tissue.

    Font RL, Ferry AP: Carcinoma metastatic to the eye and orbit III. A clinicopathologic study of 28 cases metastatic to the orbit. Cancer 38:1326–1335, 1976.
    Goldberg RA, Rootman J: Clinical characteristics of metastatic orbital tumors. Ophthalmology 97:620–624, 1990.
    Shields CL, Shields JA, Peggs M: Tumors metastatic to the orbit. Ophthal Plast Reconstr Surg 4:73–80, 1988.

14. **What is the appropriate work-up for orbital lymphoma and lymphoid hyperplasia?**
    Regardless of the histopathology, any lymphoproliferative lesion of the orbit or ocular adnexa requires a systemic work-up, as follows:
    - Complete blood count is performed.
    - Serum protein electrophoresis is performed.
    - Imaging of the neck, thorax, and abdomen, which should be repeated every 6 months for at least 2 years, is performed.
    - Some specialists also perform bone marrow biopsy on initial presentation.

    Medeiros LJ, Andrade RE, Harris NL, Cossman J: Lymphoid infiltrates of the orbit and conjunctiva: Comparison of immunologic and gene rearrangement data [abstract]. Lab Invest 60:61A, 1989.
    Medeiros LJ, Harmon DC, Linggood RM, Harris NL: Immunohistologic features predict clinical behavior of orbital and conjunctival lymphoid infiltrates. Blood 74:2121–2129, 1989.
    Medeiros JL, Harris NL: Lymphoid infiltrates of the orbit and conjunctiva: A morphologic and immuno-phenotypic study of 99 cases. Am J Surg Pathol 13:459–471, 1989.

15. **What are the important facts about orbital lymphoproliferative lesions?**
   - Inflammatory orbital pseudotumor is *not* a lymphoproliferative disorder because, histopathologically, the reaction is not limited to lymphocytes. It is *not* a precursor for orbital lymphoma.
   - Most orbital lymphomas are of B-cell origin, usually of the so-called MALT type (mucosa-associated lymphoid tissue).
   - The vast majority of lymphoid lesions, whether polyclonal (lymphoid hyperplasia) or monoclonal (lymphoma), are highly radiosensitive.
   - Based on their review, Knowles and Jakobiec concluded that tumor location, not histopathology, is the most important factor in determining systemic involvement (Table 52-2).

   Harris NL: Extranodal lymphoid infiltrates and mucosa-associated lymphoid tissue (MALT). A unifying concept [editorial]. Am J Surg Pathol 15:879–884, 1991.

   Knowles DM, Jakobiec FA: Orbital lymphoid neoplasms: Clinical, pathologic and immunohistochemical characteristics. In Jakobiec FA (ed): Ocular and Adnexal Immunohistochemical Characteristics. Birmingham, AL, Aesculapius Publishing, 1978, pp 806–838.

   Knowles DM, Jakobiec FA: Orbital lymphoid neoplasms: A clinicopathologic study of 60 cases. Cancer 46:576–589, 1980.

   Knowles DM, Jakobiec FA: Ocular adnexal lymphoid neoplasms: Clinical, histopathologic, electron microscopic, and immunologic characteristics. Hum Pathol 13:148–162, 1982.

TABLE 52-2. RISK OF CONCURRENT OR FUTURE SYSTEMIC LYMPHOMA BASED ON THE LOCATION OF THE PERIOCULAR LESION	
Location	Risk
Conjunctiva	20%
Orbit (including lacrimal gland)	35%
Eyelid	67%

16. **What is the differential diagnosis of a well-circumscribed orbital mass?**
   - Cavernous hemangioma
   - Schwannoma
   - Fibrous histiocytoma
   - Neurofibroma
   - Solitary fibrous tumor with fibrosis
   - Solitary fibrous tumor with cellularity (hemangiopericytoma)
   - Dermoid cyst
   - ± Lymphoma

INDEX

Page numbers in **boldface type** indicate complete chapters.

A

Abducens nerve palsy, 269–270, 272
Abduction defects, 238, 269
Abetalipoproteinemia, 248
Abney effect, 36
Abscess
    orbital subperiosteal, 295
    subconjunctival, 253
Acanthamoeba infections, corneal, 91, 92, 95
AC:A ratio. *See* Accommodative convergence:
        accommodation ratio
Accommodation
    amplitude of, 20, 21, 29
        measurement of, 32
    range of, 20
Accommodative convergence: accommodation ratio
        (AC:A), 240–241
Accommodative insufficiency, 244
Acetazolamide, as glaucoma treatment, 182
Acetylcysteine, 119
Achromatopsia, 257, 259
    electroretinographic evaluation of, 45, 46
Acid burns, 84
Acne rosacea, 80
Acquired immunodeficiency syndrome (AIDS), ocular
        manifestations of, 335–340
Acuity meters, false-positive readings with, 30
Acute retinal necrosis (ARN) syndrome, 330
Acyclovir, 79, 98, 99, 105
Adaptometer, Goldmann-Weekers, 48
Adenoid cystic carcinoma, 432
Adenopathy, preauricular, 107
Adherence syndrome, 254
Adolescents
    convergence insufficiency in, 244
    idiopathic infantile nystagmus in, 259
    myopia in, 137
Adrenergic agonists
    action mechanism of, 181
    as glaucoma treatment, 181, 182, 184–185
    side effects of, 189
African Americans, glaucoma in, 149, 152–153
Afterimages, 37, 38, 39
Albinism, 257, 258, 259
Alcohol, anticoagulant effects of, 202

Alexia, 284
Alkaline burns, 83–84
Allergic reactions
    to ophthalmic drugs, 77–78, 187
    to penicillin, 110
    as ptosis cause, 314
Alpha agonists, as hyphema treatment, 202
Altitudinal defects, 280–281
Amaurosis
    fugax, 281, 385
    Leber's congenital, 257
        achromatopsia-related, 45
        electroretinographic evaluation of, 45
        keratoconus associated with, 130
Amblyopia, **231–236**
    anisometropic, 233, 235–236, 245
    classification of, 231
    congenital esotropia-related, 238, 239
    congenital fibrosis syndrome-related, 248
    "critical" or "sensitive" period for, 231, 233, 234–235
    definition of, 231, 233
    orbital capillary hemangioma-related, 429
    smoking or alcohol use-related, 279
    treatment of, 233–236
Aminocaproic acid
    adverse effects of, 202
    contraindications to, 203
    as hyphema treatment, 202–203, 205
Aminoglycosides, 108–109, 112
    synergistic interactions of, 110
Amoxicillin, 110
Ampicillin, 110
Amsler grids, 59, 362
Anesthesia
    for cataract surgery, 219
    retrobulbar injection of, 9
    for trabeculectomy, 191
Aneurysm
    Leber's miliary, 348
    of optic chiasm, 65–66
    telangiectatic-like, 348, 349
    third-nerve palsy-associated, 266, 267
Angiography
    carotid, 56
    computed tomography, 266

Angiography *(Continued)*
  fluorescein
    for age-related macular degeneration
        evaluation, 364
    for choroid visualization, 14
    for Coats disease evaluation, 348
    for diabetic retinopathy evaluation, 378, 379, 381
    for differentiation of melanoma from
        hemorrhage, 413
  magnetic resonance, 56, 266
Angiomatosis retinae. *See* von Hippel-Lindau syndrome
Angle recession, 199, 201
  gonioscopic appearance of, 208–209
  gonioscopic diagnosis of, 208
Aniridia, 179
Aniseikonia, 266
Anisocoria, 262, 272
Anisometropia
  alleviation of, 23
  as amblyopia cause, 233
  cataracts-related, 218
  Prentice's rule of, 22, 23
  treatment of, 236
Ankylosing spondylitis, 322, 323
Annulus of Zinn, 9, 10, 16
Anterior chamber
  anatomy of, 157
  in angle-closure glaucoma, 161, 168
  angle of
    closure classification of, 160–161
    gonioscopic classification of, 159
    gonioscopic visualization of, 11, 157–160
    landmarks of, 157
    recession of, 169–170
  blood in. *See* Hyphema
  effect of pilocarpine on, 186
  flat
    cataract surgery-related, 226
    differential diagnosis of, 197
    management of, 197
    trabeculectomy-related, 193
  in herpetic keratitis, 78–79
  reformation of, 171
Anterior chamber tap, 93
Anterior inferior cerebellar artery syndrome, 270
Anterior membrane dystrophy, 120, 121–122
Anterior segment
  blunt trauma to, 199
  ischemia of, 254–255
  in plateau iris, 170
Antibiotics. *See also names of specific antibiotics*
  topical, 106–110, 112
Anticholinergic drugs, contraindication in narrow-angle
        glaucoma, 168–169
Anticoagulation
  as disc hemorrhage cause, 155
  discontinuation of, prior to trabeculectomy, 191
Antifibrinolytic agents, as hyphema treatment, 202

Antiglaucoma medications. *See* Glaucoma, medical
        treatment of; *names of specific antiglaucoma
        medications*
Antihistamines, 77
Antimetabolites
  as orbital inflammation treatment, 307
  use in trabeculectomy patients, 194–195, 196
Antinuclear antibodies, 394
Antiphospholipid antibodies, 394
Antireflective coatings, on spectacle lens, 29
Antiviral therapy
  for cytomegalovirus retinitis, 336–338
  resistance to, 337
Apert's syndrome, 243
Aphakia, 215, 222
Apoplexy, pituitary, 65–66, 249
Apraclonidine
  allergic reactions to, 187
  as glaucoma treatment, 181, 182, 187
Apraxia, congenital ocular motor, 249
Aqueous misdirection syndrome. *See* Glaucoma,
        malignant/ciliary block
Aqueous suppressants, 171
Arden ratio, 46
Arnold-Chiari malformations, 13
Arteritis, giant cell, 281, 386, 387
Arthritis. *See also* Rheumatoid arthritis
  Lyme disease-related, 330
  neonatal conjunctivitis-related, 104
  psoriatic, 322, 323
Asian Americans, glaucoma in, 89, 161
Aspergillosis, as retinitis cause, 330
Aspiration, of subretinal exudates, 350
Aspirin, anticoagulant effects of, 202
Asthenopia, 31–32, 244
  convergence insufficiency-related, 271
Asthma, keratoconus associated with, 130
Astigmatism
  acquired, 31
  contact lens-related, 129
  definition of, 137
  as diplopia cause, 266
  of oblique incidence, 24–26
  post-corneal transplant, 146
  surgical treatment of, 146
  with-the-rule *versus* against-the-rule, 24
Astrocytoma, juvenile pilocytic, 295
Atopy, 130
Atropine, 29, 193
Avellino dystrophy, 124
Axenfeld's anomaly, 179

B
Bacillus cereus infections, 358
Bacitracin, 78, 104, 107, 112
Bartonella henselae infections, 331
Basal cell carcinoma, of the eyelid, 316–318
  metastatic, 317

Basal cell carcinoma, of the eyelid *(Continued)*
  "rodent cell," 316
Basal cell nevus syndrome, 318
Bassen-Kornzweig syndrome, 248
Batten-Mayou (Vogt-Spielmeyer) disease, 386
Behçet's disease, 326, 329, 330, 331
Bell's palsy, 79, 116, 117, 118
Benedikt's syndrome, 270
Bergmeister's papilla, 13
Best's disease, 47
Beta blockers
  action mechanism of, 181
  as glaucoma treatment, 181, 182, 183–184
    in children, 188
  as hyphema treatment, 202, 203
  side effects of, 189
Betaxolol
  as glaucoma treatment, 182, 187
  secretion in breast milk, 187
Bezold-Brucke phenomenon, 36
Bietti's peripheral crystalline dystrophy, 123
Bifocals, 259
  with low-vision aids, 27
  prismatic effect of, 23
Bimatoprost, as glaucoma treatment, 182
Biomicroscopy, ultrasound, 53
Biopsy
  conjunctival, 329
  corneal, 95
  fine-needle aspiration
    retinoblastoma as contraindication to, 407
    of uveal melanoma, 413
  lacrimal, 329
  orbital, 306
  of sebaceous gland carcinoma, 319
  of the temporal artery, 17, 281
Bleb needling, 197
Blebs, 191, 192, 195, 196
Bleeding disorders, 201
Blepharitis, 80, 116
  as red eye cause, 77
  as superficial punctate keratopathy, 79
  treatment of, 107
Blepharochalasis, as ptosis cause, 314
Blepharophimosis syndrome, 311
Blepharoplasty
  as dry eye exacerbation cause, 117
  in thyroid-related ophthalmopathy patients, 303
Blepharoptosis, topical steroids-related, 111
Blepharotomy, transverse, 17
Blindness. *See also* Vision loss
  cataracts-related, 213
  major cause of, 323
  onchocerciasis-related, 323
  retinopathy of prematurity-related, 370
Blind spot, physiologic, 59
Blink reflex, 116
Bloch-Sulzberger syndrome, 374

Blood-retinal barrier, 12
Blunt trauma, ocular, 199
Blurred vision
  age-related macular degeneration-related, 362
  chelating agents-related, 346
  convergence insufficiency-related, 244
  keratoconus-related, 130
  xanthopsia-related, 346
Botulinum toxin (Botox)
  as abducens nerve palsy treatment, 269
  as ptosis cause, 314
Bowman's layer, 11
  corneal dystrophies of, 120, 121, 122
"Boxcarring," 386
Brain stem tumors, 250
Breast cancer, metastatic, 421, 433
Brightness, of colors, 35
Brimonidine
  allergic reactions to, 187
  contraindication in infants and children, 188
  as glaucoma treatment, 166, 181, 183, 185, 187–188
  secretion in breast milk, 187–188
Brinzolamide, as glaucoma treatment, 182
Brow lift, 303
Brown's syndrome, 245, 246, 253
Bruch's membrane, 11–12
  tears of, 354–355
Bruckner test, 232
Bull's-eye deposits, 175
Burns
  phacoemulsification-related, 225
  ultraviolet, 79
Busacca nodules, 321, 322

C
Calcification, imaging of, 53, 54, 55
Canaliculo-dacryocystorhinostomy, 290
Canaliculus, obstruction of, 289, 290
Cancer. *See also specific types of cancer*
  imaging of, 56
Canthaxanthin, as retinopathy cause, 344
"Capsular bag,", 216–217
Capsular tension rings, 230
Capsulorrhexis, 216
Capsulotomy, 217, 221, 229–230
Carbachol, as glaucoma treatment, 182
Carbonic anhydrase inhibitors
  action mechanisms of, 181
  discontinuation of, prior to trabeculectomy, 191
  as glaucoma treatment, 166, 181, 182, 183, 185, 187
    in children, 188
  as hyphema treatment, 202, 203
  secretion in breast milk, 187
  side effects of, 189
Carteolol hydrochloride, as glaucoma
    treatment, 182
Cataracts, **213–217**
  Coats disease-related, 348

Cataracts *(Continued)*
  congenital, 214
    nystagmus associated with, 257
  as diplopia cause, 266
  effect on electroretinographic findings, 45
  Fuchs' heterochromic iridocyclitis-related, 177–178
  glassblowers', 214
  morgagnian, 176–177, 214
  nonsurgical management of, 218
  nuclear sclerotic, 213
  posterior subscapular, 213, 214, 218
  radiation therapy-related, 318, 408
  "ripeness" of, 215
  sympathetic ophthalmia-related, 359
  topical steroids-related, 111
  traumatic, 199, 201, 215
  ultrasound evaluation of, 50
Cataract surgery
  complications of, 177, 178, **225–230**
  extracapsular, 217, 220–221
  in Fuchs' dystrophy patients, 127
  indications for, 215, 218
  intracapsular, 217, 220
  for pseudoexfoliation glaucoma, 175
  as retinal detachment risk factor, 397
  techniques of, **218–224**
Cat-scratch disease, as uveitis cause, 324
Cavernous sinus
  injury to, 249
  thrombosis of, 249
Cavernous sinus syndrome, 270
Cefazolin, 110
Ceftriaxone, 78, 104
Cellulitis
  orbital, 295, 307–308, 429
  strabismus surgery-related, 253
Central cloudy dystrophy of François, 124
Central retinal artery, occlusion of
  electroretinographic evaluation of, 45–46
  as giant cell arteritis cause, 281
Central retinal vein, occlusion of, electroretinographic
    evaluation of, 45–46
Cephalosporins, 108, 109
Cephalosporium acremonium, 109
Cephazolin, 109
Cerebellopontine angle tumors, 270
Chalazion, 31, 266, 318–319
Chalcosis, 179, 358
Chandler's syndrome, 161, 179
Chelating agents, as maculopathy cause, 346
Chemical injuries, as open-angle glaucoma cause, 179
Chemosis, 77, 78, 108, 293
Cherry-red spots, 386
Chest trauma, as fundus abnormalities cause, 359
Chiasm. *See* Optic chiasm
Child abuse, ocular manifestations of, 360
Children. *See also* Infants; Neonates
  amblyopia in, 231–233, 235–236

Children *(Continued)*
  amblyopia screening in, 232
  astigmatism in, spectacle prescription for, 29
  Coats disease in, 348
  developmentally-delayed, rectus muscle recession in, 9
  glaucoma medication use in, 188
  leukemia in, 332
  nonspecific orbital inflammation in, 306
  optic nerve glioma in, 295
  orbital cellulitis in, 295, 308
  orbital tumors in, 429
  Parinaud's syndrome in, 249
  retinoblastoma in, 332, 406, 407
  rhabdomyosarcoma in, 296
  rheumatoid arthritis-related uveitis in, 322–323
  sarcoidosis in, 329
  secondary open-angle glaucoma in, 179
  spontaneous hyphema in, 323
Chin-down head position, 258
Chin-up head position, 247–248, 258
Chlamydia trachomatis infections, 101, 102, 103, 104
Chloramphenicol, 112
Chlorolabe, 34
Chloroquine, 278–279
  effect on ophthalmic test findings, 47
  as retinopathy cause, 341–342
Chlorpromazine, as retinopathy cause, 342
Chorioretinitis, birdshot, 329
Choroid
  detachment of, 52
  fluorescein angiography visualization of, 14
  hemangioma of, 51, 52, 417, 422
  hemorrhage from, 51
  leukemic infiltrate of, 334
  melanoma of, 50–51, 415
  melanosomes in, 12
  neovascularization of, 361, 362, 363, 366–367
    occult, 363, 364
  nevus of, 51, 412, 413, 415
  rupture of, 199, 201, 354–355
  tumors of, 417
Choroidal effusions
  filtering procedures-related, 11
  trabeculectomy-related, 197–198
Choroiditis
  fungal, as uveitis cause, 324
  multifocal, 329, 331
    as uveitis cause, 325
  serpiginous, 326, 331
  syphilis-related, 329
  tuberculosis-related, 330
Chromatic aberrations, 25
Chronic progressive external ophthalmoplegia (CPEO),
    248–249
Ciliary bodies
  anterior, angle recession of, 199
  gonioscopic appearance of, 11
  medulloepithelioma of, 427

Ciliary bodies *(Continued)*
  melanoma of, 414, 415
  swelling or anterior rotation of, 160
  as trabeculectomy site blockage cause, 196
Ciliary body band, 157
Ciliary nerves, 14
Ciliochoroidal effusions, 173
Cilioretinal arteries, 13
  in central retinal artery obstruction, 385
  oral contraceptives-related occlusion of, 346
Ciprofloxacin, 109, 110, 112
Circle of least confusion, 23–24
Clear lens extraction, 139, 145, 147
Clotting disorders, 200
Coats disease, **348–352**, 426–427
  differential diagnosis of, 55, 349–350, 406, 407
Cocaine abuse, as retinopathy cause, 343
Cocaine test, for Horner's syndrome, 264
Cogan-Reese syndrome, 161, 179
Cogan's lid twitch, 311
Cold sores, 96
Collaborative Ocular Melanoma Study, 420
Collagenase inhibitors, 84
Collier's sign, 249
Coloboma
  as bitemporal field defect mimic, 278
  of optic nerve, 66
Color, attributes and properties of, 35–39
Color vision, **33–40**
  defects of, 39–40
    amblyopia-related, 235
    inheritance of, 40
Color wheel, 35–36
Coma, 24–25
Commotio retinae, 353
Computed tomography (CT)
  for Coats disease diagnosis, 350
  for intraocular foreign body detection, 357
  of optic nerve lesions, 57
  of optic nerve sheath lesions, 57
  orbital, 55, 430–431
    for calcification evaluation, 54
  of orbital tumors, 56
  of retinoblastoma, 410
  of thyroid-related ophthalmopathy, 300
Computed tomography (CT) angiography, 266
  for third-nerve palsy evaluation, 266
Cone dystrophy
  electroretinographic evaluation of, 45, 46
  progressive, 45
Cones, 34, 37, 39, 40, 42, 43
Confrontation visual fields, 59
Congenital fibrosis syndrome, 247–248
Congenital hereditary endothelial dystrophy, 125, 126–127
Congenital rubella syndrome, 45
Conjunctiva
  foreign bodies in, 82–83

Conjunctiva *(Continued)*
  Kaposi's sarcoma of, 340
  scarring of, as dry eye cause, 116
  squamous cell carcinoma of, in AIDS patients, 340
  tarsal follicles of, 78
  traumatic hyphema-related injuries to, 199
Conjunctivitis
  bacterial, 84, 108
  chlamydial inclusion, 84–85
  chronic, 84–85, 108, 315
  follicular, 96, 315
  giant papillary, 81, 82
  gonococcal, 78, 96, 108
  herpes simplex, 98
  neonatal (ophthalmia neonatorum), **101–105**
  Parinaud's oculoglandular, 84, 85
  as "pink eye" cause, 78
  as red eye cause, 77, 86
  Reiter's disease-related, 323
  toxic, 85
  verna, keratoconus associated with, 130
  viral, 78, 84, 107–108
Connective tissue disorders, keratoconus associated with, 130
Contact lens
  corneal infiltrates associated with, 95–96
  as corneal ulcer cause, 91, 108–109
  corrective power of, 20
  deposits on, 81, 82
  as dry eye cause, 117, 118
  effect on nystagmus, 260
  gas-permeable, 132
  as keratoconus cause, 129, 132
  as keratoconus treatment, 129–130, 134
  Koeppe, 158
  prismatic effect alleviation with, 23
  as ptosis cause, 314
  as red eye cause, 80–81, 82
  retinal detachment through, 354
  steepening the fit of, 31
  use after cataract surgery, 222
Contact lens solutions, sterile reaction to, 96
Contact lens warpage syndrome, 129
Contrast sensitivity test, 274
Contrecoup mechanism, 353
Convergence insufficiency, 31, 243, 244, 271–272
Copper foreign bodies, 358
Cornea
  abrasions of, 199
    in neonates, 103
    as recurrent corneal erosion cause, 82
    as red eye cause, 81, 82
  disease of, as red eye cause, 77
  dystrophies of, 82, **120–128,** 130
  edema of
    angle closure glaucoma-related, 161, 162, 167
    cataract surgery-related, 227, 228

Cornea *(Continued)*
  endothelial cells of, effects of refractive
    surgery on, 147
  erosion of, 121
  foreign bodies in, 82–83
    in neonates, 103
  infections of, **90–100**
    gonococcal, 96
    herpetic, 96–99
    laser in-situ keratomileusis (LASIK)-related, 98,
      99–100
    predisposing conditions for, 91
  infiltrates of, 95–96
  innervation of, 14
  keratometric measurement of, 28
  opacity of
    effect on electroretinographic findings, 45
    as false-positive field defect cause, 60
    in neonates, 14
  perforation of, neonatal conjunctivitis-related
    101, 105
  refractive function of, 137
  scarring of
    corneal ulcer-related, 110
    herpetic keratitis-related, 98
    neonatal conjunctivitis-related, 105
    topical steroid treatment for, 112–114
  scratches to, 80
  thickness of, in glaucoma, 153
  topography of, in refractive surgery patients, 138
  traumatic hyphema-related injuries to, 199
  ulcers of. *See* Ulcers, corneal
Cornea guttata, 128
  differentiated from Fuchs' dystrophy, 125
Corneal blood staining, 204
Corneal haze, post-photorefractive keratectomy, 148
Corneal transplantation, 135–136
  as astigmatism cause, 146
  as corneal dystrophy treatment, 127
Corticosteroids
  as glaucoma cause, 331
  as herpes simplex keratitis treatment, 98
  as optic neuritis treatment, 275
  as orbital capillary hemangioma treatment, 429
  as orbital inflammation treatment, 307
  as uveitis treatment, 331
Cotton-wool spots, 334, 335, 359, 378, 390, 392–393
Couching, 217, 219
Coumadin, anticoagulant effects of, 202
Covering test, 247
Cranial nerve palsies
  eighth, 270
  fifth, 249, 270
  fourth, 245, 249, 267, 269, 270
  as giant cell arteritis cause, 281
  localization of symptom complexes of, 270
  multiple, 249
  second, 270

Cranial nerve palsies *(Continued)*
  seventh, 270
  sixth, 238, 270, 283
  third, 243, 249, 262–263, 266, 267, 270, 271, 272,
    310
Cranial nerves
  fifth, divisions of, 16
  location within the superior orbital fissure, 9
Craniopharyngioma, of optic chiasm, 65–66
Credé prophylaxis, for neonatal conjunctivitis, 102
Critical angle, 21
Cross-fixation, 238
Crouzon syndrome, 243
Crowding phenomenon, 235
Cryoglobulins, 394
Cryotherapy
  for basal cell carcinoma, 317
  for blepharitis, 80
  for retinopathy of prematurity, 370–371
Cryptococcal infections, in AIDS patients, 339
Cultures, corneal, 91, 92, 94
Cyanolabe, 34
Cyclodestruction, 172
Cyclodialysis, 199, 208
Cyclodialysis cleft, 199, 201, 208–209
Cyclogyl, 29
Cycloplegic agents
  as aqueous misdirection syndrome treatment, 171
  as corneal ulcer treatment, 94
  as hyphema treatment, 202
  length of effectiveness of, 29
  as systemic intoxication cause, 29
Cyclosporine, as dry eye treatment, 118, 119
Cyst
  "chocolate,", 429
  dermoid, 434
    imaging of, 56
    ruptured, 429
Cystinosis, 123
Cytomegalovirus infections, in AIDS patients, 335,
  336–338, 339

D
Dacryoadenitis, 306
Dacryocystitis, 85, 103, 108
  acute, 290–291
  silent, 84
Dacryocystorhinostomy, 290, 291, 292
Dalen-Fuchs' nodules, 330
Dark adaptation, 48
Decompression
  optic nerve sheath, 280–281
  orbital, 301, 302, 303
Decongestants, 77
Dellen, 83
Dendrites, 113
  corneal, 97
  herpetic keratitis-related, 78–79

Dermatitis, radiation therapy-related, 318
Dermatochalasis, 310
Descemet's membrane, 11, 179
  corneal dystrophies of, 120
Desferrioxamine, as maculopathy cause, 346
Deuteranopes, 39
Deuteranopia, 39
Dexamethasone, 111–112, 113, 114
Diabetes mellitus. *See also* Retinopathy diabetic
  as cataract cause, 214
  maternal, 283
  oculomotor palsies associated with, 271, 272
  as open-angle glaucoma cause, 149
  ophthalmologic screening in, 377
  as optic disc hemorrhage cause, 155
  as retinal vein occlusion cause, 393
  as third-nerve palsy cause, 272
Dialysis
  iris, 199, 201
  retinal, 199, 201
    inferotemporal, 399
Dichromatism, congenital, 39
Dilation, for anterior chamber angle
    visualization, 160
Diopters, 22
  relationship to meters, 20
Diphenhydramine (Benadryl), 77
Dipivefrin hydrochloride, as glaucoma treatment, 181,
    182, 183, 185, 187
Diplopia, **266–273**
  binocular, 266, 282
  cataract surgery-related, 227
  definition of, 266
  elevated intracranial pressure-related, 282, 283
  intermittent, 266
  monocular, 30, 31, 266
  multiple ocular motor nerve palsy-related, 249
  myasthenia gravis-related, 271
  proptosis-related, 293, 295
Distortion, thick lens-related, 25
Divergence insufficiency, 244
Divergence paresis, 272
Dorsal midbrain syndrome. *See* Parinaud's
    oculoglandular syndrome
Dorzolamide, as glaucoma treatment, 182, 183,
    185, 186
Double elevator palsy, 246
Double ring sign, 283
Double vision. *See* Diplopia
Down syndrome, 130
Doxycycline, 78, 103
Driving, by nystagmus patients, 260
Drugs. *See also* names of specific drugs
  allergic reactions to, 77–78
  as dry eye cause, 119
  as hyphema risk factor, 202
  as optic neuropathy cause, 278–279
Drusen, 53, 66, 279–280, 362, 415
Dry eyes. *See* Keratoconjunctivitis sicca

Duane's retraction syndrome, 238, 243, 244–245
Dye disappearance test, 290
Dyschromatopsia, 284
Dyschromoplasia, 279
Dysproteinemia, 123
Dystrophy
  cone, 45, 46
  corneal, 82, **120–128**
    keratoconus associated with, 130
  differentiated from degeneration, 120
  ocular pharyngeal, 248–249
  pattern, 47
  posterior polymorphous, 179

E
Ear, music perception ability of, 36
Early receptor potentials (ERPs), 41
Early Treatment Diabetic Retinopathy Study (ETDRS),
    379–380
Echothiophate iodide, as glaucoma
    treatment, 182
Ectasia, progressive corneal, 144
Ectropion, 289
  as dry eye cause, 117
  ophthalmic medications-related, 78
  upper-eyelid, 312–313
Eczema, keratoconus-associated, 130
Edema
  corneal, 98
    Fuchs' dystrophy-related, 127
    posterior polymorphous dystrophy-related, 179
  of eyelids, 295, 296
  macular, 30
    clinically significant, 379–380
    cystic, 227, 229, 344
    diabetic, 376, 377, 379–380, 382–383
    nicotinic acid-related, 344
    refractory, 382
    retinal vein occlusion-related, 390, 391,
        393–394
    treatment for, 394
  of optic disc, 359, 392–393
Edinger-Westphal nucleus, 261
Edrophonium chloride. *See* Tensilon test
Ehlers-Danlos syndrome, 130
Elderly patients
  ocular ischemic syndrome in, 332
  steroid-resistant panuveitis in, 332
Electromagnetic spectrum, 33
Electro-oculography (EOG), 46–47
  Arden ratio in, 46
  for toxic retinopathy evaluation, 342, 343
Electrophoresis, 394
Electroretinography (ERG), 41–46
  extinguished, 45
  full field, 41–43, 45
  new variations of, 46
  for toxic retinopathy evaluation, 342, 343
  wave amplitudes in, 41, 45–46

Embolism, as retinal artery occlusion cause, 385
Emmetropia, far point in, 19
Endophthalmitis, 93
  foreign body-related, 358
  infectious, 227, 228
  neonatal conjunctivitis-related, 101, 105
  postoperative
    cataract surgery-related, 177
    chronic, as uveitis cause, 324
    refractive surgery-related, 147
    strabismus surgery-related, 253–254
  posttraumatic, 358–359
    antibiotic prophylaxis against, 359
Enophthalmos, 310
Enterobacter infections, 110
Entropion, 289
  involutional, 17
  radiation therapy-related, 318
  as superficial punctate keratopathy, 79
Enucleation
  as choroidal melanoma treatment, 415
  as Coats disease treatment, 351
  as retinoblastoma treatment, 408
  as uveal melanoma treatment, 419
EOG. See Electro-oculography (EOG)
Epicanthus inversus, 311
Epikeratophakia, 135
Epinephrine
  as glaucoma treatment, 181, 182, 183, 185
  as hyphema treatment, 203
Epiphora. See Tearing
Episcleral venous pressure, elevated, 178
Episcleritis
  differentiated from scleritis, 86
  nodular, 86–87
  as red eye cause, 77
Epithelial basement membrane dystrophy, 120, 121
Epithelioid cells, 419
Epitheliopathy, acute posterior multifocal placoid pigment, 326, 329
ERG. See Electroretinography (ERG)
Erythema, orbital inflammation-related, 305
Erythema migrans, 330
Erythema multiforme, 328
Erythema nodosum, 330
Erythrolabe, 34
Erythromycin, 103, 105, 107, 112
Esodeviations, 237–242
Esophoria, 237
Esotropia, 237
  accommodative, 239–240
    as amblyopia cause, 235
    early-onset, 238
    nonrefractive, 240, 241–242
    partial or decompensated, 240, 242
    refractive, 240, 241
    relationship with congenital esotropia, 241

Esotropia (Continued)
  acute acquired comitant (AACE), 242
  congenital, 235, 237–239, 241
  congenital fibrosis syndrome-related, 247–248
  cyclic, 242
  Duane's syndrome-related, 244–245
  left, 237
Ethmoid bone, 9, 16
Ethylene glycol, as retinopathy cause, 344
Exenteration, of recurrent eyelid tumors, 317
Exfoliation syndrome, 214
Exophoria, 244
Exotropia
  congenital fibrosis syndrome-related, 247–248
  congenital/neonatal, 243
  constant, 235
  convergence insufficiency-related, 271–272
  differential diagnosis of, 243
  Duane's syndrome-related, 244–245
  intermittent, 235, 243–244
  internuclear ophthalmoplegia associated with, 282
  sensory, 243
Eye
  clinical anatomy of, 9–15
  color perception ability of, 36
  schematic, 22
Eye drops 106 See also Topical medications
  as dry eye cause, 119
  as glaucoma treatment, 155, 186, 187
  improper administration of, 109
Eyelashes
  as blepharitis cause, 80
  epilation of, 80
Eyelid crutches, 312
Eyelids
  allergic reactions in, 77–78
  anatomy of, 11, 17–18
  crease of, 309, 310, 312–313
    height of, 312
  edema of, 295, 296
  lag of, 294
  laxity of, as tearing cause, 287, 288
  lower
    lacerations to, 17–18
    laxity of, 287, 288
    retractors of, 17–18
  orbital inflammation-related deformities of, 305
  retraction of, 310
    thyroid-related ophthalmopathy-related, 294–295, 299, 300, 302, 303
  rubbing of, as ptosis cause, 314
  schematic cross-section of, 11
  sensory nerve supply to, 17
  swollen, 77
  tear drainage path in, 287, 288
  tumors of, 315–319
  upper, fat pads of, 18

F

Familial amyloid type IV polyneuropathy, 123
Farber syndrome, 386
Far point, 19
Fat pads, of upper eyelid, 18
Fetal alcohol syndrome, 344
Fetal hyaloid vasculature, 13
Fiber layer of Henle, 12
Fibrohistiocytoma, 296
Fibrosis syndrome, congenital, 247–248
Filters, neutral density, 235
Fistulas
    arteriovenous, 249
    carotid, 178
    dural, 178
Fixation, eccentric, 235
Fixation errors, 60, 235
Fleischer rings, 132
Fleurettes, 424
Flexner-Wintersteiner rosettes, 408
Floaters, 336, 390
Floppy eyelid syndrome, 79, 130
Floppy iris syndrome, 230
Floppy lens syndrome, intraoperative (IFIS), 216
Fluorescein stain, differentiated from rose Bengal
        stain, 117
Fluorometholone, 114, 176
Fluoroquinolones, 108, 111, 112
5-Fluorouracil, 194, 195, 196
Focal points, 19, 20
    of schematic eye, 22
Forced ductions, 251
Foreign bodies, intraocular
    conjunctival, 82
    copper, 358
    corneal, 82–83
        in neonates, 103
    imaging of, 53, 55, 357
    iron, 346
    metallic, 82–83, 179
    orbital, 55, 83
    removal of, 357–358
    as superficial punctate keratopathy, 79
    as uveitis mimic, 333, 335
    wooden, imaging detection of, 55
Foreign-body sensation, 79, 80
    anterior membrane corneal dystrophy-related, 121
    corneal ulcer-related, 108–109
    herpetic keratitis-related, 113
    intraocular implants-related, 227
Foster-Kennedy syndrome, 284
Fovea
    anatomy of, 14
    in intraretinal hemorrhage, 390
Foveal avascular zone, 381
Foville's syndrome, 270
Fractures
    blowout, 9, 16, 246

Fractures *(Continued)*
    medial wall, 243
Frontal bone, 9
Frontal nerve, 16
Fuchs' corneal dystrophy, 125, 126, 128
Fuchs' heterochromic iridocyclitis, 177–178, 322, 325
Full-threshold testing, 59
Functio laesa, 304
Fundus
    pigmentation/pigmented lesions of, 12, **412–415**
    traumatic injury to, **353–360**
Fundus examination, in anterior uveitis patients, 322
Fungal infections
    corneal, 91
    orbital, 307

G

β-Galactosidase deficiency, 386
Ganciclovir, intraocular implant of, 337
Ganglion cell disease, retinal, 43
Gangliosidase GM1, type 2, 386
Gases, intraocular use of, 403
Gaucher's disease, 386
Geneva lens clock, 28
Gentamycin, 112
Ginkgo biloba, as glaucoma treatment, 189
Glands of Krause, 13
Glands of Wolfring, 13
Glare/contrast sensitivity testing, 218
Glaucoma, **149–156**
    acute, as red eye cause, 77
    angle-closure, **157–173**
        in Asian Americans, 89
        chronic, 162
        inflammation-related, 172
        intermittent, 162
        primary, 161–169, 170
        secondary, 172, 208
        subacute, 162
        treatment of, 163–166
    angle-recession, 174, 208, 209–210
    average-pressure (low-tension), 149, 155–156
    as branch retinal vein occlusion risk factor, 390
    in cataract patients, 230
    classification of, 149
    closed-angle, 149
    Coats disease-related, 348
    congenital, 103
    definition of, 149
    elevated episcleral venous pressure-related, 178
    end-stage, 279
    ghost-cell, 179, 208
    hemolytic, 179, 208
    hemosiderotic, 208
    herpes zoster ophthalmicus-related, 97
    hyphema-related, 204, 206, 208
    juvenile, 188
    lens-particle, 177

Glaucoma *(Continued)*
  low-tension, 155
  malignant/ciliary block, 160, 171, 178
  medical treatment of, **181–189**
  melanomalytic, 334–335
  narrow-angle, 168–169
  neovascular, 160, 172, 179, 388
    retinal vein occlusion-related, 393–394
  open-angle, 149
    primary, 149–150, 154
    secondary, **174–180**
  phacoanaphylactic, 177
  phacolytic, 177, 214
  phacomorphic, 214
  postoperative, 178, 179
  prevalence of, 149
  pseudoexfoliation, 174–175
  as retinal vein occlusion risk factor, 393
  retinoblastoma-associated, 406
  secondary, 149
  sympathetic ophthalmia-related, 359
  topical steroids-related, 111
  trabeculectomy surgery for, **190–198**
  traumatic, **199–211**
  treatment for, 154–155
  uveitis-related, 331
  visual field findings in, 62, 69–71
Glaukomflecken, 161, 162
Glioma
  of optic chiasm, 65–66, 258
  of optic nerve, 56, 295
Globe
  Coats disease-related loss of, 351
  inferior displacement of, 296
  perforation/rupture of, 199, 356
    blunt trauma-related, 11
    cataract surgery-related, 225
    scleral suture-related, 254
Glycerin, as glaucoma treatment, 166, 176–177, 182
Goldberg's syndrome, 386
Goldenhar's syndrome, 283
Goldmann gonioscope, 158
Goldmann lens, 29
Goldmann perimetry, 63
Goldmann visual field, 59, 72
Goniolens, 157–158
Gonioscopes, types of, 158
Gonioscopy, 157–160
  for angle recession evaluation, 208–209
  for anterior chamber angle visualization, 11, 157–160
  for hyphema evaluation, 206, 208–209
  indentation, 162–163, 170
  for primary angle-closure glaucoma evaluation, 161
  technique of, 158
Goniosynechialysis, 167
Gonococcal infections, 78, 96, 101, 102, 103, 104, 108
Gradenigo's syndrome, 270
Gram-negative organisms, as corneal infection cause, 91

Granular-lattice dystrophy, 124
Granuloma
  choroidal, 324
  eosinophilic, 56
Granulomatosis, Wegener's, 274, 308, 331, 429
Graves' disease, 294, 429
Green light rays, refraction by plus lens, 25
Guarded filtering procedure (GFP), 167, 172
Guillain-Barré syndrome, 249

H
HAART (highly-active antiretroviral therapy), 337–338
Haemophilus infections, as corneal infection
    cause, 92, 93
Haemophilus influenzae infections
    as conjunctivitis cause, 84
    as orbital cellulitis cause, 295, 308
Hallervorden-Spatz disease, 386
Hallucinations, 283, 284
Harada-Ito procedure, 269
Hay fever, 77, 130
Headaches, 278, 282
  migraine, 149, 155, 262, 310
Head injury, as fundus abnormalities cause, 359
Hemangioma
  as astigmatism cause, 31
  capillary, 430
    differentiated from retinoblastoma, 407
    imaging of, 56
    orbital, 429
  cavernous, 296, 429–430, 434
    imaging of, 56
  choroidal, 417, 422
Hemangiopericytoma, 296, 430, 434
  imaging of, 56
Hemianopia, 62, 63, 64
  binasal, 67
  bitemporal, 65–66
  definition of, 61
Hemoglobin A_1C, 377
Hemorrhage
  of anterior segment, 199
  cataract surgery-related, 225, 226
  choroidal
    expulsive, 225, 226
    ultrasound evaluation of, 51
  of optic disc, 155
  of optic nerve sheath, 225
  recurrent, hyphema-related, 204, 205
  retinal, 390
    retinal arterial obstruction-related, 386
    retinal venous obstruction-related, 392, 393
  retrobulbar, 225
  subconjunctival, 82, 85, 199
    as red eye cause, 77
  subretinal, 412
    choroidal rupture-related, 355
    differentiated from choroidal melanoma, 412–413

Hemorrhage *(Continued)*
    suprachoroidal, post-trabeculectomy, 195
    vitreous
        diabetic retinopathy-related, 377, 380, 382
        as hemolytic glaucoma risk factor, 179
        magnetic resonance imaging of, 55
        melanoma-related, 335
        retinal vein occlusion-related, 391
Hering's law, 312
Herpes simplex virus infections, 78–79
    corneal, 91, 96, 97
    as corneal infection cause, 91
    as keratouveitis cause, 113, 114
    as neonatal conjunctivitis cause, 105
    as ophthalmia neonatorum cause, 103
    topical steroid therapy for, 111
    as uveitis cause, 331
Herpesvirus infections
    as acute retinal necrosis cause, 330
    as ophthalmia neonatorum cause, 101, 102, 104
    as uveitis cause, 323
Herpes zoster virus infections
    AIDS-related, 335–336, 338
    corneal, 97
    topical steroid therapy for, 111
    trigeminal nerve distribution of, 11
    as uveitis cause, 331
Heterochromia, 177–178
Highly-active antiretroviral therapy (HAART), 337–338
Histamine₁ receptor antagonists, 77
Histiocytoma, fibrous, 430, 434
    imaging of, 56
Histoplasmosis, ocular, 324, 329
HLA-B27-associated conditions, 322, 323, 325, 328
Homatropine, 29
Homer Wright rosettes, 423–424
Homocystinuria, 214, 394
Horner's syndrome, 263, 264, 270, 272, 310, 313
Horseshoe tears, retinal, 353, 354, 398, 401
Hruby lens, 29
Hue, 35, 36
Humphrey perimetry, 63
Hurler's syndrome, 386
Hutchinson's sign, 11
Hyaloidotomy, laser, 171
Hydrops, acute, 133
Hydroxychloroquine
    effect on ophthalmic test findings, 47
    as retinopathy cause, 341–342
Hypercholesterolemia, 123–124, 315–316
Hyperemia, 108
Hyperlipidemia, 123–124
Hyperopia
    absolute, 32
    accommodative requirements in, 26
    acquired, 30
    amplitude of accommodation in, 20
    corrective lens for, 20

Hyperopia *(Continued)*
    definition of, 137
    direct ophthalmoscope image size in, 27
    facultative, 32
    far point in, 19
    latent, 32
    manifest, 32
    near point in, 20
    round-top *versus* flat-top reading lens for, 23
    surgical treatment for, 141–142, 147
    total, 32
    undercorrection of, 31–32
Hyperosmotic agents
    action mechanism of, 181
    as aqueous misdirection syndrome treatment, 171
    as glaucoma treatment, 166, 181, 182
    as hyphema treatment, 202
Hyperplasia, lymphoid, 433–434
Hypertension
    as branch retinal vein occlusion risk factor, 390
    as diabetic retinopathy risk factor, 377
    idiopathic intracranial. *See* Pseudotumor cerebri
    as open-angle glaucoma risk factor, 149
    as retinal vein occlusion risk factor, 393
Hyperthyroidism, 298
Hypertropia, three-step test for, 267–269
Hyphema, **199–211**, 226
    cataract surgery-related, 226
    classification of, 200
    definition of, 199
    eight-ball, 205–206
    spontaneous, in children, 323
Hypopyon
    corneal ulcer-associated, 93
    layered, 227
Hypothyroidism, 298
Hypotony, 195, 205, 225–226
Hypotropia, 310
Hysteria, 279–280

I
ICE (iridocorneal endothelial) syndrome, 126, 161, 179
Ice test, 272, 313, 314
Image displacement, 23
Image jump, 23
Image point, 22
Imaging, ophthalmic. *See also* Computed tomography;
        Magnetic resonance imaging; Ultrasonography
    orbital, for thyroid-related ophthalmopathy
        evaluation, 299
Immunosuppression. *See also* Acquired
        immunodeficiency syndrome (AIDS)
    as corneal infection risk factor, 91
Immunosuppressive agents, as uveitis
        treatment, 331, 332
Incontinentia pigmenti, 374
Infants. *See also* Neonates
    cataracts in, 214

Infants *(Continued)*
Coats disease in, 348
myopia in, 137
nystagmus in, 239, 256–258, 259
premature, retinopathy in, **368–375**
strabismus in, 237
visual acuity in, 14
Infarction, vaso-occlusive, 266
Infection
of radial keratotomy incision, 140
strabismus surgery-related, 253
Inferior oblique overaction, 239
Inferior oblique palsy, 246
Infiltrates, leukemic
choroidal, 334
imaging of, 56
intraocular lens implants-related, 230
of optic nerve, 334
Inflammation
definition of, 304
granulomatous, 359
of lacrimal glands, 306
melanoma-related, 334–335
of the optic nerve. *See* Neuritis, optic
orbital, **304–308**
idiopathic, imaging of, 56
nonspecific, 304–307
specific, 307
postoperative, 227
Inflammatory bowel disease, 322, 323
Interferon, 276, 346, 429
Intracorneal ring segments (Intacs), 135, 139, 144–145
complications of, 145
Intracranial pressure, elevated, 282, 283
Intraocular lens implants, 222
accommodative, 145
complications of, 230
dislocation of, 214
foreign-body reactions to, 227
multifocal, 216
new developments in, 223
phakic, 139, 145
as hyperopia treatment, 147
Verisyse, 145
power calculations for, 26, 215–216, 222–223
Intraocular pressure
effect of corneal thickness on, 153
elevated
angle-closure glaucoma-related, 161, 162–163, 164–165
differential diagnosis of, 175–176
Fuchs' heterochromic iridocyclitis-related, 177–178
in glaucoma, 149, 150, 152, 155–156, 188
optic nerve resistance to, 155
post-cataract surgery, 178
post-peripheral iridotomy, 169
steroids-related, 114, 175–176

Intraocular pressure *(Continued)*
elevated *(Continued)*
trabecular meshwork obstruction-related, 175
uveitis-related, 331
fluctuations in, in glaucoma, 152
measurement of, 154
medically uncontrolled, 203–204
normal, 150
in glaucoma, 153
post-trabeculectomy, 190
Intraoperative floppy lens syndrome (IFIS), 216
Iodine, radioactive, 298–299
Iridectomy
corneal peripheral, 167
during trabeculectomy surgery, 192
Iridocorneal endothelial (ICE) syndrome, 126, 161, 179
Iridocyclectomy, as ciliary body melanoma treatment, 415
Iridocyclitis, Fuchs' heterochromic, 177–178, 322, 325
Iridodialysis, 199
Iridoplasty, laser peripheral, 170
Iridotomy, laser peripheral, 163
as angle-closure glaucoma treatment, 164, 165, 166–167, 168
complications of, 167
intraocular pressure elevation after, 169
as plateau iris treatment, 170
Iris
in angle-closure glaucoma, 168
as anterior chamber angle landmark, 157
atrophy of
as diplopia cause, 266
essential, 179
progressive, 161
heterochromia of, 335
injuries to, cataract surgery-related, 225
melanoma of, 421
neovascularization of, 200, 388
in diabetic patients, 381
peripheral configuration of, 160
plateau, 160, 169–171
in primary angle-closure glaucoma, 161
prolapse of, cataract surgery-related, 226
sphincter tears of, 199
trabeculectomy site blockage by, 195
Iris bombé, 172
Iritis, 321
bilateral chronic granulomatous, 329
Iron, as siderosis cause, 358
Iron intraocular foreign bodies, 346
Irrigation, ocular
as gonococcal conjunctivitis treatment, 78
of lye burns, 83–84
Ischemia
anterior segment, 254–255
posterior segment, 172
retinal arterial obstruction-related, 385

Ischemia *(Continued)*
    retinal venous obstruction-related, 391–392, 393,
        394, 395
Ischemic vascular disease, 250

J

Jackson cross, 31
Jones, Lester, 18
Jones dye tests, primary or secondary, 290

K

Kaiser Fleischer rings, 358
Kaposi's sarcoma, 339, 340
Kawasaki disease, 325
Kearns-Sayre syndrome, 248
Kellman, Charles, 220
Keratectomy
    photorefractive, 139, 140–141
        drug therapy with, 147–148
        hyperopic excimer laser, 147
    phototherapeutic, 122
Keratic precipitates, 90, 321, 322
Keratitis
    Acanthamoeba-related, 91, 92
    contact lens-related, 91
    diffuse lamellar, 99, 143–144
    fungal, 91
    herpetic, 78–79, 90, 91, 96, 97, 98, 99, 113
    necrotizing, 98
Keratoacanthoma, 316
Keratoconjunctivitis
    atopic, 130
    sicca, 79, **116–119**
        as corneal ulcer cause, 91
        definition of, 116
        radiation therapy-related, 318, 408
        as red eye cause, 77
        as tearing cause, 287, 288
        topical medications-related, 187
        types of, 117
    superior limbic, 86
Keratoconus, 128, **129–136**
    as contraindication to refractive surgery, 137
    as diplopia cause, 266
    "forme fruste," 144
    surgical treatment of, 144
    topographic signs of, 130, 131–132
Keratometers, 28
Keratometry, 26
Keratomileusis, laser in-situ (LASIK), 139, 141–143
    comparison with
        photorefractive keratectomy, 142
        radial keratotomy, 142
    complications of, 143–144
    as corneal infection risk factor, 98, 99–100
    definition of, 141
    as dry eye exacerbation cause, 117
    Epi-LASIK, 144

Keratomileusis, laser in-situ (LASIK) *(Continued)*
    hyperopic, 147
    techniques in, 141–142
    wavefront-guided, 143
Keratopathy
    exposure, proptosis-related, 293
    neurotrophic, 90
    superficial punctate, 79, 80, 84
        Thygeson's, 79
Keratoplasty
    conductive, 147
    deep anterior lamellar, 125
    Descemet-stripping endothelial, 125, 127
    lamellar (partial-thickness), 135
    penetrating, 124, 125, 134–135
Keratosis
    actinic, 315, 316
    seborrheic, 315
Keratotomy, radial, 139–140
    comparison with photorefractive keratectomy, 141
Keratouveitis
    chronic, 98
    herpetic, 113, 114
Knapp's rules, 269
Koeppe gonioscope, 158
Koeppe nodules, 321, 322
Kollner's rule, 40
Krukenberg spindles, 176

L

Lacrilube, 118
Lacrimal bone, 9, 16
Lacrimal glands
    accessory, 13
    inflammation of, 306
    tumors of, 432–433
        benign differentiated from malignant, 433
        "the rule of 50's" for, 432
Lacrimal nerve, 16
Lacrimal pump mechanism, 18
Lacrimal sac, obstructions of, 289, 290
Lacrimal system, **287–292**
    anatomy of, 287
    obstruction of, 289, 290
        congenital, 291
        radiation therapy-related, 318
Lacrisert, 118
Lagophthalmos, 13, 295
    differentiated from red eye, 79
Laser in-situ keratomileusis (LASIK). *See*
    Keratomileusis, laser in-situ (LASIK)
Laser (light amplification by stimulated emission
    of radiation)
    as age-related macular degeneration treatment, 365
    as angle-closure glaucoma treatment, 165, 166–167
    definition of, 31, 217
    femtosecond, 144
    as malignant/ciliary block glaucoma treatment, 171

Laser (light amplification by stimulated emission of radiation) *(Continued)*
  use in capsulotomy, 217, 229–230
  use in cataract surgery, 221–222
  use in corneal dystrophy treatment, 122
  use in photocoagulation
    as age-related macular degeneration treatment, 365–366
    differentiated from photodynamic therapy, 365–366
    as macular edema treatment, 391
    as retinal vein occlusion treatment, 391–392, 394, 395
    as retinopathy of prematurity treatment, 372–373
  use in photorefractive keratectomy, 140
  use in trabeculectomy surgery, 190
Latanoprost, 177, 182, 183
Lateral inhibition, 37
Lattice degeneration, 397–398
"Leash effect," 244
Leber's congenital amaurosis, 257
  achromatopsia-related, 45
  electroretinographic evaluation of, 45
  keratoconus associated with, 130
Leber's hereditary optic neuropathy, 279, 284
Leber's miliary aneurysm, 348
Leber's neuroretinitis, 331
Leber's optic atrophy, 67
Lens. *See also* Spectacles, lens of
  as angle-closure glaucoma cause, 177
  anterior chamber, 216
  corrective power of, 20
  extraction of, as aqueous misdirection syndrome treatment, 171
  Goldmann, 29
  Hruby, 29
  lack of innervation of, 14
  opacity of, as false-positive field defect cause, 60
  in phacolytic glaucoma, 177
  posterior chamber, 216
  in primary angle-closure glaucoma, 161, 162
  refractive function of, 19, 137
  retained material in, 227
  spontaneously dislocated, 214–215
  subluxated, 15, 199
  Volk, 29
Leukemia, 332, 334
Leukemic infiltrates
  choroidal, 334
  imaging of, 56
  intraocular lens implants-related, 230
  of optic nerve, 334
Leukocoria
  imaging studies of, 54, 55
  retinoblastoma-related, 55, 406
Levator muscle
  aponeurosis dehiscence of, 314
  congenital maldevelopment of, 310–311

Levator muscle *(Continued)*
  in ptosis, 310
    function measurement of, 311–312
Levobunolol hydrochloride, as glaucoma treatment, 182
Light
  fluorescent, 38
  incandescent, 38
  refractive index-related bending of, 21
  spectrum of, 33
  transmission to the brain, 35
  visual perception of, 33
  wavelengths of, 29
Light/near dissociation, 264
Light rays
  refraction by plus lens, 25
  vergence of, 21–22
Light reflex test, 247
Limbus, surgical, 11
Liver, as uveal melanoma metastasis site, 419
Loratadine (Claritin), 77
Loteprednol, 77, 114, 176
Loupes, as low-vision aids, 28
Lower lid retractors, 17
Low-vision aids, 27–28, 367
Lung cancer, metastatic, 421, 433
Lupus anticoagulants, 394
Lye burns, 83–84
Lyme disease, 274, 323, 324, 330
Lymphadenopathy, 331
Lymphangioma, 56, 429
Lymphatics, absence of, from the orbit, 10
Lymphoma
  imaging of, 56
  MALT (mucosa-associated lymphoid tissue), 434
  orbital, 293, 296, 433–434
  as papilledema cause, 339
  primary intraocular, 332, 334
  as retinitis cause, 330
Lymphoproliferative disorders
  imaging of, 56
  orbital, 434
Lysergic acid diethylamide (LSD), 283

M
Macula
  anatomy of, 14
  cherry-red spots of, 386
  differentiation of, 14
  edema of, effect on potential acuity readings, 30
  hole in, 15
  optical coherence tomography of, 381
  scars of, as amblyopia cause, 231
  vertically displaced, 247
  in the visual cortex, 15
Macular degeneration, age-related, **361–367**
  as Bruch's membrane defect cause, 12
  dry, 361, 362
  electroretinographic evaluation of, 43

Macular degeneration, age-related *(Continued)*
  exudative (wet), 361, 362–363, 365
  nonexudative (dry), 361, 362, 363
Macular Photocoagulation Study (MPS), 365
Macular sparing, 64, 284
Macular splitting, 65, 284
Macular translocation, 366
Maculopathy
  bull's-eye, 341
  ischemic, 391, 393–394
  toxic, 346
Magnetic resonance angiography, 56
Magnetic resonance imaging (MRI)
  of idiopathic infantile nystagmus, 258
  of intraocular foreign bodies, 357
  metallic foreign bodies as contraindication to, 358
  of normal orbital tissues, 57
  of optic nerve lesions, 57
  of optic nerve sheath lesions, 57
  orbital, 56. 54, 431
  of orbital tumors, 56
  of retinoblastoma, 410
  for third-nerve palsy evaluation, 266
Magnification, 26
Magnification formulae
  for axial magnification, 26
  for telescopes, 27
  for transverse magnification, 26
Magnifiers, handheld, 27–28
Malingering, 279–280
MALT (mucosa-associated lymphoid tissue)
    lymphoma, 434
Mannitol, 177, 182
Marcus-Gunn jaw-winking syndrome, 310, 313
Mare's-tail sign, 120
Marfan's syndrome, 214
Marginal reflex distance, 311
Masquerade syndromes, 332–335
Mast cell inhibitors, 77
Maxillary bone, 9, 16
Maxillary nerve, 17
McLean, Ian, 418
Medial wall fractures, 243
Medulloepithelioma, 427, 428
Meesmann's juvenile epithelial dystrophy, 120, 121
Meibomian glands, 116
Meibomianitis, 80
Melanin, 431
Melanocytoma, 414
Melanocytosis
  congenital ocular, 414
  oculodermal, 414
Melanoma, 417
  cell types in, 418–419
  choroidal, 412, 415, 420–421
    differentiated from subretinal hemorrhage,
        412–413
    malignant, 417

Melanoma *(Continued)*
  choroidal *(Continued)*
    metastatic, 421
    shape of, 417
    TFSOM mnemonic for, 420–421
    ultrasound evaluation of, 50–51
  of ciliary bodies, 414, 415
  of the eyelid, 319
  inflammatory signs of, 334–335
  of the iris, 421
  retinoblastoma-associated, 406
  uveal, 413, 414, 417–420
    Callender classification of, 418
    malignant, 417
    metastatic, 419
    posterior, 420
    Zimmerman hypothesis of, 419–420
  as uveitis mimic, 333
Melanosomes, choroidal, 12
Meningioma, 249
  of olfactory groove, 62
  of optic chiasm, 65–66
Meningitis
  cryptococcal, 339
  neonatal conjunctivitis-related, 104
Meniscus
  low tear, 79, 86
  normal appearance of, 79
Meretoja's syndrome, 123
Metallosis, extinguished electroretinogram in, 45
Metals, ocular toxicity of, 358
Metamorphopsia, 266, 362
Metastases
  imaging of, 56
  of pigmented choroidal lesions, 414
  uveal, 417
Methazolamide, as glaucoma treatment, 182
Methoxyflurane anesthesia, as retinopathy
    cause, 344
Methylphenidate hydrochloride, as retinopathy
    cause, 344–345
Methylprednisone, as giant cell arteritis
    treatment, 281
Metipranolol, as glaucoma treatment, 182
Meyer's loop, 283
Microaneurysm, diabetic retinopathy-related, 378
Micropsia, 362
Migraine, ophthalmic, 149, 155, 262, 310
Millard-Gruber syndrome, 270
Minus cylinder form, 24
Miotics
  action mechanism of, 181
  contraindication in trabecular meshwork
      blockage, 175
  as glaucoma treatment, 166, 181, 182, 183
  as plateau iris treatment, 170–171
  use in narrow-angle glaucoma patients, 169
Mirrors, convex and concave, vergence of, 28

Mitomycin C, 194, 195, 196
  use in photorefractive keratectomy patients, 148
Mittendorf's dot, 13
Möbius syndrome, 238, 247
Mohs' lamellar resection, 317
Molluscum contagiosum, 84, 85, 315
Motility disorders, congenital esotropia-related, 239
Moxifloxacin, 112
Mucin, as tear film component, 288
Mucocele, 249
Mucormycosis, 249
Müller's muscle contraction, in ptosis, 312
Multiple evanescent white dot syndrome, 326
Multiple sclerosis
  as internuclear ophthalmoplegia
    cause, 250, 282
  optic neuritis as risk factor for, 274,
    275–276
  as ptosis cause, 310
  as uveitis cause, 326, 329
Myasthenia gravis, 243
  as abduction deficit cause, 269
  diagnosis of, 313
  as hypertropia cause, 245
  as internuclear ophthalmoplegia cause, 282
  as multiple cranial nerve palsy mimic, 249
  as ptosis cause, 310–311
  signs and symptoms of, 271, 311
  work-up for, 271
Mycobacterium avium infections, AIDS-related,
  335–336
Mydriasis, 199
Myeloma, 123
Myopathy, as diplopia cause, 266
Myopia
  accommodative requirements in, 26
  acquired, 30
  age factors in, 137
  amplitude of accommodation in, 21
  axial, 20
  cataracts-related, 213, 218
  corrective lens for, 20
    power of, 25–26
  definition of, 137
  direct ophthalmoscope image size in, 27
  far point in, 19
  near point in, 21
  as open-angle glaucoma risk factor, 149
  refractive, 20
  residual, post-refractive surgery, 146–147
  as retinal detachment risk factor, 397, 398
  round-top *versus* flat-top reading lens for, 23
  surgical treatment for, 139–142, 144–145
Myositis
  as diplopia cause, 266
  orbital, 306, 307
    differentiated from thyroid-associated
     orbitopathy, 307
Myotonic dystrophy, 45–46

N
Nanophthalmos, 173, 196
Nasolacrimal duct, 287
  obstructions of, 289, 290
    congenital, 103, 291
Nasopharyngeal carcinoma, 249
Near point, 20, 21
Near point exercises, 244
Near reflex, spasm of, 269
Nearsightedness. *See* Myopia
Necrosis
  progressive outer retinal, 338, 339
  retinal, 330
Neisseria gonorrhoeae infections, as ophthalmia
  neonatorum cause, 101, 102, 103, 104
Neisseria infections, as corneal infection cause, 92, 93
Neomycin, 112
  toxicity of, 110
Neonates
  conjunctivitis in, **101–105**
  corneal opacification in, 14
  retinopathy of prematurity in, **368–375**
Neosynephrine test, 312
Neovascularization
  anterior segment, 394
  choroidal, 361, 362, 363, 364, 366–367
    occult, 363, 364
  of the iris, in diabetic patients, 381
  of the optic disc, 394
  retinal, 394
    diabetic retinopathy-related, 376, 381
    retinal arterial occlusion-related, 388
    retinal vein occlusion-related, 390, 391–392
    talc-related, 344–345
Neurilemoma, 56
Neuritis, optic, 67, **274–277**
  definition of, 274
  retrobulbar, in AIDs patients, 339
  visual outcome in, 274, 275
Neurofibroma, 296, 434
  imaging of, 56
  plexiform, 56
Neurofibromatosis, 179, 295
Neurologic disturbances, **278–285**
Neuromuscular junction disorders, as diplopia cause, 266
Neuropathy, optic
  cataract surgery-related, 227
  ischemic, 227, 280–281
  metabolic, 278–279
  miscellaneous, **278–285**
  radiation therapy-related, 318
  syphilis-related, 329
  toxic/nutritional, 67, 278–279
Neuroretinitis, diffuse unilateral subacute, 45, 324
Neurotomy, radial optic, 394
Nevus
  choroidal, 51, 412, 413, 415
  of Ota, 414
Nicotinic acid, as cystoid macular edema cause, 344

Niemann-Pick disease, 386
Nightblindness, stationary
  central, electroretinographic evaluation of, 45
  congenital
    achromatopsia-related, 45
    electro-oculographic evaluation of, 47
    electroretinographic evaluation of, 45
Night vision, 34
Nitric oxide synthase inhibitors, as glaucoma
    treatment, 189
Nodal point (np), of schematic eye, 22
Nonsteroidal anti-inflammatory drugs, 77
  anticoagulant effects of, 202
  as scleritis treatment, 88
  use in photorefractive keratectomy patients, 148
Norfloxacin, 112
Null zone, in idiopathic infantile nystagmus, 257, 258
Nutritional supplements, as macular degeneration
    treatment, 365
Nystagmus, **256–260**
  achromatopsia-related, 45
  amaurotic, 256
  bidirectional jerk, 257
  congenital esotropia-related, 239
  definition of, 256
  downbeat, 13
  idiopathic infantile, 256–258, 259
  latent, 256
  periodic alternating, 258–259
  torsional, 258
  upbeat, 282
  vertical, 258
  vestibular, 256
Nystagmus blockage syndrome, 238, 242

O
Obesity, as pseudotumor cerebri cause, 283
Oblique muscles, in strabismus surgery, 251
Occipital lobe, lesions of, 284
Ocular coherence tomography (OCT), 15, 364, 381
Ocular deviations, miscellaneous, **243–250**
Ocular ischemic syndrome, as uveitis mimic, 332, 333
Oculocerebrorenal syndrome, 179
Oculomotor nerve palsies. See Cranial nerve
    palsies, third
Ofloxacin, 109, 112
Oguchi's disease, 45–46
Ointments, 107
Olfactory groove, meningioma of, 62
Omega fatty acids, as macular degeneration
    treatment, 365
Onchocerciasis, 323, 324
Opacification
  as false-positive field defect cause, 60
  posterior capsular, 216–217
Ophthalmia, sympathetic, 326, 330, 331
Ophthalmia neonatorum, **101–105**
Ophthalmic artery, occlusion of, 45
Ophthalmic nerve, 17

Ophthalmicus, herpetic, 97
Ophthalmoplegia
  chronic progressive external (CPEO), 248–249
  internuclear, 243, 249–250, 270, 282
Ophthalmoscope/ophthalmoscopy
  direct, 26, 27, 29
  indirect, 29, 358, 402
Optical coherence tomography (OCT), 15, 364, 381
Optic atrophy, sympathetic ophthalmia-related, 359
Optic chiasm
  crossed and uncrossed fibers in, 13
  lesions of, 65–66, 278
Optic disc
  edema of, 359, 392–393
  glaucoma-like, differential diagnosis of, 156
  hemorrhage of, 155
  hypoplasia of, 257
  neovascularization of, 394
  pallor of, 278, 279
  tilted, 60, 278
Optic nerve
  in angle-closure glaucoma, 168
  avulsion of, 353
  coloboma of, 66
  compression of, 293, 302
  cupping of, 175
  drusen of, 279–280
  glioma of, 56, 295
  hypoplasia of, 283
  injury to, 152
    glaucoma-related, 150, 151, 152, 155
    traumatic hyphema-related, 199, 201
  intraocular pressure resistance in, 155
  lesions of
    differentiated from optic nerve sheath
      lesions, 57
    imaging of, 57
  leukemic infiltrates of, 334
  melanocytoma of, 414
  papillitis of, 339, 340
  retinoblastoma invasion of, 407, 408
Optic nerve sheath
  hemorrhage from, 225
  lesions of, differentiated from optic nerve
    lesions, 57
Optic Neuritis Treatment Trial (ONTT), 274, 275, 276
Optic pits, 67
  glaucoma-related, 151
Optics, **19–32**
Optic-tract syndrome, 69
Optociliary shunt vessels, 281
Oral contraceptives
  as dry eye cause, 117
  as retinal arterial occlusion cause, 346
Orbicularis oculi muscle
  in involutional entropion, 17
  in lacrimal pump mechanism, 18
  myasthenia gravis-related weakness of, 311
  three portions of, 18

Orbit
  adnexal trauma to, 355
  anatomy of, 10, 11, 16
  anterior, schematic cross-section of, 11
  bones of, 9, 16
  cellulitis of, 307–308
  fat/fat pads of, 10, 11, 17
  inflammatory conditions of, **304–308**
    idiopathic, imaging of, 56
    nonspecific, 304–307
    specific, 307
  lymphoma of, 293, 433–434
  lymphoproliferative lesions of, 434
  septum of, 10, 11, 17
  thyroid-related ophthalmopathy of, **298–303**
  trauma to, 245
  tumors/cancer of, 296, **429–434**
    imaging of, 56
  vasculitis of, 308
Orbital apex syndrome, 306
Orbital fissures, superior, injury to, 249
Orbital inflammatory pseudotumor, 243, 245
Orbital rim, weak areas of, 16
Orthophoria, 247, 248
Oscillopsia, 256
Osteosarcoma, 406
Otitis, neonatal conjunctivitis-related, 104
Oxalosis, 344

P
Pachymeters, 29
Pain
  optic neuritis-related, 274
  orbital, 305
Palatine bone, 9, 16
Palpebral fissure width, in ptosis, 312
Panuveitis, 321, 329
  steroid-resistant, 332, 334
Papilledema, 282, 339
  differentiated from pseudopapilledema, 283
Papillitis, 339, 340
Paracentesis, 177, 178, 192, 194, 387
Paramagnetic agents, 54
Parasitic infections, orbital, 307
Parinaud's oculoglandular syndrome, 249, 265, 331
Pars plana, vitrectomy of, 401, 402–403
Pars planitis
  treatment of, 327
  as uveitis cause, 325
  as vision loss cause, 327
Patching
  alternatives to, 234
  as amblyopia treatment, 233–234
  as hyphema treatment, 202
  risks of, 234
Penalization, as amblyopia treatment, 233–234, 236
"Pencil push-ups," 244
Penicillin, allergic reactions to, 110

Peribulbar injection, of anesthesia, 219
Perimetry
  Goldmann, 63
  Humphrey, 63
  kinetic, 59
  short wavelength automated, 73–74
  static, 59
Peripheral vision, in glaucoma, 150
Phacodonesis, 215
Phacoemulsification, 220–221
Phenothiazines, as retinopathy cause, 342–343
Phimosis, of the eyelid, 311
Photocoagulation
  in darkly pigmented fundi, 12
  laser
    as age-related macular degeneration treatment,
      365–366
    differentiated from photodynamic therapy,
      365–366
    as macular edema treatment, 391
    as retinal vein occlusion treatment, 391–392,
      394, 395
    as retinopathy of prematurity treatment, 372–373
  panretinal, 380, 381
    as constricted visual field cause, 279–280
Photodynamic therapy, for macular degeneration,
  365–366
Photons, 33, 35, 37, 38
Photophobia
  anterior membrane corneal dystrophy-related, 121
  anterior uveitis-related, 88
  corneal ulcer-related, 108–109
  herpetic keratitis-related, 78–79
  nystagmus-related, 259
  superior limbic keratoconjunctivitis-related, 86
Photoreceptor response, 42–43, 397
Photoreceptors, 34, 35, 37, 38, 397
  traumatic injury to, 353
Phthisis bulbi, 53, 310, 348
Physiologic blind spot, 59
Physostigmine, 29
"Pie-in-the-sky" lesions, 67, 68, 283
"Pie-on-the-floor" defect, 284
Pigmentary dispersion syndrome, 176
Pigmentation, fundal, 12
Pigments, 38
Pilocarpine
  as glaucoma treatment, 182, 183, 186
  as symblepharon cause, 187
Pinealoblastoma, 406
Pingueculum, 83
Pinhole diameter, most effective, 29
"Pink eye," 78, 108
Pituitary tumors, 65–66, 278
Plateau iris, 160, 169–171
Plateau iris configuration (PIC), 169–170
Plus cylinder form, 24
"Plus disease," 370

Pneumonitis, neonatal conjunctivitis-related, 104
Polycoria, as diplopia cause, 266
Polymyxin, toxicity of, 110
Polymyxin B, 107, 112
Polyneuropathy, familial amyloid type IV, 123
Polysporin, 107
PORN (progressive outer retinal necrosis), 338, 339
Posner gonioscope, 158
Posner-Schlossman syndrome, 177
Posterior capsular
    opacification of, 216–217
Posterior capsule
    cataract surgery-related rupture of, 225, 226
Posterior crocodile shagreen, 124
Posterior membrane corneal dystrophy, 120, 125–127
Posterior polymorphous dystrophy, 125, 126–127
Power (P), of schematic eye, 22
Preauricular nodes, 77, 78, 84
Prednisolone, 113, 114, 175, 177
Prednisone, 275, 281
Pregnancy
    as aminocaproic acid contraindication, 203
    diabetic retinopathy during, 377
    glaucoma medication use during, 187–188
    as tetracycline contraindication, 104
Prematurity, retinopathy of, 247, **368–375**
    differential diagnosis of, 55, 247, 349–350, 406, 407
Prentice's law, 22, 23
Presbyopia, 137, 138
Pressure patches, contraindications to, 81
Primary focal point (F₁), 19, 22
Prince rule, 32
Principal plane, of schematic eye, 22
Prisms, 33–34
    base-in, 244
    calculation of power of, 22
    as thyroid-related ophthalmopathy treatment, 302
Progressive supranuclear palsy, 249, 272
Prolactinoma, 278
Propionibacterium acnes infections, 323
Proptosis, **293–297**
    bilateral, 9, 294–295
    computed tomography evaluation of, 55
    definition of, 293
    magnetic resonance imaging evaluation of, 55, 56
    thyroid-related ophthalmopathy-related, 299, 300
    unilateral, 9, 294–295, 296
Prosopagnosia, 284
Prostaglandin agonists, 175
Prostaglandin analogs, 175
    action mechanism of, 181
    as glaucoma treatment, 181, 182, 184, 186
    side effects of, 189
Prostaglandins, 147–148
Proteinuria, as diabetic retinopathy risk factor, 377
Proteus infections, treatment for, 110
Pseudoabduction defects, differentiated from true
    abduction defects, 238

Pseudoesotropia, 237
Pseudoexfoliation, 214
Pseudoexfoliation syndrome, 174–175
Pseudo-Foster Kennedy syndrome, 284
Pseudohypertropia, 245, 247
Pseudohypopyon, 179
Pseudomembranes, 78
Pseudomonas infections
    as corneal infection cause, 91
    as red eye cause, 81
    treatment for, 109, 110
Pseudopapilledema, differentiated from
    papilledema, 283
Pseudophakia, 215
Pseudoptosis, 310
Pseudostrabismus, 243
Pseudotumor, 266, 295, 304, 429
Pseudotumor cerebri, 282, 283
Pseudoxanthoma elasticum, 12
Pterygium, 83
Ptosis, **309–314**
    acquired, 309, 314
    aponeurotic, 309
    as astigmatism cause, 31
    bilateral, 248, 311
    classification of, 309
    congenital, 309–310
    congenital fibrosis syndrome-related, 248
    as false-positive field defect cause, 60
    Horner's syndrome-related, 264
    intraocular surgery-related, 310
    myogenic causes of, 310–311
    nonsurgical correction of, 312
    orbital capillary hemangioma-related, 429
    preoperative examination of, 311–312
    surgical correction of, 312
        complications of, 312–313
    unilateral, as amblyopia cause, 233
Ptosis surgery, eye closure difficulties after, 79
Puncta, tear drainage through, 287
Punctal occlusion
    as dry eye treatment, 118
    during topical medication administration, 106, 107,
        111, 186
Pupil, **261–265**
    Adie's tonic, 244, 262, 263
    afferent defects of, 235, 261–262
    Argyll Robertson, 329
    Flomax, 216
    innervation of, 261
    muscular control of, 261
    nonreactive, as diplopia cause, 266
    small, as false-positive field defect cause, 60
    in third-nerve palsy, 263
    unilateral dilated, poorly reactive, 262
Pupillary block, 208
    anterior chamber angle in, 160
    relative. *See* Glaucoma, angle-closure, primary

Pupillary dilation, of cataracts, 218
Pupillary light reflex, 261

Q

Quadrantanopia, 62, 66, 67, 68
Quinine intoxication, 45–46
Quinine sulfate, as retinopathy cause, 343, 344

R

Radiation therapy
  for basal cell carcinoma, 317
  complications of, 117, 279, 318, 408
  for thyroid-related ophthalmopathy, 301
Raynaud's phenomenon, 149, 155
Recess-resect procedures, 251
Rectus muscles
  inferior, entrapment of, 245, 246
  lateral, excessively resected, 243
  medial
    resection of, 247
    restricted, 269
    slipped or lost, 243, 247
  recession of, 9, 247
  in strabismus surgery, 251
  in thyroid-related ophthalmopathy, 299, 300
Red eye, **77–89**
  retinal vein occlusion-related, 392
  treatment of, 108
Red light rays, refraction by plus lens, 25
Reflection, total internal, 21
Refraction, **19–32**
  in against-the-rule astigmatism, 24
  as cataract treatment, 218
  critical angle of, 21
  cycloplegic, 29
  plus cylinder conversion to minus cylinder
    version of, 24
  postoperative, 24
  spherical equivalents in, 24
Refractive components, of the eye, 137
Refractive errors
  congenital esotropia-related, 238
  types of, 137
Refractive indices, 22
Refractive surgery, **137–148**
  contraindications to, 137–138
  as pediatric anisometropic amblyopia treatment,
    235–236
Refsum's syndrome, 248
Reis-Bücklers corneal dystrophy, 122
Reiter's disease, 322, 323
Relative luminosity curves, 37
Reticulum cell sarcoma, 332
Retina
  AIDS-related microvasculopathy of, 335, 339
  anatomic layers of, 12
  in angle-closure glaucoma, 161, 168
  attachment mechanisms of, 397

Retina *(Continued)*
  breaks/tears of 353, 398–401. *See also* Retinal
    detachment
    blunt trauma-related, 353, 354, 355
    dialysis-related, 353, 354, 355
    horseshoe tears, 353, 354, 398, 401
    scleral buckling of, 402
    traumatic hyphema-associated, 199, 201
  cells of, 12
  degenerative diseases of, 44
  leukemic infiltrates of, 334
  necrosis of, 330, 338, 339
  neovascularization of, 394
    diabetic retinopathy-related, 376, 381
    retinal arterial occlusion-related, 388
    retinal vein occlusion-related, 390, 391–392
    talc-related, 344–345
  pigmentation of, 34
    in Kearns-Sayre syndrome, 248
  separation from ora serrata, 199
Retinal arterial obstruction, **384–389**
  as altitudinal defect cause, 74
  branch-type, 13, 384, 386, 387
    symptoms of, 385
  causes of, 384–385
  central-type, 384, 386, 387
    arteritis-associated, 281
    cilioretinal artery in, 13
    emergency treatment for, 388
    symptoms of, 385
  differentiated from retinal venous obstruction, 388
  oral contraceptives-related, 346
  prevention of, 387
  systemic diseases associated with, 386
  treatment for, 387–388
Retinal arteries, central, structure of, 14–15
Retinal arterioles, structure of, 14–15
Retinal detachment, **396–404**
  acute retinal necrosis syndrome-related, 330
  in AIDS patients, 338
  cataract surgery-related, 227, 228
  in children, imaging studies of, 54
  Coats disease-related, 348, 351
  definition of, 396
  extinguished electroretinogram in, 45
  exudative, 335, 396, 397
  infectious retinitis-related, 338
  peripheral, as uveitis mimic, 332, 333
  repair of, 400–404
  retinal dialysis-related, 354, 355
  retinopathy of prematurity-related, 370, 373
  rhegmatogenous, 396, 397–398, 399–400, 402–403
    diabetes-related, 377, 382
    electro-oculography evaluation of, 47
    as uveitis mimic, 335
  sympathetic ophthalmia-related, 359
  tractional, 396–397, 403–404
    diabetes-related, 377, 382

Retinal detachment *(Continued)*
  traumatic hyphema-associated, 199, 201
  ultrasound evaluation of, 52
  visual-field defects associated with, 73
Retinal pigment epithelium
  congenital hypertrophy of, 412
  desferrioxamine-related changes in, 346
  role in retinal attachment, 397
  tamoxifen-related changes in, 346
  thioridazine-related changes in, 346
  tumors of, 412
Retinal veins, tortuous, 392, 393
Retinal venous occlusive disease, **390–395**
  branch-type, 390–392
  central-type, 392–395
    anterior chamber angle in, 160
  as disc hemorrhage cause, 155
Retinitis
  cytomegalovirus, in AIDS patients, 335, 336–338
  necrotizing, in AIDS patients, 335, 336
  syphilic, 329, 336
Retinitis pigmentosa
  as bitemporal field defect mimic, 278
  Coats disease-associated, 351
  as constricted visual field cause, 279
  electro-oculographic evaluation of, 46–47
  electroretinographic evaluation of, 44–45, 46–47
  keratoconus associated with, 130
  as uveitis mimic, 333, 335
  X-linked, electroretinographic evaluation of, 44–45
Retinoblastoma, **405–411,** 417, 422–427
  bilateral, 409, 411
  classification of, 409–410
  clinical features of, 332
  definition of, 405
  differentiated from Coats disease, 55, 349–350
  endophytic, 407
  exophytic, 407, 422–423, 427
  familial, 425–426
  fleurettes in, 424
  genetic factors in, 406, 409, 425, 426
  germline mutation, 406
  imaging of, 410
  laterality of, 405
  low-magnification light microscopic appearance
    of, 423
  magnetic resonance imaging of, 54
  as mortality cause, 425
  prognostic features of, 424
  rosettes in, 423–424
  secondary cancers associated with, 406
  somatic mutation, 406
  spontaneous regression of, 407
  sporadic, 426
  syndromes associated with, 405
  treatment of, 408, 411
  trilateral, 406, 426
  unifocal, 426

Retinoblastoma *(Continued)*
  unilateral, 411, 425, 426
  as uveitis mimic, 332, 333
Retinoblastoma gene, 425, 426
Retinochoroiditis, necrotizing, 327–328
Retinocytoma, 407
Retinoma, 407
Retinopathy
  crystalline, 344
  decompression, 168
  diabetic, **376–383**
    cataract surgery-related exacerbation
      of, 230
    microvasculopathy of, 376
    nonproliferative, 376, 378
    proliferative, 376, 377, 378, 380, 404
  of prematurity, 247, **368–375**
    differentiated from Coats disease, 55, 349–350,
      406, 407
  radiation, 318
  toxic, **341–347**
Retinopexy, pneumatic, 400–401, 403
Retinoschisis
  degenerative, 400
  X-linked, 374
    electro-oculographic evaluation of, 47
    electroretinographic evaluation of, 45–46
Retinoscopy, "with" movement during, 28
Retrobulbar injection, of anesthesia, 9, 219
Retrobulbar tumors, 178
Rhabdomyosarcoma, 296, 429
  histologic classification of, 431–432
  imaging of, 56
Rheumatoid arthritis, 87
  juvenile, 322–323, 325
  as vasculitis cause, 331
Rhodopsin, 34
Rieger's anomaly, 179
Rifabutin, ocular toxicity of, 340
Rim defects, as false-positive field defect
  cause, 60, 62
Rimexolone, 114
Ritalin abuse, as retinopathy cause, 344–345
"Rodent ulcers," 316
Rods, 34, 39, 42–43
Rose Bengal stain, 79
  differentiated from fluorescein stain, 117
Rosettes, in retinoblastoma, 423–424
Rubella syndrome, congenital, 45, 179
"Rule of 50's," 432

S
Salicylates, as retinopathy cause, 344
Sampolesi's line, 174, 175
Sandhoff's disease, 386
"Sand in the eyes" sensation, 80
"Sands of the Sahara syndrome." *See* Keratitis,
  diffuse lamellar

Sarcoidosis, 175, 429
  clinical features of, 328–329
  diagnosis of, 329
  as optic neuritis cause, 274
  as uveitis cause, 323, 325, 328–329, 331
Sarcoma
  Kaposi's, 339
  retinoblastoma-associated, 406
Saturation, of colors, 35
Scheie system, of anterior chamber angle
    classification, 159
Schirmer test, 79, 118, 288–289
Schlemm's canal, 157
  blood in, 178
Schnyder's crystalline stromal dystrophy, 123–124
Schwalbe's line, 11, 157, 174
Schwannoma, 296, 430, 434
Sclera
  blunt trauma to, 353
  in globe rupture, 199
  rupture of, 355–356
  thinnest area of, 11
Scleral buckling, 401, 402, 403
  as myopia cause, 31
Scleral flaps, 192, 193, 194
Scleral spur, 157
Scleritis
  anterior, 87
  differentiated from episcleritis, 86
  posterior, 87–88
  as red eye cause, 77, 87–88
  systemic disease associated with, 88
Scleromalacia perforans, 88
Scopolamine, 29, 177
Scotoma
  bilateral arcuate, 67
  cecocentral, 66
  central, 66, 72–73
    age-related macular degeneration-related, 362
    bilateral, 278
  centrocecal, 278
  definition of, 60
  junctional, 68, 69, 278
  macular, 30
  paracentral, 346
  parafoveal, 341–342
  ring, 72
Sebaceous gland carcinoma, 318–319
Secondary focal point (F$_2$), 19, 20, 22
Secondary membrane, 216–217, 227, 229–230
"Second sight,", 213, 218
Secrets, Top 100, 1–7
Sepsis, neonatal conjunctivitis-related, 104
Sickle cell disease, 201, 202, 203
Siderosis, 179
Siderosis bulbi, 358
Sildenafil (Viagra), as retinopathy
    cause, 343

Silver nitrate drops, as neonatal conjunctivitis
    prophylaxis, 102
Sjögren's syndrome, 117
Skew deviation, 245, 272
Skin cancer, metastatic, 249
Sky, color of, 39
Slab-off, 23
Slit-lamp examination
  for keratoconus evaluation, 132–133
  for nystagmus evaluation, 258
Smears, for corneal ulcer evaluation, 91, 92, 94
Smoking, as thyroid-related ophthalmopathy risk
    factor, 298, 302
Snellen visual acuity test, 27, 31, 218
Snell's law, 21
Solumedrol, as optic neuritis treatment, 275
Spaeth system, of anterior chamber angle
    classification, 159
Spasmus nutans, 257, 258
Spectacles
  aphakic, 215, 222
  bifocal, 259
    with low-vision aids, 27
    prismatic effect of, 23
  for cataract patients, 218, 222
  for children with astigmatism, 29
  corrective power of, 20
  lens of
    antireflective coatings on, 29
    bifocal, 27
    bifocal high-power single-vision, 27
    as low-vision aids, 27
    minus, 25–26
    plus, 23, 25, 26, 27
    round-top versus flat-top, 23
    strabismic deviation measurement of, 23
    thick, aberrations of, 24–25
  new, patients' dissatisfaction with, 30
  for nystagmus correction, 259
  power of
    comparison with contact lens, 20
    lensmeter measurement of, 28
  for ptosis correction, 312
  as refractive accommodative esotropia
      treatment, 241
  vertex distance and, 29
Sphenoid bone, 9, 16
Spherical aberration, of thick lens, 24
Spherical equivalent, 24
Sphingolipidosis, 386
Spindle cells, 419
Spiral of Tillaux, 9
Squamous cell carcinoma, 318, 340
SRK formula, for intraocular lens implant calculation, 26
Staphylococcal hypersensitivity, as corneal infiltrate
    cause, 95
Staphylococcus aureus
  methicillin-resistant, 109, 110

Staphylococcus aureus (Continued)
  penicillin-resistant, 110
Staphylococcus aureus infections
  as conjunctivitis cause, 84
  endophthalmitis, 228, 358
  as orbital cellulitis cause, 307
Staphylococcus epidermis, penicillin-resistant, 110
Staphylococcus epidermis infections, 228
Steroids. *See also* Corticosteroids
  as giant cell arteritis treatment, 281
  low-dose, as red eye treatment, 77
  as open-angle glaucoma treatment, 175, 176
  post-trabeculectomy use of, 193
  subjunctival injections of, 88
  as thyroid-related ophthalmopathy treatment, 299,
    300–301
  topical, 110–114
    generic and brand names of, 114
    as glaucoma treatment, 166
    side effects of, 111–112
    use in photorefractive keratectomy patients, 148
Stevens-Johnson syndrome, 328
Strabismus
  alternating, 237
  as amblyopia cause, 231
  congenital ocular motor apraxia-related, 249
  cycloplegic refraction in, 29
  in infants, 237
  measurement of, Prentice's rule of, 23
  retinoblastoma-related, 406
  surgical treatment of, **251–255**
    in amblyopia patients, 236
    complications of, 253–255
Streptococcal infections, as orbital cellulitis cause, 307
Streptococcus faecalis, methicillin-resistant, 110
Stroke, occipital, 279–280
Stromal corneal dystrophy, 120, 122–125
STUMPED mnemonic, for neonatal cloudy corneas, 14
Sturge-Weber syndrome, 178, 179
Subarachnoid space, retinoblastoma invasion of, 425
Sulfacetamide, 108, 112
Sulfisoxazole, 112
Sulfur hexafluoride, 403
Sunset, color of, 39
Superior oblique palsy, 267–269
Superior orbital fissure, 9, 16
Superior orbital fissure syndrome, 270
Superior vena cava syndrome, 178
Suprathreshold testing, 59
Suspensions, 106–107, 113
Sussman four-mirror gonioscope, 158
Sutures
  adjustable, 252
  releasable, 192
  scleral, as globe perforation cause, 254
Swinging flashlight test, 261–262
Symblepharon, 105
Sympathetic ophthalmia, 326, 359

Sympathomimetic drugs, contraindication in
    narrow-angle glaucoma, 168–169
Synechiae
  as open-angle glaucoma risk factor, 175, 176
  peripheral angle, 172
  peripheral anterior, 157, 161, 162, 208, 321, 326
  posterior, 175, 321, 322
Syphilis
  diagnostic tests for, 329
  ocular manifestations of, 329
    in AIDS patients, 336, 338
    Argyll-Robertson pupil, 264
    optic neuritis, 274
    orbital, 307
    retinitis, 330
    uveitis, 323, 324, 329, 331
Systemic lupus erythematosus, 274

T
Talc, as retinopathy cause, 344–345, 346
Tamoxifen, as retinopathy cause, 344, 346
Tamsulosin (Flomax), 216, 230
Tarsal conjunctival follicles, 78
Tay-Sachs disease, 386
Tear break-up time, measurement of, 117
Tear film
  abnormalities of, 288
  components of, 116
  in dry eyes, 116, 117
  layers of, 14, 116, 288
  normal, 116
Tearing
  causes of, 13, 79, 121, 287
  congenital, 291
Tear pump, 287–288
Tear replacement therapy, 118
Tears
  adequate volume of, 288–289
  artificial, 107, 118
    preservative-free, 118
  composition of, 288
    inadequate, 289
  drainage path of, 287–288
Telangiectasia, 80
  retinal, Coats disease-related, 348, 349, 351
Telecanthus, 311
Telescopes, 27, 28
Temporal artery
  biopsy of, 17, 281
  superficial, surgical landmarks of, 17
Temporal lobe, "pie-in-the-sky" defects of, 283
Tenon's capsule
  in strabismus surgery, 251
  in trabeculectomy, 191
Tensilon test, 271
Testing, ophthalmic and orbital, **41–58**
Tetracycline, 80, 103, 112
  contraindications to, 103

Thermokeratoplasty, 135
  holmium laser, 147
Thiel-Behnke corneal dystrophy, 122
Thioridazine (Mellaril), as retinopathy cause, 342, 343
Third-nerve palsy. *See* Cranial nerve palsies, third
13q deletion syndrome, 405
Three-step test, 267–269
Thromboembolism, retinal, drug-related, 346
Thrombophlebitis, Behçet's disease-related, 330
Thrombosis, as retinal artery occlusion cause, 384–385
Thyroid-related ophthalmopathy, 86, **298–303.**
     See also Graves' disease
  as constricted visual field cause, 279–280
  definition of, 298
  differentiated from Brown's syndrome, 246
  as diplopia cause, 266
  as elevated episcleral venous pressure cause, 178
  as hypertropia cause, 245
  as orbital inflammation cause, 307
  as proptosis cause, 9, 294–295
Thyroid-stimulating hormone, 299
Thyroid-stimulating hormone receptors, 9
Tight lens syndrome, 81
Timolol, 114
  as glaucoma treatment, 182, 183, 186
TINU syndrome, 325
Tobramycin, 110, 112
Tolosa-Hunt syndrome, 249
Topical anesthesia, for cataract surgery, 219
Topical medications, **106–115**
  allergic reactions to, 187
  antibiotics, 106–110, 112
  as red eye treatment, 77–78
  steroids, 110–114
  as superficial punctate keratopathy, 79
Topiramate, as angle-closure glaucoma cause, 173
Topographic mapping, for keratoconus diagnosis, 130,
    131–132
Top 100 Secrets, **1–7**
Torticollis, 258
Toxins, as retinopathy cause, **341–347**
Toxocariasis, ocular, 247, 426
  differentiated from retinoblastoma, 406
  as uveitis cause, 324
Toxoplasmosis, ocular
  AIDS-related, 335–336
  as papilledema cause, 339
  as retinitis cause, 330
  treatment for, 328
  as uveitis cause, 327–328, 331
Trabecular meshwork
  anterior, nonpigmented, 157
  inflammatory cell blockage of, 175–176
  obstruction of, 176–177, 208
  tears to, 199
Trabeculectomy, 167, 172, **190–198**
  antimetabolite use in, 194–195, 196
  failure of, 190

Trabeculectomy *(Continued)*
  flaps in, 192, 193, 194
  fornix *versus* limbal-conjunctival approach to, 191
  indications for, 190
  wound leaks associated with, 193
Trabeculectomy site, blockage of, 195, 196
Trabeculoplasty, argon laser, 11, 174
Trachoma, 84, 85
Tranexamic acid, 202
Transillumination, of uveal melanoma, 413
Transposition procedures, 252
Transverse magnification, formula for, 26
Trauma, ocular
  as angle-recession glaucoma cause, 174
  to the fundus, **353–360**
  initial examination of, 356
  to the optic chiasm, 66
  orbital, computed tomography evaluation of, 55
  treatment algorithm for, 207
  ultrasound evaluation of, 53
Travoprost, as glaucoma treatment, 182
Treponemal antibody absorption test, 394
Triamcinolone, 392, 394
Trichiasis, 79, 80
Trichromatism, anomalous, 40
Trichromats, 39
Trifluorothymidine, 78–79
Trifluridine, 113
Trigeminal nerve, herpes zoster lesions of, 11
Trimethoprim, 108
Tritanopes, 39
Trochlear nerve, 16
Trochlear nerve palsy. *See* Cranial nerve palsies, fourth
Trophozoites, 95
Tropicamide (Mydriacyl), 29
Tuberculosis, ocular
  clinical features of, 330
  orbital, 307
  as uveitis cause, 323, 324
Tumors, ocular, **417–428**
  of the eyelid, **315–319**
  imaging of, 55, 56
  as open-angle glaucoma cause, 179
  orbital, **429–434**
    soft-tissue, 433
  ultrasound evaluation of, 53

U
UGH (uveitis-glaucoma-hyphema) syndrome, 178
Ulcers
  Behçet's disease-related, 330
  corneal, 90
    antibiotic therapy for, 92–93, 108–110, 111
    biopsy of, 95
    in contact lens wearers, 80–81, 82
    dendritic, 96
    diagnostic smears and cultures of, 91, 92, 94
    infections of, 80

Ulcers *(Continued)*
  corneal *(Continued)*
    perforated, 94
    ptosis surgery-related, 312
    as red eye cause, 80–81, 82
    sequelae of, 94
    sterile, 80, 90
    topical steroid therapy for, 95, 111
   dendritic, 78–79
   genital, 330
   oral, 330
Ultrasonography, ophthalmic, 48–54
  biomicroscopy method in, 53
  of calcification, 53, 54
  of choroidal hemangioma, 51, 52
  of choroidal melanoma, 50–51
  for Coats disease evaluation, 350
  color-Doppler, 53–54
  of foreign bodies, 53, 357
  of intraocular tumors, 50
  of ocular trauma, 53
  of orbital lesions, 56
  for preoperative cataract evaluation, 50
  of retinal detachment, 52, 54
  of uveal melanoma, 413
Uvea, tumors of, 417–418
  melanoma, 413, 414, 417
Uveitis, **321–340**
  anterior, 88–89, 321
    granulomatous, 321, 322, 323, 327
    nongranulomatous, 321, 322
    as red eye cause, 77
  anterior chamber angle in, 160
  autoimmune, 331
  cataract surgery-related, 227
  definition of, 321
  as glaucoma cause, 331
  granulomatous, 321
  herpes zoster ophthalmicus-related, 97
  in immunocompetent patients, 321–332
  infectious causes of, 323, 324
  intermediate, 321, 327
  masquerade syndromes as mimics of, 332–335
  noninfectious causes of, 321–323, 325–326
  orbital inflammation-related, 306
  phacoanaphylactic, 325
  posterior, 321, 327–328
    Behçet's disease-related, 330
  syphilitic, 329
  treatment for, 331
Uveitis-glaucoma-hyphema (UGH) syndrome, 178
Uveoscleral outflow inhibitors, 163, 166

V
Valsalva maneuver, 85
Valve of Rosenmüller, 288
Vancomycin, 110
Van Herrick technique, 159

Varicella-zoster virus infections, 97
Varices, orbital, 178
Vascular endothelial growth factor inhibitors, 365, 366
Vasculitis, orbital, 308
Vasoconstrictors, as red eye cause, 87
Venous occlusion. *See also* Retinal venous occlusive
    disease
  as altitudinal defect cause, 72
Vergence
  of convex mirrors, 28
  formula for, 21
  of parallel light rays, 22
Vertex distance, 29
Vertical deviation, dissociated, 239
Vidarabine, 78–79, 105, 113
Videoangiography, indocyanine green, 364
Vigabatrin, as retinopathy cause, 344
Viscoelastic, retained, 178
Vision loss
  cataracts-related, 213
  diabetic retinopathy-related, 376, 377
  glaucoma-related, 150
  macular degeneration-related, 361, 364
  optic neuritis-related, 274, 276
  papillitis-related, 339
  pars planitis-related, 327
  retinal vein occlusion-related, 391, 392
  sympathetic ophthalmia-related, 359
Visual acuity
  in amblyopia, 231, 232, 235
  in nystagmus, 259
  preoperative evaluation of, 218
Visual acuity testing
  in nystagmus patients, 260
  potential, 218
Visual cortex
  location of, 13
  macular function in, 15
Visual development, delayed, 257
Visual fields, **59–76**
  constricted, 279–280
  defects of, 283, 284
    bitemporal, conditions which simulate, 278
    congruous, 61
    description of, 62–65
    false, 60, 61
    glaucoma-related, 151, 152, 153, 156
    homonymous, 61, 62
    neuro-ophthalmologic disorders-related, 65–66
    optic neuritis-related, 274
  with glaucomatous-appearing optic nerves, 156
Visual field testing, 59
  developments in, 73–74
  false-negative and false-positive errors in, 60, 61
Visual pathway, 65
Visual pigments, 34
Vitamin A deficiency, 279–280
Vitamin B_{11} deficiency, 279

Vitamin B$_{12}$ deficiency, 278–279
Vitamins, as macular degeneration
    treatment, 365
Vitrectomy
    as diabetic retinopathy treatment, 382
        complications of, 382
    "dry," 194
    as endophthalmitis treatment, 93
    familial exudative, 374
    for foreign body removal, 357–358
    pars plana, 171, 401, 402–403
        contraindication in retinoblastoma, 410
    as retinal vein occlusion treatment, 392
    retinoblastoma as contraindication to, 407, 410
Vitreoretinopathy
    familial exudative
        differentiated from Coats disease, 350
        differentiated from retinoblastoma, 407
    proliferative, 403, 404
Vitreous
    detachment of, 199, 201
    loss of
        cataract surgery-related, 226, 228
        posterior capsule rupture-related, 226
        trabeculectomy-related, 194
    opacity of, as false-positive field defect
        cause, 60
    persistent hyperplastic primary, 426
    posterior, detachment of, ultrasound
        evaluation of, 52
    prolapse of, 199, 201
Vitreous tap, 93
Vitritis
    steroids-resistant panuveitis-related, 334
    syphilis-related, 329
Vogt-Koyanagi-Harada syndrome, 326, 329, 331, 334

Volk lens, 29
von Hippel-Lindau syndrome, 350

W
Waldenstrom's macroglobulinemia, 123
"Wall-eyed," 243
Wavefront ablations, 143
Weber's syndrome, 270
Wegener's granulomatosis, 274, 308, 331, 429
White dot syndrome, retinal, 331
Whitnall's superior suspensory ligament
    bony attachments of, 18
    in ptosis, 313
Willebrand's knee, 13, 68
Wilm's tumor, 179
Women
    Coats disease incidence in, 348
    optic neuritis in, 274

X
Xanthelasma, 315–316
Xanthogranuloma, juvenile, 323, 325, 327
Xanthopsia, 346

Y
Yellow vision, 346

Z
Zeaxanthin, 365
Zeiss gonioscope, 158
Zimmerman hypothesis, of uveal
    melanoma, 419–420
Zonules
    in angle-closure glaucoma, 168
    tears of, 199
Zygomatic bone, 9, 16